Nutraceutical, Nutrition Supplements and Human Health

Nutraceutical, Nutrition Supplements and Human Health

Special Issue Editors

Rafat A. Siddiqui
Mohammed H. Moghadasian

MDPI • Basel • Beijing • Wuhan • Barcelona • Belgrade • Manchester • Tokyo • Cluj • Tianjin

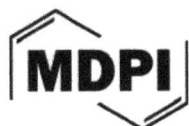

Special Issue Editors
Rafat A. Siddiqui   Mohammed H. Moghadasian
Virginia State University   St. Boniface Hospital
USA   Canada

Editorial Office
MDPI
St. Alban-Anlage 66
4052 Basel, Switzerland

This is a reprint of articles from the Special Issue published online in the open access journal *Nutrients* (ISSN 2072-6643) (available at: https://www.mdpi.com/journal/nutrients/special_issues/Nutraceutica_Nutrition).

For citation purposes, cite each article independently as indicated on the article page online and as indicated below:

LastName, A.A.; LastName, B.B.; LastName, C.C. Article Title. *Journal Name* **Year**, *Article Number*, Page Range.

ISBN 978-3-03936-555-5 (Hbk)
ISBN 978-3-03936-556-2 (PDF)

© 2020 by the authors. Articles in this book are Open Access and distributed under the Creative Commons Attribution (CC BY) license, which allows users to download, copy and build upon published articles, as long as the author and publisher are properly credited, which ensures maximum dissemination and a wider impact of our publications.

The book as a whole is distributed by MDPI under the terms and conditions of the Creative Commons license CC BY-NC-ND.

Contents

About the Special Issue Editors ix

Rafat A. Siddiqui and Mohammed H. Moghadasian
Nutraceuticals and Nutrition Supplements: Challenges and Opportunities
Reprinted from: *Nutrients* **2020**, *12*, 1593, doi:10.3390/nu12061593 1

Kazuya Toda, Yuki Yamauchi, Azusa Tanaka, Tetsuya Kuhara, Toshitaka Odamaki, Shin Yoshimoto and Jin-zhong Xiao
Heat-Killed *Bifidobacterium breve* B-3 Enhances Muscle Functions: Possible Involvement of Increases in Muscle Mass and Mitochondrial Biogenesis
Reprinted from: *Nutrients* **2020**, *12*, 219, doi:10.3390/nu12010219 5

Dina C. Simes, Carla S. B. Viegas, Nuna Araújo and Catarina Marreiros
Vitamin K as a Diet Supplement with Impact in Human Health: Current Evidence in Age-Related Diseases
Reprinted from: *Nutrients* **2020**, *12*, 138, doi:10.3390/nu12010138 19

Yair Olovaldo Santiago-Saenz, Rebeca Monroy-Torres, Diana Olivia Rocha-Amador and Alma Delia Hernández-Fuentes
Effect of a Supplementation with Two *Quelites* on Urinary Excretion of Arsenic in Adolescents Exposed to Water Contaminated with the Metalloid in a Community in the State of Guanajuato, Mexico
Reprinted from: *Nutrients* **2020**, *12*, 98, doi:10.3390/nu12010098 43

Alessandra Durazzo, Emanuela Camilli, Laura D'Addezio, Raffaela Piccinelli, Angelika Mantur-Vierendeel, Luisa Marletta, Paul Finglas, Aida Turrini and Stefania Sette
Development of Dietary Supplement Label Database in Italy: Focus of FoodEx2 Coding
Reprinted from: *Nutrients* **2020**, *12*, 89, doi:10.3390/nu12010089 65

Se-Chun Liao, Wei-Hsiang Hsu, Zi-Yi Huang, Kun-Lin Chuang, Kuan-Ting Lin, Chia-Ling Tseng, Tung-Hu Tsai, Anh-Hoang Dao, Chun-Li Su and Chi-Ying F. Huang
Bioactivity Evaluation of a Novel Formulated Curcumin
Reprinted from: *Nutrients* **2019**, *11*, 2982, doi:10.3390/nu11122982 75

Mohammed H. Moghadasian, Ramandeep Kaur, Kayla Kostal, Akhila A. Joshi, Mahboubeh Molaei, Khuong Le, Gabor Fischer, Francesca Bonomini, Gaia Favero, Rita Rezzani and et al.
Anti-Atherosclerotic Properties of Wild Rice in Low-Density Lipoprotein Receptor Knockout Mice: The Gut Microbiome, Cytokines, and Metabolomics Study
Reprinted from: *Nutrients* **2019**, *11*, 2894, doi:10.3390/nu11122894 97

Ye Jin Kim, Eun-Young Kwon, Ji-Won Kim, Youngmi Lee, Ri Ryu, Jongbok Yun, Manheun Kim and Myung-Sook Choi
Intervention Study on the Efficacy and Safety of *Platycodon grandiflorus* Ethanol Extract in Overweight or Moderately Obese Adults: A Single-Center, Randomized, Double-Blind, Placebo-Controlled Trial
Reprinted from: *Nutrients* **2019**, *11*, 2445, doi:10.3390/nu11102445 111

Michael Schmiech, Sophia J. Lang, Judith Ulrich, Katharina Werner, Luay J. Rashan, Tatiana Syrovets and Thomas Simmet
Comparative Investigation of Frankincense Nutraceuticals: Correlation of Boswellic and Lupeolic Acid Contents with Cytokine Release Inhibition and Toxicity against Triple-Negative Breast Cancer Cells
Reprinted from: *Nutrients* **2019**, *11*, 2341, doi:10.3390/nu11102341 123

Melanie S. Trudeau, Robyn F. Madden, Jill A. Parnell, W. Ben Gibbard and Jane Shearer
Dietary and Supplement-Based Complementary and Alternative Medicine Use in Pediatric Autism Spectrum Disorder
Reprinted from: *Nutrients* **2019**, *11*, 1783, doi:10.3390/nu11081783 141

Chyn Boon Wong, Noriyuki Iwabuchi and Jin-zhong Xiao
Exploring the Science behind *Bifidobacterium breve* M-16V in Infant Health
Reprinted from: *Nutrients* **2019**, *11*, 1724, doi:10.3390/nu11081724 153

Lidiani F. Santana, Aline C. Inada, Bruna Larissa Spontoni do Espirito Santo, Wander F. O. Filiú, Arnildo Pott, Flávio M. Alves, Rita de Cássia A. Guimarães, Karine de Cássia Freitas and Priscila A. Hiane
Nutraceutical Potential of *Carica papaya* in Metabolic Syndrome
Reprinted from: *Nutrients* **2019**, *11*, 1608, doi:10.3390/nu11071608 177

Sandramara Sasso, Priscilla Cristovam Sampaio e Souza, Lidiani Figueiredo Santana, Claudia Andréa Lima Cardoso, Flávio Macedo Alves, Luciane Candeloro Portugal, Bernardo Bacelar de Faria, Anderson Fernandes da Silva, Ana Rita Coimbra Motta-Castro, Luana Silva Soares and et al.
Use of an Extract of *Annona muricata* Linn to Prevent High-Fat Diet Induced Metabolic Disorders in C57BL/6 Mice
Reprinted from: *Nutrients* **2019**, *11*, 1509, doi:10.3390/nu11071509 197

Faten A. Alsolmei, Haiwen Li, Suzette L. Pereira, Padmavathy Krishnan, Paul W. Johns and Rafat A. Siddiqui
Polyphenol-Enriched Plum Extract Enhances Myotubule Formation and Anabolism while Attenuating Colon Cancer-induced Cellular Damage in C2C12 Cells
Reprinted from: *Nutrients* **2019**, *11*, 1077, doi:10.3390/nu11051077 219

Virginia Martín, Nivia Cárdenas, Sara Ocaña, María Marín, Rebeca Arroyo, David Beltrán, Carlos Badiola, Leónides Fernández and Juan M. Rodríguez
Rectal and Vaginal Eradication of *Streptococcus agalactiae* (GBS) in Pregnant Women by Using *Lactobacillus salivarius* CECT 9145, A Target-specific Probiotic Strain
Reprinted from: *Nutrients* **2019**, *11*, 810, doi:10.3390/nu11040810 237

Bill J. Gurley, Isabelle R. Miousse, Intawat Nookaew, Laura E. Ewing, Charles M. Skinner, Piroon Jenjaroenpun, Thidathip Wongsurawat, Stefanie Kennon-McGill, Bharathi Avula, Ji-Yeong Bae, Mitchell R. McGill, David Ussery, Ikhlas A. Khan and Igor Koturbash
Decaffeinated Green Tea Extract Does Not Elicit Hepatotoxic Effects and Modulates the Gut Microbiome in Lean B6C3F$_1$ Mice
Reprinted from: *Nutrients* **2019**, *11*, 776, doi:10.3390/nu11040776 259

Amine Allaoui, Sonia Gascón, Souhila Benomar, Javier Quero, Jesús Osada, Moncef Nasri, María Jesús Rodríguez-Yoldi and Ahmed Boualga
Protein Hydrolysates from Fenugreek (*Trigonella foenum graecum*) as Nutraceutical Molecules in Colon Cancer Treatment
Reprinted from: *Nutrients* **2019**, *11*, 724, doi:10.3390/nu11040724 273

Alessio Martucci, Delia Reurean-Pintilei and Anamaria Manole
Bioavailability and Sustained Plasma Concentrations of CoQ10 in Healthy Volunteers by a
Novel Oral Timed-Release Preparation
Reprinted from: *Nutrients* **2019**, *11*, 527, doi:10.3390/nu11030527 289

Sung Ho Lim and Chang-Ik Choi
Pharmacological Properties of *Morus nigra* L. (Black Mulberry) as A Promising Nutraceutical
Resource
Reprinted from: *Nutrients* **2019**, *11*, 437, doi:10.3390/nu11020437 303

**Nivia Cárdenas, Virginia Martín, Rebeca Arroyo, Mario López, Marta Carrera,
Carlos Badiola, Esther Jiménez and Juan M. Rodríguez**
Prevention of Recurrent Acute Otitis Media in Children Through the Use of *Lactobacillus salivarius* PS7, a Target-Specific Probiotic Strain
Reprinted from: *Nutrients* **2019**, *11*, 376, doi:10.3390/nu11020376 321

About the Special Issue Editors

Rafat A. Siddiqui, Associate Professor. Dr. Rafat Siddiqui is currently working as Associate Professor and Director of the Nutrition Science Food Chemistry Laboratory at Virginia State University, Petersburg, Virginia, United States. Dr. Siddiqui earned his BSc and MSc degrees in Biochemistry from the University of Karachi in Karachi, Pakistan. He obtained his Ph.D. from the Australian National University in Canberra, Australia. Dr. Siddiqui served as a postdoctoral fellow at Massey University in Palmerton North, New Zealand. He immigrated to America in 1989 and worked as a Howard Hughes Research Fellow at Vanderbilt University Medical Center in Nashville. Dr. Siddiqui began his work as a researcher at Methodist Hospital/Methodist Research Institute in 1993 and served as the Director of Cellular Biochemistry and Lipid Biology programs from 2000–2015. He is an internationally recognized expert in nutrition in many areas, including cancer, cardiovascular disease, inflammation, and neurosciences. He has published over 100 scientific papers in peer-reviewed journals and has written several invited review articles, book chapters, commentaries, and editorials on emerging issues. He has been invited as a keynote speaker at several national and international conferences. Dr. Siddiqui's research has been supported by funding from National Institutes of Health (NCI), United States Department of Agriculture (USDA), the American Heart Association (AHA), the Showalter Foundation, the Clinical and Translational Sciences Institute (CTSI, Indiana), and the pharmaceutical companies, including Baxter and Abbott Laboratories. Dr. Siddiqui's research has been featured on BBC, FOX TV, and WTHR broadcasts, as well as in the Sun, Telegraph, Indianapolis Star newspapers, and several other media outlets. He is on the editorial board of numerous journals, including the British Journal of Nutrition. His recent work focuses on the health benefits of grape pomace, green papaya, pomegranate, plums, ginger, and turmeric extracts. At present, Dr. Siddiqui's research interests are in cancer, inflammation, and cardiovascular diseases. His research emphasis is on the synergistic modulation of chronic diseases by a combination of nutrients and drugs.

Mohammed H. Moghadasian, Professor. Dr. Moghadasian completed a master's program in Pharmacology and Therapeutics and a PhD program in Pathology and Laboratory Medicine at the University of British Columbia, Vancouver, Canada. After extensive post-doctoral training, Dr. Moghadasian was appointed as a Clinical Assistant Professor in the Department of Pathology and Laboratory Medicine, Faculty of Medicine and St. Paul's Hospital, the University of British Columbia in 2000. Dr. Moghadasian moved to the University of Manitoba in 2003. He is currently a full-time tenured Professor in the Department of Human Nutritional Sciences, and a Principal Investigator within the Canadian Centre for Agri-Food Research in Health and Medicine (CCARM). Dr. Moghadasian is known for his excellent contribution to the understanding of the pathogenesis of dyslipidemia and atherosclerosis using well-established animal models, namely, apolipoprotein E-deficient and LDL-receptor knockout mice. His laboratory has received funding from several granting agencies including CIHR, the Heart and Stroke Foundation of Canada, NSERC, Manitoba Health Research Council, Manitoba Medical Services Foundation, University of Manitoba, and others to further investigate the pathogenesis of atherogenesis and dyslipidemia. The impact of dietary intervention on these disorders is another focus of Dr. Moghadasian's research team. His studies have resulted in over one hundred peer-reviewed publications in high-impact journals, one book entitled "Functional Foods and Cardiovascular Disease" and many book chapters. His outstanding contributions have been recognized by the international scientific community and made him an authority in the area of Functional Foods and Cardiovascular Disorders.

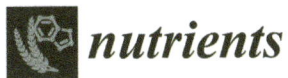 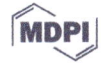

Editorial

Nutraceuticals and Nutrition Supplements: Challenges and Opportunities

Rafat A. Siddiqui [1],* and Mohammed H. Moghadasian [2,3]

1. Food Chemistry and Nutrition Science Laboratory, Agricultural Research Station, Virginia State University, Petersburg, VA 23806, USA
2. Department of Food and Human Nutritional Sciences, University of Manitoba, Winnipeg, MB R3T 2N2, Canada; mmoghadasian@sbrc.ca
3. Canadian Center for Agri-food Research in Health and Medicine, St. Boniface Hospital Research Center, Winnipeg, MB R2H 2A6, Canada
* Correspondence: rsiddiqui@vsu.edu; Tel.: +(804)-524-5957

Received: 26 May 2020; Accepted: 27 May 2020; Published: 29 May 2020

The term "nutraceuticals" is derived from "nutrition" and "pharmaceuticals" and is used for nutrition products that are also used as medicine [1]. "Nutraceuticals" often contain modified/unmodified whole food, plant extracts alone or in combination, semipurified and purified phytochemicals, or a combination of different phytochemicals. On the other hand, nutritional supplements are nutritional compounds that supplement one's diet by increasing one's total daily intake. Nutritional supplements also contain substances alone or in combination with vitamins and minerals, with or without other herbal products, with or without zoochemicals (creatinine, glucosamine, melatonin, bee pollens) and with or without probiotics.

Nutraceuticals and nutrition supplements are collectively referred to as "dietary supplements," intended to be taken orally [2]. The use of supplements is suggested to (but may not claim to) diagnose, cure, mitigate, treat, or prevent diseases. Often, background information suggests that they are intended to affect the structure or function of the body [3]. However, they do not undergo premarket approval. The common reasons for using dietary supplements are to improve conditions such as overall health and disease prevention, performance (athletics, sports, sex, etc.) and appearance (weight loss, sex appeal) [4]. These are often perceived as "safe" and less likely to have side effects. The scientific research on nutraceuticals and nutrition supplements is frequently misinterpreted or overstretched for commercial interests because of high consumer demands. The manufacturing and marketing of supplements are full of challenges.

Several challenges associated with the development of nutraceuticals are often ignored because of a lack of authoritative control. These challenges include identification of the authentic source of raw materials, purity of the compound, presence of other active compounds, quality, lack of experimental evidence, false advertising, contamination with heavy metals, and interactions between supplements and drugs. For example, a common herb "ginseng" has several varieties [5] such as California ginseng, wild ginseng, prickly ginseng, Pacific ginseng, Malaysian ginseng, Indian ginseng, Peruvian ginseng, Southern ginseng, Brazilian ginseng, and wild-red ginseng. All of these are sold as ginseng, but none of these belongs to the genus *Panax*, which contains real ginseng including Korean ginseng (*P. ginseng*), South China ginseng (*P. notoginseng*) and American ginseng (*P. quinquefolius*). Some varieties of star anise have several hundred-fold anisatin, a neurotoxin, that the authentic star anise (*Illicium verum*) has [6]. The supplements that are not prepared under strict GMP conditions may have unintentional contamination [7], including microbes (pathogens/nonpathogens), pesticides, mycotoxin (aflatoxin), heavy metals (seaweeds), zinc (cadmium), and calcium (lead). In addition, some supplements such as those commonly used for weight loss, body building, and sex enhancement are spiked with prohibited drugs to improve efficacy [8]. Some manufacturers also try to use a closely related herb, which may or may not have the active ingredients. For example, goldenseal (*Hydrastis canadensis*), used for berberine/hydrastine content, is often substituted with goldthread (*Coptis chinensis*) or Oregon grape (*Mahonia aquifolium*), which may have low or no berberine/hydrastine [9].

Besides, maintaining the quality of nutraceuticals is another challenge, as phytochemistry is inherently variable due to seasonal and geographical variations [10]. It is challenging to measure and maintain consistency in finished products and limit undesirable constituents. Interaction of herbal supplements with medicinal drugs is also a big concern [11]. For example, St. John's wort (*Hypericum perforaum*) is used as an effective antidepressant, but it also activates several cytochrome P450 isoenzymes, which make a large number of medicinal drugs ineffective [12,13]. Among all the major concerns for using the nutraceuticals is the lack of scientific evidence [14]. Some are never tested under properly controlled experimental conditions, and unlike pharmaceuticals, most nutraceuticals do not undergo "randomized controlled clinical studies."

The purpose of this Special Issue on "Nutraceuticals, Nutrition Supplements, and Human Health" is to comprehensively review the data from basic and clinical research to discuss the benefits as well as potential adverse effects of "functional food-derived" products. We have invited international experts, researchers and authors to submit original research and review articles that address the progress and our current understanding of nutraceuticals/supplements from in vitro and in vivo studies, as well as from clinical trials describing the benefits/adverse effects with underlying mechanisms. This Special Issue presents a compendium of excellent laboratory and clinical studies using plant extracts [15–20], purified compounds [21–23], modified formulations [22,24], and probiotics [25–28] to improve many health conditions, including metabolic disorders [17,20], cardiovascular disease [29], muscle metabolism [18,25], obesity [16,17,20], neurological disorders [30], infectious diseases [26,27], aging [23], and cancers [18,21,24,31].

This Special Issue's overall goal is to present readers with high-quality scientific evidence for the use of dietary supplements, nutraceuticals, and functional foods that can be appropriately used to improve health parameters in various stages of one's lifecycle. We thank all the contributors for their contributions and for their dedication to making a difference in human health with low-cost remedies.

Author Contributions: R.A.S. and M.H.M. equally contributed in the preparation of this editorial. All authors have read and agreed to the published version of the manuscript.

Funding: None.

Acknowledgments: The authors greatly acknowledge the contribution of all authors for this Special Issue.

Conflicts of Interest: The authors declare no conflict of interest.

References

1. Kalra, E.K. Nutraceutical-definition and introduction. *AAPS Pharm. Sci.* **2003**, *5*, 27–28. [CrossRef]
2. US National Institutes of Health. *Dietary Supplements: Background Information*; Office of Dietary Supplements, US National Institutes of Health: Bethesda, MD, USA, 2011.
3. FDA. *Small Entity Compliance Guide on Structure/Function Claims*; Docket Number: FDA-2013-S-0610; Center for Food Safety and Applied Nutrition: College Park, MD, USA, 2002.
4. Dickinson, A.; Blatman, J.; El-Dash, N.; Franco, J.C. Consumer usage and reasons for using dietary supplements: Report of a series of surveys. *J Am. Coll. Nutr.* **2014**, *33*, 176–182. [CrossRef] [PubMed]
5. Foster, S. Towards an understanding of ginseng adulteration: The tangled web of names, history, trade, and perception. *HerbalGram* **2016**, *3*, 36–57.
6. Mathon, C.; Bongard, B.; Duret, M.; Ortelli, D.; Christen, P.; Bieri, S. Analysis of the neurotoxin anisatin in star anise by LC-MS/MS. *Food Addit. Contam. Part A* **2013**, *30*, 1598–1605. [CrossRef] [PubMed]
7. Costa, J.G.; Vidovic, B.; Saraiva, N.; Do Céu Costa, M.; Favero, G.D.; Marko, D.; Oliveira, N.G.; Fernandes, A.S. Contaminants: A dark side of food supplements? *Free Radic. Res.* **2019**, *53*, 1113–1135. [CrossRef]
8. Mathews, N.M. Prohibited contaminants in dietary supplements. *Sports Health* **2018**, *10*, 19–30. [CrossRef]
9. Edwards, D.J.; Draper, E.J. Variations in alkaloid content of herbal products containing goldenseal. *J. Am. Pharm. Assoc.* **2003**, *43*, 419–423.

10. Dhami, N.; Mishr, A.D. Phytochemical variation: How to resolve the quality controversies of herbal medicinal products? *J. Herb. Med.* **2015**, *5*, 118–127.
11. Brazier, N.C.; Levine, M.A.H. Drug-herb interaction among commonly used conventional medicines: A compendium for health care professionals. *Am. J. Ther.* **2003**, *10*, 163–169.
12. Mills, E.; Montori, V.M.; Wu, P.; Gallicano, K.; Clarke, M.; Guyatt, G. Interaction of St John's wort with conventional drugs: Systematic review of clinical trials. *Br. Med. J.* **2004**, *329*, 27.
13. Henderson, L.; Yue, Q.Y.; Bergquist, C.; Gerden, B.; Arlett, P. St John's wort (Hypericum perforatum): Drug interactions and clinical outcomes. *Br. J. Clin. Pharmacol.* **2002**, *54*, 349–356. [CrossRef] [PubMed]
14. Santini, A.; Cammarata, A.M.; Capone, G.; Ianaro, A.; Tenore, G.C.; Pani, L.; Novellino, E. Nutraceuticals: Opening the debate for a regulatory framework. *Br. J. Clin. Pharmacol.* **2018**, *84*, 659–672. [CrossRef] [PubMed]
15. Santiago-Saenz, Y.O.; Monroy-Torres, R.; Rocha-Amador, D.O.; Hernández-Fuentes, A.D. Effect of a supplementation with two quelites on urinary excretion of arsenic in adolescents exposed to water contaminated with the metalloid in a community in the state of guanajuato, Mexico. *Nutrients* **2020**, *12*, 98. [CrossRef] [PubMed]
16. Kim, Y.J.; Kwon, E.Y.; Kim, J.W.; Lee, Y.; Ryu, R.; Yun, J.; Kim, M.; Choi, M.S. Intervention study on the efficacy and safety of platycodon grandiflorus ethanol extract in overweight or moderately obese adults: A single-center, randomized, double-blind, placebo-controlled trial. *Nutrients* **2019**, *11*, 2445. [CrossRef] [PubMed]
17. Sasso, S.; Sampaio e Souza, P.C.; Santana, L.F.; Cardoso, C.A.L.; Alves, F.M.; Portugal, L.C.; De Faria, B.B.; Da Silva, A.F.; Motta-Castro, A.R.C.; Soares, L.S.; et al. Use of an extract of annona muricata linn to prevent high-fat diet induced metabolic disorders in C57BL/6 Mice. *Nutrients* **2019**, *11*, 1509. [CrossRef]
18. Alsolmei, F.A.; Li, H.; Pereira, S.L.; Krishnan, P.; Johns, P.W.; Siddiqui, R.A. Polyphenol-enriched plum extract enhances myotubule formation and anabolism while attenuating colon cancer-induced cellular damage in C2C12 Cells. *Nutrients* **2019**, *11*, 1077. [CrossRef]
19. Gurley, B.J.; Miousse, I.R.; Nookaew, I.; Ewing, L.E.; Skinner, C.M.; Jenjaroenpun, P.; Wongsurawat, T.; Kennon-McGill, S.; Avula, B.; Bae, J.Y.; et al. Decaffeinated green tea extract does not elicit hepatotoxic effects and modulates the gut microbiome in lean B6C3F1 mice. *Nutrients* **2019**, *11*, 776. [CrossRef]
20. Santana, L.F.; Inada, A.C.; Espirito Santo, B.L.S.; Filiú, W.F.O.; Pott, A.; Alves, F.M.; Guimarães, R.C.A.; Freitas, K.C.; Hiane, P.A. Nutraceutical potential of carica papaya in metabolic syndrome. *Nutrients* **2019**, *11*, 1608. [CrossRef]
21. Schmiech, M.; Lang, S.J.; Ulrich, J.; Werner, K.; Rashan, L.J.; Syrovets, T.; Simmet, T. Comparative investigation of frankincense nutraceuticals: Correlation of boswellic and lupeolic acid contents with cytokine release inhibition and toxicity against triple-negative breast cancer cells. *Nutrients* **2019**, *11*, 2341. [CrossRef]
22. Martucci, A.; Reurean-Pintilei, D.; Manole, A. Bioavailability and sustained plasma concentrations of CoQ10 in healthy volunteers by a novel oral timed-release preparation. *Nutrients* **2019**, *11*, 527. [CrossRef]
23. Simes, D.C.; Viegas, C.S.B.; Araújo, N.; Marreiros, C. Vitamin K as a diet supplement with impact in human health: Current evidence in age-related diseases. *Nutrients* **2020**, *12*, 138. [CrossRef] [PubMed]
24. Liao, S.C.; Hsu, W.H.; Huang, Z.Y.; Chuang, K.L.; Lin, K.T.; Tseng, C.L.; Tsai, T.H.; Dao, A.H.; Su, C.L.; Huang, C.Y.F. Bioactivity evaluation of a novel formulated curcumin. *Nutrients* **2019**, *11*, 2982. [CrossRef] [PubMed]
25. Toda, K.; Yamauchi, Y.; Tanaka, A.; Kuhara, T.; Odamaki, T.; Yoshimoto, S.; Xiao, J.Z. Heat-killed bifidobacterium breve B-3 Enhances Muscle Functions: Possible involvement of increases in muscle mass and mitochondrial biogenesis. *Nutrients* **2020**, *12*, 219. [CrossRef] [PubMed]
26. Martín, V.; Cárdenas, N.; Ocaña, S.; Marín, M.; Arroyo, R.; Beltrán, D.; Badiola, C.; Fernández, L.; Rodríguez, J.M. Rectal and vaginal eradication of streptococcus agalactiae (GBS) in pregnant women by using lactobacillus salivarius CECT 9145, a target-specific probiotic strain. *Nutrients* **2019**, *11*, 810. [CrossRef] [PubMed]
27. Cárdenas, N.; Martín, V.; Arroyo, R.; López, M.; Carrera, M.; Badiola, C.; Jiménez, E.; Rodríguez, J.M. Prevention of recurrent acute otitis media in children through the use of lactobacillus salivarius PS7, a target-specific probiotic strain. *Nutrients* **2019**, *11*, 376. [CrossRef]
28. Wong, C.B.; Iwabuchi, N.; Xiao, J.Z. Exploring the science behind bifidobacterium breve M-16V in infant health. *Nutrients* **2019**, *11*, 1724. [CrossRef]

29. Moghadasian, M.H.; Kaur, R.; Kostal, K.; Joshi, A.A.; Molaei, M.; Le, K.; Fischer, G.; Bonomini, F.; Favero, G.; Rezzani, R.; et al. Anti-atherosclerotic properties of wild rice in low-density lipoprotein receptor knockout mice: The gut microbiome, cytokines, and metabolomics study. *Nutrients* **2019**, *11*, 2894.
30. Trudeau, M.S.; Madden, R.F.; Parnell, J.A.; Gibbard, W.B.; Shearer, J. Dietary and supplement-based complementary and alternative medicine use in pediatric autism spectrum disorder. *Nutrients* **2019**, *11*, 1783.
31. Allaoui, A.; Gascón, S.; Benomar, S.; Quero, J.; Osada, J.; Nasri, M.; Rodríguez-Yoldi, M.J.; Boualga, A. Protein hydrolysates from fenugreek (trigonella foenum graecum) as nutraceutical molecules in colon cancer treatment. *Nutrients* **2019**, *11*, 724. [CrossRef]

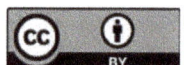

© 2020 by the authors. Licensee MDPI, Basel, Switzerland. This article is an open access article distributed under the terms and conditions of the Creative Commons Attribution (CC BY) license (http://creativecommons.org/licenses/by/4.0/).

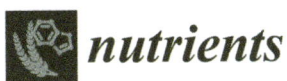

Article

Heat-Killed *Bifidobacterium breve* B-3 Enhances Muscle Functions: Possible Involvement of Increases in Muscle Mass and Mitochondrial Biogenesis

Kazuya Toda *, Yuki Yamauchi, Azusa Tanaka, Tetsuya Kuhara, Toshitaka Odamaki, Shin Yoshimoto and Jin-zhong Xiao

Next Generation Science Institute, Morinaga Milk Industry Co., Ltd., Kanagawa 252-8583, Japan; yuki-yamauchi045@morinagamilk.co.jp (Y.Y.); ad-tanaka@morinagamilk.co.jp (A.T.); t_kuhara@morinagamilk.co.jp (T.K.); t-odamak@morinagamilk.co.jp (T.O.); shin-yoshimoto923@morinagamilk.co.jp (S.Y.); j_xiao@morinagamilk.co.jp (J.-z.X.)
* Correspondence: kazuya-toda983@morinagamilk.co.jp; Tel.: +81-462-52-3067; Fax: +81-462-52-3077

Received: 11 November 2019; Accepted: 11 January 2020; Published: 15 January 2020

Abstract: A previous clinical study on pre-obesity subjects revealed that *Bifidobacterium breve* B-3 shows anti-obesity effects and possibly increases muscle mass. Here, we investigated the effects of B-3 on muscle function, such as muscle strength and metabolism, and some signaling pathways in skeletal muscle. Male rodents were orally administered live B-3 (B-3L) or heat-killed B-3 (B-3HK) for 4 weeks. We found that administration of B-3 to rats tended to increase muscle mass and affect muscle metabolism, with stronger effects in the B-3HK group than in the B-3L group. B-3HK significantly increased muscle mass and activated Akt in the rat soleus. With regard to muscle metabolism, B-3HK significantly increased phosphorylated AMP-activated protein kinase (AMPK), peroxisome proliferator-activated receptor gamma coactivator (PGC)-1α and cytochrome *c* oxidase (CCO) gene expression in the rat soleus, suggesting an effect on the AMPK-PGC1α-mitochondrial biogenesis pathway. Furthermore, B-3HK promoted oxidative muscle fiber composition in the gastrocnemius. We also observed a significantly higher level of murine grip strength in the B-3HK group than in the control group. These findings suggest the potential of heat-killed B-3 in promoting muscle hypertrophy and modifying metabolic functions, possibly through the Akt and AMPK pathways, respectively.

Keywords: skeletal muscles; probiotics; *Bifidobacterium breve* B-3; muscle mass; mitochondria

1. Introduction

Bifidobacterium breve B-3 (B-3), a probiotic strain originating from the gut of an infant, has been demonstrated to exert anti-obesity effects [1,2] through mechanisms speculated to include improvement of intestinal barrier function; adiponectin and colonic proglucagon production; and the production of B-3-derived metabolites with anti-obesity activity (e.g., acetic acids and conjugated linoleic acids) [1,3]. In a clinical study on mild obesity subjects, body fat mass was significantly lower in the B-3 group than in the placebo group. Remarkably, B-3 administration also significantly increased muscle mass [2], suggesting potential effects of B-3 on muscle.

Accumulating evidence has indicated that gut microbiota are associated with host health conditions in numerous ways [4], including through energy metabolism and mitochondrial function [5,6]. Moreover, the cross-talk pathway between the gut microbiota and skeletal muscle, i.e., the gut-muscle axis, has been extensively studied, and microbiota composition and the intestinal environment have been suggested to influence muscle mass and function, possibly by modification of microbiota composition, immune function, energy metabolism and oxidative stress [7,8].

However, studies on the effects of probiotics on muscle mass and function have been scarcely reported, and the potential effects of probiotics on physical performance and their underlying mechanisms remain unclear. Few studies have suggested the potential impact of probiotics on the gut microbiomes of athletes [9], and the possible involvement of metabolites of gut microbiota, such as acetic acid, in the stimulation of muscular energy metabolism [10], and the enhancement of endurance performance [11].

Recently, heat-killed microorganisms have attracted attention as postbiotics [12]. Numerous studies have indicated the effects of the cell components of probiotic bacteria in modulating the immune functions and enhancing the intestinal barrier [13,14]. Piqué et al. showed that non-viable bacteria and bacterial fractions could pass through the mucus and stimulate epithelial cells more efficiently compared with viable bacteria [15]. In addition, although the use of probiotic bacteria has been demonstrated to meet safety concerns, some uses of probiotic strains have been pointed at regarding risks such as systemic infections due to translocation, particularly in vulnerable patients and pediatric populations [15]. Therefore, from a safety point of view, there is an increasing interest in non-viable beneficial microbes to be used as functional ingredients. Furthermore, heat-killed bacteria are generally easier and more suitable for industrial applications in different types of foods and dietary supplements.

We investigated whether B-3 influences muscle mass and muscle metabolism using rodents fed a regular chow diet. To understand the mechanisms, the activations of Akt and AMPK involved in the signalling pathway related to muscle mass and muscle metabolism in skeletal muscle, respectively, were evaluated [16,17]. Moreover, animals were treated with heat-killed B-3 to evaluate the potential effects of heat-killed bacteria and to understand the underlying mechanisms of the effects of B-3 on skeletal muscle.

2. Materials and Methods

2.1. Preparation of the Samples

B-3 (MCC1274) lyophilized powder was obtained from the Morinaga Milk Industry (Tokyo, Japan). The live B-3 (B-3L) were suspended in saline just before daily administration. The heat-killed B-3 (B-3HK) were prepared as previously described with slight modifications [18], by heating B-3 lyophilized powder suspended in saline at 90 °C for 30 min. A lack of viable bacteria was confirmed with anaerobic culture methods using TOS propionate agar (Eiken Chemical, Tokyo, Japan). B-3HK was stored at −20 °C until an administration.

2.2. Animal Experiments

All animal studies were approved by the Animal Research Committee of Morinaga Milk Industry (approval dates: 22 February 2018 and 21 September 2018) and performed in accordance with the relevant guidelines and regulations. Male, 8-week-old Crl:CD (SD) rats and C57BL/6J mice (CRJ, Inc., Kanagawa, Japan) were housed in individual cages under controlled lighting conditions (12 h light/dark cycle; lights on from 8:00 to 20:00) at a constant temperature (25 °C) and were provided Labo MR Stock food (NOSAN Corporation, Kanagawa, Japan) and water ad libitum.

In Experiment 1 (rearing date: 6 March to 19 April 2018), rats were used for evaluation of the effects of B-3 on the anabolic and catabolic signaling pathways. Fifty rats were divided into the following four groups (n = 12 or 13): a control group (given saline), a positive control group for mTOR activation (given leucine at 1 mmol/kg/day), a B-3L group (given 1×10^9 cfu/rat) and a B-3HK group (given an amount of B-3HK equivalent to the number of cells given to the B-3L group). Each ingredient was orally administered six days a week for 28 days with the exception of the dissection date. Body weight and food intake per day were monitored weekly (Figure 1).

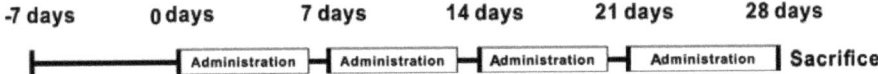

Figure 1. Protocol for the In Vivo test. Fifty male rats were acclimatized to the environmental conditions for 7 d after receipt and were then divided into four groups (n = 12 or 13). Each treatment (e.g., B-3L or B-3HK) was orally administered for 4 weeks. Body weight and food intake were monitored weekly. After administration for 4 weeks, the tissues were collected in order to evaluate the effects on muscle.

In Experiment 2 (rearing date: 2 October to 22 November 2018), mice were evaluated for fitness performance. Thirty-six mice were divided into 2 groups (n = 18): a control group (given saline) and a B-3HK group (given the same dosage as in experiment 1). The treatments were orally administered for 4 weeks, as in Experiment 1, and then a grip test was conducted at 2 and 4 weeks.

2.3. Western Blotting

The left solei of the rats (20 mg) were stored at −80 °C after freezing with liquid nitrogen. The frozen tissues were homogenized for 2 min on ice with RIPA buffer (Cell Signaling Technology [CST], Danvers, MA, USA), protease inhibitor (Invitrogen, Carlsbad, CA, USA) and 1 mM phenylmethylsulfonyl fluoride (PMSF, Nacalai Tesque, Inc., Kyoto, Japan) using a BioMasher (Nippi, Inc., Tokyo, Japan). After centrifugation at 13,000× g for 15 min at 4 °C, the protein in the supernatant was measured with a bicinchoninic acid (BCA) assay (Thermo Fisher Scientific, Waltham, MA, USA). After heat treatment for 5 min at 95 °C, the lysate samples were loaded (10 μg of protein per well) with SDS sample buffer (250 mM Tris-HCl (pH 6.8), 5% glycerol, 5% 2-mercaptoethanol, 2% SDS and 0.01% bromophenol blue) onto NuPAGE gels with MOPS buffer (Invitrogen) and separated. After SDS-PAGE, the proteins were transferred to PVDF membranes using an iBlot system (Invitrogen). The membranes were blocked for 1 h at RT with Blocking One buffer (Nacalai Tesque, Inc., Kyoto, Japan), and then incubated overnight at 4 °C with phosphorylated Akt (pAkt, catalogue number 2965, CST, Boston, MA, USA), Akt (catalogue number 2966, CST), phosphorylated mammallian target of rapamycin (pmTOR, catalogue number 5536, CST), mTOR (catalogue number 4517, CST), phosphorylated p70 S6 kinase (pp70S6K, catalogue number 9206, CST), p70S6K (catalogue number 2708, CST), phosphorylated AMP-activated protein kinase (pAMPK, catalogue number 2535, CST) and AMPK (catalogue number 2793, CST) or β-actin (catalogue number sc-47778, Santa Cruz Biotechnology, Inc., Dallas, TX, USA) antibodies at 1:1000 dilutions. The membranes were washed with TBS buffer with 1% Tween 20 and incubated for 1 h at RT with anti-rabbit or anti-mouse horseradish peroxidase-conjugated secondary antibodies (catalogue number 074-1516 or 074-1806, KPL, Gaithersburg, MD, USA) at a concentration of 0.1 μg/mL. After washing, the immunoreactive bands were visualized using ECL Prime Western Blotting Detection Reagent (GE Healthcare, Tokyo, Japan), and the band intensities were measured with a ChemiDoc™ MP Imaging System (Bio-Rad Laboratories, Hercules, CA, USA).

2.4. Quantitative Real-Time PCR (qPCR) Analysis

Total RNA was extracted from 20 mg rat soleus samples stored with RNAlater (Thermo Fisher Scientific) at −20 °C using a TissueLyser and RNeasy Mini Kit with DNase (Qiagen, Valencia, CA, USA). qPCR was performed using an ABI PRISM 7500 Fast Real-Time PCR system (Thermo Fisher Scientific K.K., Uppsala, Sweden) with SYBR Premix Ex Taq (TaKaRa Bio, Shiga, Japan) following reverse transcription of the RNA into cDNA using a PrimeScript™ RT Reagent Kit (TaKaRa Bio). The primer sets used in this study are shown in Supplementary Table S1. The expression levels of the target mRNAs were normalized to those of GAPDH mRNA.

2.5. Histological Analysis

After scarification, the right gastrocnemius of rats was fixed in 4% paraformaldehyde (Wako, Tokyo, Japan) at 4 °C for 2 days and then placed in 70% ethanol for storage. The thickest part of the fixed tissues was cut out, embedded in paraffin block, and sliced to 3 μm using a microtome. The sliced tissues were adhered to silane-coated slide glass (Muto Pure Chemicals Co., Ltd., Tokyo, Japan), which was used for immunohistochemistry (IHC) against SERCA2 ATPase. The deparaffinizing tissues with xylene and ethanol were incubated in Histo VT One (Nacalai tesque, Inc., Kyoto, Japan), heated antigen retrieval solution for 30 min at 90 °C, and reacted with the first antibody against SERCA2 ATPase (ab2861, Abcam, Cambridge, UK) overnight at 4 °C after blocking with 5% normal goat serum (Nichirei bioscience, Inc., Tokyo, Japan) for 1 h at room temperature (RT). After washing with PBS, the slides were reacted with Histofine Simple Stain Rat MAX-PO (M) (Nacalai tesque, Inc.) for 30 min at RT. After washing with Tris-buffered saline (TBS) buffer, ImmPACT™ DAB (Vector Laboratories, Inc., Burlingame, CA, USA) and hematoxylin were used for staining. The 450 fibers in a medial head of gastrocnemius were randomly counted and SERCA2 ATPase positively stained fibers were viewed using a stereoscopic microscope BX53 and Olympus cellSens Dimension software (Olympus, Tokyo, Japan). This counting was carried out under the blind. The images are provided in Supplementary Figure S1.

2.6. Grip Test

The fitness performance of the treated mice was determined at 2 and 4 weeks by testing whole-body grip strength using 4 limbs with a grip strength machine (MELQUEST Co., Ltd., Toyama, Japan), as described previously with slight modifications [19]. The grip tests were repeated five times, and all replicates were conducted within 5 min. The median was used as a representative value.

2.7. Statistical Analysis

The data are presented as means and standard errors (SEs). One-way ANOVA was used for parametric analyses, and followed by a Student's t-test or Tukey–Kramer test. The Mann–Whitney U test and Steel–Dwass test were used as the non-parametric analysis methods.

2.8. Data Availability

The datasets generated and analyzed during the current study are available from the corresponding author, K.T., upon reasonable request.

3. Results

To verify the beneficial effect of B-3 administration on muscle tissue and muscle function, we used two different animals. Rats were used to examine the muscle mass and some activated signaling pathways (Experiment 1). On the other hand, mice were used for functional evaluation of B-3HK on the muscle strength (Experiment 2).

Experiment 1

3.1. The Effects of B-3 Administration on Body and Tissue Weight in Rats

We first evaluated changes in muscle mass in rats after B-3 administration according to the schedules described (Figure 1). A significant increase in the weight of the soleus (a slow oxidative (SO) fiber-dominant muscle) per total body weight was observed in the B-3HK group compared with the control group. In addition, the weights of the plantaris and gastrocnemius (fast glycolytic (FG) fiber-dominant muscles) per total body weight tended to be higher in the B-3HK group than in the control group (Table 1), but without statistical significance. Although the masses of these muscles were also higher in the B-3L group and the leucine (a muscle hypertrophy promoting nutrients) group than in the control group, the differences were not significant. A significant difference in food intake was observed at week 1 between the control and B-3HK groups, but there were no significant differences afterwards. There were no significant differences in body weight at each time point, or in liver weights at week 4, between each group (Table 1).

Table 1. The effects of B-3 on body and tissue weights in rats.

		Control	Leucine	B-3L	B-3HK
Body weight (g)	initial	311.2 ± 2.7	307.3 ± 3.5	302.1 ± 2.9	303.8 ± 3.6
	1 week	361.1 ± 4.6	356.9 ± 5.5	358.4 ± 3.3	354.1 ± 5.1
	2 weeks	408.0 ± 6.3	397.3 ± 9.5	400.5 ± 4.8	393.2 ± 7.5
	3 weeks	430.7 ± 9.6	418.1 ± 9.7	425.9 ± 6.5	417.9 ± 9.0
	4 weeks	433.2 ± 9.4	430.6 ± 10.7	430.1 ± 6.2	421.3 ± 9.4
Food intake (g)	initial	31.8 ± 0.6	30.7 ± 0.8	30.5 ± 0.5	31.0 ± 0.9
	1 week	33.7 ± 1.1	31.6 ± 1.3	31.4 ± 0.7	29.8 ± 1.1 *
	2 weeks	31.2 ± 0.9	30.3 ± 1.0	30.7 ± 1.5	29.5 ± 1.1
	3 weeks	30.8 ± 1.1	28.5 ± 1.2	30.7 ± 1.5	30.0 ± 1.3
	4 weeks	33.5 ± 1.2	32.1 ± 1.4	31.8 ± 0.7	32.2 ± 1.1
Liver weight (g)		12.0 ± 0.4	11.5 ± 0.4	11.7 ± 0.3	11.3 ± 0.4
Liver weight/body weight (mg/g)		27.6 ± 0.8	26.5 ± 0.5	27.2 ± 0.5	26.8 ± 0.4
Soleus weight (mg)		193.3 ± 5.8	203.5 ± 5.7	205.4 ± 5.7	209.7 ± 5.4
Soleus weight/body weight (mg/g)		0.45 ± 0.01	0.47 ± 0.01	0.48 ± 0.01	0.50 ± 0.01 *
Plantaris weight (mg)		415.0 ± 21.6	431.4 ± 12.4	440.3 ± 12.4	456.4 ± 24.4
Plantaris weight/body weight (mg/g)		0.96 ± 0.05	1.00 ± 0.02	1.03 ± 0.03	1.08 ± 0.05
Gastrocnemius weight (mg)		2242.9 ± 50.3	2253.3 ± 48.1	2303.5 ± 44.8	2274.2 ± 53.4
Gastrocnemius weight/body weight (mg/g)		5.19 ± 0.09	5.26 ± 0.13	5.37 ± 0.12	5.40 ± 0.06

The data are presented as the means and SEs. Asterisks (*) denote significant differences from the control group at * $p < 0.05$ (Tukey–Kramer test).

3.2. B-3HK Promoted Phosphorylation of Akt in the Rat Soleus

To clarify the mechanisms by which B-3HK increased muscle mass, we investigated the activation of Akt, one of the key regulators of protein synthesis in skeletal muscle [20]. The western blot results indicate that the levels of activated Akt in the soleus were significantly increased by B-3HK administration (Figure 2). It is well known that activated Akt in skeletal muscle induces the mTOR signaling pathway, which is a critical pathway regulating protein synthesis, leading to increased muscle mass. We observed that B-3HK tended to induce phosphorylation of mTOR and its downstream molecule p70S6K in soleus, similarly to leucine (Figure 3), indicating that the possible involvement of the Akt-mTOR-p70S6K signaling pathway in increased muscle mass by B-3HK administration.

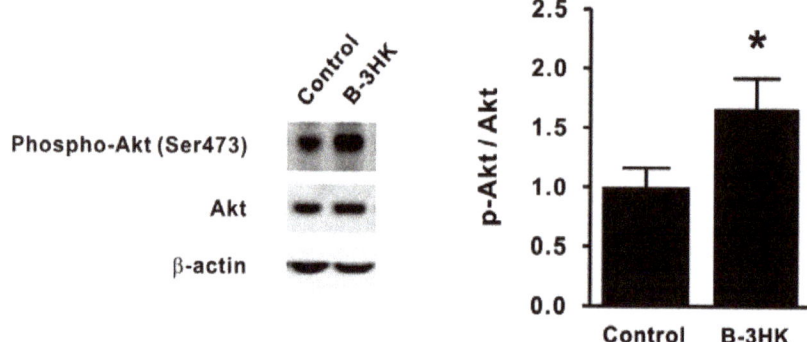

Figure 2. The effects of B-3 on Akt activation in the soleus. Representative bands and the expression ratio of pAkt to Akt in the soleus are shown (n = 9, 10). Difference was analyzed for statistical significance using Mann–Whitney U test (* $p < 0.05$). The data are expressed as the means and SEs.

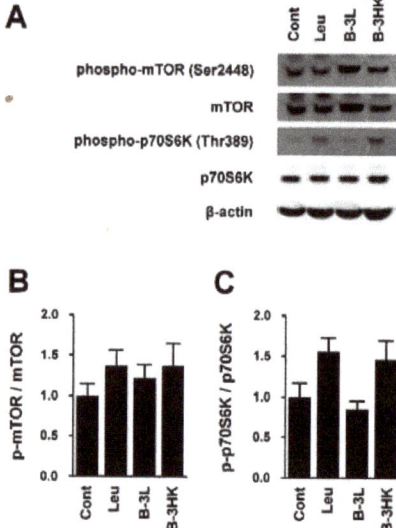

Figure 3. The effects of B-3 on mTOR signaling in soleus. Western blotting was used for the signaling pathways related protein synthesis in rat soleus muscle. (**A**) Representative bands and the expression ratio of (**B**) p-mTOR to mTOR and (**C**) p-p70S6K to p70S6K are shown (n = 6). Leucine was used as a positive control for induction of mTOR. The data are expressed as the means and SEs. Abbreviations: Cont, control; Leu, leucine; B-3L, live B-3; B-3HK, heat-killed B-3.

3.3. The Effects of B-3 on the AMPK-PGC-1α-Mitochondrial Biogenesis Pathway in the Rat Soleus

We then examined the effects of B-3 administration on muscle metabolism, which is related to energy productivity and consumption [21]. B-3HK significantly promoted the activation of AMPK (Figure 4A,B), which regulates energy balance at both the cellular and physiological levels as a master regulator of metabolism [22,23]. No change was observed in the group treated with leucine, a well-known muscle hypertrophy-promoting nutrient. Moreover, B-3HK also significantly increased the mRNA expression of peroxisome proliferator-activated receptor gamma coactivator (PGC)-1α, a master regulator of mitochondrial biogenesis [24], and cytochrome c oxidase (CCO), which has been reported to control enzymes related to the mitochondrial oxidative phosphorylation system (OXPHOS) at the mitochondrial membrane [25,26], in the soleus (Figure 4C,D). Although the expression of these genes was also higher in the B-3L group than in the control group, the differences were not significant.

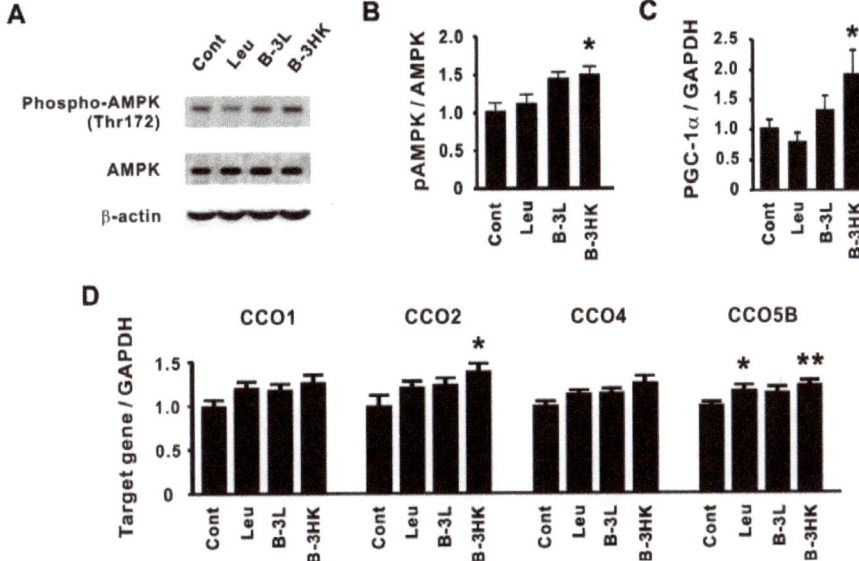

Figure 4. B-3 enhanced the AMPK-PGC-1α-mitochondrial biogenesis signaling pathway in the soleus. (**A**) Representative bands and (**B**) the expression ratio of pAMPK to AMPK in the soleus are shown ($n = 6$). (**C,D**) qPCR was used to evaluate the relative mRNA expressions of PGC-1α, CCO1, CCO2, CCO4 and CCO5B in the soleus ($n = 12$–13). Statistical differences were analyzed for significance using the Steel–Dwass test (* $p < 0.05$, ** $p < 0.01$, versus control). The data are expressed as means and SEs. Abbreviations: Cont, control; Leu, leucine; B-3L, live B-3; B-3HK, heat-killed B-3.

3.4. B-3HK Promoted the Distribution of Oxidative Fibers in the Gastrocnemius in Rats

A high expression of PGC-1α is well known to be involved in shifting muscle fiber type distribution toward oxidative fibers [27]. To examine the enhancing effect of B-3HK on the oxidative fiber composition in the gastrocnemius, an FG fiber-dominant muscle adjoining soleus was evaluated by counting the number of sarco-/endoplasmic reticulum Ca^{2+} (SERCA)2 ATPase-positive fibers (Figure 5A). The administration of B-3HK significantly increased the relative abundance of type I muscle fibers (the most oxidative fibers) compared with saline administration (Figure 5B). B-3HK had a greater effect than B-3L in promoting the distribution of oxidative fibers. This finding indicates that B-3HK induced PGC-1α expression in the gastrocnemius as well as in the soleus.

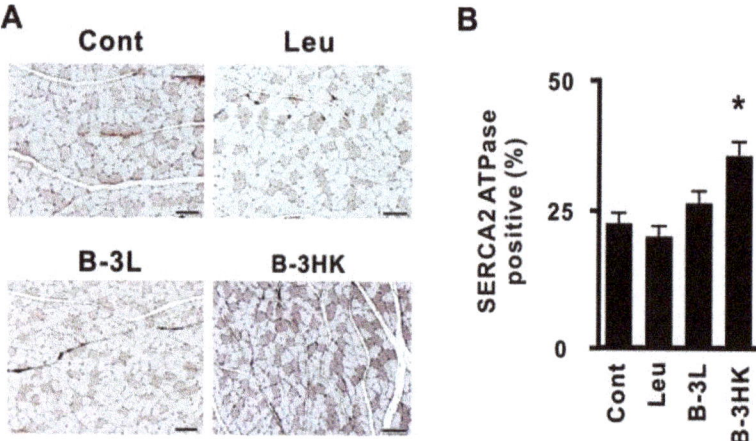

Figure 5. B-3 promoted the switching of type 1 fibers through the AMPK signaling pathway in rats. (**A**) Representative results of immunohistochemistry against SERCA2 ATPase in the rat medial gastrocnemius. The scale bar represents 100 μm. (**B**) The percentage of SERCA2 ATPase-positive fibers was determined among 450 fibers in three sections per rat ($n = 7$). Statistical differences were analyzed for significance using the Steel–Dwass test (* $p < 0.05$, versus control). The data are expressed as the means and SEs.

Experiment 2

3.5. B-3HK-Enhanced Fitness Performance in Mice

Since increasing muscle mass was expected to enhance muscle strength, we used a murine model to evaluate the effects of B-3HK on muscle function. We observed a significantly higher level of grip strength in the B-3HK group compared to the control group at both two and four weeks (Figure 6), in addition to significantly increased muscle mass in the mice's solei (Supplementary Table S2).

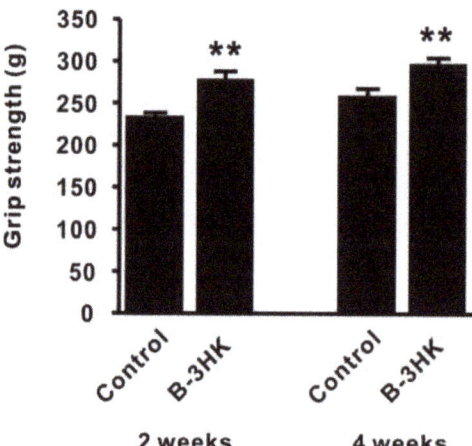

Figure 6. The effect of B-3 on whole-body grip strength in mice. Physical performance was analyzed by the grip strength test at 2 and 4 weeks ($n = 18$). Differences with the control group were analyzed for significance using Student's t-test (** $p < 0.01$). The data are expressed as the means and SEs.

4. Discussion

Skeletal muscle is the largest organ in the body; in most mammals, it makes up ~45%–55% of the body mass and is a major determinant of the basal metabolic rate [28–30]. Our previous clinical results in mild obesity subjects indicated that B-3 administration both decreases body fat percentage and increases muscle mass [2]. Thus, we hypothesized that B-3 exerts beneficial effects on muscle mass and function related to basal muscle metabolism that might contribute to its anti-obesity effects.

Indeed, in the present study, we found that daily administration of B-3 to rats for a prolonged period tended to increase muscle mass and activate AMPK, a well-known master metabolic regulator, in the soleus [22,23]. Furthermore, the gene expression of PGC-1α and CCO was higher in the B-3 administration group than in the control group. The increase in PGC-1α and CCO gene expression indicates a possibility of the enhancement of basal metabolism through mitochondrial biogenesis and OXPHOS [24–26]. Thus, these results suggest that B-3 induces mitochondrial biogenesis in skeletal muscle through the AMPK-PGC-1α signaling pathway, which might be a mechanism by which B-3 exerts its anti-obesity effects.

Intriguingly, B-3HK had a greater effect than B-3L in eliciting some muscle improvements. For example, B-3HK activated Akt-mTOR-protein synthesis signaling, and consequently increased muscle mass. Through its beneficial effects, B-3HK was observed for the possible enhancement of grip strength in a murine model. In addition, B-3HK was suggested to enhance mitochondrial biogenesis (e.g., increase CCO gene expression) through AMPK-PGC-1α signaling pathways, probably leading to increased mitochondrial energy productivity, and induced an oxidative fiber type composition in the gastrocnemius.

In general, AMPK is well known to inhibit protein synthesis through the suppression of the mTOR, a critical regulator of anabolic pathways [22,23], which indicates that the co-activation of both anabolic and catabolic pathways does not occur in the skeletal muscle at the same time. However, we observed the co-activation of Akt and AMPK in response to B-3HK by western blotting analysis. These results suggest that several independent pathways from B-3HK might activate both Akt and AMPK. Since the bacterial cells of B-3HK might contain various components, such as lipoteichoic acid, peptide glycans and nucleotides, each component might separately activate the Akt and/or AMPK signaling pathway with various strengths in the skeletal muscle. As a result, the mTOR-protein synthesis pathway might be positively influenced in response to B-3HK for muscle hypertrophy, in spite of AMPK activation. To unravel the reasons for this, further studies are required for the identification of bioactive factors.

Similarly to our observation, it has been reported that *Lactobacillus plantarum* TWK10 increases muscle mass and promotes type I fibers (slow muscle) in murine gastrocnemius muscle [31]. Moreover, TWK10 has shown potential as an ergogenic aid to improve aerobic endurance performance via physiological adaptation effects in amateur runners and healthy humans [32,33].

Furthermore, the way in which heat-killing treatment enhances the effects of B-3 remains to be elucidated. *Plovier* et al. reported that heat-killed *Akkermansia muciniphila* exerted stronger anti-obesity effects than live *A. muciniphila* in high-fat diet-fed mice [34,35]. In addition, another study reported that although the administration of heat-killed *A. muciniphila* improved several metabolic parameters, such as insulin sensitivity and plasma total cholesterol, in obese insulin-resistant volunteers, it did not change the gut microbiome structure [36]. Therefore, it has been suggested that the mechanism by which heat-killed *A. muciniphila* exerts its effects involves the modulation of host immune responses and the intestinal barrier function by an outer membrane protein (Amuc_1100 protein) through activation of TLR2 and TLR4 [34,35]. It is also well known that *Bifidobacterium* has cell components that can regulate TLR signaling pathways [37,38]. Thus, we speculate that certain cell component(s) of B-3HK might exhibit enhanced ligand binding with targeted receptors to activate signaling pathways in intestinal cells (e.g., intestinal epithelial cells or intestinal immune cells), and then induce the production of some bioactive factors. Notably, the administration of serum from B-3HK-treated rats activated AMPK in a differentiated L6 rat myoblast cell line (Supplementary Figure S2), indicating that bioactive factors such as cytokines and hormones could have been present in the serum. In addition, some reports suggested that live and heat-killed probiotics strains had different immune responses, such as cytokine secretion profiles [39,40], which may be one of the possible mechanisms by which heat-killed B-3 is more effective on muscle functions. To clarify the differences in activity between B-3L and B-3HK, further studies are needed to elucidate the specific B-3HK-affected signaling pathway and to identify the bioactive factors in B-3HK-treated rat serum.

Recent studies have suggested that *Bifidobacterium* is recognized as a key taxon for physical frailty and sarcopenia in elderly individuals [8]; however, it remains unclear whether the decreases in bifidobacterial abundance that occur with age influence muscle health [7,41]. The present study explored the positive relationships between *Bifidobacterium* and muscle health. Although further studies using ageing models [42] are required, B-3HK was expected to be useful for improving muscle atrophy, such as that occurring in sarcopenia according to the increase in muscle mass by B-3HK.

There are some limitations in this study. Firstly, we used leucine as a positive control for activation of mTOR signaling pathway. Leucine tended to promote phosphorylation mTOR and p70S6K (Figure 3b,c), but the effect appeared to be weaker than expected. Moreover, owing to the limits of administrated volume and the solubility of leucine in saline, leucine was administrated at 0.131 g/kg/day, which was lower compared to previous study (>0.675 g/kg/day) by Fumiaki et al. [43]. The low dosage of leucine used in the present study might have influenced the degree of mTOR phosphorylation induction. Secondly, the mechanisms of the effects of B-3, and the reason why heat-killed B-3 was more effective, were not clarified. Moreover, since the results were observed in animal models, translation of the effects to humans remains unknown. These issues need to be addressed in future studies.

5. Conclusions

Daily administration of B-3, a probiotic strain for anti-obesity, promoted mitochondrial biogenesis through the AMPK-PGC-1α signaling pathway in skeletal muscle, and the distribution of oxidative muscle fibers through increasing in PGC-1α gene expression; and induced muscle hypertrophy through the Akt signaling pathway in rats. Remarkably, it was observed that heat-killing treatment enhanced the activities of B-3. In addition, B-3HK also showed potential in increasing grip strength in a mouse model. These findings may contribute to the understanding of the mechanism of the anti-obesity effects of B-3 and suggest its potential benefits for improving physical fitness and ameliorating physical fatigue and muscle atrophy; in particular, after heat-killing treatment.

Supplementary Materials: The following are available online at http://www.mdpi.com/2072-6643/12/1/219/s1. Figure S1. Histopathological images. Figure S2. The effects of the rat serum on AMPK activation in vitro. Table S1. List of primer sets. Table S2. The effects of B-3 on body and tissue weight in the treated mice at 4 weeks.

Author Contributions: The corresponding author is K.T., who contributed to study conception and design; conducted most of the experiments; analyzed and interpreted the data; and wrote the manuscript. Y.Y. and A.T. performed some of the animal experiments. T.K. contributed to study conception and design. T.O. and S.Y. contributed to study design, data interpretation and writing of the manuscript. J.-z.X. designed and supervised the entire project, including data interpretation, and revised the manuscript. All authors have read and agreed to the published version of the manuscript.

Funding: This study was funded by Morinaga Milk Industry Co., Ltd. All the authors are employees of Morinaga Milk Industry Co., Ltd. The funders had no role in the study design, data collection and analysis, decision to publish, or preparation of the manuscript.

Acknowledgments: We thank Yutaka Matsunaga for technical advice pertaining to the animal experiments.

Conflicts of Interest: All the authors are employees of Morinaga Milk Industry Co., Ltd., which is a commercial company that sells dairy products such as milk, yogurt and infant formula.

References

1. Kondo, S.; Xiao, J.; Satoh, T.; Odamaki, T.; Takahashi, S.; Sugahara, H.; Yaeshima, T.; Iwatsuki, K.; Kamei, A.; Abe, K. Antiobesity effects of Bifidobacterium breve strain B-3 supplementation in a mouse model with high-fat diet-induced obesity. *Biosci. Biotechnol. Biochem.* **2010**, *74*, 1656–1661. [CrossRef]
2. Minami, J.; Iwabuchi, N.; Tanaka, M.; Yamauchi, K.; Xiao, J.Z.; Abe, F.; Sakane, N. Effects of Bifidobacterium breve B-3 on body fat reductions in pre-obese adults: A randomized, double-blind, placebo-controlled trial. *Biosci. Microbiota Food Health* **2018**, *37*, 67–75. [CrossRef] [PubMed]
3. Kurose, Y.; Minami, J.; Sen, A.; Iwabuchi, N.; Abe, F.; Xiao, J.; Suzuki, T. Bioactive factors secreted by Bifidobacterium breve B-3 enhance barrier function in human intestinal Caco-2 cells. *Benef. Microbes* **2019**, *10*, 89–100. [CrossRef] [PubMed]
4. Marchesi, J.R.; Adams, D.H.; Fava, F.; Hermes, G.D.A.; Hirschfield, G.M.; Hold, G.; Quraishi, M.N.; Kinross, J.; Smidt, H.; Tuohy, K.M.; et al. The gut microbiota and host health: A new clinical frontier. *Gut* **2016**, *65*, 330–339. [CrossRef] [PubMed]
5. Levy, M.; Kolodziejczyk, A.A.; Thaiss, C.A.; Elinav, E. Dysbiosis and the immune system. *Nat. Rev. Immunol.* **2017**, *17*, 219–232. [CrossRef] [PubMed]
6. Belizário, J.E.; Faintuch, J.; Garay-Malpartida, M. Gut Microbiome Dysbiosis and Immunometabolism: New Frontiers for Treatment of Metabolic Diseases. *Mediat. Inflamm.* **2018**, *2018*, 2037838. [CrossRef] [PubMed]
7. Grosicki, G.J.; Fielding, R.A.; Lustgarten, M.S. Gut Microbiota Contribute to Age-Related Changes in Skeletal Muscle Size, Composition, and Function: Biological Basis for a Gut-Muscle Axis. *Calcif. Tissue Int.* **2018**, *102*, 433–442. [CrossRef]
8. Ticinesi, A.; Nouvenne, A.; Cerundolo, N.; Catania, P.; Prati, B.; Tana, C.; Meschi, T. Gut Microbiota, Muscle Mass and Function in Aging: A Focus on Physical Frailty and Sarcopenia. *Nutrients* **2019**, *11*, 1633. [CrossRef]
9. Wosinska, L.; Cotter, P.D.; O'Sullivan, O.; Guinane, C. The Potential Impact of Probiotics on the Gut Microbiome of Athletes. *Nutrients* **2019**, *11*, 2270. [CrossRef]
10. Maruta, H.; Yoshimura, Y.; Araki, A.; Kimoto, M.; Takahashi, Y.; Yamashita, H. Activation of AMP-Activated Protein Kinase and Stimulation of Energy Metabolism by Acetic Acid in L6 Myotube Cells. *PLoS ONE* **2016**, *11*, e0158055. [CrossRef]
11. Pan, J.H.; Kim, J.H.; Kim, H.M.; Lee, E.S.; Shin, D.H.; Kim, S.; Shin, M.; Kim, S.H.; Lee, J.H.; Kim, Y.J. Acetic acid enhances endurance capacity of exercise-trained mice by increasing skeletal muscle oxidative properties. *Biosci. Biotechnol. Biochem.* **2015**, *79*, 1535–1541. [CrossRef] [PubMed]
12. Wegh, C.A.M.; Geerlings, S.Y.; Knol, J.; Roeselers, G.; Belzer, C. Postbiotics and Their Potential Applications in Early Life Nutrition and Beyond. *Int. J. Mol. Sci.* **2019**, *20*, 4673. [CrossRef] [PubMed]
13. Sakai, F.; Hosoya, T.; Ono-Ohmachi, A.; Ukibe, K.; Ogawa, A.; Moriya, T.; Kadooka, Y.; Shiozaki, T.; Nakagawa, H.; Nakayama, Y.; et al. Lactobacillus gasseri SBT2055 induces TGF-β expression in dendritic cells and activates TLR2 signal to produce IgA in the small intestine. *PLoS ONE* **2014**, *9*, e105370. [CrossRef] [PubMed]
14. Murata, K.; Tomosada, Y.; Villena, J.; Chiba, E.; Shimazu, T.; Aso, H.; Iwabuchi, N.; Xiao, J.Z.; Saito, T.; Kitazawa, H. Bifidobacterium breve MCC-117 Induces Tolerance in Porcine Intestinal Epithelial Cells: Study of the Mechanisms Involved in the Immunoregulatory Effect. *Biosci. Microbiota Food Health* **2014**, *33*, 1–10. [CrossRef]
15. Piqué, N.; Berlanga, M.; Miñana-Galbis, D. Health Benefits of Heat-Killed (Tyndallized) Probiotics: An Overview. *Int. J. Mol. Sci.* **2019**, *20*, 2534. [CrossRef]
16. Yoon, M.S. mTOR as a Key Regulator in Maintaining Skeletal Muscle Mass. *Front. Physiol.* **2017**, *8*, 788. [CrossRef]
17. Mihaylova, M.M.; Shaw, R.J. The AMPK signalling pathway coordinates cell growth, autophagy and metabolism. *Nat. Cell Biol.* **2011**, *13*, 1016–1023. [CrossRef]
18. Arai, S.; Iwabuchi, N.; Takahashi, S.; Xiao, J.Z.; Abe, F.; Hachimura, S. Orally administered heat-killed Lactobacillus paracasei MCC1849 enhances antigen-specific IgA secretion and induces follicular helper T cells in mice. *PLoS ONE* **2018**, *13*, e0199018. [CrossRef]
19. Tanaka, M.; Yoshino, Y.; Takeda, S.; Toda, K.; Shimoda, H.; Tsuruma, K.; Shimazawa, M.; Hara, H. Fermented Rice Germ Extract Alleviates Morphological and Functional Damage to Murine Gastrocnemius Muscle by Inactivation of AMP-Activated Protein Kinase. *J. Med. Food* **2017**, *20*, 969–980. [CrossRef]

20. Egerman, M.A.; Glass, D.J. Signaling pathways controlling skeletal muscle mass. *Crit. Rev. Biochem. Mol. Biol.* **2014**, *49*, 59–68. [CrossRef]
21. Frontera, W.R.; Ochala, J. Skeletal muscle: A brief review of structure and function. *Calcif. Tissue Int.* **2015**, *96*, 183–195. [CrossRef] [PubMed]
22. Mounier, R.; Lantier, L.; Leclerc, J.; Sotiropoulos, A.; Pende, M.; Daegelen, D.; Sakamoto, K.; Foretz, M.; Viollet, B. Important role for AMPKalpha1 in limiting skeletal muscle cell hypertrophy. *FASEB J.* **2009**, *23*, 2264–2273. [CrossRef] [PubMed]
23. Thomson, D.M. The Role of AMPK in the Regulation of Skeletal Muscle Size, Hypertrophy, and Regeneration. *Int. J. Mol. Sci.* **2018**, *19*, 3125. [CrossRef] [PubMed]
24. Fernandez-Marcos, P.J.; Auwerx, J. Regulation of PGC-1α, a nodal regulator of mitochondrial biogenesis. *Am. J. Clin. Nutr.* **2011**, *93*, 884S–890S. [CrossRef]
25. Diaz, F. Cytochrome c oxidase deficiency: Patients and animal models. *Biochim. Biophys. Acta* **2010**, *1802*, 100–110. [CrossRef]
26. Pacelli, C.; Latorre, D.; Cocco, T.; Capuano, F.; Kukat, C.; Seibel, P.; Villani, G. Tight control of mitochondrial membrane potential by cytochrome c oxidase. *Mitochondrion* **2011**, *11*, 334–341. [CrossRef]
27. Zhang, L.; Zhou, Y.; Wu, W.; Hou, L.; Chen, H.; Zuo, B.; Xiong, Y.; Yang, J. Skeletal Muscle-Specific Overexpression of PGC-1α Induces Fiber-Type Conversion through Enhanced Mitochondrial Respiration and Fatty Acid Oxidation in Mice and Pigs. *Int. J. Biol. Sci.* **2017**, *13*, 1152–1162. [CrossRef]
28. Janssen, I.; Heymsfield, S.B.; Wang, Z.M.; Ross, R. Skeletal muscle mass and distribution in 468 men and women aged 18–88 yr. *J. Appl. Physiol.* **2000**, *89*, 81–88. [CrossRef]
29. Zurlo, F.; Nemeth, P.M.; Choksi, R.M.; Sesodia, S.; Ravussin, E. Whole-body energy metabolism and skeletal muscle biochemical characteristics. *Metabolism* **1994**, *43*, 481–486. [CrossRef]
30. Zurlo, F.; Larson, K.; Bogardus, C.; Ravussin, E. Skeletal muscle metabolism is a major determinant of resting energy expenditure. *J. Clin. Investig.* **1990**, *86*, 1423–1427. [CrossRef]
31. Chen, Y.M.; Wei, L.; Chiu, Y.S.; Hsu, Y.J.; Tsai, T.Y.; Wang, M.F.; Huang, C.C. Lactobacillus plantarum TWK10 Supplementation Improves Exercise Performance and Increases Muscle Mass in Mice. *Nutrients* **2016**, *8*, 205. [CrossRef] [PubMed]
32. Huang, W.C.; Hsu, Y.J.; Li, H.; Kan, N.W.; Chen, Y.M.; Lin, J.S.; Hsu, T.K.; Tsai, T.Y.; Chiu, Y.S.; Huang, C.C. Effect of Lactobacillus Plantarum TWK10 on Improving Endurance Performance in Humans. *Chin. J. Physiol.* **2018**, *61*, 163–170. [CrossRef]
33. Huang, W.; Lee, M.C.; Lee, C.; Ng, K.; Hsu, Y.; Tsai, T.Y.; Young, S.L.; Lin, J.S.; Huang, C.C. Effect of Lactobacillus plantarum TWK10 on Exercise Physiological Adaptation, Performance, and Body Composition in Healthy Humans. *Nutrients* **2019**, *11*, 2836. [CrossRef] [PubMed]
34. Ottman, N.; Reunanen, J.; Meijerink, M.; Pietilä, T.E.; Kainulainen, V.; Klievink, J.; Huuskonen, L.; Aalvink, S.; Skurnik, M.; Boeren, S.; et al. Pili-like proteins of Akkermansia muciniphila modulate host immune responses and gut barrier function. *PLoS ONE* **2017**, *12*, e0173004. [CrossRef] [PubMed]
35. Plovier, H.; Everard, A.; Druart, C.; Depommier, C.; Van Hul, M.; Geurts, L.; Chilloux, J.; Ottman, N.; Duparc, T.; Lichtenstein, L.; et al. A purified membrane protein from Akkermansia muciniphila or the pasteurized bacterium improves metabolism in obese and diabetic mice. *Nat. Med.* **2017**, *23*, 107–113. [CrossRef]
36. Depommier, C.; Everard, A.; Druart, C.; Plovier, H.; Van Hul, M.; Vieira-Silva, S.; Falony, G.; Raes, J.; Maiter, D.; Delzenne, N.M.; et al. Supplementation with Akkermansia muciniphila in overweight and obese human volunteers: A proof-of-concept exploratory study. *Nat. Med.* **2019**, *25*, 1096–1103. [CrossRef]
37. Villena, J.; Aso, H.; Kitazawa, H. Regulation of toll-like receptors-mediated inflammation by immunobiotics in bovine intestinal epitheliocytes: Role of signaling pathways and negative regulators. *Front. Immunol.* **2014**, *5*, 421. [CrossRef]
38. Plantinga, T.S.; Van Maren, W.W.C.; Van Bergenhenegouwen, J.; Hameetman, M.; Nierkens, S.; Jacobs, C.; De Jong, D.J.; Joosten, L.A.B.; Van't Land, B.; Garssen, J.; et al. Differential toll-like receptor recognition and induction of cytokine profile by Bifidobacterium breve and Lactobacillus strains of probiotics. *Clin. Vaccine Immunol.* **2011**, *18*, 621–628. [CrossRef]
39. Donkor, O.N.; Ravikumar, M.; Proudfoot, O.; Day, S.L.; Apostolopoulos, V.; Paukovics, G.; Vasiljevic, T.; Nutt, S.L.; Gill, H. Cytokine profile and induction of T helper type 17 and regulatory T cells by human peripheral mononuclear cells after microbial exposure. *Clin. Exp. Immunol.* **2012**, *167*, 282–295. [CrossRef]

40. Sugahara, H.; Yao, R.; Odamaki, T.; Xiao, J.Z. Differences between live and heat-killed bifidobacteria in the regulation of immune function and the intestinal environment. *Benef. Microbes* **2017**, *8*, 463–472. [CrossRef]
41. Picca, A.; Fanelli, F.; Calvani, R.; Mulè, G.; Pesce, V.; Sisto, A.; Pantanelli, C.; Bernabei, R.; Landi, F.; Marzetti, E. Gut Dysbiosis and Muscle Aging: Searching for Novel Targets against Sarcopenia. *Mediat. Inflamm.* **2018**, *2018*, 7026198. [CrossRef] [PubMed]
42. Dalle, S.; Rossmeislova, L.; Koppo, K. The Role of Inflammation in Age-Related Sarcopenia. *Front. Physiol.* **2017**, *8*, 1045. [CrossRef] [PubMed]
43. Yoshizawa, F.; Mochizuki, S.; Sugahara, K. Differential dose response of mTOR signaling to oral administration of leucine in skeletal muscle and liver of rats. *Biosci. Biotechnol. Biochem.* **2013**, *77*, 839–842. [CrossRef] [PubMed]

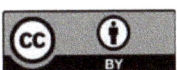

© 2020 by the authors. Licensee MDPI, Basel, Switzerland. This article is an open access article distributed under the terms and conditions of the Creative Commons Attribution (CC BY) license (http://creativecommons.org/licenses/by/4.0/).

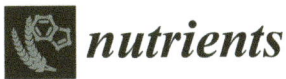

Review

Vitamin K as a Diet Supplement with Impact in Human Health: Current Evidence in Age-Related Diseases

Dina C. Simes [1,2,*], Carla S. B. Viegas [1,2], Nuna Araújo [1] and Catarina Marreiros [1]

1. Centre of Marine Sciences (CCMAR), University of Algarve, Campus de Gambelas, 8005-139 Faro, Portugal; caviegas@ualg.pt (C.S.B.V.); naraujo@ualg.pt (N.A.); cimarreiros@ualg.pt (C.M.)
2. GenoGla Diagnostics, Centre of Marine Sciences (CCMAR), University of Algarve, Campus de Gambelas, 8005-139 Faro, Portugal
* Correspondence: dsimes@ualg.pt; Tel.: +351-289-800100

Received: 5 December 2019; Accepted: 31 December 2019; Published: 3 January 2020

Abstract: Vitamin K health benefits have been recently widely shown to extend beyond blood homeostasis and implicated in chronic low-grade inflammatory diseases such as cardiovascular disease, osteoarthritis, dementia, cognitive impairment, mobility disability, and frailty. Novel and more efficient nutritional and therapeutic options are urgently needed to lower the burden and the associated health care costs of these age-related diseases. Naturally occurring vitamin K comprise the phylloquinone (vitamin K1), and a series of menaquinones broadly designated as vitamin K2 that differ in source, absorption rates, tissue distribution, bioavailability, and target activity. Although vitamin K1 and K2 sources are mainly dietary, consumer preference for diet supplements is growing, especially when derived from marine resources. The aim of this review is to update the reader regarding the specific contribution and effect of each K1 and K2 vitamers in human health, identify potential methods for its sustainable and cost-efficient production, and novel natural sources of vitamin K and formulations to improve absorption and bioavailability. This new information will contribute to foster the use of vitamin K as a health-promoting supplement, which meets the increasing consumer demand. Simultaneously, relevant information on the clinical context and direct health consequences of vitamin K deficiency focusing in aging and age-related diseases will be discussed.

Keywords: vitamin K; diet supplement; age-related diseases; vitamin K-dependent proteins; pathological calcification; inflammation

1. Introduction

Historically recognized as a key factor for the synthesis of blood clotting factors in the liver, vitamin K is currently known to be involved in a wide range of biological processes and is associated with many pathological conditions. Since its discovery in 1936 [1], the most well-known function of vitamin K is as a cofactor for the γ-glutamyl carboxylase (GGCX) enzyme responsible for the post-translational modification of vitamin K-dependent proteins (VKDPs) through the conversion of specific glutamic acid (Glu) into calcium binding γ-carboxyglutamic acid (Gla) residues [2,3]. In humans, at least 17 different VKDPs, which are also known as Gla proteins, have been identified to date, and are generally referred to as hepatic and extra-hepatic VKDPs, according to the synthesis location (Table 1). The hepatic group of VKDPs synthetized in the liver are essential for regulating blood coagulation and comprise the coagulation factors II, VII, IX, and X, and the anti-coagulation proteins C, S, and Z. Extra-hepatic VKDPs include matrix Gla protein (MGP), osteocalcin (OC), Gla-rich protein (GRP), growth arrest-specific protein 6 (Gas6), proline-rich Gla proteins (PRGP1 and 2), transmembrane Gla proteins (TMG3 and 4), periostin, and the GGCX enzyme. These extra-hepatic VKDPs, which are mostly known for their protective role in the bone and cardiovascular system, exhibit a broad tissue distribution and are involved in a wide range of biological functions such as bone homeostasis, ectopic calcification, cell differentiation and proliferation, inflammation, and signal transduction. γ-carboxylation has been shown essential for the correct function of VKDPs. In addition, vitamin K deficiency has been linked to several pathological conditions such as cardiovascular diseases (CVD), chronic kidney disease (CKD) [4], osteoarthritis (OA) [5], rheumatoid arthritis (RA), osteoporosis, cancer, dementia, certain skin pathologies, functional decline, and disability [6]. Most of these chronic health conditions are associated with pathological calcification and inflammation, where the role of VKDPs and vitamin K is being highlighted. Since both inflammation and pathological mineralization are associated with the aging process and these diseases are highly prevalent in the elderly, a new concept on the involvement of vitamin K in *inflammation* is growing. In addition, novel roles have been disclosed for vitamin K independent of its activity as a cofactor for GGCX, such as an antioxidant, anti-inflammatory, promoter of cognition, inhibition of tumor progression, and transcriptional regulator of osteoblastic genes. However, in clinical practice, vitamin K is mainly used in blood clotting-associated prophylaxis. The number of in vitro, in vivo, and clinical data showing the beneficial effects of vitamin K without adverse effects or documented toxicity raised increasing interest on the use of vitamin K as a health promoting supplement. In fact, aging societies represent a major economic challenge for health care systems, and diet supplements promoting healthy aging and improving the prognosis of age-related diseases, are required to be implemented in clinical practice.

In this context, it is crucial to highlight that naturally occurring vitamin K comprise the vitamin K1 (also known as phylloquinone or phytonadione), and a series of menaquinones (MKs), designated as vitamin K2 [3,6]. A growing amount of scientific evidence has demonstrated differences between vitamin K1 and K2 in terms of source, function, and target activity. While vitamin K1 and K2 from different sources are currently commercially available and are becoming popular as health supplements, novel tactics for more efficient and affordable attainment of both vitamers are currently being explored. However, it is important to clearly establish a specific cause-effect for each of the vitamin K vitamers to increase efficacy and disease-target specificity.

This work thoroughly reviews available data regarding differences between vitamin K1 and K2, contextualized with clinical aspects of vitamin K deficiency, including their sources, functions, target activity, and involvement in age-related diseases. Processes for the chemical and biological production of vitamin K1 and K2 will be briefly addressed. Additionally, novel sources with potential biotechnological application, and new formulations to improve vitamin K absorption and bioavailability are presented.

Table 1. Vitamin K-dependent proteins.

	Designation	Function
Hepatic	Factor II (Prothrombin)	Pro-coagulant [7]
	Factor VII	Pro-coagulant [7]
	Factor IX	Pro-coagulant [7]
	Factor X (Stuart Factor)	Pro-coagulant [7]
	Protein C	Anti-coagulant, anti-inflammatory, anti-apoptotic [7–10]
	Protein S	Co-factor for activated protein C, anti-coagulant, bone turnover, anti-inflammatory [7,8,11,12]
	Protein Z	Regulation of coagulation, anti-thrombotic [13,14]
Extra Hepatic	OC	Negative regulator of bone formation, regulator of mineral maturation rate, mechanical stabilizer of bone matrix, regulator of glucose metabolism [15,16]
	MGP	Inhibitor of soft tissue calcification, modulator of angiogenesis and tumorigenesis [17–19]
	Gas6	Signal transduction, regulator of proliferation, migration, differentiation, adhesion, and apoptosis, anti-inflammatory, platelet activation, thrombus stabilization [20–22]
	GRP	Inhibitor of soft tissue calcification, inhibitor of mineral crystal maturation and growth in blood, anti-inflammatory [23–26]
	Periostin (isoforms 1–4)	Regulator of cell-matrix interactions, adhesion, proliferation, and differentiation processes, tissue remodelling and wound repair, angiogenesis [27–29]
	PRGP1/PRGP2	Signal transduction [30,31]
	TGM3/TGM4	Signal transduction [32]
Endoplasmic Reticulum/Golgi Apparatus	GGCX	γ-carboxylation of VKDPs [33]

VKDPs, Vitamin K-dependent Proteins. OC, Osteocalcin. MGP, Matrix Gla-Protein. Gas6, growth arrest-specific protein-6. GRP, Gla-Rich Protein. PRGP, proline-rich Gla protein. TGM, transmembrane Gla protein. GGCX, γ-glutamyl carboxylase.

2. Clinical Context of Vitamin K

2.1. Vitamin K Deficiency

Vitamin K deficiency is clinically characterised by a bleeding tendency due to the loss of function of vitamin K-dependent hepatic clotting factors. Vitamin K deficiency is not very common in adults and is usually associated with specific conditions, such as malabsorption disorders, antibiotics, and drug interactions, especially with coumarin-based anticoagulants, or an extremely poor vitamin K-content diet. Anticoagulant treatment with coumarin derivatives is widely prescribed to prevent thromboembolic events or stroke in patients with atrial fibrillation or cardiac disease. Clinical evaluation of the vitamin K status is assessed only in specific conditions, such as individuals with bleeding disorders or under anticoagulants. 4-hydroxycoumarin anticoagulant drugs such as warfarin, acenocoumarol, and phenprocoumon are widely used oral anticoagulants acting as vitamin K antagonists (VKAs). In these cases, prothrombin time, which is indicative of the time necessary for blood clotting and known as the International Normalized Ratio (INR), is usually the parameter used for a drug dosage. Treatment with VKAs inhibits the recycling of vitamin K and the synthesis of the vitamin K-dependent biologically active clotting factors II, VII, IX, and X. Patients' warfarin dose is adapted based on INR scores so that it remains in the therapeutic range to prevent thrombosis or haemorrhagic complications [34].

Gastrointestinal disorders can compromise the pancreatic/biliary functions and trigger fat absorptive mechanisms, such as in the case of celiac disease, cystic fibrosis, ulcerative colitis, cholestasis, short bowel syndrome, or in a situation of bariatric surgical intervention. These conditions might lead to a situation of inadequate absorption of vitamin K and, ultimately, to a status of vitamin K deficiency.

Antibiotics also interfere with vitamin K levels since they generally contribute to a decrease of vitamin K-producing bacteria in the gut [35]. Vitamin K deficiency is currently observed in patients with prolonged oral broad-spectrum antibiotic therapy. Antibiotics such as cephalosporins, which include the N-methylthiotetrazole side chain, are suggested as inhibitors of hepatic vitamin K epoxide reductase [36–38]. A nested case-control study performed in a cohort of 6191 patients concluded that patients receiving cephalosporins and other antibiotics for more than 48 h had an increased risk of haemorrhagic events [39].

Some medications are also reported to interfere with vitamin K absorption. These are drugs prescribed to reduce cholesterol in a dyslipidemia scenario, or drugs that interfere with lipases activity used for obesity treatment such as orlistat, or bile acid sequestrants, such as colesevelam and cholestyramine. Overall, these medications can affect the absorption of fat-soluble vitamins and lead to a decrease in the vitamin K status [40,41]. In these situations, monitoring and supplementation might be recommended.

Newborns might experiment with vitamin K deficiency during the first few weeks of life as a consequence of a combination of factors that contribute to low levels of vitamin K [42]. Poor vitamin K carriage through placenta, low content of vitamin K1 in breast milk, and liver immaturity that leads to an inefficient use of vitamin K and recycling represent part of the conditions that could lead to a situation known as vitamin K deficiency bleeding (VKDB) [43,44]. To reduce the incidence of VKDB, oral vitamin K prophylaxis with phytomenadione, or administration of a single intramuscular (IM) dose of 0.5–1 mg at birth is recommended by the World Health Organization (WHO) [45].

In the last decade, the bulk of research on vitamin K has shifted beyond coagulation, which further explores its physiological role in skeletal, CVD, and brain health [46,47]. Vitamin K deficiency has been associated with a higher risk of age-related chronic diseases such as osteoporosis, CVD, RA, and OA, which contributes to its onset and progression [5,48–50]. Several extra-hepatic VKDPs such as MGP, GRP, and OC are well described to be of vital importance in the pathophysiology of these age-related diseases. More recently, several in vitro and in vivo studies, as well as clinical data, have highlighted the role of vitamin K in cognitive performance, particularly associated with Alzheimer's disease. The action of vitamin K in brain cells' development and survival has been linked with its role in the synthesis of sphingolipids, and through the function of the VKDPs, Gas6, and protein

S [51]. Although the association between vitamin K deficiency and cognitive impairment is still not definitively established, several works have shown a direct correlation between low levels of vitamin K and deterioration of cognitive and behavioural performances (recently reviewed in Reference [47]).

In fact, the current use of oral anticoagulants acting as VKAs, has also been associated with adverse clinical outcomes in extra-hepatic tissues such as bone, cartilage, the vascular tree, and brain [52–55].

2.2. Vitamin K Antagonists (VKAs)

The role of vitamin K in arterial calcification has been associated with its function as a co-factor for carboxylation of MGP and GRP. The role of MGP as an inhibitor of vascular calcification (VC) is strictly dependent on its γ-carboxylation status [56]. In addition, only the carboxylated form of GRP was shown to have calcification inhibitory properties [26]. Preclinical studies clearly demonstrate that the use of VKAs induces a vitamin K deficiency status, which enhances medial and intimal calcification in the vascular tree. Vitamin K treatment was shown not only to be able to inhibit mineralization in warfarin-treated rats, but even to promote the regression of the pre-formed medial elastocalcinosis [57]. This is in line with several studies demonstrating negative effects of warfarin treatment in cardiovascular health [58]. In humans, the detrimental effect of VKAs on extra-coronary calcification has been shown on a small cross-sectional study in patients on long-term oral coumarin treatment [59]. In another cohort study assessing 430 patients, the presence of calcification in peripheral arteries was compared between warfarin patient users and non-users. In this study, the prevalence of arterial calcification was 44% greater in patients on warfarin therapy versus without warfarin use [60].

Several [61–63] clinical studies, but not all [64] clinical studies, give indications that warfarin promotes atherosclerotic calcification, since an increase in coronary calcification, which is predominantly atherosclerotic, was observed in patients using VKAs. An observational study reported that the use of VKAs is related with increased aortic stiffness in end-stage CKD patients undergoing haemodialysis (HD) [65]. In a retrospective clinical study including patients on haemodialysis who developed calciphylaxis, 6/8 patients were on VKAs therapy. This suggests VKAs therapy as one of the factors involved in the development of calciphylaxis [66], which is a rare but fatal complication in CKD patients, characterized by ischemic skin ulceration due to mineralization affecting subcutaneous small arterioles.

Recently, a large population-based cohort study including individuals from the Gutenberg health study comprising 287 VKAs users and 14,564 VKAs non-users demonstrated that patients on VKAs therapy had a higher cardiovascular burden. In this cross-sectional study, although no cause-effect interpretation could be made, the authors suggest a relation between VKAs use and several parameters of clinical and subclinical CVD, such as with increased arterial stiffness, decreased cardiac systolic function, and higher left ventricular mass. This study also shows an association and dose-response effect of VKAs intake with low grade systemic inflammation. This was shown by the high levels of high-sensitivity C-reactive protein (hsCRP) found in long-term VKAs users when compared with short-term VKAs intake users [67]. A post hoc analysis used serial coronary intravascular ultrasound examinations and involved eight prospective randomized trials. Changes in coronary atheroma burden were compared between patients with coronary artery disease patients treated with (n = 171) and without (n = 4129) warfarin for 18 to 24 months. In this study, the authors concluded that warfarin use was independently associated with serial coronary calcification with no association with renal function, statin therapy, or changes in atheroma volume [68].

Overall, the available studies and the information on the detrimental side effects of VKAs reinforces the notion that special care should be given on their clinical use. This is even more relevant for patients requiring long-time anticoagulant therapy and for those considered to be at higher atherosclerotic risk. Furthermore, new direct oral anticoagulants (DOACs) drugs that do not inhibit vitamin K recycling and target different factors in the coagulation cascade, specifically factor Xa and thrombin, such as dabigatran, rivaroxaban, apixaban, and edoxaban, are now available as medications. More recently, a cross-sectional observational study including 236 atrial fibrillation patients were divided in three groups, according to the type of anticoagulation therapy (no oral anticoagulation, VKAs or DOACs).

The main findings of this study pointed toward an increased prevalence of calcification of the thoracic aorta in patients treated with VKAs when compared to patients with DOACs treatment, with no effect on calcification observed in DOACs-treated patients compared with no oral anticoagulation group [69].

DOACs are recognized as an attractive alternative option to VKAs for short-term and long-term coagulation due to their single-dose oral administration without the need for repeated blood monitoring, their proven safety, and short half-life [70]. This will allow the safe use of vitamin K as a supplement to prevent soft tissue pathological mineralization in aging diseases such as osteoporosis, OA, CKD, and CVD. Nevertheless, randomized controlled trials addressing causality of VKAs and DOACs on VC are still warranted.

3. Vitamin K1 and K2: Similar Function but Different Absorption, Storage, Bioavailability, and Targets

3.1. Vitamin K Chemical Structure

Vitamin K are fat-soluble vitamins that occur and function in the membranes of living organisms and comprise vitamin K1 and vitamin K2. Both forms share a 2-methyl-1,4-naphtoquinone double ring structure in their chemical backbone (menadione, vitamin K3) but differ in their lipophilic side chain (Figure 1). While vitamin K1 has a phytyl substituted chain, vitamin K2 contains unsaturated isoprenyl side chains, designated as MK-4 through to MK-13, depending on its length [71,72]. Vitamin K1 is present in vegetables, mainly in green leafy vegetables, vegetable oils, and some fruits and it is the main source of vitamin K in diet. Vitamin K2 is found in animal-based and fermented foods or produced by bacteria in the human gut. MK-4 is an exception since is not a common product of bacterial synthesis but considered to be of animal origin based on its tissue-specific conversion from vitamin K1 [73,74]. On the other hand, although often referred to as vitamin K3, menadione is not a natural component of foods but is considered a product of catabolism of vitamin K1 and a circulating precursor of tissue MK-4 [72,74]. For this reason, it should, more adequately, be known as a pro-vitamin.

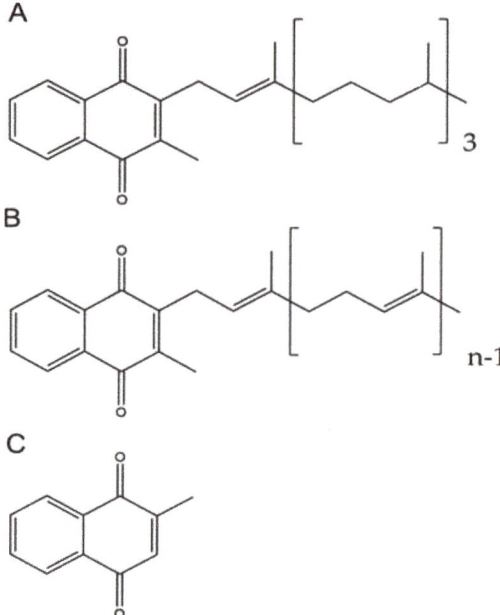

Figure 1. Chemical Structure of Vitamin K vitamers. Phylloquinone or vitamin K1 (**A**), menaquinone-n (MKn), or vitamin K2 (**B**) and menadione or vitamin K3 (**C**).

3.2. Vitamin K Functions

Both vitamin K1 and K2 can act as cofactors in the carboxylation process of VKDPs. The reduced form of vitamin K (vitamin K hydroquinone, KH_2) is the active cofactor for the γ-glutamyl carboxylase (GGCX) enzyme, which modifies Glu residues to Gla residues in VKDPs. The reaction also requires carbon dioxide and oxygen. During the carboxylation reaction, vitamin K 2,3-epoxide (KO) is continuously recycled by vitamin K epoxide reductase (VKOR) and vitamin K reductase (VKR), to its quinone (K) and KH_2 forms in a process known as the vitamin K cycle [75–77]. Due to this efficient cell recycling process, the organism can preserve limited nutritional stores of vitamin K depending on minimal vitamin K amounts to cover its daily diet requirements [78]. Of note, a higher bioactivity of MK-7 relative to K1 as a cofactor of GGCX-mediated protein carboxylation in both hepatic and extra-hepatic tissues is supported by several in vitro and in vivo studies. An in vitro study demonstrated that cofactor activity of vitamin K increased with the length of the aliphatic side chain [79].

In addition to the proposed involvement of some VKDPs in inflammation processes, vitamin K has been proposed to act as an anti-inflammatory and antioxidant agent independent of its GGCX cofactor activity. Several in vitro and animal studies have shown that vitamin K reduced the activation of nuclear factor kappa B (NFκB) and inhibited IkappaB kinase (IKB) α/β phosphorylation, with a consequent decrease in the production of pro-inflammatory cytokines [80–82]. This action was proposed to be mediated through the naphthoquinone ring of vitamin K, and it is not surprising that both vitamin K1 and K2 (MK-3, MK-4, and MK-7) were found to suppress a liposaccharide (LPS)-induced inflammatory state in vitro and in vivo in the mouse model. In addition, a role for vitamin K as an antioxidant agent has been proposed. The reduced form of vitamin K (KH_2) was shown to protect phospholipid membranes from peroxidation by direct reactive oxygen species (ROS) uptake [83,84]. An important player in this antioxidant activity is the paralogous enzyme of the vitamin K epoxide reductase complex subunit 1 (VKORC1), which is the vitamin K epoxide reductase complex subunit 1 (VKORC1)-like 1 (VKORC1L1), responsible for increasing KH_2 intracellularly and limiting the amount of intracellular ROS [85]. In cultured neurons and oligodendrocytes, vitamin K was shown to prevent cell death caused by oxidative stress by inhibiting the activation of 12-lipoxygenase (12-LOX). Both vitamin K1 and K2 have been shown to have antioxidant properties [86,87]. Recently, a study aiming to evaluate the effect of vitamin K on the redox metabolism of human osteoblasts cultured in the presence of hydroxyapatite-based biomaterials showed that vitamin K prevented a redox imbalance by decreasing ROS levels. The highest effect was obtained with MK-7 [88].

The involvement of vitamin K with sphingolipids metabolism, although known for some decades, has recently gained renewed attention due to suggested implications of alterations in sphingolipid metabolism with the aging process [89] and neurodegenerative disorders such as Alzheimer's and Parkinson's diseases [90,91]. It has been shown that vitamin K activates 3-ketodihydrosphingosine (3-KDS) synthase (also known as serine palmitoyltransferase), which is the enzyme involved in the initial step of sphingolipid biosynthesis [92], and the sulfotransferase responsible for sulfatide synthesis [93]. In rats, warfarin treatments were associated with decreased activity of 3-KDS synthase and sulfotransferase, and significant reductions in brain sulfatides, sphingomyelin, and cerebrosides [93,94]. Data on the association of specific vitamin K vitamers with sphingolipid metabolism in humans is still scarce and warrants further investigation. The predominant form of vitamin K in the brain of rats and humans is MK-4 [95,96]. In rats, the stimulatory effect of vitamin K on the activity of sphingolipids metabolism enzymes was observed with either K1 or MK-4 as a source of vitamin K [97]. In addition, the concentration of MK-4 in the rat brain was shown to positively correlate with the concentration of sphingolipids, particularly with sulfatides and sphingomyelin, and both K1 and MK-4 increased with K1 intake [96]. This is in line with our knowledge that MK-4 is a result of K1 conversion, and that cerebral MK-4 originates from K1 intake [98]. In humans, a few studies have shown a relationship between low levels of K1 and Alzheimer's disease and impaired memory performance in older adults [99,100]. However, specific relationships between higher K1 or MK-4 levels and sphingolipid synthesis requires further elucidation. A currently active field of research around vitamin K relates to its potential anti-cancer effect. Although this topic will not be explored in this review, vitamin K has been implicated with the inhibition of several neoplastic cell lines mainly by inducing apoptosis and cell cycle arrest of cancer cells through various mechanisms [101]. Among the different forms of vitamin K tested, vitamin K2 was shown to inhibit several cancer cell lines without side effects and has been selected as a promising agent for cancer prevention and clinical therapy. Clinical trials have demonstrated the potential of vitamin K2 to improve the prognosis of cancer patients [102,103].

3.3. Vitamin K1 and K2 Absorption, Storage, and Bioavailability

Although both vitamin K1 and K2 are involved in γ-carboxylation of VKDPs, these molecular forms act differently in processes such as absorption, transport, cellular uptake, tissue distribution, and turnover [78]. Despite sharing a similar structure (Figure 1) and physicochemical characteristics, natural vitamin K forms have different lipophilicity. The longer-chain menaquinones, including MK7, are much more hydrophobic and have longer half-times. Although there are many studies reporting different results, it seems clear that the length and degree of saturation of the isoprene side chain influences their clearance from circulation and bioavailability [72]. In healthy adults, absorption of MKs (MK-4, MK-7, and MK-9) has been compared with K1. The results indicate that MK-7 is the most efficiently absorbed form of vitamin K [104–106]. Although K1 is the major type (>90%) of dietary vitamin K, it is poorly retained in the organism. Its concentrations in animal tissues are remarkably low when compared with those of MKs, especially MK-4, which is the major form (>90%) of vitamin K found in animal tissues [74,107].

Both vitamin K1 and K2 forms follow a similar and well-established intestinal absorption pathway. Following their packing into chylomicrons, they are further transported in circulation to their target tissues by lipoproteins [78,106]. While vitamin K1 in circulation is mostly associated with triacylglycerol-rich lipoproteins (TLR), vitamin K2 is mainly transported by low-density lipoproteins (LDL). This difference could also justify the higher half-life time, bioavailability, and higher bioactivity of MK-7 when compared with vitamin K1. A study comparing vitamin K1 and MK-7 shows that MK-7 had a half-life time of 68 h compared with only 1–2 h for K1 [105]. This results in more stable blood levels and a higher bioavailability of MK-7, while vitamin K1 is rapidly removed from circulation, accumulated in the liver, and excreted in urine and bile. In the Japanese population, known for its higher K2 diet intake, mainly due to natto consumption, MK-7 was found to be the predominant circulation form of vitamin K [108]. The concept that long-chain MKs are available longer in circulation than K1 for cell uptake supports the suggestion that vitamin K2 represent a more adequate form of vitamin K delivery to extra-hepatic tissues such as bone and the vasculature. In fact, using equimolar amounts of both vitamin K forms as supplements, a cross-over study showed that circulating levels of carboxylated OC were higher in subjects taking MK-7 when compared to the vitamin K1 supplemented group [105]. In the same study population, another cross-over study shows that MK-7 was almost three times more potent than K1 in counteracting the effect of coumarin anticoagulants [105]. This rationale might explain the reported prevalent association of vitamin K2 and not K1 intake, with a reduced risk of CVD [109]. In fact, although several studies have demonstrated a relation between vitamin K1 and cardiovascular health, studies aiming to compare the effects of K1 and K2 clearly highlight the prevalence of K2 as a cardiovascular protective agent. In the prospective, population-based Rotterdam Study, comprising 4807 subjects free from myocardial infarction at baseline, followed up for 7 years, low levels of vitamin K2 but not K1 were associated with a significant risk in coronary heart disease (CHD), all-cause mortality, and severe aortic calcification [109]. In the Prospect-EPIC cohort study, enrolling 16,057 women free from CVD at baseline, with a mean follow-up of 8.1 years, an inverse association between vitamin K2 (particularly MK-7, MK-8, and MK-9) and risk of CHD was found with an 85%–100% reduction in coronary events for every 10 μg increase in vitamin K2 intake [110]. Again, vitamin K1 intake was not significantly associated with cardiovascular outcomes [110,111].

In relation to bone health, although vitamin K2 has been suggested as the vitamer with the highest bone-protecting effects, available clinical data is still conflicting in this subject. In fact, the effect of vitamin K supplementation has been evaluated in several clinical trials using either K1 or K2, with results pointing for a protective effect of both vitamers through the improvement of bone quality with increased strength and reduced turnover, and a reduction in fractures (reviewed in Reference [6]). Several inconsistent results are found in the literature concerning the specific effects of each vitamin K vitamer. This might be explained by the small sample number in interventional studies and the heterogeneity associated with these studies specifically related to different evaluation methods for vitamin K status, supplementation doses, and specific types of vitamin K. Importantly, simultaneous comparisons between the effects of K1 and different MKs such as MK-4 and MK-7 on bone outcomes should help the clarification of the most suitable vitamer for improving bone health.

4. Dietary Sources of Vitamin K1 and K2

Vertebrates, including humans, do not synthesise vitamin K and depend on dietary sources to obtain the required daily allowance. Moreover, vitamin K body storage is rapidly depleted in the absence of a regular dietary intake [112]. Comprehensive reviews addressing both vitamers content in a variety of foods have recently become available [104,113–115]. However, only a few national food composition databases including vitamin K content are available, and most of them do not include specific information on K1 and K2 content in each food item.

Vitamin K1 is a final product of the shikimate pathway in the photosynthesis process, and, therefore, can be found in all photosynthetic organisms, including plants, algae, and cyanobacteria [116,117]. The main sources of dietary vitamin K are green leafy vegetables such as kale, romaine lettuce, broccoli, cabbage, and spinach [115]. Vegetable oils such as soybean, sunflower, olive, and canola are the next best dietary source of K1 [118,119]. Lower amounts of K1 can also be found in fruits, cereals, meat, and dairy products [120]. High levels of vitamin K1 can be found in common Japanese food items such as in vegetables, with the highest value found in perilla (raw, 1007 µg/100 g), in edible seaweed such as hijiki (*Sargassum fusiform*, dried, 175 µg/100 g) and wakame (*Undaria pinnatifida* dried, 1293 µg/100 g) [121]. Different vitamin K contents have been reported for the edible red algae *Porphyra* sp., commonly known as laver or nori, describing levels of around 2600 µg/100 g on a dry basis in the dried nori, with a significant reduction found in toasted dry nori (approximately 390 µg/100 g on a dry basis) [122] and in roasted and seasoned laver (dried 413 µg/100 g) [121]. Additionally, different types of vegetable fats and oils such as soybean oil (234 µg/100 g) and green powdered tea (3049 µg/100 g), which are widely consumed in Japan, are reported to contain high amounts of K1 [108].

Vitamin K2 is mainly produced by bacteria, except for MK-4, which can be produced by tissue-specific conversion from vitamin K1 in animals. This reaction is catalysed by the UbiA prenyltransferase domain-containing 1 enzyme [74], which involves the menadione form as an intermediate. In fact, MK-4 formed from vitamin K1 can be found in higher amounts in animal organs not commonly consumed in the diet (liver, brain, pancreas, or kidney) [95]. Vitamin K2, such as MK-7, MK-8, and MK-9, which is the most recognized forms in terms of nutrition value [123], are biosynthesized by several obligate and facultative anaerobic bacteria [113,124]. In addition, the bacterial flora in the human gut is described to produce several long-chain MKs. In the human large intestine, the major forms of K2 found to be present, including MK-6, MK7, MK-8, MK-10, and MK11, are produced by several types of enterobacteria such as *Bacteroides*, *Enterobacteria*, *Eubacterium lentum*, and *Veillonella* [125,126]. Although intestinal bacteria synthesis is described to contribute to vitamin K requirements [127], it is not yet clear its true contribution to human vitamin K2 nutrition, and there is a need for further progress in this area [123].

The use of bacteria in food production processes has greatly increased in the last decade [128] along with the interest in the production of food products enriched with vitamin K2. Several lactic acid bacteria commonly used for making fermented food products, and generally recognized as safe (GRAS), have been used for the biosynthetic production of MKs for the last few decades, with significant production amounts of MKs (MK-7 to MK-10) [129]. Nevertheless, some genera of bacteria widely used in the food industry, including *Lactobacillus* and *Streptococcus*, have lost the functional ability to produce vitamin K2. Due to this, the K2 content of food products using these bacteria is almost undetectable [130]. A study examining the capacity of several bacterial strains to produce K compounds selected three strains of *Lactococcus lactis ssp. cremoris*, two strains of *Lactococcus lactis ssp. lactis*, and *Leuconostoc lactis* as high producers able to deliver more than 230 nmol/g dried cells of MK-7 to MK-10 [129]. In fact, several other bacterial species including *Brevibacterium linens, Brochontrix thermosphacta, Hafnia alvei, Staphylococcus xylosus, Staphylococcus equorum*, and *Arthrobacter nicotinae*, which are commonly used in industrial food fermentations, are well-known to produce several forms of K2, from MK-5 to MK-9, in different amounts [113].

Other major sources of vitamin K2 are meat, especially chicken, bacon, and ham [120]. In addition, egg yolks and high-fat dairy products, such as hard cheeses, provide appreciated amounts of this vitamer [73]. Of note, cheese was found to be the most important source of dietary long-chain MKs (MK-8 and MK-9) [131]. In particular, propionibacteria-fermented cheese, such as Norwegian Jarlsberg cheese and Swiss Emmental cheese, were shown to have the highest concentration of vitamin K2 in the form of tetrahydromenaquinone-9 [132]. Another important dietary source of vitamin K2, with interest for the industry, are fermented plant foods, such as natto. Natto is a traditional Japanese soybean food produced by fermenting cooked soybean with *Bacillus subtilis natto* and considered one of the most relevant dietary sources of MK-7 (around 1000 µg/100 g natto) [104,121,133].

5. Vitamin K1 and K2 Chemical and Biotechnological Production Methods

The health benefits of vitamin K [46,134], together with the growing trend for sustainable and natural health products, has led to a high interest on the search for sustainable and cost-effective processes to produce natural vitamin K. Both chemical and biochemical synthetic strategies for vitamin K are currently being explored. Chemical synthesis processes for both vitamin K forms, either vitamin K1 or vitamin K2, have been developed in the past few years [135–137], while biosynthetic production methods have been mostly explored for MKs (MK-4/MK-7). In addition, the continuous discovery of vitamin K vitamers in aquatic organisms, widely recognized as a valuable source of bioactive compounds and with biotechnological potentialities, might open new perspectives for novel vitamin K sources and production methods.

5.1. Vitamin K1

Currently, a chemical synthesis process for vitamin K1 is well established [138,139] and used in a wide range of commercial applications, from human nutrition to pharmaceutical products [140–142], but not in cosmetics where vitamin K1 formulations were banned from use in 2009 [143]. Improvements on the chemical synthesis methods of vitamin K1 have been mainly focused on the reduction of the inactive Z-isomer formation [141], and in decreasing the use of toxic chemicals that are hazardous to both the environment and humans [142,144]. One of the major chemical synthesis challenges resides in eliminating menadione traces [138,144]. In fact, menadione and its derivates such as menadione sodium bisulfite and menadione sodium diphosphate were banned from human products since 1963 due to evidence of toxicity, even though they are still used for animal feed as pro-vitamins [145]. Research on the biotechnological production of vitamin K1 is still quite incipient but constitute a promising route to increase the quality of the final product (active trans(E)-isomer), and to reduce the costs associated with the inclusion of this vitamin in diet supplements [146].

5.2. Vitamin K2

Chemical synthesis of vitamin K2, although described almost 40 years ago [147], remains challenging due to the need of stereoselective synthesis of the bioactive all-trans configuration. Despite traditional high cost and low yield, chemically synthetized vitamin K2 has gained renewed interest with new and optimized methods for an efficient and stereoselective production of high pure (99.9%)

all-trans vitamin MK-7 with a moderate yield (11% starting from menadione) [148]. Additionally, chemical approaches have been used to synthetize novel vitamin K2 analogues, reported to have higher bioactivities when compared with their natural counterparts [136,149–151]. These new compounds, with vitamin K activity but different pharmacological properties compared with the natural homologues, might reveal novel and interesting biological activities for commercialization as active diet supplements.

Compared to chemical synthesis, biosynthetic production methods for natural vitamin K2 using bacterial fermentation have been the most studied and reported production systems for this vitamer [152–154]. This is mainly due to the advantage of selective production of the all-trans isomer by microorganisms, and the easy manipulation and culture conditions optimization of many bacterial strains. Over recent years, research on vitamin K2 biotechnological production has moved from the identification of bacterial types producing K2, to screening of K2 high-producing bacterial strains, often combined with genetic mutations and resistant mutants leading to improved K2 yields. More recently, bioengineered K2 metabolic pathways using high-producing bacterial strains and improved culture conditions have been described.

Biotechnological strategies using either liquid and solid state fermentation processes (LSF and SSF), and modifications in culture conditions such as media composition and carbon source, temperature, shaking speed, and time in culture, have been developed for vitamin K2 production in several bacterial types such as *Flavobacterium* sp., Lactic acid bacteria, *Bacillus subtilis*, *Bacillus subtilis natto*, *Bacillus amyloliquefaciens*, and *Bacillus licheniformis* (reviewed in [155]). In general, the highest levels of vitamin K2 are produced by *Bacillus* species. Since *Bacillus subtilis* has been granted the status of GRAS [156], and several methods to improve vitamin K2 bacterial productivity have resulted in high yield, these are positioned among the most important industrial vitamin K producers for its use as diet supplements providing human health benefits. Particularly, *Bacillus subtilis natto* has been shown to produce a range of vitamin K2 homologues (MK-4, MK-5, MK-6, MK-7, and MK-8) with the major component being MK7 and accounting for more than 90% of total vitamin K2 production [157]. Depending on the strategy employed, *Bacillus subtilis natto* has been reported to produce MK-7 with yields of 3.6 mg/L in a mutant strain resistant to 1-hydroxy-2-naphthoic acid (HNA) [158], 32.2 mg/L in an isolated strain from the traditional Japanese food natto fermented for 72 h [159], 35.0 mg/L in a menadione-resistant mutant strain isolated from natto cultivated for four days [160], and 1719 µg/100 g natto [161] in a multiple resistant mutant strain. More recently, approaches of metabolic engineering to enhance MK-7 production in *Bacillus subtilis* have been reported [162]. This strategy is based on the overexpression of different combinations of rate-limiting enzymes involved in MK-7 biosynthetic pathways. Using these approaches in the *B. subtilis* 168 strain, yields of 50 mg/L [163] and 69.5 mg/L [164] of MK-7 were reported. This represents a considerable improvement on vitamin K2 production, and further optimization may open the perspective for new and affordable manufacturing processes allowing a considerable reduction of costs that will benefit the final consumer.

5.3. Aquatic Organisms as Sources of Vitamin K with a Potential Biotechnological Application

In recent years, an increasing interest is given to aquatic organisms, as a source of useful and sustainable bioproducts meeting the increasing market and consumer demands for nutritional supplements, with benefits in human health promotion and disease prevention [165]. Freshwater and marine organisms, especially macroalgae, microalgae, and several species of cyanobacteria, have been widely recognised as a valuable source of diet supplements and functional ingredients with great health benefits [166,167]. In this area, a considerable amount of research efforts has been focused on improving the biomass supply and bioactive extraction by developing safe, sustainable, and environmentally-friendly processes [168].

The ability to synthesise vitamin K has been already described for several marine organisms such as macroalgae, microalgae, and cyanobacteria. In particular, the synthesis of vitamin K1 is reported in different species of macroalgae and microalgae such as *Porphyra* sp. (Rhodophyta), *Sargassum muticum*, *Sargassum fusiforme*, *Undaria pinnatifida*, *Nannochloropsis oculata* (Ochrophyta),

Tetraselmis suecica, Dunaliella salina, Desmodesmus asymmetricus, Chlorella vulgaris, Chlamydomonas reinhardtii (Chlorophyta), *Isochrysis galbana, Pavlova lutheri* (Haptophyta), and *Skeletonema costatum* (Bacillariophyta) [121,122,169,170]. Additionally, several species of cyanobacteria are described to be able to biosynthesise and produce vitamin K1 such as *Anabaena cylindrica, Anabena variabilis, Spirulina* sp., and *Nostoc muscorum, Synechocytis* sp. PCC 6803 [124,171]. Biosynthesis of phylloquinone has been mainly associated with oxygenic photosynthetic organisms such as plants, algae, and cyanobacteria. MKs are described to be synthetized by a limited number of obligate and facultative anaerobic bacteria. Nevertheless, several species of cyanobacteria and microalgae, such as the cyanobacteria *Gloeobacter violaceus* [172] and *Synechococcus* sp. PCC 7002 [173], the diatom *Chaetoceros gracilis* [174], and the red algae *Cyanidium caldarium* [175] have been shown to synthetize MK-4. Moreover, evidence from the literature describes several aquatic species with different content in vitamin K1 [169]. This suggests that algae should be an attractive and potential source of biomass for biosynthesis of vitamin K production with potential for biotechnological applications [146]. In fact, vitamin K1 has been found in variable amounts in several species of macroalgae, microalgae, and cyanobacteria, as summarized in Table 2. In a recent study analysing seven different microalgae species, the cyanobacteria *Anabaena cylindrica* was identified as the richest source of the active E-isomer of vitamin K1 (200 µg/g dry weight) [170] (Table 2). This concentration was around six times higher when compared with parsley (*Petroselinum crispum*) [170], which is a known rich dietary source of K1, and higher than any other previously reported phylloquinone dietary source [115,175–177]. Additionally, the method proposed in this study uses low temperatures, low pressures, and sustainable feedstocks, precluding great prospects for biotechnological and industrial application. Furthermore, the cyanobacteria *Spirulina* sp. was found to have a content of 0.255 µg/g dry weight [170], and, in the marine green microalgae *Tetraselmis suecica*, the concentration of vitamin K1 on a dry weight basis was 28 µg/g [169].

Table 2. Vitamin K1 content in algae.

	Phylum	Species Designation	Content (µg/g)
Macroalgae	Ochrophyta	*Undaria pinnatifida* *1	12.9 [121]
		Sargassum fusiforme *2	1.75 [121]
		Sargassum muticum	750 [169]
	Rhodophyta	*Porphyra* sp. *3	26 [122,169]
Microalgae	Bacillariophyta	*Skeletonema costatum*	5.5 [169]
	Chlorophyta	*Tetraselmis suecica*	28 [169]
		Dunaliella salina	0.1 [170]
		Desmodesmus asymmetricus	0.46 [170]
		Chlorella vulgaris	0.73 [170]
	Cyanobacteria	*Anabaena cylindrica*	200.25 [170]
		Spirulina sp.	12.70 [170]
	Haptophyta	*Isochrysis galbana*	8 [169]
		Pavlova lutheri	6.5 [169]
	Ochrophyta	*Nannochloropsis oculata*	0.17 [171]

*1 Also known as Wakame. *2 Also known as Hijiki. *3 Also known as Nori.

Within macroalgae, two species of edible seaweeds native to Japan, *Sargassum muticum* and *Undaria pinnatifida* are considered highly invasive species with negative economic and ecological impacts for the region [178,179]. Both macroalgae species were tested as biomass for the extraction and quantification of vitamin K1 and shown to have different contents with 12.9 µg/g dry mass in *Undaria pinnatifida* [121] as well as a remarkably high content in *Sargassum muticum* (750 µg/g dry matter) [169].

The exploitation of this biomass as a vitamin K1 source should encourage its harvesting and control, bringing a potential economic and environmental interest.

Macroalgae species have been described as a potential alternative for the biosynthetic production of vitamin K1 due to its higher vitamin K1 content when compared to terrestrial plants. On the other hand, microalgae and cyanobacteria represent an interesting alternative for the biotechnological industrial production of vitamin K1 due to their easy cell manipulation when compared with plant cell cultures. Another advantage of using microalgae for industrial production of products intended for human consumption is the fact that many species are considered as GRAS.

6. Vitamin K Formulations and Impact on Absorption and Bioavailability

Recently, a few studies have addressed the production of novel and more stable vitamin K formulations to improve vitamin K absorption and bioavailability. This is of crucial importance for patients with cholestasis due to extremely low level of bile salts in the intestine. Konakion® (phytomenadione) mixed micelles (MM) is a formulation composed of phytomenadione in clear bile acid/lecithin MM solution, for oral or parenteral administration, used for the prophylaxis and treatment of VKDB [180]. Nevertheless, some reports describe that these formulations do not increase vitamin K bioavailability because they are unstable and tend to aggregate in gastric pH conditions [181]. Strategies to increase its stability, absorption, and bioavailability include mixed formulations with poly (ethylene glycol) [182] and saponins [183], which are preferred components due to its natural plant origin (such as quillaja bark and soybean) and consist of a hydrophobic polycyclic aglycone tail, attached to one or more saccharide moieties. Saponin-containing Konakion® MM were shown to be a promising oral formulation for vitamin K due to its increased stability at low pH, cytocompatibility, and cell uptake capacity [183].

Intramuscular administration of vitamin K1, although effective, has raised concerns related with the administration, such as injection pain, skin bruising, and toxic ingredients, which compromise therapy compliance [183,184]. Recently, an innovative drug delivery mechanism was developed as an alternative to the hypodermic conventional needles drug administration, consisting of drug-loaded microneedles (MNs). MNs matrix or baseplate are impregnated with the required molecule/drug. After dermic application, the interstitial fluid is able to dissolve the MNs and allow the content release, which represents a micro-dimensional and less invasive method. Several substances were already successfully delivered using this system by enabling the transdermal delivery of drugs that can be absorbed directly into the systemic circulation [185–188]. A recent study was developed to investigate the production of microneedles for the delivery of vitamin K [189]. The in vitro results showed that vitamin K in a microneedle array was successfully delivered in neonatal porcine skin over 24 h. This methodology, even though it still needs to be clinically validated, anticipates great potential for improvement of patient compliance in vitamin K prophylaxis in developed countries and might contribute to reduce VKDB cases in undeveloped countries [189].

7. Conclusions

Overall, the concept of multifunctional vitamins associated with vitamin K has been growing in recent decades with evidence showing its involvement in a wide range of biological functions with a pivotal role in several highly prevalent low-grade inflammatory diseases. Several age-related diseases such as skeletal and CVD, Alzheimer's disease, and dementia are becoming a major social and economic burden in our aging society. Compelling clinical evidence combined with a strong scientific biological rational clearly support a beneficial health effect of vitamin K and has led to an increased procurement of vitamin K as a health promoting supplement. Interestingly, some scientific evidence from in vitro and in vivo models, as well as from clinical studies, suggests a synergistic effect of vitamin K combined with vitamin D, with beneficial effects of joint supplementation at optimal concentrations of both vitamins, particularly for bone health [190,191]. However, although the benefits of vitamin D in bone health are well established, high levels of vitamin D might promote hypercalcemia and soft tissue calcification with consequent detrimental effects on the cardiovascular system [192]. While additional studies are required to establish the optimal concentration of a combined supplementation with vitamins K and D, high levels of K1, MK4, or MK7 have no documented toxicity or adverse health effect. No hypercoagulable state was observed in individuals consuming doses above the recommended daily allowance of 75 micrograms vitamin K (Commission Directive 2008/100/EC) [193]. Additional specific cases of extremely high levels of vitamin K intake have also been reported without adverse effects [194,195]. However, the current and increasing knowledge on the different types of vitamin K vitamers and their specific biological activity imply a clearer differentiation between the potential health effect and target specificity for each vitamer. It is well accepted that both K1 and K2 can play an important role in the pathogenesis and progression of many diseases. Nevertheless, the K2 vitamer (MK-7) has been shown to have advantages given its superior bioavailability and higher half-life in circulation when compared with other K vitamers. In addition, the vast majority of available clinical studies are still related to the effects of vitamin K1 in health, while K2 has been shown to have a prevalent function in extra-hepatic tissues with a protective role in the vascular system reducing the risk of CVD, mitigating cognitive diseases, and suppressing inflammation. Although both vitamin K1 and K2 are commercially available, optimized production methods and more efficient formulations for each vitamer are needed to meet the increasing customer requirements at affordable prices. Additionally, marine diet supplements and functional products are already well represented in the global market and the exploitation of new aquatic-derived sources for vitamin K should represent a benefit for human health with a potential economic and environmental interest.

Funding: The Portuguese Society of Nephrology (SPN) through project funding 2016 and the Portuguese national funds from FCT-Foundation for Science and Technology through the transitional provision DL57/2016/CP1361/CT0006, project UID/Multi/04326/2019, and the Project 0055 ALGARED+ 5E-INTERREG V-A España-Portugal project funded this research.

Acknowledgments: N Araújo is the recipient of the Portuguese Science and Technology Foundation (FCT) fellowship SFRH/BD/111824/2015. C Marreiros is the recipient of a 0055 ALGARED+5E fellowship.

Conflicts of Interest: Dina Simes and Carla Viegas are cofounders of Genogla Diagnostics. The authors declare that there is no conflict of interest regarding the publication of this paper.

Abbreviations

CHD	Coronary heart disease
CKD	Chronic kidney disease
CRP	C-reactive protein
CVD	Cardiovascular disease
DOACs	Direct oral anticoagulants
GGCX	γ-glutamyl carboxylase
Gas6	Growth arrest-specific protein 6
Gla	γ-carboxyglutamic acid
Glu	Glutamic acid
GRAS	Generally recognized as safe
GRP	Gla-rich protein
HD	Haemodialysis
IKB	IkappaB kinase
INR	International normalized ratio
KH2	Vitamin K hydroquinone
KO	Vitamin K 2,3-epoxide
LDL	Low-density lipoproteins
12-LOX	12-lipoxygenase
LPS	Liposaccharide

LSF	Liquid-state fermentation process
MGP	Matrix-Gla protein
MKs	Menaquinones
MM	Mixed micelles
NF-κB	Nuclear factor kappa B
OA	Osteoarthritis
OC	Osteocalcin
PRGP1	Proline-rich Gla proteins
RA	Rheumatoid arthritis
ROS	Reactive oxygen species
SSF	Solid-state fermentation process
TLR	Triacylglycerol-rich lipoproteins
TMG	Transmembrane Gla proteins
VC	Vascular calcification
VKAs	Vitamin K antagonists
VKDB	Vitamin K deficiency bleeding
VKDPs	Vitamin K-dependent proteins
VKORC1	Vitamin K epoxide reductase complex subunit 1
VKORC1L1	Vitamin K epoxide reductase complex subunit 1-like 1
WHO	World Health Organization

References

1. Dam, B.Y.H.; Schnheyder, F. The occurence and chemical nature of vitamin k. *Biochem. J.* **1936**, *30*, 897–901. [PubMed]
2. Nelsestuen, G.L.; Suttie, W. Mode of Action of Vitamin K. Calcium Binding Properties of Bovine Prothrombint. *Biochem. J.* **1972**, *11*, 4961–4964. [CrossRef] [PubMed]
3. Willems, B.A.G.; Vermeer, C.; Chris, P.; Reutelingsperger, M.; Schurgers, L.J. The realm of vitamin K dependent proteins: Shifting from coagulation toward calcification. *Mol. Nutr. Food Res.* **2014**, *58*, 1620–1635. [CrossRef] [PubMed]
4. Cranenburg, E.C.M.; Schurgers, L.J.; Uiterwijk, H.H.; Beulens, J.W.J.; Dalmeijer, G.W.; Westerhuis, R.; Magdeleyns, E.J.; Herfs, M.; Vermeer, C.; Laverman, G.D. Vitamin K intake and status are low in hemodialysis patients. *Kidney Int.* **2012**, *82*, 605–610. [CrossRef]
5. Misra, D.; Booth, S.L.; Tolstykh, I.; Felson, D.T.; Nevitt, M.C.; Lewis, C.E.; Torner, J.; Neogi, T. Vitamin K Deficiency Is Associated with Incident Knee Osteoarthritis. *Am. J. Med.* **2013**, *126*, 243–248. [CrossRef]
6. Simes, D.C.; Viegas, C.S.B.; Araujo, N.; Marreiros, C. Vitamin K as a Powerful Micronutrient in Aging and Age-Related Diseases: Pros and Cons from Clinical Studies. *IJMS* **2019**, *20*, 4150. [CrossRef]
7. Lippi, G.; Favaloro, E.J. Laboratory hemostasis: From biology to the bench. *Clin. Chem. Lab. Med.* **2018**, *56*, 1035–1045. [CrossRef]
8. Dahlbäck, B. Blood coagulation and its regulation by anticoagulant pathways: Genetic pathogenesis of bleeding and thrombotic diseases. *J. Intern. Med.* **2005**, *257*, 209–223. [CrossRef]
9. Van De Wouwer, M.; Collen, D.; Conway, E.M. Thrombomodulin-protein C-EPCR system integrated to regulate coagulation and inflammation. *Arter. Thromb. Vasc. Biol. Biol.* **2004**, *24*, 1374–1383. [CrossRef]
10. Riewald, M.; Petrovan, R.J.; Donner, A.; Mueller, B.M.; Ruf, W. Activation of endothelial cell protease activated receptor 1 by the protein C pathway. *Science* **2002**, *296*, 1880–1882. [CrossRef]
11. Maillard, C.; Berruyer, M.; Serre, C.; Dechavanne, M.; Delmas, P. Protein-S, a vitamin K-dependent protein, is a bone matrix component synthesized and secreted by osteoblasts. *Endocrinology* **1992**, *130*, 1599–1604.
12. Rezende, S.M.; Simmonds, R.E.; Lane, D.A. Coagulation, inflammation, and apoptosis: Different roles for protein S and the protein S-C4b binding protein complex. *Blood* **2004**, *103*, 1192–1201. [CrossRef]
13. Vasse, M. Protein Z, a protein seeking a pathology. *Thromb. Haemost.* **2008**, *100*, 548–556. [CrossRef]
14. Almawi, W.Y.; Al-Shaikh, F.S.; Melemedjian, O.K.; Almawi, A.W. Protein Z, an anticoagulant protein with expanding role in reproductive biology. *Reproduction* **2013**, *146*, R73–R80. [CrossRef] [PubMed]
15. Neve, A.; Corrado, A.; Cantatore, F.P. Osteocalcin: Skeletal and extra-skeletal effects. *J. Cell. Physiol.* **2013**, *228*, 1149–1153. [CrossRef] [PubMed]

16. Zoch, M.L.; Clemens, T.L.; Riddle, R.C. New Insights into the Biology of Osteocalcin. *Bone* **2016**, *27*, 915–918. [CrossRef] [PubMed]
17. Bjorklund, G.; Svanberg, E.; Dadar, M.; David, J.C.; Salvatore, C.; Dominic, J.H.; Jan, A. The role of matrix Gla protein (MGP) in vascular calcification. *Curr. Med. Chem.* **2018**. [CrossRef] [PubMed]
18. Gheorghe, S.R.; Craciun, A.M. Matrix Gla protein in tumoral pathology. *Clujul Med.* **2016**, *89*, 319–321. [CrossRef]
19. Boström, K.; Zebbondj, A.F.; Yao, Y.; Lin, T.S.; Torres, A. Matrix GLA protein stimulates VEGF expression through increased transforming growth factor-β1 activity in endothelial cells. *J. Biol. Chem.* **2004**, *279*, 52904–52913. [CrossRef]
20. Fernández-Fernández, L.; Bellido-Martín, L.; De Frutos, P.G. Growth arrest-specific gene 6 (GAS6): An outline of its role in haemostasis and inflammation. *Thromb. Haemost.* **2008**, *100*, 604–610. [CrossRef]
21. Cosemans, J.M.E.M.; Van Kruchten, R.; Olieslagers, S.; Schurgers, L.J.; Verheyen, F.K.; Munnix, I.C.A.; Waltenberger, J.; Angelillo-Scherrer, A.; Hoylaerts, M.F.; Carmeliet, P.; et al. Potentiating role of Gas6 and Tyro3, Axl and Mer (TAM) receptors in human and murine platelet activation and thrombus stabilization. *J. Thromb. Haemost.* **2010**, *8*, 1797–1808. [CrossRef] [PubMed]
22. Hasanbasic, I.; Rajotte, I.; Blostein, M. The role of γ-carboxylation in the anti-apoptotic function of gas6. *J. Thromb. Haemost.* **2005**, *3*, 2790–2797. [CrossRef] [PubMed]
23. Viegas, C.S.B.; Costa, R.M.; Santos, L.; Videira, P.A.; Silva, Z.; Araújo, N.; Macedo, A.L.; Matos, A.P.; Vermeer, C.; Simes, D.C. Gla-rich protein function as an anti-inflammatory agent in monocytes/macrophages: Implications for calcification-related chronic inflammatory diseases. *PLoS ONE* **2017**, *12*, e0177829. [CrossRef] [PubMed]
24. Viegas, C.S.B.; Rafael, M.S.; Enriquez, J.L.; Teixeira, A.; Vitorino, R.; Luís, I.M.; Costa, R.M.; Santos, S.; Cavaco, S.; Neves, J.; et al. Gla-Rich Protein acts as a Calcification Inhibitor in the Human Cardiovascular System. *Arter. Thromb. Vasc. Biol.* **2015**, *35*, 399–408. [CrossRef]
25. Cavaco, S.; Viegas, C.S.B.; Rafael, M.S.; Ramos, A.; Magalhães, J.; Blanco, F.J.; Vermeer, C.; Simes, D.C. Gla-rich protein is involved in the cross-talk between calcification and inflammation in osteoarthritis. *Cell. Mol. Life Sci.* **2016**, *73*, 1051–1065. [CrossRef]
26. Viegas, C.S.B.; Santos, L.; Macedo, A.L.; Matos, A.A.; Silva, A.P.; Neves, P.L. Chronic Kidney Disease Circulating Calciprotein Particles and Extracellular Vesicles Promote Vascular Calcification: A Role for GRP (Gla-Rich Protein). *Arter. Thromb. Vasc. Biol.* **2018**, *38*, 575–587. [CrossRef]
27. Hamilton, D.W. Functional role of periostin in development and wound repair: Implications for connective tissue disease. *J. Cell Commun. Signal.* **2008**, *2*, 9–17. [CrossRef]
28. Kim, B.R.; Kwon, Y.W.; Park, G.T.; Choi, E.J.; Seo, J.K.; Jang, I.H.; Kim, S.C.; Ko, H.C.; Lee, S.C.; Kim, J.H. Identification of a novel angiogenic peptide from periostin. *PLoS ONE* **2017**, *12*, e0187464. [CrossRef]
29. Kühn, B.; Del Monte, F.; Hajjar, R.J.; Chang, Y.S.; Lebeche, D.; Arab, S.; Keating, M.T. Periostin induces proliferation of differentiated cardiomyocytes and promotes cardiac repair. *Nat. Med.* **2007**, *13*, 962–969. [CrossRef]
30. Kulman, J.D.; Harris, J.E.; Xie, L.; Davie, E.W. Proline-rich Gla protein 2 is a cell-surface vitamin K-dependent protein that binds to the transcriptional coactivator Yes-associated protein. *Proc. Natl. Acad. Sci. USA* **2007**, *104*, 8767–8772. [CrossRef]
31. Kulman, J.D.; Harris, J.E.; Haldeman, B.A.; Davie, E.W. Primary structure and tissue distribution of two nove proline-rich γ-carboxyglutamic acid proteins. *Proc. Natl. Acad. Sci. USA* **1997**, *94*, 9058–9062. [CrossRef] [PubMed]
32. Khazi, F.R.; Chu, K.C.; High, K.A. Transmembrane Gla Protein 4 as a Novel Modulator of ERK2. *Blood* **2006**, *108*, 544. [CrossRef]
33. Presnell, S.R.; Stafford, D.W. The Vitamin K-dependent Carboxylase. *Thromb. Haemost.* **2002**, *87*, 937–946. [CrossRef] [PubMed]
34. Shikdar, S.; Bhattacharya, P.T. International Normalized Ratio (INR) [Updated 2019 Mar 25]. In *StatPearls [Internet]*; StatPearls Publishing: Treasure Island, FL, USA, 2019. Available online: https://www.ncbi.nlm.nih.gov/books/NBK507707/ (accessed on 12 December 2019).
35. Conly, J.; Stein, K.; Worobetz, L.; Rutledge-Harding, S. The contribution of vitamin K2 (menaquinones) produced by the intestinal microflora to human nutritional requirements for vitamin K. *Am. J. Gastroenterol.* **1994**, *89*, 915–923.

36. Aziz, F.; Patil, P. Role of Prophylactic Vitamin K in Preventing Antibiotic Induced Hypoprothrombinemia. *Indian J. Pediatr.* **2015**, *82*, 363–367. [CrossRef]
37. Shevcbuk, Y.M.; Conly, J.M. Antibiotic-Associated Hypoprothrombinemia: A Review of Prospective Studies, 1966–1988. *Rev. Infect. Dis.* **1990**, *12*, 1109–1126. [CrossRef]
38. Cinaz, S.Y.; Tavi, B.; Sarı, S.; Cinaz, P. Vitamin k deficiency because of ceftriaxone usage and prolonged diarrhoea. *JPCH* **2011**, *47*, 314–315.
39. Chen, L.; Hsiao, F.; Shen, L.; Wu, F.L.; Tsay, W. Use of Hypoprothrombinemia-Inducing Cephalosporins and the Risk of Hemorrhagic Events: A Nationwide Nested Case-Control Study. *PLoS ONE* **2016**, *27*, e0158407. [CrossRef]
40. Vroonhof, K.; Van Rijn, H.J.M.; Van Hattum, J. Vitamin K deficiency and bleeding after long-term use of cholestyramine. *Neth. J. Med.* **2003**, *61*, 19–21.
41. MacWalter, R.; Fraser, H.; Armstrong, K. Orlistat Enhances Warfarin Effect. *Ann. Pharmacother.* **2003**, *37*, 510–512. [CrossRef]
42. Sutor, A.; von Kries, R.; Cornelissen, E.; McNinch, A.; Andrew, M. Vitamin K deficiency bleeding (VKDB) in infancy. ISTH Pediatric/Perinatal Subcommittee. International Society on Thrombosis and Haemostasis. *Thromb. Haemost.* **1999**, *81*, 456–461. [PubMed]
43. American Academy of Pediatrics Committee on Fetus and Newborn. Controversies concerning vitamin K and the newborn. *Pediatrics* **2003**, *112*, 191–192.
44. Pichler, E.; Pichler, L. The neonatal coagulation system and the vitamin K deficiency bleeding—A mini review. *Wien. Med. Wochenschr.* **2008**, *158*, 385–395. [CrossRef] [PubMed]
45. Schulte, R.; Jordan, L.C.; Morad, A.; Naftel, R.P.; Iii, J.C.W.; Sidonio, R. Rise in Late Onset Vitamin K Deficiency Bleeding in Young Infants Because of Omission or Refusal of Prophylaxis at Birth. *Pediatr. Neurol.* **2014**, *50*, 564–568. [CrossRef] [PubMed]
46. Wen, L.; Chen, J.; Duan, L.; Li, S. Vitamin K-dependent proteins involved in bone and cardiovascular health. *Mol. Med. Rep.* **2018**, *18*, 3–15. [CrossRef]
47. Alisi, L.; Cao, R.; De Angelis, C.; Cafolla, A.; Caramia, F.; Cartocci, G.; Librando, A.; Fiorelli, M. The Relationships Between Vitamin K and Cognition: A Review of Current Evidence. *Front. Neurol.* **2019**, *10*, 239. [CrossRef]
48. Shea, M.K.; Kritchevsky, S.B.; Hsu, F.; Nevitt, M.; Booth, S.L.; Kwoh, C.K.; Mcalindon, T.E.; Drummen, N.; Harris, T.B.; Womack, C.; et al. The association between vitamin K status and knee osteoarthritis features in older adults: The Health, Aging and Body Composition Study. *Osteoarthr. Cartil.* **2016**, *23*, 370–378. [CrossRef]
49. Shea, M.K.; Booth, S.L.; Weiner, D.E.; Brinkley, T.E.; Kanaya, A.M.; Murphy, R.A.; Simonsick, E.M.; Wassel, C.L.; Vermeer, C.; Kritchevsky, S.B. Circulating Vitamin K Is Inversely Associated with Incident Cardiovascular Disease Risk among Those Treated for Hypertension in the Health, Aging, and Body Composition Study (Health ABC) 1–3. *J. Nutr.* **2017**, *147*, 888–895. [CrossRef]
50. Zhang, S.; Guo, L.; Bu, C. Vitamin K status and cardiovascular events or mortality: A meta-analysis. *Eur. J. Prev. Cardiol.* **2019**, *26*, 549–553. [CrossRef]
51. Ferland, G. Vitamin K, an emerging nutrient in brain function. *Biofactors* **2012**, *38*, 151–157. [CrossRef]
52. Chatrou, M.L.; Winckers, K.; Hackeng, T.M.; Reutelingsperger, C.P.; Schurgers, L.J. Vascular calcification: The price to pay for anticoagulation therapy with vitamin K-antagonists. *Blood Rev.* **2012**, *26*, 155–166. [CrossRef] [PubMed]
53. Dinicolantonio, J.J.; Bhutani, J.; Keefe, J.H.O. The health benefits of vitamin K. *Open Heart* **2015**, *2*, e000300. [CrossRef] [PubMed]
54. Namba, S.; Yamaoka-tojo, M.; Hashikata, T.; Ikeda, Y.; Kitasato, L.; Hashimoto, T.; Shimohama, T.; Tojo, T.; Takahira, N.; Masuda, T.; et al. Long-term warfarin therapy and biomarkers for osteoporosis and atherosclerosis. *BBA Clin.* **2015**, *12*, 76–80. [CrossRef] [PubMed]
55. Van Gorp, R.H.; Schurgers, L.J. New Insights into the Pros and Cons of the Clinical Use of Vitamin K Antagonists (VKAs) Versus Direct Oral Anticoagulants (DOACs). *Nutrients* **2015**, *7*, 9538–9557. [CrossRef] [PubMed]
56. Schurgers, L.J.; Uitto, J.; Reutelingsperger, C.P. Vitamin K-dependent carboxylation of matrix Gla-protein: A crucial switch to control ectopic mineralization. *Trends Mol. Med.* **2013**, *19*, 217–226. [CrossRef]

57. Schurgers, L.J.; Spronk, H.M.H.; Soute, B.A.M.; Schiffers, P.M.; Demey, J.G.R.; Vermeer, C. Regression of warfarin-induced medial elastocalcinosis by high intake of vitamin K in rats. *Blood* **2007**, *109*, 2823–2831. [CrossRef]
58. Lerner, R.G.; Aronow, W.S.; Sekhri, A.; Palaniswamy, C.; Ahn, C.; Singh, T.; Sandhu, R. Warfarin use and the risk of valvular calcification. *J. Thromb. Haemost.* **2009**, *7*, 2023–2027. [CrossRef]
59. Rennenberg, R.J.M.W.; Van Varik, B.J.; Schurgers, L.J.; Hamulyak, K.; Cate, H.; Leiner, T.; Vermeer, C.; De Leeuw, P.W.; Kroon, A.A. Chronic coumarin treatment is associated with increased extracoronary arterial calcification in humans. *Blood* **2010**, *115*, 5121–5123. [CrossRef]
60. Han, K.H.; O'Neill, W.C. Increased Peripheral Arterial Calcification in Patients Receiving Warfarin. *J. Am. Heart Assoc.* **2016**, *5*, e002665. [CrossRef]
61. Schurgers, L.J.; Joosen, I.A.; Laufer, E.M.; Chatrou, M.L.L.; Herfs, M.; Winkens, M.H.M.; Westenfeld, R.; Veulemans, V.; Krueger, T.; Shanahan, C.M.; et al. Vitamin K-Antagonists Accelerate Atherosclerotic Calcification and Induce a Vulnerable Plaque Phenotype. *PLoS ONE* **2012**, *7*, e43229. [CrossRef]
62. Koos, R.; Mahnken, A.H.; Mühlenbruch, G.; Brandenburg, V.; Pflueger, B.; Wildberger, J.E.; Kühl, H.P. Relation of Oral Anticoagulation to Cardiac Valvular and Coronary Calcium Assessed by Multislice Spiral Computed Tomography. *Am. J. Cardiol.* **2005**, *96*, 747–749. [CrossRef] [PubMed]
63. Weijs, B.; Blaauw, Y.; Rennenberg, R.; Schurgers, L.; Timmermans, C.; Pison, L.; Nieuwlaat, R.; Hofstra, L.; Kroon, A.; Wildberger, J.; et al. Patients using vitamin K antagonists show increased levels of coronary calcification: An observational study in low-risk atrial fibrillation patients. *Eur. Heart J.* **2011**, *32*, 2555–2562. [CrossRef] [PubMed]
64. Villines, T.C.; Malley, P.G.O.; Feuerstein, I.M.; Thomas, S.; Taylor, A.J. Does Prolonged Warfarin Exposure Potentiate Coronary Calcification in Humans? Results of the Warfarin and Coronary Calcification Study. *Calcif. Tissue Int.* **2009**, *85*, 494–500. [CrossRef] [PubMed]
65. Mac-Way, F.; Poulin, A.; Utescu, M.S.; De Serres, S.A.; Marquis, K.; Douville, P.; Desmeules, S.; Larivière, R.; Lebel, M.; Agharazii, M. The impact of warfarin on the rate of progression of aortic stiffness in hemodialysis patients: A longitudinal study. *Nephrol. Dial. Transpl.* **2014**, *29*, 2113–2120. [CrossRef]
66. Verdalles Guzmán, Ú.; De La Cueva, P.; Verde, E.; De Vinuesa, S.G.; Goicoechea, M.; Mosse, A.; López Gómez, J.M.; Luño, J. Calciphylaxis: Fatal complication of cardiometabolic syndrome in patients with end stage kidney disease. *Nefrologia* **2008**, *28*, 32–36.
67. Eggebrecht, L.; Prochaska, H.; Schulz, A.; Arnold, N.; Junger, C.; Gobel, S.; Laubert-reh, D.; Binder, H.; Beutel, M.E.; Pfeiffer, N.; et al. Intake of Vitamin K Antagonists and Worsening of Cardiac and Vascular Disease: Results From the Population-Based Gutenberg Study. *J. Am. Heart Assoc.* **2018**, *7*, e008650. [CrossRef]
68. Andrews, J.; Psaltis, P.J.; Bayturan, O.; Shao, M.; Stegman, B.; Elshazly, M.; Kapadia, S.R.; Tuzcu, E.M.; Nissen, S.E.; Nicholls, S.J.; et al. Warfarin Use Is Associated With Progressive Coronary Arterial Calcification: Insights From Serial Intravascular Ultrasound. *JACC Cardiovasc. Imaging* **2018**, *11*, 1315–1323. [CrossRef]
69. Peeters, F.; Dudink, E.; Kimenai, D.; Weijs, B.; Altintas, S.; Heckman, L.; Mihl, C.; Schurgers, L.; Wildberger, J.; Meex, S.; et al. Vitamin K Antagonists, Non-Vitamin K Antagonist Oral Anticoagulants, and Vascular Calcification in Patients with Atrial Fibrillation. *TH Open* **2018**, *2*, e391–e398. [CrossRef]
70. Schwarb, H.; Tsakiris, D.A. New Direct Oral Anticoagulants (DOAC) and Their Use Today. *Dent. J.* **2016**, *4*, 5. [CrossRef]
71. Shearer, M.; Newman, P. Metabolism and cell biology of vitamin K. *Thromb. Haemost.* **2008**, *100*, 530–547.
72. Shearer, M.J.; Newman, P. Recent trends in the metabolism and cell biology of vitamin K with special reference to vitamin K cycling and MK-4 biosynthesis. *J. Lipid Res.* **2014**, *55*, 345–362. [CrossRef] [PubMed]
73. Booth, S.L. Vitamin K: Food composition and dietary intakes. *Food Nutr. Res.* **2012**, *1*, 1–5. [CrossRef] [PubMed]
74. Nakagawa, K.; Hirota, Y.; Sawada, N.; Yuge, N.; Watanabe, M.; Uchino, Y.; Okuda, N.; Shimomura, Y.; Suhara, Y.; Okano, T. Identification of UBIAD1 as a novel human menaquinone-4 biosynthetic enzyme. *Nature* **2010**, *468*, 117–121. [CrossRef] [PubMed]
75. Tie, J.; Stafford, D. Structural and functional insights into enzymes of the vitamin K cycle. *J. Thromb. Haemost.* **2016**, *14*, 236–247. [CrossRef] [PubMed]
76. Stafford, D.W. The vitamin K cycle. *J. Thromb. Haemost.* **2005**, *3*, 1873–1878. [CrossRef]

77. Rishavy, M.A.; Berkner, K.L. Vitamin K Oxygenation, Glutamate Carboxylation, and Processivity: Defining the Three Critical Facets of Catalysis by the Vitamin K-Dependent Carboxylase. *Adv. Nutr.* **2012**, *3*, 135–148. [CrossRef]
78. Shearer, M.J.; Fu, X.; Booth, S.L. Vitamin K Nutrition, Metabolism, and Requirements: UBIAD and Future Research. *Adv. Nutr.* **2012**, *3*, 182–195. [CrossRef]
79. Buitenhuis, H.; Soute, B.; Vermeer, C. Comparison of the vitamins K1, K2 and K3 as cofactors for the hepatic vitamin K-dependent carboxylase. *Biochim. Biophys. Acta* **1990**, *1034*, 170–175. [CrossRef]
80. Ohsaki, Y.; Shirakawa, H.; Hiwatashi, K.; Furukawa, Y.; Mizutani, T.; Komai, M. Vitamin K Suppresses Lipopolysaccharide-Induced Inflammation in the Rat. *Biosci. Biotechnol. Biochem.* **2006**, *70*, 926–932. [CrossRef]
81. Ohsaki, Y.; Shirakawa, H.; Miura, A.; Giriwono, P.E.; Sato, S.; Ohashi, A.; Iribe, M.; Goto, T.; Komai, M. Vitamin K suppresses the lipopolysaccharide-induced expression of inflammatory cytokines in cultured macrophage-like cells via the inhibition of the activation of nuclear factor κB through the repression of IKKα/β phosphorylation. *J. Nutr. Biochem.* **2010**, *21*, 1120–1126. [CrossRef]
82. Fujii, S.; Shimizu, A.; Takeda, N.; Oguchi, K.; Katsurai, T. Systematic synthesis and anti-inflammatory activity of x-carboxylated menaquinone derivatives. Investigations on identified and putative vitamin K2 metabolites. *Bioorg. Med. Chem.* **2015**, *23*, 2344–2352. [CrossRef] [PubMed]
83. Mukai, K.; Shingo, I.; Morimoto, H. Stopped-flow Kinetic Study of Vitamin E Regeneration Reaction with Biological Hydroquinones (Reduced Forms of Ubiquinone, Vitamin K and Tocopherolquinone) in Solution. *Biol. Chem.* **1992**, *267*, 22277–22281.
84. Vervoort, L.M.T.; Ronden, J.E.; Thijssen, H.H.W. The Potent Antioxidant Activity of the Vitamin K Cycle in Microsomal Lipid Peroxidation. *Biochem. Pharmacol.* **1997**, *54*, 871–876. [CrossRef]
85. Westhofen, P.; Watzka, M.; Marinova, M.; Hass, M.; Kirfel, G.; Mu, J.; Bevans, C.G.; Mu, C.R.; Oldenburg, J. Human Vitamin K 2,3-Epoxide Reductase Complex Subunit 1-like 1 (VKORC1L1) Mediates Vitamin K-dependent Intracellular Antioxidant Function. *Biol. Chem.* **2011**, *286*, 15085–15094. [CrossRef]
86. Li, J.; Lin, J.C.; Wang, H.; Peterson, J.W.; Furie, B.C.; Furie, B.; Booth, S.L.; Volpe, J.J.; Rosenberg, P.A. Novel Role of Vitamin K in Preventing Oxidative Injury to Developing Oligodendrocytes and Neurons. *J. Neurosci.* **2003**, *23*, 5816–5826. [CrossRef]
87. Li, J.; Wang, H.; Rosenberg, P.A. Vitamin K Prevents Oxidative Cell Death by Inhibiting Activation of 12-Lipoxygenase in Developing Oligodendrocytes. *J. Neurosci. Res.* **2009**, *87*, 1997–2005. [CrossRef]
88. Ambrożewicz, E.; Muszyńska, M.; Tokajuk, G.; Grynkiewicz, G.; Žarković, N.; Skrzydlewska, E. Beneficial Effects of Vitamins K and D3 on Redox Balance of Human Osteoblasts Cultured with Hydroxypatite-Based Biomaterials. *Cells* **2019**, *8*, 325. [CrossRef]
89. Cutler, R.G.; Kelly, J.; Storie, K.; Pedersen, W.A.; Tammara, A.; Hatanpaa, K.; Troncoso, J.C.; Mattson, M.P. Involvement of oxidative stress-induced abnormalities in ceramide and cholesterol metabolism in brain aging and Alzheimer's disease. *Proc. Natl. Acad. Sci. USA* **2004**, *101*, 2070–2075. [CrossRef]
90. Jana, A.; Hogan, E.L.; Pahan, K. Ceramide and neurodegeneration: Susceptibility of neurons and oligodendrocytes to cell damage and death. *J. Neurol. Sci.* **2009**, *278*, 5–15. [CrossRef]
91. De Chaves, E.P.; Sipione, S. Sphingolipids and gangliosides of the nervous system in membrane function and dysfunction. *FEBS Lett.* **2010**, *584*, 1748–1759. [CrossRef]
92. Lev, M.; Milford, A. The 3-Ketodihydrosphingosine melaninogenicus: Synthetase of Bacteroides melaninogenicus: Induction by Vitamin K. *Arch. Biochem. Biophys.* **1973**, *157*, 500–508. [CrossRef]
93. Sundaram, K.S.; Lev, M. Regulation of sulfotransferase activity by vitamin k in mouse brain. *Arch. Biochem. Biophys.* **1990**, *277*, 109–113. [CrossRef]
94. Sundaram, K.S.; Lev, M. Warfarin administration reduces synthesis of sulfatides and other sphingolipids in mouse brain. *J. Lipid Res.* **1988**, *29*, 1475–1479. [PubMed]
95. Thijssen, H.; Drittij-Reijnders, M. Vitamin K status in human tissues: Tissue-specific accumulation of phylloquinone and menaquinone-4. *Br. J. Nutr.* **1996**, *75*, 121–127. [CrossRef]
96. Carrie, I.; Portoukalian, J.; Vicaretti, R.; Rochford, J.; Potvin, S.; Ferland, G. Menaquinone-4 Concentration Is Correlated with Sphingolipid Concentrations in Rat Brain. *J. Nutr.* **2004**, *134*, 167–172. [CrossRef]
97. Sundaram, K.S.; Engelke, J.A.; Foley, A.L.; Suttie, J.; Lev, M. Vitamin K Status Influences Brain Sulfatide Metabolism in Young Mice and Rats. *J. Nutr.* **1996**, *126*, 2746–2751.

98. Okano, T.; Shimomura, Y.; Yamane, M.; Suhara, Y.; Kamao, M.; Sugiura, M.; Nakagawa, K. Conversion of Phylloquinone (Vitamin K1) into Menaquinone-4 (Vitamin K2) in Mice. Two Possible Routes for Menaquinone-4 Accumulation in Cerebra of Mice. *J. Biol. Chem.* **2008**, *25*, 11270–11279. [CrossRef]
99. Presse, N.; Shatenstein, B.; Kergoat, M.J.; Ferland, G. Low Vitamin K Intakes in Community-Dwelling Elders at an Early Stage of Alzheimer's Disease. *J. Am. Diet. Assoc.* **2008**, *108*, 2095–2099. [CrossRef]
100. Presse, N.; Belleville, S.; Gaudreau, P.; Greenwood, C.E.; Kergoat, M.; Morais, J.A.; Payette, H.; Shatenstein, B.; Ferland, G. Vitamin K status and cognitive function in healthy older adults. *Neurobiol. Aging* **2013**, *34*, 2777–2783. [CrossRef]
101. Xv, F.; Chen, J.; Duan, L.; Li, S. Research progress on the anticancer effects of vitamin K2. *Oncol. Lett.* **2018**, *15*, 8926–8934. [CrossRef]
102. Hitomi, M.; Yokoyama, F.; Nonomura, T.; Masaki, T.; Yosiji, H.; Inoeu, H.; Kinekawa, F.; Kurokohchi, K.; Uchida, N.; Watanabe, S.; et al. Antitumor effects of vitamins K1, K2 and K3 on hepatocellular carcinoma in vitro and in vivo. *Int. J. Oncol.* **2005**, *26*, 713–720. [CrossRef] [PubMed]
103. Dasari, S.; Ali, S.M.; Zheng, G.; Chen, A.; Dontaraju, V.S.; Bosland, M.C.; Kajdacsy-balla, A.; Gnanasekar, M. Vitamin K and its analogs: Potential avenues for prostate cancer management. *Oncotarget* **2017**, *8*, 57782–57799. [CrossRef] [PubMed]
104. Schurgers, L.J.; Vermeer, C. Determination of Phylloquinone and Menaquinones in Food. Effect of Food Matrix on Circulating Vitamin K Concentrations. *Haemostasis* **2000**, *30*, 298–307. [PubMed]
105. Schurgers, L.J.; Teunissen, K.J.F.; Hamulya, K.; Knapen, M.H.J.; Vik, H.; Vermeer, C. Vitamin K- containing dietary supplements: Comparison of synthetic vitamin K1 and natto-derived menaquinone-7. *Blood* **2007**, *109*, 3279–3283. [CrossRef] [PubMed]
106. Schurgers, L.J.; Vermeer, C. Differential lipoprotein transport pathways of K-vitamins in healthy subjects. *Biochim. Biophys. Acta* **2002**, *1570*, 27–32. [CrossRef]
107. Hirota, Y.; Tsugawa, N.; Nakagawa, K.; Suhara, Y.; Tanaka, K.; Uchino, Y.; Takeuchi, A.; Sawada, N.; Kamao, M.; Wada, A.; et al. Menadione (Vitamin K3) Is a Catabolic Product of Oral Phylloquinone (Vitamin K1) in the Intestine and a Circulating Precursor of Tissue Menaquinone-4 (Vitamin K2) in Rats. *J. Biol. Chem.* **2013**, *288*, 33071–33080. [CrossRef]
108. Tsugawa, N.; Shiraki, M.; Suhara, Y.; Kamao, M.; Tanaka, K.; Okano, T. Vitamin K status of healthy Japanese women: Age-related vitamin K requirement for gamma-carboxylation of osteocalcin. *Am. J. Clin. Nutr.* **2006**, *83*, 380–386. [CrossRef]
109. Geleijnse, J.M.; Vermeer, C.; Grobbee, D.E.; Schurgers, L.J.; Knapen, M.H.J.; Van Der Meer, I.M.; Hofman, A.; Witteman, J.C.M. Dietary Intake of Menaquinone Is Associated with a Reduced Risk of Coronary Heart Disease: The Rotterdam Study. *J. Nutr.* **2004**, *134*, 3100–3105. [CrossRef]
110. Gast, G.C.; de Roos, N.M.; Sluijs, I.; Bots, M.L.; Beulens, J.W.; Geleijnse, J.M.; Witteman, J.C.; Grobbee, D.E.; Peeters, P.H.; van der Schouw, Y.T. A high menaquinone intake reduces the incidence of coronary heart disease. *Nutr. Metab. Cardiovasc. Dis.* **2009**, *19*, 504–510. [CrossRef]
111. Shea, M.K.; Booth, S.L.; Miller, M.E.; Burke, G.; Chen, H.; Cushman, M.; Tracy, R.P.; Kritchevsky, S.B. Associations between circulating vitamin K1 and coronary calcium progression in community-dwelling adults: the Multi-Etcnic Study of Atherosclerosis. *Am. J. Clin. Nutr.* **2013**, *98*, 197–208. [CrossRef]
112. Usui, Y.; Tanimura, H.; Nishimura, N.; Kobayashi, N.; Okanou, T.; Zawa, K. Vitamin K concentrations in the plasma and liver of surgical patients. *Am. J. Clin. Nutr.* **1990**, *51*, 846–852. [CrossRef] [PubMed]
113. Walther, B.; Karl, J.P.; Booth, S.L.; Boyaval, P. Menaquinones, Bacteria, and the Food Supply: The Relevance of Dairy and Fermented Food Products to Vitamin K Requirements. *Adv. Nutr.* **2013**, *4*, 463–473. [CrossRef] [PubMed]
114. Shearer, M.J.; Bolton-Smith, C. The UK food data-base for vitamin K and why we need it. *Food Chem.* **2000**, *68*, 213–218. [CrossRef]
115. Bolton-smith, C.; Price, R.J.G.; Fenton, S.T.; Harrington, D.J.; Shearer, M.J. Compilation of a provisional UK database for the phylloquinone (vitamin K1) content of foods. *Br. J. Nutr.* **2000**, *83*, 389–399. [PubMed]
116. Ben-shem, A.; Frolow, F.; Nelson, N. Crystal structure of plant photosystem I. *Nature* **2003**, *426*, 630–635. [CrossRef] [PubMed]
117. Gross, J.; Cho, W.K.; Lezhneva, L.; Falk, J.; Krupinska, K.; Shinozaki, K.; Seki, M.; Herrmann, R.G.; Meurer, J. A Plant Locus Essential for Phylloquinone (Vitamin K1) Biosynthesis Originated from a Fusion of Four Eubacterial Genes. *J. Biol. Chem.* **2006**, *281*, 17189–17196. [CrossRef]

118. Piironen, V.; Koivu, T.; Tammisalo, O.; Mattila, P. Determination of phylloquinone in oils, margarines and butter by high-performance liquid chromatography with electrochemical detection. *Food Chem.* **1997**, *59*, 473–480. [CrossRef]
119. Peterson, J.W.; Muzzey, K.L.; Haytowitz, D.; Exler, J.; Lemar, L.; Booth, S.L. Phylloquinone (vitamin K1) and Dihydrophylloquinone Content of Fats and Oils. *JAOCS* **2002**, *79*, 641–646. [CrossRef]
120. Elder, S.J.; Haytowitz, D.B.; Howe, J.; Peterson, J.W.; Booth, S.L. Vitamin K Contents of Meat, Dairy, and Fast Food in the U.S. Diet. *J. Agric. Food Chem.* **2006**, *54*, 463–467. [CrossRef]
121. Kamao, M.; Yoshitomo, S.; Tsuwaga, N.; Uwano, M.; Yamaguchi, N.; Uenishi, K.; Ishida, H.; Sasaki, S.; Okano, T. Vitamin K Content of Foods and Dietary Vitamin K Intake in Japanese Young Women. *J. Nutr. Sci. Vitaminol.* **2007**, *53*, 464–470. [CrossRef]
122. Bito, T.; Teng, F.; Watanabe, F. Bioactive Compounds of Edible Purple Laver Porphyra sp. (Nori). *J. Agric. Food Chem. Agric. Food Chem.* **2017**, *65*, 10685–10692. [CrossRef] [PubMed]
123. Suttie, J. The importance of menaquinones in human nutrition. *Ann. Rev. Nutr.* **1995**, *15*, 399–417. [CrossRef] [PubMed]
124. Collins, M.D.; Jones, D. Distribution of isoprenoid quinone structural types in bacteria and their taxonomic implications. *Microbiol. Rev.* **1981**, *45*, 316–354. [PubMed]
125. Fernandez, F.; Collins, M.D. Vitamin K composition of anaerobic gut bacteria. *FEMS Microbiol. Lett.* **1987**, *41*, 175–180. [CrossRef]
126. Conly, J.; Stein, K. Quantitative and qualitative measurements of K vitamins in human. *Am. J. Gastroenterol.* **1992**, *87*, 311–316.
127. Conly, J.; Stein, K. The production of menaquinones (vitamin K2) by intestinal bacteria and their role in maintaining coagulation homeostasis. *Prog. Food Nutr. Sci.* **1992**, *16*, 307–343.
128. Bourdichon, F.; Casaregola, S.; Farrokh, C.; Frisvad, J.C.; Gerds, M.L.; Hammes, W.P.; Harnett, J.; Huys, G.; Laulund, S.; Ouwehand, A.; et al. Food fermentations: Microorganisms with technological beneficial use. *Int. J. Food Microbiol.* **2012**, *154*, 87–97. [CrossRef]
129. Morishita, T.; Tamura, N.; Makino, T.; Kudo, S. Production of Menaquinones by Lactic Acid Bacteria. *J. Dairy Sci.* **1999**, *82*, 1897–1903. [CrossRef]
130. Manoury, E.; Jourdon, K.; Boyaval, P.; Fourcassié, P. Quantitative measurement of vitamin K2 (menaquinones) in various fermented dairy products using a reliable high-performance liquid chromatography method. *J. Dairy Sci.* **2013**, *96*, 1335–1346. [CrossRef]
131. Vermeer, C.; Raes, J.; Van Hoofd, C.; Knapen, M.H.J.; Xanthoulea, S. Menaquinone Content of Cheese. *Nutrients* **2018**, *10*, 446. [CrossRef]
132. Hojo, K.; Watanabe, R.; Mori, T.; Taketomo, N. Quantitative measurement of tetrahydromenaquinone-9 in cheese fermented by propionibacteria. *J. Dairy Sci.* **2007**, *90*, 4078–4083. [CrossRef] [PubMed]
133. Kaneki, M.; Hedges, S.J.; Hosoi, T.; Fujiwara, S.; Lyons, A.; Crean, S.J.; Ishida, N.; Nakagawa, M.; Takechi, M.; Sano, Y.; et al. Japanese Fermented Soybean Food as the Major Determinant of the Large Geographic Difference in Circulating Levels of Vitamin K2: Possible Implications for Hip-Fracture Risk. *Nutrition* **2001**, *4*, 315–321. [CrossRef]
134. Villa, J.K.; Diaz, M.A.; Pizziolo, V.R.; Martino, H.S. Effect of vitamin K in bone metabolism and vascular calcification: A review of mechanisms of action and evidences. *Crit. Rev. Food Sci. Nutr.* **2017**, *57*, 3959–3970. [CrossRef] [PubMed]
135. Sakane, R.; Kimura, K.; Hirota, Y.; Ishizawa, M.; Takagi, Y.; Akimori, W.; Shigefumi, K.; Makoto, M.; Suhara, Y. Synthesis of novel vitamin K derivatives with alkylated phenyl groups introduced at the ω-terminal side chain and evaluation of their neural differentiation activities. *Bioorg. Med. Chem.* **2017**, *27*, 4881–4884. [CrossRef] [PubMed]
136. Kimura, K.; Hirota, Y.; Kuwahara, S.; Takeuchi, A.; Tode, C.; Wada, A.; Osakabe, N.; Suhara, Y. Synthesis of Novel Synthetic Vitamin K Analogues Prepared by Introduction of a Heteroatom and a Phenyl Group That Induce Highly Selective Neuronal Differentiation of Neuronal Progenitor Cells. *J. Med. Chem.* **2017**, *60*, 2591–2596. [CrossRef] [PubMed]
137. Fujii, S.; Kagechika, H. Medicinal Chemistry of Vitamin K Derivatives and Metabolites. *Vital Health Wellbeing* **2017**, 239–255. [CrossRef]
138. Isler, O.; Doebel, K.; Hoffman-La Roche Inc. Synthesis of Vitamin K1 Using Boron Trifluoride Catalysts. U.S. Patent 2,683,176, 6 July 1954.

139. Fieser, L.F. Synthesis of Vitamin K1. *J. Am. Chem. Soc.* **1939**, *61*, 3467–3475. [CrossRef]
140. Afanasjeva, J. Administration of Injectable Vitamin K Orally. *Hosp. Pharm.* **2017**, *52*, 645–649. [CrossRef]
141. Daines, A.M.; Payne, R.J.; Humphries, M.E.; Abell, A.D. The Synthesis of Naturally Occurring Vitamin K and Vitamin K Analogues. *Org. Chem.* **2003**, *7*, 1–15. [CrossRef]
142. Coman, S.M.; Parvulescu, V.I.; Wuttke, S.; Kemnitz, E. Synthesis of Vitamin K1 and K1-Chromanol by Friedel–Crafts Alkylation in Heterogeneous Catalysis. *ChemCatChem* **2010**, *2*, 92–97. [CrossRef]
143. European Commission. *Opinion on Vitamin K1 (Phytonadione)*; SCCP/1105/07; Scientific Committee on Consumer Safety: Brussels, Belgium, 2007; pp. 1–31.
144. Tien, J.-H.; Pang, C.-Y.; Hsu, N.-H.; Sunny Pharmatec Inc. Method of Making Vitamin K1. U.S. Patent Application WO2016060670A1, 21 April 2016.
145. EFSA FEEDAP Panel (EFSA Panel on Additives and Products or Substances used in Animal Feed). Scientific Opinion on the safety and efficacy of vitamin K3 (menadione sodium bisulphite and menadione nicotinamide bisulphite) as a feed additive for all animal species. *EFSA J.* **2014**, *12*, 3532.
146. Tarento, T.D.C.; Mcclure, D.D.; Talbot, A.M.; Regtop, H.L.; Biffin, J.R.; Valtchev, P.; Dehghani, F.; Kavanagh, J.M.; Tarento, T.D.C.; Mcclure, D.D.; et al. A potential biotechnological process for the sustainable production of vitamin K1. *Crit. Rev. Biotechnol.* **2019**, *39*, 1–19. [CrossRef] [PubMed]
147. Snyder, C.D.; Rapoport, H. Synthesis of Menaquinones. *J. Am. Chem. Soc.* **1974**, *96*, 8046–8054. [CrossRef]
148. Baj, A.; Wa, P.; Kutner, A.; Morzycki, J.W.; Witkowski, S. Convergent synthesis of menaquinone-7 (MK-7). *Org. Process Res. Dev.* **2016**, *20*, 1026–1033. [CrossRef]
149. Suhara, Y.; Watanabe, M.; Motoyoshi, S.; Nakagawa, K.; Wada, A.; Takeda, K.; Takahashi, K.; Tokiwa, H.; Okano, T. Synthesis of new vitamin K analogues as steroid and xenobiotic receptor (SXR) agonists: Insights into the biological role of the side chain part of vitamin K. *J. Med. Chem.* **2011**, *54*, 4918–4922. [CrossRef] [PubMed]
150. Suhara, Y.; Hanada, N.; Okitsu, T.; Sakai, M.; Watanabe, M.; Nakagawa, K.; Wada, A.; Takeda, K.; Takahashi, K.; Tokiwa, H.; et al. Structure-activity relationship of novel menaquinone-4 analogues: Modification of the side chain affects their biological activities. *J. Med. Chem.* **2012**, *55*, 1553–1558. [CrossRef]
151. Vermeer, C.; van't Hoofd, C.; Knapen, M.H.J.; Xanthoulea, S. Synthesis of 2-methyl-1,4-naphthoquinones with higher gamma-glutamyl carboxylase activity than MK-4 both in vitro and in vivo. *Bioorg. Med. Chem.* **2017**, *27*, 208–211. [CrossRef]
152. Mahanama, R.; Berenjian, A.; Valtchev, P.; Talbot, A.; Biffin, R.; Regtop, H.; Dehghani, F.; Kavanagh, J.M. Enhanced production of menaquinone 7 via solid substrate fermentation from Bacillus subtilis. *Int. J. Food Eng.* **2011**, *7*. [CrossRef]
153. Berenjian, A.; Mahanama, R.; Talbot, A.; Regtop, H.; Kavanagh, J.; Dehghani, F. Advances in menaquinone-7 production by bacillus subtilis natto: Fed-batch glycerol addition. *Am. J. Biochem. Biotechnol.* **2012**, *8*, 105–110.
154. Singh, R.; Puri, A.; Panda, B.P. Development of menaquinone-7 enriched nutraceutical: Inside into medium engineering and process modeling. *J. Food Sci. Technol.* **2015**, *52*, 5212–5219. [CrossRef]
155. Berenjian, A.; Mahanama, R.; Kavanagh, J.; Dehghani, F.; Berenjian, A.; Mahanama, R.; Kavanagh, J.; Dehghani, F. Critical Reviews in Biotechnology Vitamin K series: Current status and future prospects. *Crit. Rev. Biotechnol.* **2015**, *35*, 199–208. [CrossRef] [PubMed]
156. Schallmey, M.; Singh, A.; Ward, O.P. Developments in the use of Bacillus species for industrial production. *Can. J. Microbiol.* **2004**, *50*, 1–17. [CrossRef] [PubMed]
157. Sato, T.; Yamada, Y.; Ohtani, Y.; Mitsui, N.; Murasawa, H.; Araki, S. Production of menaquinone (vitamin K2)-7 by Bacillus subtilis. *J. Biosci. Bioeng.* **2001**, *91*, 16–20. [CrossRef]
158. Song, J.; Liu, H.; Wang, L.; Dai, J.; Liu, Y.; Liu, H.; Zhao, G.; Wang, P.; Zheng, Z. Enhanced Production of Vitamin K2 from Bacillus subtilis (natto) by Mutation and Optimization of the Fermentation Medium. *Braz. Arch. Biol. Technol.* **2014**, *57*, 606–612.
159. Berenjian, A.; Chan, N.L.C.; Mahanama, R.; Talbot, A.; Regtop, H.; Kavanagh, J.; Dehghani, F. Effect of biofilm formation by Bacillus subtilis natto on menaquinone-7 biosynthesis. *Mol. Biotechnol.* **2013**, *54*, 371–378. [CrossRef]
160. Sato, T.; Yamada, Y.; Ohtani, Y.; Mitsui, N.; Murasawa, H.; Araki, S. Efficient production of menaquinone (vitamin K2) by a menadione-resistant mutant of Bacillus subtilis. *J. Ind. Microbiol. Biotechnol.* **2001**, *26*, 115–120. [CrossRef]

161. Tsukamoto, Y.; Kasai, M.; Kakuda, H. Construction of a Bacillus subtilis (natto) with High Productivity of Vitamin K2 (Menaquinone-7) by Analog Resistance. *Biosci. Biotechnol. BioChem.* **2001**, *65*, 2007–2015. [CrossRef]
162. Nishito, Y.; Osana, Y.; Hachiya, T.; Popendorf, K.; Toyoda, A.; Fujiyama, A.; Itaya, M.; Sakakibara, Y. Whole genome assembly of a natto production strain Bacillus subtilis natto from very short read data. *BMC Genom.* **2010**, *11*, 243. [CrossRef]
163. Ma, Y.; McClure, D.D.; Somerville, M.V.; Proschogo, N.W.; Dehghani, F.; Kavanagh, J.M.; Coleman, N.V. Metabolic Engineering of the MEP Pathway in Bacillus subtilis for Increased Biosynthesis of Menaquinone-7. *ACS Synth. Biol.* **2019**, *8*, 1620–1630. [CrossRef]
164. Yang, S.; Cao, Y.; Sun, L.; Li, C.; Lin, X.; Cai, Z.; Zhang, G.; Song, H. Modular Pathway Engineering of Bacillus subtilis to Promote de Novo Biosynthesis of Menaquinone-7. *ACS Synth. Biol.* **2019**, *8*, 70–81. [CrossRef]
165. Sanghvi, A.; Lo, Y. Present and potential industrial applications of macro- and microalgae. *Recent Pat. Food Nutr. Agric.* **2010**, *2*, 187–194. [CrossRef] [PubMed]
166. Collins, K.G.; Fitzgerald, G.F.; Stanton, C.; Ross, R.P. Looking beyond the terrestrial: The potential of seaweed derived bioactives to treat non-communicable diseases. *Mar. Drugs* **2016**, *14*, 60. [CrossRef] [PubMed]
167. Romano, G.; Costantini, M.; Sansone, C.; Lauritano, C.; Ruocco, N.; Ianora, A. Marine microorganisms as a promising and sustainable source of bioactive molecules. *Mar. Environ. Res.* **2017**, *128*, 58–69. [CrossRef] [PubMed]
168. Stengel, D.B.; Connan, S. Marine Algae: A Source of Biomass for Biotechnological Applications. *Methods Mol. Biol.* **2015**, *1308*, 1–37. [PubMed]
169. De Roeck-holtzhauer, Y.; Quere, I.; Claire, C. Vitamin analysis of five planktonic microalgae and one macroalga. *J. Appl. Phycol.* **1991**, *3*, 259–264. [CrossRef]
170. Tarento, T.D.C.; Mcclure, D.D.; Vasiljevski, E.; Schindeler, A.; Dehghani, F.; Kavanagh, J.M. Microalgae as a source of vitamin K1. *Algal Res.* **2018**, *36*, 77–87. [CrossRef]
171. Johnson, T.W.; Shen, G.; Zybailov, B.; Kolling, D.; Reategui, R.; Beauparlant, S.; Vassiliev, I.R.; Bryant, D.A.; Jones, A.D.; Golbeck, J.H.; et al. Recruitment of a foreign quinone into the A1 site of photosystem I. I. Genetic and physiological characterization of phylloquinone biosynthetic pathway mutants in Synechocystis sp. PCC 6803. *J. Biol. Chem.* **2000**, *275*, 8523–8530. [CrossRef]
172. Mimuro, M.; Tsuchiya, T.; Inoue, H.; Sakuragi, Y.; Itoh, Y.; Gotoh, T.; Miyashita, H.; Bryant, D.A.; Kobayashi, M. The secondary electron acceptor of photosystem I in Gloeobacter violaceus PCC 7421 is menaquinone-4 that is synthesized by a unique but unknown pathway. *FEBS Lett.* **2005**, *579*, 3493–3496. [CrossRef]
173. Sakuragi, Y.; Zybailov, B.; Shen, G.; Bryant, D.A.; Golbeck, J.H.; Diner, B.A.; Karygina, I.; Pushkar, Y.; Stehlik, D. Recruitment of a foreign quinone into the A1 site of photosystem I: Characterization of a menB rubA double deletion mutant in Synechococcus sp. PCC 7002 devoid of FX, FA, and FB and containing plastoquinone or exchanged 9,10-anthraquinone. *J. Biol. Chem.* **2005**, *280*, 12371–12381. [CrossRef]
174. Ikeda, Y.; Komura, M.; Watanabe, M.; Minami, C.; Koike, H.; Itoh, S.; Kashino, Y.; Satoh, K. Photosystem I complexes associated with fucoxanthin-chlorophyll-binding proteins from a marine centric diatom, Chaetoceros gracilis. *Biochim. Biophys. Acta* **2008**, *1777*, 351–361. [CrossRef]
175. Yoshida, E.; Nakamura, A.; Watanabe, T. Reversed-phase HPLC determination of chlorophyll a' and naphthoquinones in photosystem I of red algae: Existence of two menaquinone-4 molecules in photosystem I of Cyanidium caldarium. *Anal. Sci.* **2003**, *19*, 1001–1005. [CrossRef] [PubMed]
176. Koivu, T.J.; Piironen, V.I.; Henttonen, S.K.; Mattila, P.H. Determination of Phylloquinone in Vegetables, Fruits, and Berries by High-Performance Liquid Chromatography with Electrochemical Detection. *J. Agric. Food Chem. Food Chem.* **1997**, *45*, 4644–4649. [CrossRef]
177. Booth, S.L.; Sadowski, J.A.; Penningtont, J.A.T. Phylloquinone (Vitamin K1) Content of Foods in the US. Food and Drug Administration's Total Diet Study. *J. Agric. Food Chem. Food Chem.* **1995**, *43*, 1574–1579. [CrossRef]
178. Salvaterra, T.; Green, D.S.; Crowe, T.P.; O'Gorman, E.J. Impacts of the invasive alga Sargassum muticum on ecosystem functioning and food web structure. *Biol. Invasions* **2013**, *15*, 2563–2576. [CrossRef]
179. Epstein, G.; Smale, D.A. Undaria pinnatifida: A case study to highlight challenges in marine invasion ecology and management. *Ecol. Evol.* **2017**, *7*, 8624–8642. [CrossRef]
180. von Kries, R.; Hachmeister, A.; Gobel, U. Oral mixed micellar vitamin K for prevention of late vitamin K deficiency bleeding. *Arch. Dis Child. Fetal Neonatal Ed.* **2003**, *88*, 109–112. [CrossRef]

181. Hasselt, P.M.; Van Janssens, G.E.P.J.; Slot, T.K.; Van Der Ham, M.; Minderhoud, T.C.; Talelli, M.; Akkermans, L.M.; Rijcken, C.J.F.; Van Nostrum, C.F. The influence of bile acids on the oral bioavailability of vitamin K encapsulated in polymeric micelles. *J. Control. Release* **2009**, *133*, 161–168. [CrossRef]
182. Leiro, V.; Moreno, P.; Sarmento, B.; Durão, J.; Gales, L.; Pêgo, A.; Barrias, C. 1-Design and preparation of biomimetic and bioinspired materials. In *Bioinspired Materials for Medical Applications*; Rodrigues, L., Mota, M., Eds.; Woodhead Publishing: Cambridge, UK, 2017; pp. 1–44.
183. Sun, F.; Ye, C.; Thanki, K.; Leng, D.; Van Hasselt, P.M.; Hennink, W.E.; van Nostrum, C.F. Mixed micellar system stabilized with saponins for oral delivery of vitamin K. *Colloids Surf. B Biointerfaces* **2018**, *170*, 521–528. [CrossRef]
184. Hamrick, H.J.; Gable, K.; Freeman, H.; Dunn, L.; Zimmerman, P.; Rusin, M.M.; Linthavong, R.; Wright, E.; Moss, A.; Skinner, C. Reasons for Refusal of Newborn Vitamin K Prophylaxis: Implications for Management and Education. *Hosp. Pediatr.* **2019**, *6*, 15–21. [CrossRef]
185. Gomaa, Y.A.; Garland, M.J.; Mcinnes, F.; El-khordagui, L.K.; Wilson, C.; Donnelly, R.F. Laser-engineered dissolving microneedles for active transdermal delivery of nadroparin calcium. *Eur. J. Pharm. Biopharm.* **2012**, *82*, 299–307. [CrossRef]
186. Quinn, H.L.; Bonham, L.; Hughes, C.M.; Donnelly, R.F. Design of a Dissolving Microneedle Platform for Transdermal Delivery of a Fixed-Dose Combination of Cardiovascular Drugs. *J. Pharm. Sci.* **2015**, *104*, 3490–3500. [CrossRef] [PubMed]
187. Sullivan, S.P.; Koutsonanos, D.G.; Martin, P.; Lee, J.; Zarnitsyn, V.; Murthy, N.; Compans, R.W.; Skountzou, I.; Prausnitz, R. Dissolving Polymer Microneedle Patches for Influenza Vaccination. *Nat. Med.* **2010**, *16*, 915–920. [CrossRef] [PubMed]
188. González-vázquez, P.; Larrañeta, E.; Mccrudden, M.T.C.; Jarrahian, C.; Rein-weston, A.; Quintanar-solares, M.; Zehrung, D.; Mccarthy, H.; Courtenay, A.J.; Donnelly, R.F. Transdermal delivery of gentamicin using dissolving microneedle arrays for potential treatment of neonatal sepsis. *J. Control. Release* **2017**, *265*, 30–40. [CrossRef] [PubMed]
189. Hutton, A.R.J.; Quinn, H.L.; Mccague, P.J.; Jarrahian, C.; Rein-weston, A.; Co, P.S.; Gerth-guyette, E.; Zehrung, D.; Larrañeta, E.; Donnelly, R.F. Transdermal delivery of vitamin K using dissolving microneedles for the prevention of vitamin K deficiency bleeding. *Int. J. Pharm.* **2018**, *541*, 56–63. [CrossRef]
190. Kidd, P.M. Vitamins D and K as pleiotropic nutrients: Clinical importance to the skeletal and cardiovascular systems and preliminary evidence for synergy. *Altern. Med. Rev.* **2010**, *15*, 199–222.
191. Van Ballegooijen, A.J.; Pilz, S.; Tomaschitz, A.; Grübler, M.R.; Verheyen, N. The Synergistic Interplay between Vitamins D and K for Bone and Cardiovascular Health: A Narrative Review. *Int. J. Endocrinol.* **2017**, *2017*, 7454376. [CrossRef]
192. Viegas, C.; Araújo, N.; Marreiros, C.; Simes, D. The interplay between mineral metabolism, vascular calcification and inflammation in Chronic Kidney Disease (CKD): Challenging old concepts with new facts. *Aging* **2019**, *11*, 4274–4299. [CrossRef]
193. Theuwissen, E.; Cranenburg, E.C.; Knapen, M.H.; Magdeleyns, E.J.; Teunissen, K.J.; Schurgers, L.J.; Smit, E.; Vermeer, C. Low-dose menaquinone-7 supplementation improved extra-hepatic vitamin K status, but had no effect on thrombin generation in healthy subjects. *Br. J. Nutr.* **2012**, *108*, 1652–1657. [CrossRef]
194. Schulman, S.; Furie, B. How I treat poisoning with vitamin K antagonists. *Blood* **2015**, *125*, 438–442. [CrossRef]
195. Spahr, J.E.; Maul, J.S.; Rodgers, G.M. Superwarfarin Poisoning: A Report of Two Cases and Review of the Literature. *Am. J. Hematol.* **2007**, *82*, 656–660. [CrossRef]

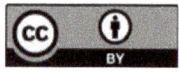

© 2020 by the authors. Licensee MDPI, Basel, Switzerland. This article is an open access article distributed under the terms and conditions of the Creative Commons Attribution (CC BY) license (http://creativecommons.org/licenses/by/4.0/).

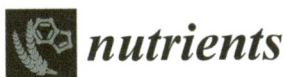

Article

Effect of a Supplementation with Two *Quelites* on Urinary Excretion of Arsenic in Adolescents Exposed to Water Contaminated with the Metalloid in a Community in the State of Guanajuato, Mexico

Yair Olovaldo Santiago-Saenz [1], Rebeca Monroy-Torres [2,*], Diana Olivia Rocha-Amador [3] and Alma Delia Hernández-Fuentes [1,*]

1. Área Académica de Ingeniería Agroindustrial e Ingeniería en Alimentos, Instituto de Ciencias Agropecuarias, Universidad Autónoma del Estado de Hidalgo, Tulancingo 43600, Mexico; y.sant.sanz@gmail.com
2. Departamento de Medicina y Nutrición, División de Ciencias de la Salud, Universidad de Guanajuato, León 37670, Mexico
3. Departamento de Farmacia, División de Ciencias Naturales y Exactas, Universidad de Guanajuato, Guanajuato 36050, Mexico; olivia2000_mx@hotmail.com
* Correspondence: rmonroy79@gmail.com (R.M.-T.); hfad@hotmail.com (A.D.H.-F.); Tel.: +(477)-267-4900 (ext. 3677) (R.M.-T.); +775-75-606-78 (A.D.H.-F.)

Received: 4 November 2019; Accepted: 12 December 2019; Published: 30 December 2019

Abstract: *Quelites* are Mexican wild plants, reported as excellent sources of nutritional compounds such as amino acids (serine, glycine, and cysteine), minerals (Mg, Fe, and Zn), and phytochemicals, as phenolic acids (chlorogenic acid) and flavonoids (phloridzin and naringenin); on the other hand, high biological activity has been shown in these compounds. This work aimed to evaluate the effect of a supplementation with two endemic *quelites* of Mexico (*Chenopodium berlandieri* L. and *Portulaca Oleracea* L.); in addition to supplementation, a nutritional intervention was performed; the biomarkers of hemoglobin (Hb), urinary malondialdehyde (UMDA), and urinary arsenic (UAs) were measured in adolescents exposed to arsenic. A clinical intervention study was conducted in 27 adolescents ages 11 to 12 years for 4 weeks. Weekly anthropometric and dietary evaluations were carried out, as well as the concentration of Hb; the UMDA and UAs were performed by plate-based colorimetric measurement and atomic absorption spectrophotometry with the hydrides generation system, respectively. The results showed that UMDA concentrations had a significant improvement in the supplemented group (SG) vs. control group (CG) (SG = 1.59 ± 0.89 µM/g creatinine vs. CG = 2.90 ± 0.56 µM/g creatinine) in the second week of intervention; on the other hand, the supplemented group showed an increase in Hb levels (15.12 ± 0.99 g/dL) in the same week; finally after the second week, an increase in UAs levels was observed significantly compared to the baseline value (Baseline: 56.85; Week 2: 2.02 µg/g creatinine). Therefore, the results show that the mixture of *quelites* (a rich source of phytochemicals and nutrients) improved hemoglobin and UMDA levels, and urinary arsenic excretion from the second week in the exposed population.

Keywords: *quelites*; supplementation; arsenic

1. Introduction

Arsenic (As) is an element that is naturally distributed on the surface of the earth's crust, it can be filtered to groundwater reserves, due to soil drilling, water movements, and when there is mining activity. In other cases, depending on the composition of the rock, water can dissolve and drag these elements, producing natural pollution and increasing the concentration in ground and surface waters [1,2], which become the main source of drinking water in rural areas. There are many other types of pollution of As, including chemical pollution into bodies of water and soil through improper disposal practices and agricultural activities, due for use of pesticides and fertilizers, among other factors that compromise human health.

In countries such as Thailand, India, China, Argentina, and Mexico, concentrations of As have been found in ranges from 0.5 to 5000 µg/L [3,4]. As for Mexico, the highest concentrations of As are found in the northeast and central parts of the country [5], generally in arid and semi-arid areas, including Coahuila, Zacatecas, Hidalgo, San Luis Potosí, and Guanajuato [6]. Particularly in the state of Guanajuato, in the northeast region, given its location in the vicinity of three geological provinces, combined with volcanic activity alternated with periods of intense erosion and sedimentation, give rise to different dissolved elements [1,7]. But in the central area of the state of Guanajuato, since 2004, they have been identified in several communities with high levels of As in water [8].

According to the World Health Organization (WHO) [9], As, due to its ubiquity characteristic, is classified as one of the chemicals of greatest concern worldwide, which, if not handled properly, can be very dangerous for the environment and health. Chronic exposure to As can cause hyperkeratosis, dermatitis, respiratory diseases, cancer, adverse thyroid effects, and neurotoxicity [8–11].

Few studies have shown that a high intake of antioxidants and fructooligosaccharides (FOS) identified in the Mexican diet foods such as beans, lentils, bananas, and onions can prevent or reverse some of the effects involved in the development of cancer and cardiovascular diseases and chronic, caused by this pollutant, by avoiding bioaccumulate in the organism and thus an improvement in the excretion in the urine [12,13]; therefore, the consumption of foods rich in phytochemicals with adequate nutritional contributions and with high antioxidant capacity, has been considered a strategy to reduce the effects of this element when people have acute or chronic exposure, by providing the requirements of various nutrients such as cysteine, methionine, vitamin C [14,15], and phenolic compounds [16–18], essential for arsenic detoxification [19], to increase antiradical effects (ROS), and reduce the production of malondialdehyde (MDA) in the body [17,18].

Mexico has a wide variety of wild edible plants found in rural areas referred to as *quelites* [20]; between them, we can differentiate two important species, *Chenopodium berlandieri* L. and *Portulaca oleraceae* L., which naturally grow in abundance in mountains, flat fields, or near corn or bean crops of Mexican territory [21]. The leaves and stems of these species have a high nutritional contribution (dietary fiber, proteins, minerals) and bioactive compounds (carotenoids, chlorophyll, phenolic acids, and flavonoids) [22], as well as a high antioxidant capacity and provide biological effects of interest in human health [21,22]. Recent studies have found excellent results when using plants that belong to the genera of *Chenopodium* spp., reporting a reduction in MDA and increased activity of antioxidant enzymes in rats induced with toxic agents [23] or decreasing levels of lipid peroxidation in lines of cancer cells [24]. Finally, when using *Portulaca* spp. in animal models, the potential effect of its bioactive compounds on the integrity of the CNS (Central Nervous System) [25], hepatoprotective capacity [26], and the reduction of damage by stress mechanisms against external factors such as pollutants (rotenone) [27] have been observed.

In Mexico, there is evidence that shows that the administration of supplements that incorporate vegetables such as broccoli and fruits such as grapes, as well as minerals and vitamins essential for the detoxification process [14–19], promote better arsenic excretion and improve the nutritional status, in this case, by inducing an increase in hemoglobin (Hb) levels of participants [28]. However, given these bases and the nutritional contribution of these *quelites*, the aim of this research was to evaluate the effect of a supplement made with two novelty ingredients (*Portulaca oleraceae* L. and *Chenopodium berlandieri* L.), economical, accessible, and with sufficient evidence of its antioxidant and nutritional potential, on hemoglobin (Hb), urinary arsenic excretion (UAs), and urinary malondialdehyde (UMDA) concentration, which will be biomarkers of interest to know the positive effect of this supplement provided in adolescents from a rural area in Guanajuato, Mexico, exposed to arsenic.

2. Materials and Methods

2.1. Reagents and Equipments

Nitric acid, perchloric acid, sodium borohydride, potassium iodide, sodium hydroxide, hydrochloric acid, and ascorbic acid were purchased from J.T Baker (Avantor Performance Materials, Ecatepec, Estado de Mexico, Mexico) and Fermont (Rye S.A de C.V, Tlalnepantla, Estado de Mexico, Mexico). The microcuvettes for hemoglobin determination (Hb-201) were purchased from HemoCue (HemoCue, Ciudad de Mexico, Mexico). The TBARS assay kit (MDA) was purchased from Cayman Chemical (Cayman Chemical, Ann Arbor, MI, USA). The arsenic standard was purchased from Agilent (Agilent, Santa Clara, CA, USA). The quality control for As (ClinChek®-urine control lyophilised for trace elements, level II) was purchased from Iris Tech (IRIS Technologies International GmbH, Olathe, KS, USA). The concentration of arsenic (As) in drinking water with Arsenator®-Digital Arsenic Test Kit from Wagtech WTD, Palintest, CO, USA). All solutions were prepared using deionized water.

2.2. Intervention Design, Study Groups, and Acquisition of Data

A clinical intervention study was conducted in 27 participants (13 men and 14 women) ages 11 to 12 years belonging to the rural area of Valencianita, Irapuato, in the state of Guanajuato, Mexico. It was a randomized study to assess the effect of supplementation on UAs excretion. The random assignment code was generated using a randomized block design with SAS® (Cary, NC, USA). All participants were randomly assigned in into two groups referred to as control and supplemented (4 g of supplement). The details of the study are mentioned by section and in Figure 1.

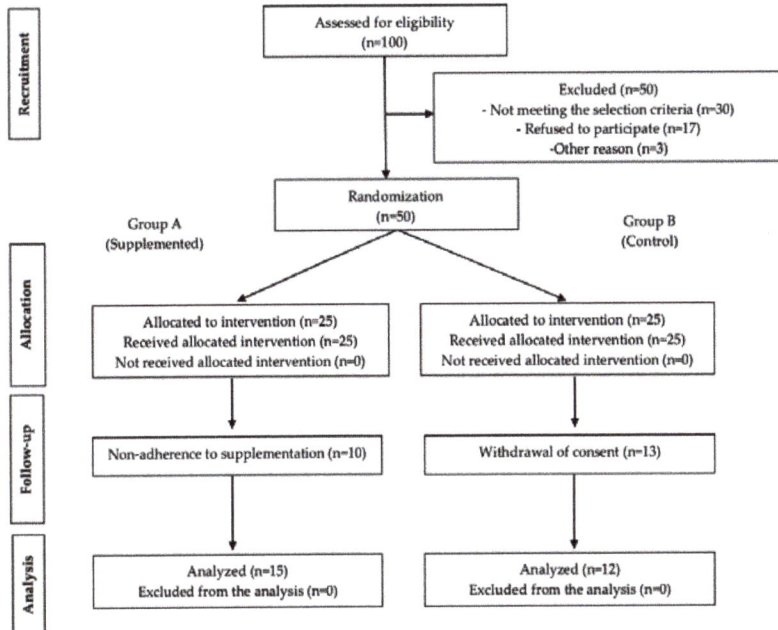

Figure 1. Flow diagram of patient progress through the phases of the randomized trial.

2.2.1. Eligibility Criteria

Inclusion criteria: High school students #117 of the community of Valencianita, Irapuato in the state of Guanajuato, men and women with a minimum residence of three years in the community, arsenic concentrations in drinking water above 25 µg/L (hydroarsenism) [29].

Exclusion criteria: Participants who are taking a supplement (trademarks of natural products), or drug (treatment or over-the-counter), participants with some type of kidney or liver damage confirmed by the clinical history, participants who did not want to join the study, and participants who provided a single urine sample or were evaluated only once.

2.2.2. Pre-Selection Phase and Ethical Statement

Parents and adolescents received verbal and written information about the study, informed parental consent, and consent from the adolescents were obtained before they participated in the study. The study was free, anonymous, and voluntary, was conducted in accordance with the Declaration of Helsinki, and approved by the institutional research bioethics committee of the University of Guanajuato (Code-CIBIUG-P34-2018).

2.2.3. Selection Phase and Clinical Intervention

Participants who met the inclusion criteria were incorporated into the study. It was confirmed that the adolescents included in the research did not have acute or chronic diseases, their liver function was normal, and they were not taking drugs or supplements before and during the intervention.

The adolescents were divided into two groups: the supplemented group with 15 participants (9 men and 6 women) and the control group with 12 participants (4 men and 8 women).

Before beginning treatment and during the intervention, parents and adolescents were informed of the importance of consuming treated and purified water to observe a better recovery process. In addition, a questionnaire was applied to the mothers of the participants for the acquisition of information concerning drinking water, and later these data were confirmed with the analysis of water samples consumed at the participants' homes and provided by the mothers during the intervention.

The clinical intervention was carried out according to Monroy-Torres et al. [28]. A detailed nutritional history was obtained for each child and a physical examination was performed, which included anthropometric parameters.

2.3. Supplement of Quelites

In this research a powder supplement made with two endemic vegetable ingredients from Mexico was used; these plants contained, in dietary supplement, belong to the species of *Chenopodium berlandieri* L. and *Portulaca Oleraceae* L. In addition, each species was characterized [22], and also the nutritional and functional evaluation of the supplement was performed [30]; the research considered the nutritional profile [macronutrients and micronutrients (minerals and amino acids)] and antioxidant properties (antioxidant compounds and antioxidant activity) [30].

2.4. Dietary Supplementation

Parents and adolescents belonged to the supplemented group were informed about storage and intake of the supplement before the beginning of the study; two units of 60 g each of supplement were delivered to the parents for the total period of the intervention. The dose of the treatment was 4 g per day for 4 consecutive weeks (November 2018) and with a single dose 1 h before the intake of any food during morning hours, considering taking it at the same time every day; on the other hand, no placebo was administered to the control group because of the social and cultural factors previously identified in the rural community. The adolescents included in this work were not provided an orientation about an adequate diet, allowing them to maintain their diet as usual during the study. The supplement intake monitoring was evaluated by adherence questionnaires once a week at the school and by telephone two days per week. At the end of the study, the participants were asked to return any pouches not consumed. The dose of the supplement was selected by extrapolated calculations on the basis of a previous animal studies [23,27] and a previous clinical intervention [28].

2.5. Urine Sample

The urine samples were collected in polyethylene containers previously washed with HNO_3 (10%) and being the first urine in the morning. These samples were requested from the participant minutes before the corresponding evaluation and stored in refrigeration at 4 °C until the end of the day indicators measurement. Later, samples were transported inside thermal containers. Before submitting the samples to the freezing process, a 1 mL aliquot of urine was extracted from each container and stored in previously labeled microtubes, which were taken to ultra-freezing (−76 °C) (Thermo-Scientific, 703, Outside, USA) for the subsequent MDA assay; the samples collected in the polyethylene containers were stored in freezing at −20 °C until the moment of analysis. The creatinine content of the samples was determined within the week of collection of each batch and according to the Jaffe reaction method [31]. The results of the urinary biomarkers were adjusted per grams of creatinine.

2.6. Anthropometric Assessment

Weight (Kg), fat mass (%), and lean body mass (%) were obtained with the impedance technique (bioimpedance analyzer, InBody® R20); waist (cm) and abdominal (cm) circumferences (metal tape measure, Lufkin) were measured; also height (cm) (stadiometer, Seca®) of each participant was measured. The anthropometric measurements were obtained according to Lohman et al. [32]. With the weight and height, the body mass index (BMI) was calculated and they were classified in obesity, overweight, or normal weight; in addition, height-for-age (H/A) was obtained; WHO reference tables [33] and WHO Anthro Plus® software were used for data interpretation. A BMI with thinness (malnutrition) with <−2 standard deviation (SD), normal between −2 to +1 (SD), overweight with >+1 (SD), and obesity with >+2 (SD) was considered. On the other hand, low height-for-age [<−2 (SD)] and normal height [−2 to +3 (SD)] were estimated. The measurements were being made weekly by nutritionists.

2.7. Dietary Assessment

A food frequency questionnaire (FFQ) was carried out, as well as a 24-h dietary recall (24 DR) [34]. The quantification of the average energy consumption (kcal), proteins (g), carbohydrates (g), fats (g), sugars (g), fiber (g), vitamin A (µg), B1 (mg), B2 (mg), B6 (mg), B12 (µg), C (mg), folic acid (µg), niacin (mg), vitamin E (mg), Ca (mg), Fe (mg), K (mg), Mg (mg), Na (mg), P (mg), Se (µg), and Zn (mg) were determined with NutriKcal® (nutritional software based on food composition tables in Mexico and derived from 24-h dietary recall); on the other hand, adherence questionnaires and treatment monitoring were applied. The register was made and monitored weekly by nutritionists.

2.8. Hemoglobin Concentration

The concentration of hemoglobin (Hb) in capillary blood was carried out by photometry; participant was stung on a finger with a sterile lancet and Hb was measured from a drop of blood (preferably the third drop) using a microcuvette and deposited in the portable Hb analyzer (HemoCue®, 201, Brea, CA, USA), with a detection range of 0 to 24.6 g/dL. Hb was used to evaluate the absorption of nutrients from the diet during the intervention. The results were expressed as grams of hemoglobin per deciliter (g Hb/dL).

2.9. Urine Malondialdehyde Concentration

According to the most recent study carried out in the rural community of Valencianita where the first effects of a supplement were reported in the first month [28], it was decided to include 3 measurements, taking into account a Baseline measurement (week 0), at week 2 and at the end of the study (week 4).

The concentration of malondialdehyde in urine (UMDA) was carried out with a TBARS assay kit purchased from Cayman Chemical (Cayman Chemical, Ann Arbor, MI, USA) and according to the recommendations described by the manufacturer. Briefly, an aliquot of the urine sample (100 µL) was mixed with SDS solution (100 µL) and color reagent (4 mL) in a screw cap tube glass, and allowed to stand in a water bath at constant temperature (90 °C) for 1 h; later, tubes were removed and taken to an ice bath for 10 min to stop the reaction. After, samples were poured into 15 mL tubes to centrifuge for 10 min at 1600× g at 4 °C. Finally, 150 µL aliquots of the supernatant (duplicate) were taken and placed on clear plates (96-well solid plate) and read at an absorbance of 530–540 nm in a plate reader (Biotek instruments, ELx800, VT, USA). The concentration of the lipid peroxidation product was calculated from a standard MDA curve. The results were expressed as micromole of malondialdehyde per gram of creatinine (µM MDA/g creatinine).

2.10. Concentrations of Arsenic in Drinking Water and Urine

2.10.1. Water

The concentration of arsenic (As) in drinking water was carried out using the hydrides generation technique using an As analysis kit (Arsenator®-Digital Arsenic Test Kit from Wagtech WTD, Palintest, CO, USA) for rural communities. The detection range of the Arsenator® was 0 to 100 µg/L. Concentrations were expressed as micrograms of arsenic per liter (µg As/L). The evaluations were conducted weekly, one month prior to the study and during the intervention. School and household water sources used for consumption were analyzed. The procedure is described as follows: a 50 mL sample of water was obtained which was taken with a 250 mL flask, then a powder sachet (sulfamic acid) was added to the sample and a catalyst tablet, both provided by the kit. Then, two filter slides were used to remove (red) the excess of arsine gas and collect the arsenic gas (black) both inserted in a bung device. Immediately the bung device was pushed down firmly into the flask. Later, after 20 min, the black filter slide was removed from the bung device. The black arsenic filter slide was read into the DigiPAsS. The validation process was carried out according to the reference coloration parameters (Palintest).

2.10.2. Urine

Quantification of As in urine (UAs) was performed according to the Cox method [35]. A 5 mL of urine sample was digested with a mixture of HNO_3 and $HClO_4$ (1:6); the mixture was stirred and covered with a watch glass and placed on a low-temperature hot plate for 15 min and later the temperature was increased to 80 °C until the sample was dried; briefly, the content was resuspended in 10 mL of HCl (3%). All procedures were performed in duplicate. For the reduction of As^{+5} to As^{+3}, 5 mL of the digested sample was reduced with 1 mL of KI (3%) and 4 mL of HCl (1.5%) for 5 min at 80 °C in darkness. Before the process of reduction of the samples, the reagents for the hydrides generation were prepared; NaOH (1%) was prepared using deionized water, and later, $NaBH_4$ (3%) was prepared with the NaOH solution previously made. Reagents were made separately and then mixed. The final $NaBH_4$ solution was filtered using a #5 filter paper and a vacuum pump. The filtered solution was covered with aluminum foil and refrigerated for use on the same day. Finally, 10 mL of reduced sample was poured into a reaction flask; an average of 40 mL of $NaBH_4$ reagent for every 6 samples analyzed was used. The sample was analyzed by atomic absorption spectrophotometry (AAS) with hydrides generation system (PerkinElmer, PinAAcle900H, Wellesley, MA, USA) using the software Syngistix 2.0 and under the following conditions: the wavelength of 197.20 nm, slit 0.7, EDL lamp (energy >50), argon as the carrier gas, and as signal mode the peak height. The results were expressed as micrograms of arsenic per gram of creatinine (µg As/g creatinine).

The concentration of As was calculated from a standard curve. The curve was calculated from a standard stock solution of 1000 ppb of As, dilutions were made for 0.5, 1.0, 5.0, 10.0, and 20.0 ppb of As, as well as a blank. The slope of the resulting curve was m = 0.0135 with a correlation coefficient of $R^2 = 0.9844$.

For quality control, the ClinChek® brand was used as a reference standard, with an average As concentration of 83.3 µg/L (66.6–99.9). For the preparation, 10 mL of deionized water was added to the control urine, and then 3 mL was taken and the digestion and reduction process were the same as the urine samples. A total of eight quality controls were performed with an average recovery percentage of 102.33% ± 2.43%.

The analysis considered 2 blanks (acids) and a quality control (ClinChek®) in duplicate for each batch (intervention week) evaluated.

2.11. Statistical Analysis

For the statistical analysis, the data were grouped according to age ranges, sex, and by group of participants (supplemented and controls). They were analyzed and compared using the statistical software SPSS® 25.0. For selection of statistical tests, the Shapiro–Wilk normality test and Levene test for equality of variances were used. Comparative analysis between sex and study group was determined with the independent samples t Student and the Mann–Whitney U test for data with normality and without it respectively. The comparison of baseline and final variables was performed with paired sample t-Test and Wilcoxon signed-rank test; besides, to compare the intervention weeks, repeated measures ANOVA test was used as well as Friedman test, according to the characteristics of the variables. A $p < 0.05$ was used. To know the effect of the treatment the number needed to treat was calculated (NNT).

3. Results

3.1. Study Population

The groups formed were two, the first referred to as supplemented and the second one referred to as control, which were previously described. The indexes (height-for-age and body mass index for age) were calculated using the Z-Score for individuals ages 5–19 years. The baseline characteristics of both groups (supplemented and control group) were homogeneous (Table 1), without statistically significant differences between them (NS); only the percentage of fat mass and muscle mass showed differences, being higher in women and men respectively (Table 2).

Table 1. General characteristics of participants of the supplemented and control group.

Baseline Variables	Supplemented n = 15	Control n = 12	p-Value
Age (years)	11.80 ± 0.41	12 ± 0.36	[3] NS
Weight (kg)	47.31 ± 10.54	48.95 ± 11.33	NS
Height (cm)	150.31 ± 6.74	153.30 ± 7.21	NS
[1] H/A interpretation (Z-Score)			NS
Normal height	15 ± 82.19	12 ± 91.42	
[2] BMI interpretation (Z-Score)			NS
Obesity	2 ± 10.14	2 ± 16.05	
Overweight	5 ± 33.67	3 ± 19.36	
Normal weight	8 ± 31.94	7 ± 35.02	
Fat mass (%)	21.92 ± 14.71	23.02 ± 14.07	NS
Muscular mass (%)	33.46 ± 11.08	32.12 ± 8.95	NS
Waist circumference (cm)	71.19 ± 12.05	71.48 ± 9.44	NS
Abdominal circumference (cm)	76.28 ± 11.58	79.33 ± 10.27	NS

The table shows the mean ± standard deviation (SD) for each baseline variable and the p-value according to the independent samples t-Test ($p < 0.05$). [1] H/A: height-for-age [ages 5–19 years (Z-Score)]; [2] BMI: body mass index for age [ages 5–19 years (Z-Score)]; [3] NS: not significant.

Table 2. General characteristics for men, women, and total participants included in the supplementation study.

Baseline Variables	Total Population n = 27	Men n = 13	Women n = 14	p-Value
Age (years)	11.88 ± 0.32	11.84 ± 0.37	11.92 ± 0.26	[3] NS
Weight (kg)	48.13 ± 10.72	48.07 ± 10.89	48.19 ± 10.98	NS
Height (cm)	151.78 ± 7.01	152.56 ± 7.28	151.00 ± 6.64	NS
[1] H/A interpretation (Z-Score)				NS
Normal height	27 ± 98.42	13 ± 86.24	14 ± 93.37	
[2] BMI interpretation (Z-Score)				NS
Obesity	4 ± 31.26	1 ± 9.32	3 ± 17.21	
Overweight	8 ± 35.74	5 ± 35.11	3 ± 21.17	
Normal weight	15 ± 42.31	8 ± 32.29	7 ± 35.18	
Fat mass (%)	22.46 ± 14.16	13.98 ± 12.64	30.32 ± 10.74	<0.001
Muscular mass (%)	32.80 ± 10.03	40.47 ± 9.25	25.67 ± 2.93	<0.001
Waist circumference (cm)	71.34 ± 10.77	71.20 ± 11.77	71.47 ± 10.20	NS
Abdominal circumference (cm)	77.81 ± 10.96	75.62 ± 10.90	79.84 ± 11.01	NS

The table shows the mean ± standard deviation (SD) for each baseline variable and the p-value according to the independent samples t-Test ($p < 0.05$). [1] H/A: height-for-age in men and women ages 5–19 years (Z-Score); [2] BMI: body mass index for age in men and women ages 5–19 years (Z-Score); [3] NS: not significant.

3.2. Diet

Baseline analysis of the ingested nutrients is shown in Tables 3 and 4. Evaluations showed scarce differences between supplemented and control group pre and post-intervention, showing that the dietary patterns remained homogeneous throughout the study. There was a significant difference by group (Table 3) only in energy ($p < 0.002$) and K ($p < 0.05$) intake; however the intake by sex (Table 4), showed that the macro and micronutrients were higher in men than in women ($p < 0.002$), with the exception of vitamin C, E, and magnesium where no significant difference was found; on the other hand, the intake of fiber and sugar did not show significant differences by sex.

Regarding the dietary reference intakes by age (9–13 years) for each macro and micronutrient [36], it was observed that the values for protein were according to the DRI (Dietary Reference Intakes) for men and women (>34 g/day); however, the intake of total fats and carbohydrates were high in both sexes. On the other hand, the men's diet complied with the DRI for B vitamins, vitamin A, C, and niacin, but not for folic acid (78%) and vitamin E (24%). Regarding minerals, men showed adequate DRI for Fe, Mg, and Se, but the minimum recommended for Ca (85%), K (45%), P (60%), and Zn (75%) was not met.

High consumption of Na was reported for men (>2 g/day). On the other hand, women did not meet the minimum requirements for vitamins (16%–66%) and minerals (25%–77%) and regarding the sodium intake, did not exceed the recommended DRI (DRI: <2 g/day). Finally, according to the recommended dietary allowance of fiber, the intake was low in both sexes (DRI: 26–31 g/day).

On the other hand, according to the FFQ, the results showed a high intake (4–5 days per week) of ultra-processed food products (chips and pastries), sweets, popsicles, chocolates, cola drinks (Coke and Pepsi), and other carbonated beverages with flavorings, sweeteners, and high sugar content. Regarding meals provided at home, a preference for fried or oil foods was shown, mostly using this method and rarely roasted and steamed. Moreover, the consumption of fruits and vegetables was low, and the foods of greater preference by the participants were the banana, apple, and orange for fruits, and potatoes, onions, and tomatoes for vegetables (cooked), these with weekly consumption frequency (2–3 fruits per week; 2–4 vegetables per week); it is important to comment that the participants showed no interest in consuming raw (salad) or steamed vegetables (preference for fried and sugary foods), or as a snack due the bitter and weird flavors of these foods. Regarding animal products such as poultry and meat (beef and pork), the limitation of their frequency (1–2 times every 15 days) was observed due to costs, the egg and bean being the main source of protein (2–3 times per week), complemented with other foods, such as corn tortilla (daily) and pork rinds (1–2 times per week) to increase satiety.

Table 3. Daily intake of energy and nutrients in supplemented and control group.

Nutrients	Supplemented n = 15	Control n = 12	p-Value
Energy (kcal)	2006.04 ± 5.07	2000.12 ± 3.49	<0.002
Protein (g)	70.05 ± 27.52	69.96 ± 27.96	[1] NS
Fat (g)	70.02 ± 33.71	66.15 ± 29.66	NS
Cholesterol (mg)	284.21 ± 169.46	282.59 ± 180.64	NS
Carbohydrates (g)	290.38 ± 96.12	273.41 ± 51.34	NS
Sugar (g)	32.36 ± 31.67	30.02 ± 36.32	NS
Fiber (g)	21.09 ± 12.20	20.17 ± 8.91	NS
Vitamin A-Retinol (µg)	767.04 ± 182.09	753.62 ± 173.48	NS
Vitamin B1 (mg)	1.15 ± 0.50	1.09 ± 0.38	NS
Vitamin B2 (mg)	1.23 ± 0.57	1.21 ± 0.45	NS
Vitamin B6 (mg)	0.94 ± 0.55	0.81 ± 0.46	NS
Vitamin B12 (µg)	1.93 ± 1.12	1.91 ± 1.27	NS
Vitamin C (mg)	52.47 ± 45.74	34.03 ± 29.79	NS
Folic acid (µg)	186.39 ± 174.18	136.25 ± 88.08	NS
Niacin (mg)	12.28 ± 6.60	9.08 ± 5.67	NS
Vitamin E (mg)	2.67 ± 2.01	1.97 ± 3.73	NS
Ca (mg)	947.59 ± 361.72	937.66 ± 363.81	NS
Fe (mg)	14.82 ± 7.30	13.29 ± 4.43	NS
K (mg)	1605.14 ± 654.99	1094.35 ± 566.09	<0.05
Mg (mg)	303.39 ± 220.35	240.26 ± 184.69	NS
Na (mg)	2501.90 ± 811.04	1949.78 ± 721.42	NS
P (mg)	631.40 ± 304.63	595.08 ± 264.43	NS
Se (µg)	51.95 ± 30.00	50.06 ± 23.06	NS
Zn (mg)	4.68 ± 2.60	4.26 ± 2.00	NS

The values show the mean ± SD for each nutrient and the p-value according to the independent samples t-Test ($p < 0.05$). [1] NS: not significant.

These results show high consumption of ultra-processed foods, rich in sugars and saturated fats and low consumption of fruits and vegetables which reflects in the increase of carbohydrates, total fats, and sodium (Na) in the participants' diet.

Table 4. Daily intake of energy and nutrients of all adolescents and by group (men and women) included in the supplementation study.

Nutrients	Total Population n = 27	Men n = 13	Women n = 14	p-Value
Energy (kcal)	2003.07 ± 1.24	2345.11 ± 1.35	1490 ± 1.11	<0.001
Protein (g)	70.24 ± 32.01	87.84 ± 27.96	43.85 ± 19.88	<0.001
Fat (g)	68.19 ± 29.36	81.03 ± 26.83	48.93 ± 8.62	<0.001
Cholesterol (mg)	283.63 ± 127.38	398.28 ± 142.17	111.67 ± 101.48	<0.001
Carbohydrates (g)	281.85 ± 82.19	321.01 ± 72.98	223.13 ± 27.13	<0.001
Sugar (g)	31.07 ± 29.70	38.01 ± 36.21	20.65 ± 14.98	[1] NS
Fiber (g)	20.64 ± 8.56	22.81 ± 10.68	17.39 ± 3.81	NS
Vitamin A-Retinol (µg)	759.60 ± 128.11	877.67 ± 143.62	582.50 ± 105.69	<0.001
Vitamin B1 (mg)	1.13 ± 0.54	1.41 ± 0.52	0.69 ± 0.11	<0.001

Table 4. Cont.

Nutrients	Total Population n = 27	Men n = 13	Women n = 14	p-Value
Vitamin B2 (mg)	1.22 ± 0.65	1.60 ± 0.55	0.64 ± 0.30	<0.001
Vitamin B6 (mg)	0.87 ± 0.56	1.11 ± 0.50	0.50 ± 0.34	<0.001
Vitamin B12 (µg)	1.92 ± 1.10	2.46 ± 1.01	1.11 ± 0.88	<0.001
Vitamin C (mg)	43.30 ± 44.13	52.41 ± 50.86	29.65 ± 11.81	NS
Folic acid (µg)	161.33 ± 198.05	235.89 ± 219.80	49.49 ± 21.16	<0.002
Niacin (mg)	10.69 ± 6.75	13.97 ± 6.61	5.76 ± 1.50	<0.001
Vitamin E (mg)	2.33 ± 1.80	2.67 ± 1.80	1.82 ± 1.87	NS
Ca (mg)	942.63 ± 270.27	1133.50 ± 332.51	656.33 ± 255.79	<0.001
Fe (mg)	14.10 ± 9.59	18.31 ± 9.57	7.79 ± 2.49	<0.001
K (mg)	1349.47 ± 436.12	1597.94 ± 445.58	976.75 ± 407.24	<0.001
Mg (mg)	271.83 ± 222.07	328.83 ± 238.09	186.33 ± 164.75	NS
Na (mg)	2226.77 ± 658.33	2993.61 ± 776.12	1076.50 ± 501.16	<0.001
P (mg)	613.67 ± 307.02	754 ± 220.09	403.17 ± 225.73	<0.001
Se (µg)	51.33 ± 29.33	67.56 ± 19.44	27 ± 14.33	<0.001
Zn (mg)	4.46 ± 2.94	5.99 ± 2.49	2.15 ± 1.37	<0.001

The values show the mean ± SD for each nutrient and the p-value according to the independent samples t-Test ($p < 0.05$). [1] NS: not significant.

3.3. Hb Concentration

The Hb levels were compared, finding differences between both study groups (supplemented and control) (Figure 2a). The initial Hb averages were 13.47 ± 1.50 and 13.22 ± 1.01 g/dL for supplemented and control respectively; there were no differences in the baseline measurement and week 1, however, week 2, 3, and 4 showed statistically significant differences between supplemented group (W2: 15.12 ± 0.99; W3: 14.89 ± 0.56; W4: 14.83 ± 0.96 g/dL) and control (W2: 12.78 ± 1.08; W3: 13.02 ± 0.80; W4: 13.13 ± 0.85 g/dL) according to the independent samples t-Test ($p < 0.001$) (Figure 2a); reflecting an increase in this nutritional biomarker in the supplemented group from the second week of supplementation and later showing stable values in weeks 3 and 4.

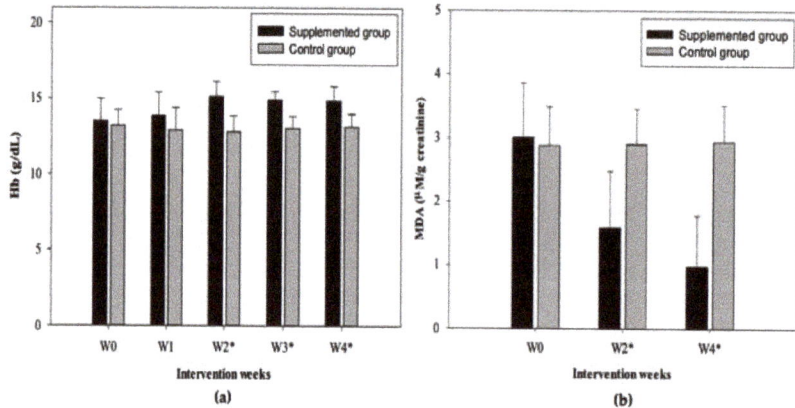

Figure 2. Concentrations of (a) Hb (Hemoglobin) (mean ± SD) and (b) UMDA (Urinary malondialdehyde) (mean ± SD) before, during, and after 4 weeks of supplementation in the supplemented and control group (W0: baseline; W1: week 1; W2: week 2; W3: week 3; W4: week 4). * Statistically significant difference between groups according to the independent samples t-Test ($p < 0.001$).

Furthermore, a comparative analysis was performed between the baseline values and values obtained at the fourth week by the group of study (supplemented and control), which show statistically significant differences in the supplemented group (W0 vs. W4) according to the paired sample t-Test ($p < 0.05$); no differences were found for the control group.

3.4. MDA Concentration

According to the results of this research, no differences were found by intragroup (supplemented) sex; however, it was presented for the control group according to the independent samples t-Test ($p < 0.05$) (Table 5). On the other hand, significant differences were found between men of the supplemented and control group and women of the supplemented and control group after two weeks of intervention (Table 6). Comparative analysis between the supplemented and control group was performed, finding statistically significant differences (Figure 2b); in addition, a significant difference was found in the means of the concentration of MDA before (week 0) and after (week 4) of the supplementation (supplemented group) according to the paired sample t-Test ($p < 0.001$); on the other hand, according to the repeated measures ANOVA test, it was observed that the levels of MDA were different throughout the treatment, rejecting the equality of the means between weeks, and showing a decrease of this compound from week 2 ($p < 0.001$); the control group did not show significant differences between weeks. The Bonferroni correction was used, confirming the results previously mentioned.

Table 5. Urinary MDA concentrations in men, women, and total participants before, during, and after 4 weeks of supplementation.

	Supplement Total Participants $n = 15$	Men $n = 9$	Women $n = 6$	p-value	Control Total Participants $n = 12$	Men $n = 4$	Women $n = 8$	p-value
Weeks	Urinary MDA concentrations (µM/g creatinine)							
Baseline	3.01 ± 0.85	3.26 ± 0.97	2.63 ± 0.48	NS	2.88 ± 0.61	3.44 ± 0.35	2.59 ± 0.51	<0.014
2	1.59 ± 0.89	1.84 ± 1.06	1.21 ± 0.36	NS	2.90 ± 0.56	3.47 ± 0.39	2.61 ± 0.38	<0.004
4	0.98 ± 0.80	1.13 ± 1.01	0.75 ± 0.28	NS	2.94 ± 0.57	3.51 ± 0.26	2.66 ± 0.44	<0.006

The values show the mean ± SD of UMDA (Urinary malondialdehyde) concentrations (µM/g creatinine) in supplemented and the control group before, during and after 4 weeks of supplementation. The week zero represents baseline. NS: no statistically significant difference between men and women of the same group per week according to the independent samples t-Test.

Table 6. Urinary MDA concentrations in men of the supplemented and control group and women of the supplemented and control group, before, during, and after 4 weeks of supplementation.

	Men Supplemented $n = 9$	Control $n = 4$	p-value	Women Supplemented $n = 6$	Control $n = 8$	p-value
Weeks	Urinary MDA concentrations (µM/g creatinine)					
Baseline	3.26 ± 0.97	3.44 ± 0.35	NS	2.63 ± 0.48	2.59 ± 0.51	NS
2	1.84 ± 1.06	3.47 ± 0.39	<0.014	1.21 ± 0.36	2.61 ± 0.38	<0.001
4	1.13 ± 1.01	3.51 ± 0.26	<0.001	0.75 ± 0.28	2.66 ± 0.44	<0.001

The values show the mean ± SD of UMDA (Urinary malondialdehyde) concentrations (µM/g creatinine) in men of supplemented and control group and women of supplemented and control group, before, during and after 4 weeks of supplementation. The week zero represents baseline. NS: no statistically significant difference between men of supplemented and control group and women of supplemented and control group per week according to the independent samples t-Test.

3.5. As Concentrations in Water and Urine

A month prior to the study, a questionnaire was applied to know the main source of water for daily intake and food preparation; later, water was monitored in the school and participants' homes (2 months), where the concentrations of As were identified. It was observed that 16% of the participants exclusively used purified water (bottle) to drink and prepare food, 15% reported consuming only drinking water to drink and prepare food, including water from the school tap during recess hours; the percentage of households that mixed water (purified water for drinking and household drinking water for food preparation) was 69%. The source and concentrations obtained of As in water samples were as follows: >100 ± 1.51 µg/L (drinking water from the school tap), 84.79 ± 17.00 µg/L (drinking water from the participants' homes) and 1.94 ± 1.73 µg/L (purified water). The values were stable the prior month and during the study.

Regarding the concentrations of urinary As, Table 7 shows the values obtained by the group, sex, and week of intervention. The results showing a lack of significant differences in the supplemented group; however, in the control group, only a difference was shown by sex at week 3, according to the Mann–Whitney U test ($p < 0.05$).

Table 7. Urinary As concentrations in the supplemented and control group during 4 weeks of supplementation.

Weeks	Supplemented Total Participants $n = 15$	Men $n = 9$	Women $n = 6$	p-value	Control Total Participants $n = 12$	Men $n = 4$	Women $n = 8$	p-value
			Urinary As concentrations (µg/g creatinine)					
0	56.85	57.42	52.09	NS	51.34	53.98	50.81	NS
1	53.60	53.90	53.48	NS	52.57	53.13	52.19	NS
2	2.02	3.95	0.45	NS	56.49	58.62	54.02	NS
3	0.29	0.27	0.30	NS	50.97	54.53	49.76	<0.05
4	0.29	0.27	0.30	NS	54.60	54.78	54.45	NS

The values show the median of UAs (Urinary arsenic) concentrations (µg/g creatinine) in the supplemented and control group. The week zero represents baseline. NS: no statistically significant difference between men and women of the same group per week according to the Mann–Whitney U test.

In addition, Figure 3 shows the maximum and minimum UAs values obtained by sex in the supplemented (Figure 3a) and control (Figure 3b) group during 4 weeks of supplementation. On the other hand, the comparative analysis between the supplemented and control group was carried out, showing statistically significant differences at week 2, 3, and 4 ($p < 0.001$) (Figure 4a); also, according to the Wilcoxon signed-rank test, significant differences were found between weeks of supplementation (supplemented group) (Figure 4b). Differences were observed between most of the weeks (W0 vs. W1: $p < 0.05$; W1 vs. W2: $p < 0.001$; W2 vs. W3: $p < 0.001$; W0 vs. W4: $p < 0.001$), but without differences between W3 vs. W4 (NS) in the supplemented group; the control group did not show significant differences. Finally, the values of the two study groups before and after the intervention (W0-W4) were compared according to the Friedman test [p-value < 0.001; x2 (2) = 58.13]. The analysis reflected differences between the weeks of supplementation (supplemented group). In addition, the UAs medians obtained before (baseline: 56.85 µg/g creatinine) and after (W4: 0.29 µg/g creatinine) indicate treatment effectiveness by decreasing the concentrations of UAs through the time. The control group did not show significant differences [x2 (2) = 4.44, NS] (Figure 4b).

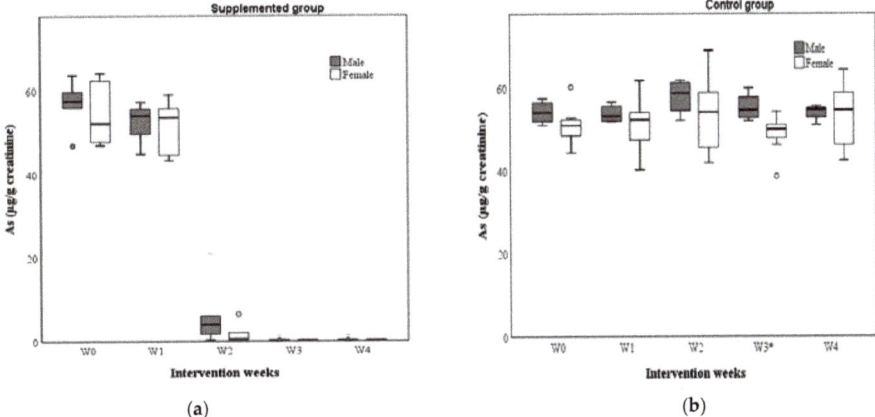

Figure 3. UAs (Urinary arsenic) (median) concentration by sex in the supplemented group (**a**) and control group (**b**) (W0: baseline; W1: week 1; W2: week 2; W3: week 3; W4: week 4). * Statistically significant difference by sex according to the Mann–Whitney U test ($p < 0.05$).

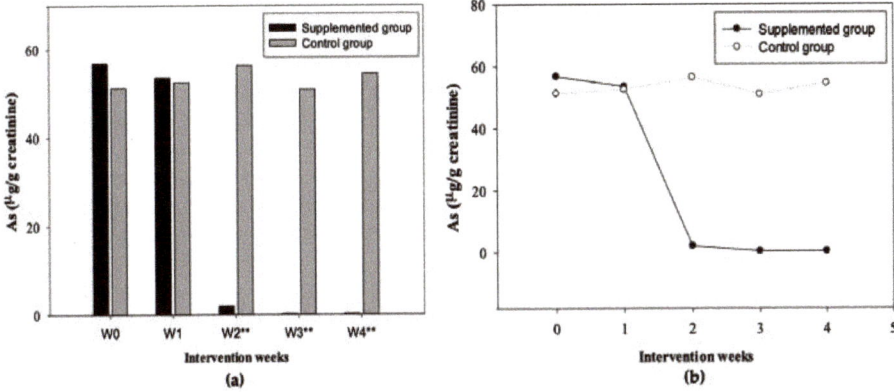

Figure 4. (**a**) Comparison of UAs (Urinary arsenic) concentrations (median) in the supplemented group and control group (W0: baseline; W1: week 1; W2: week 2; W3: week 3; W4: week 4). ** Statistically significant difference between groups according to the Mann–Whitney U test ($p < 0.001$); (**b**) Comparison of UAs concentration (median) between supplemented and control group per week of treatment. The Friedman and Wilcoxon tests were carried out to determine differences between weeks of supplementation.

3.6. NNT

The number needed to treat for second week was NNT = 2 (CI = 2 to 4), RR = 4.47 (CI = 1.47 to 16.0), which indicates that to increase the urinary arsenic excretion, treating at least two is required.

4. Discussion

4.1. As in Drinking Water

Previous studies have reported high values of As in drinking water of this population [28], which when compared with the results found in the present study, have remained unchanged through the time; the present concentrations of this element remain of concern, as they exceed the established limits [29]. This element has been recognized as one of the most serious pollutants found in drinking water, which, in addition to being ubiquitous in the environment, has a wide list of adverse health effects [9].

Although tap water samples from school and homes contain concentrations up to 3 times higher than allowed (As: >100 µg/L) of this pollutant, which has been reported through communication programs in the same community [28], the changes observed in this study have been minimal since the percentage that continues to drink drinking water is higher (84%) compared to the participants who use exclusively purified water (16%). These findings can be attributed to the fact that there is a greater proportion of families that cannot afford to supply purified water, so that drinking water is used for all needs, including water for food consumption and preparation; according to Meza-Lozano et al. [37], families having no access to an economical source of purified water, prefer not to consume it because of the high cost involved. Therefore, it is necessary to propose strategies that, in addition to understanding direct communication, and water treatment, incorporate accessible food sources (*quelites*) rich in phytochemicals, which can be incorporated into the diet in the form of mixtures or formulations, since, at the moment, there are no changes and the exposure remains.

4.2. Hb, UMDA, and UAs

4.2.1. Hb Concentration

The levels of Hb found in baseline were normal for men and women [38], however, this study showed that by incorporating a supplement with *quelites* into the diet, this nutritional biomarker can increase to 1.65 g/dL, concentrations that were higher compared to other studies. According to Egbi et al. [39] in a supplementation study with children ages 6–9 years, it was found that the consumption of green leafy vegetables, among them, plants of the genera *Amaranthus* spp., increases Hb concentrations in supplemented children (12.1 g/dL) compared to the control group (11.3 g/dL) at the end of the study, minimizing the prevalence of anemia (supplemented: 33.3%; control: 57.5%) in participants treated with the powder preparation. On the other hand, Monroy-Torres et al. [28] show that after supplementation in adolescents ages 12–15 years using a trademark based on grape, broccoli, and cranberry, Hb values increased 1 g/dL.

In this research, although both groups did not show low Hb levels, there was a significant difference from week 2 until the end of supplementation (Figure 2a). According to Egbi et al. [39], micronutrients such as Zn, Fe, and β-carotene from wild plant sources (green leafy vegetable powder), lead to an improvement in nutritional status, increasing Hb values and decreasing the proportions of anemia. Concentrations of this indicator are attributable to the quality of the diet, mainly the less varied diets with low consumption of fruits and vegetables, and mostly made up of cereals and legumes, have high concentrations of anti-nutrients such as tannins and phytates, known as inhibitors of the absorption and bioavailability of iron and zinc [39]. Another factor involved is inflammation processes, which affects red blood cells and retinol serum levels [39]. In addition, You et al. [40] report that fat consumption improves the bioavailability of carotene.

All these dietary patterns were observed in both study groups (Tables 3 and 4). Therefore, the results obtained in the supplemented group show that supplementation with *quelites* provides essential micronutrients and possibly improves their bioavailability for the increase in Hb.

4.2.2. MDA Concentration

MDA is a product of lipid peroxidation (LPO), the elevation of this in urine reflects the degree of oxidative stress, so this biomarker is usually used to evaluate LPO and DNA damage caused by exogenous free radicals or endogenous reactive oxygen species (ROS) [41]. It has been reported that the increase in MDA has a high correlation with exposure to pollutants, including As [41]. The results of MDA in both study groups (supplemented: 3.01 µM/g creatinine; control: 2.88 µM/g creatinine) (baseline), confirm the ability of this element to induce significant increases in MDA (Figure 2b; Tables 5 and 6), indicating that participants have a high level of oxidative stress due to prolonged exposure.

These values are similar to those reported by Wang et al. [41] which shows concentrations of 3.52 and 2.48 µM/g creatinine in men and women respectively (<20 years) exposed to As. Flora et al. [42] explain that the toxicity of As can be manifested directly with the attack on sulfhydryl groups or indirectly through the generation of ROS such as hydrogen peroxide, hydroxyl radical species, or superoxide anion, and where hydroxyl radicals play a role as initiators of LPO. On the other hand, according to Khuda-Bukhsh et al. [43], free radicals are electrophilic species that can react with cellular components. LPO process is initiated by the attack of a free radical, which could be emanated by As over unsaturated fats and the resulting chain reaction is terminated by the production of fat decomposition products such as alcohols and aldehydes (malondialdehyde).

On the other hand, in this study, after 4-week supplementation, the results showed a significant decrease in MDA concentrations (>50%) (Figure 2b; Tables 5 and 6). Similar results have been reported in rats induced with toxic agents [23,27]; in these trials, it was revealed that when administered varying doses of *Chenopodium* spp. and *Portulaca* spp. plants, the production of hydrogen peroxide (40%) and concentration of MDA (50%) can be reduced; in addition, an increase in the activity of antioxidant enzymes such as superoxide dismutase (SOD), catalase (CAT), and glutathione peroxidase (GPX) was reported.

Some studies show that these antioxidant enzymes can reduce the toxic effects of ROS by eliminating them since they are the first line of defense against oxidative stress, however, these can be affected if ROS production is excessive, so phytonutrients become alternatives to minimize the toxic effect of As [42,44]. It has been reported that the presence of non-enzymatic antioxidants from food (plants, vegetables, leaves, flowers) helps to neutralize or remove free radicals [42,44]. These act by reducing peroxide concentrations and even inhibiting lipid peroxidation and repairing oxidized membranes or promoting the strengthening or restoration of the antioxidant defenses of the cells; on the other hand, supplementation with non-enzymatic antioxidant molecules (phytonutrients) reduce the possibility of the metalloid interacting with biomolecules and inducing oxidative damage [42,44]. Among these compounds are some phytochemicals of the phenolic type such as phenolic acids (caffeic acid), flavonoids (quercetin, naringenin, phloretin), and non-phenolic such as carotenoids (β-carotene), chlorophylls, vitamin A, vitamin E, vitamin C, some minerals like zinc, manganese, magnesium, and selenium and amino acids like cysteine [42,44,45], nutritional compounds that were presented in high concentrations in the supplement administered [30].

In addition, according to Pace et al. [44], the ability of phenolic antioxidants to neutralize oxidants is due to the donation of a hydrogen atom from polyphenolic antioxidants, leading to the formation of phenoxy-radical, which can be stabilized through intermolecular bonds between two polyphenols or by reaction with other radicals. Therefore, the results obtained in both groups are consistent with the reported evidence.

4.2.3. UAs Concentration

Regarding UAs concentrations, the results showed that both groups had high baseline values with 51.34 µg/g creatinine and 56.85 µg/g creatinine for control and supplemented group respectively. The CDC [46] establishes diagnostic criteria for As, with concentrations greater than 50 µg/L, however, the health effects may vary depending on the acute or chronic exposure of this pollutant [9]. Subclinical complications were not evaluated in this research so their presence is not ruled out.

According to Monroy-Torres et al. [28], after supplementation in a group of adolescents ages 12–15, an increase in the excretion of UAs in the second week (53.9 µg/g creatinine) and third week (51.1 µg/g creatinine) was shown. However, our study did not register an increase in the excretion of this pollutant between weeks. The baseline values obtained were high, and later at the end of each week during the supplementation, a decrease of these concentrations was observed in the supplemented group (Table 7; Figure 4b). On the other hand, the results observed in the control group showed no significant difference between weeks, showing concentrations greater than 50 µg/g creatinine during the study (Table 7; Figure 4b). The variations found in this research regarding the literature may be due to the fact that the highest percentage of excretion of UAs may have occurred in the first days of the first and second week after supplementation, but with higher intensity in this latter week. Therefore, we infer that because the sample collection was carried out at the end of each week and not daily, the results obtained reflect the levels of this pollutant after its maximum excretion; thus, promoting an efficient balance and recovery process in the supplemented group. Nowadays, there are no clinical trials that report the biological effect of herbal remedies or the use of *quelites* as alternative recovery therapies in cases of arsenic exposure. Therefore, this research has reported interesting results. Our results showed an increase of UAs content during the first 2 weeks (high excretion and then a recovery process), and after 30 days of treatment, showing that a supplementation with *quelites* could enhance the mobilization of As during the first 15 days, observing a significant decrease (90%) of this pollutant (recovery process) (Table 7). In our study, UAs concentrations showed a fluctuation after the first week of treatment in the treated group and a notable difference being observed at week 2, resulting in an evident and periodic removal of arsenic from the body in the supplemented group. On the other hand, a decrease in the MDA level (50%) was observed (Figure 2b; Tables 5 and 6). Other investigations have been reported similar behaviors to what was observed in our study about arsenic excretion. An intervention study [47] showed that in participants aged 18, urine arsenic concentrations were stable during the day, however, variations may exist throughout the days. Hence, the evidence of our study proposes a mechanism for the excretion of As in the urine and could establish a new balance process for this pollutant.

Regarding results obtained by sex, in our research, similar values of UAs among men and women without a statistical difference (Table 7) were observed. The literature reports an absence of differences in UAs concentrations by gender [47,48]. On the other hand, the significant decrease observed in this study is attributed to the fact that growing children have a more efficient process of methylation than adults because in this latter group, the number of factors that affect methylation increases with age, such as smoking, or decreased hepatic functions [48–50]. In addition, it has been reported that children retain lower amounts of As in the body, because the second step of the methylation process is more active and allows an increase in the value of concentrations [51]; so that the results obtained in this investigation are consistent and supported by the previously reported evidence, since the supplemented group showed a surprising reduction of this pollutant after supplementation (98%). On the other hand, As can also have different excretion patterns in participants of the same group (intra-individual variability; inter-individual variability) [52] or between groups [28,51]. However, the literature reports that many factors influence arsenic metabolism and condition its efficiency, including genetic factors (example: polymorphisms of the arsenite methyltransferase), metabolic capacity, sex, hormonal mechanisms, nutritional status, and diet [28,48,52,53].

During this clinical intervention study, it was observed that the diet of the participants in both study groups remained unchanged throughout the research. Despite the fact that the DRI of some macro and micronutrients were mainly met by men, most of these were from ultra-processed products, so the diet was considered of low quality in both groups due to the high consumption of these foods, such as drinks of cola and flavored drinks, foods high in saturated fats, and with high energy content, and on the other hand, a low consumption of plant-based foods was observed. According to Monroy-Torres et al. [54], it was observed that nutrient consumption considered as antioxidants in a population exposed to As was low, while the consumption of foods that promote greater oxidation and inflammation in the body was high (sugary drinks and ultra-processed foods), showing a high baseline concentration of As. This evidence is similar to that observed in our study for both groups, regarding the diet quality and the situation of the baseline concentrations of the biomarkers evaluated, and on the other hand, the behavior of biomarkers in the control group during the research (Tables 3 and 4; Figures 2b and 4a). According to Monroy-Torres et al. [54], this dietary situation promotes the onset of obesity and pathologies directly associated with arsenic (hepatopathy and nephropathy), directly contributing to the disorders and effects caused by exposure to the metalloid.

On the other hand, according to Hervert-Hernández et al. [55], the inclusion of fruits, vegetables, even roots, stems, and leaves contributes to high consumption of antioxidants, and therefore improves to the diet quality. However, nowadays the importance of consuming these potential sources of phytochemicals such as *quelites* has been forgotten, which could be used as alternative therapies to reduce the effects of various pathophysiological conditions, including As toxicity [21]. Some studies on populations exposed to As have reported that the consumption of natural supplements or foods rich in bioactive compounds improve the processes of methylation and increase the levels of excretion of As, promoting an efficient recovery process [28,42,53,56]. On the other hand, nutritional deficiencies due to low consumption of micronutrients contribute to increasing the risk of arsenic-induced skin lesions [57]. In our study, the *quelites* included in the supplement were evaluated (each plant and mixtures) showing an excellent nutritional profile when an optimized mixture was made [22,30]. The supplement was rich in antioxidant compounds [carotenoids, chlorophyll, phenolic acids (chlorogenic acid), flavonoids (quercetin, naringenin, phloretin, and phloridzin), amino acids (methionine, cysteine, serine, and glycine), minerals (Zn, Se, Mg, and P between others), and dietary fiber [22,30].

It has been reported that the administration of vitamin C leads to the formation of complexes with heavy metals and in addition with vitamin E, promotes an efficient recovery process by decreasing As concentrations [41]. On the other hand, supplementation with essential elements such as Zn and Se, reduces the toxicity effects of As, promoting their elimination, by chelation mechanisms, with the formation of reversible compounds [42,58]. Regarding Se, an antagonistic relationship with arsenic has been demonstrated where one reduces the toxicity of the other [59]; other studies report that possibly As and Se form a complex in the lysosome (As_2Se) which is excreted in the urine [60]; in addition, As and Se compete for the union with functional proteins, thus reducing the availability of toxic metals [42]. Other studies have reported that the presence of selenium and folates increases the methylation of As in children, improving the efficiency of the 1-carbon metabolism, essential for the methylation and excretion of As. It is likely that this result in metabolism and the availability of methyl groups are particularly important in growing children to meet the production demands of creatine, proteins, phospholipids, and DNA [48].

On the other hand, other nutrients and compounds have been reported as beneficial, such as dietary fiber, carotenoids, and organic acids present in parts of plants and vegetables which reduce the toxic effects of heavy metals, including As [21,28,42]. Moreover, another study showed that low diets in green leafy vegetables and micronutrients such as calcium, folates, and vitamin C increase the probability of presenting toxic effects characteristic of As [57]. According to López-Carrillo et al. [56], the consumption of methionine, vitamin C, B6, B12, Fe, and Zn plays an important role in the metabolism of As. Each component improves the elimination of this toxic, participating in the metabolism of 1-carbon as catalyst components or donors of methyl groups. On the other hand, other studies report that vitamin C, methionine, and cysteine participate in the processes of As detoxification, promoting chelation and facilitating its removal from the body [14,42]. Finally, according to Kurzius-Spencer et al. [53], some amino acids are associated with the 1-carbon pathway such as methionine, cysteine, serine, and glycine, promoting the As methylation process. Other mechanisms have been reported to explain the beneficial effects of these nutrients and the exposure of As. Clemente et al. [61] describe that the treatments based on Fe, cysteine, flavonoids (quercetin, catechin, epigallocatechin), Mg, P, fruit, and vegetable extracts of green leaves (rich in polyphenols), reduce the transport of As through the intestinal monolayer, decreasing its absorption. Polyphenols have been reported to modulate tight junctions affecting toxic transport (paracellular permeability). On the other hand, there is possibly a relationship between the content of dietary fiber in food, the presence of As, and the interaction with the intestinal microbial ecosystem, favoring the DF-As ligand and lowering the percentage of bioaccessibility; however, this bioaccessibility will be influenced by intestinal motility, nutritional status, and genotype [62].

This evidence reinforces our results obtained in the supplemented group. As previously mentioned, during supplementation, a decrease in UAs concentrations was observed in the supplemented group and without differences in the control group, despite the content consumed of some components important for arsenic detoxification (Se, vitamin A, vitamin C, B vitamins) being similar in both study groups. On the other hand, the foods included in the diet were mostly ultra-processed. In addition, it was observed that during the entire study, other essential nutrients such as dietary fiber, vitamin E, folates, and Zn did not meet the dietary reference intakes in the supplemented and control group. Therefore, this indicates that the supplement administered provided a high-quality source of micronutrients and antioxidant compounds in the treated group that possibly allowed the reduction of the bioavailability of As, promoted the chelation and methylation process, reduced toxic effects, and finally, promoted a balancing mechanism and a recovery process.

Regarding the result of NNT being necessary to treat the observed from the second week on, it is important to compare this result with that of Monroy-Torres et al. [28], where the NNT was 7 but non confidence interval, which may lead us to demonstrate that we would be facing an advancement not only of the effects of the key nutrients that participate in arsenic excretion, but in what should be the best methodology and its intervention time.

This study approached the effect of a supplementation with two endemic *quelites* on urinary excretion of arsenic in adolescents exposed to water contaminated with the metalloid in a community in the state of Guanajuato for four weeks, which seems to increase the excretion of arsenic from the second week compared to the control group, in addition to improving other nutritional variables. Mexico is rich in plant biodiversity, where the *quelites*, in addition to being rich in nutrients, showed that they can have a beneficial effect on the urinary excretion of the metalloid.

5. Conclusions

This study showed that during supplementation based on two *quelites*, there was a significant reduction in MDA (1.59 µM/g creatinine) and UAs (2.02 µg/g creatinine) from week two; in addition to an improvement in Hb levels (15.12 g/dL). The decrease in arsenic was kept until the end of the treatment. Therefore, the incorporation in the diet of these plants high in phytochemicals could be a viable alternative therapy, by increasing the intake of macronutrients, micronutrients, and antioxidant compounds essential for detoxification, thus providing a more efficient recovery process against this pollutant. Prevention and orientation campaigns regarding consumption of tap water and the importance of a healthy diet have been carried out in this community; however, the current results show the null action to this problem, even though previous studies have reported this situation. Another reason that has also been considered, is the lack of technological solutions available to society, so it is necessary for sustainable strategies that can improve the nutritional and health status of members of rural communities exposed to arsenic, such as incorporating food with beneficial effects on the excretion of this pollutant.

Author Contributions: Conceptualization and methodology, Y.O.S.-S., D.O.R.-A., R.M.-T. and A.D.H.-F.; software, validation, analysis and investigation, Y.O.S.-S. and R.M.-T.; writing—original draft preparation and writing—review and editing, Y.O.S.-S. and R.M.-T.; supervision, A.D.H.-F., R.M.-T. and D.O.R.-A.; resources, A.D.H.-F., R.M.-T. and D.O.R.-A.

Funding: This research received no external funding.

Acknowledgments: This study was supported by The National Council of Science and Technology of Mexico (CONACYT/Ph.D. Scholarship: 273250; CVU register: 445884). Also, we thank University Observatory of Food and Nutritional Security of the state of Guanajuato (OUSANEG). We also gratefully acknowledge our volunteers and parents of this study and the principal of the High School (#117), Professor Guillermo Silva-Navarro. The authors appreciate the collaboration of the nutritionists Beatriz Roman, Marisol Serrano and Angela Castillo.

Conflicts of Interest: All authors read and approved the manuscript. The authors declare no conflict of interest.

References

1. Orteaga-Guerrero, M.A. Presencia, distribución, hidrogeoquímica y origen de arsénico, fluoruro y otros elementos traza disueltos en agua subterránea, a escala de cuenca hidrológica tributaria de Lerma-Chapala, México. *Rev. Mex. Cienc. Geol.* **2009**, *26*, 143–161.
2. Agency for Toxic Substances and Disease Registry (ATSDR). Toxicological Profile for Arsenic. ATSDR: U.S. Department of Health and Human Services Public. Health Service. 2007. Available online: https://www.atsdr.cdc.gov/toxprofiles/tp.asp?id=22&tid=3 (accessed on 15 September 2019).
3. Mandal, B.K.; Suzuki, K.T. Arsenic round the world: A review. *Talanta* **2002**, *58*, 201–235. [CrossRef]
4. Van Halem, D.; Bakker, S.A.; Amy, G.L.; Van Dijk, J.C. Arsenic in drinking water: Not just a problem for Bangladesh. *Drink. Water Eng. Sci. Discuss.* **2009**, *2*, 51–64. [CrossRef]
5. Sepúlveda-Saa, R. El arsénico en la contaminación de aguas subterráneas. *Ciencia UANL* **2009**, *12*, 239–244.
6. Méndez, M.; Armienta, M.A. Arsenic phase distribution in Zimapán mine tailings, Mexico. *Geofísica Int.* **2003**, *42*, 131–140.
7. Arreguín-Cortés, F.I.; Chávez-Guillén, R.; Soto-Navarro, P.R. *Una Revisión de la Presencia de Arsénico en el Agua Subterránea en México*; Comisión Nacional del Agua (CONAGUA), Secretaría de Medio Ambiente y Recursos Naturales (SEMARNAT): Ciudad de México, México, 2013.
8. Monroy-Torres, R.; Macías, A.E.; Gallaga-Solorzano, J.C.; Santiago-García, E.J.; Hernández, I. Arsenic in mexican children exposed to contaminated well water. *Ecol. Food Nutr.* **2009**, *48*, 59–75. [CrossRef]
9. World Health Organization (WHO). Arsenic. WHO, 2018. Available online: https://www.who.int/news-room/fact-sheets/detail/arsenic (accessed on 15 September 2019).
10. Chávez-Capilla, T.; Beshai, M.; Maher, W.; Kelly, T.; Foster, S. Bioaccessibility and degradation of naturally occurring arsenic species from food in the human gastrointestinal tract. *Food Chem.* **2016**, *212*, 189–197. [CrossRef]
11. Cubadda, F.; Jackson, B.; Cottingham, K.L.; Ornelas-Van Horne, Y.; Kurzius-Spencer, M. Human exposure to dietary inorganic arsenic and other arsenic species: State of knowledge, gaps and uncertainties. *Sci. Total Environ.* **2016**, *579*, 1228–1239. [CrossRef]
12. Denny, A.; Buttriss, J. *Plant Foods and Health: Focus on Plant Bioactives*; European Food Information Resource (EuroFIR): Norwich, UK, 2007.
13. Martins, N.; Barros, L.; Ferreira, I.C.F.R. In Vivo antioxidant activity of phenolic compounds: Facts and gaps. *Trends Food Sci. Technol.* **2016**, *48*, 1–12. [CrossRef]
14. Nandi, D.; Patra, R.C.; Swarup, D. Effect of cysteine, methionine, ascorbic acid and thiamine on arsenic-induced oxidative stress and biochemical alterations in rats. *Toxicology* **2005**, *211*, 26–35. [CrossRef]
15. Nandi, D.; Patra, R.C.; Swarup, D. Oxidative stress indices and plasma biochemical parameters during oral exposure to arsenic in rats. *Food Chem. Toxicol.* **2006**, *44*, 1579–1584. [CrossRef] [PubMed]
16. Farombi, E.O.; Fakoya, A. Free radical scavenging and antigenotoxic activities of natural phenolic compounds in dried flowers of *Hibiscus saidariffa* L. *Mol. Nutr. Food Res.* **2005**, *49*, 1120–1128. [CrossRef] [PubMed]
17. Das, A.K.; Sahu, R.; Dua, T.K.; Bag, S.; Gangopadhyay, M.; Sinha, M.K.; Dewanjee, S. Arsenic-induced myocardial injury: Protective role of *Corchorus olitorius* leaves. *Food Chem. Toxicol.* **2010**, *48*, 1210–1217. [CrossRef] [PubMed]
18. Alamolhodaei, N.S.; Shirani, K.; Karimi, G. Arsenic cardiotoxicity: An overview. *Environ. Toxicol. Pharmacol.* **2015**, *40*, 1005–1014. [CrossRef] [PubMed]
19. Spratlen, M.J.; Gamble, M.V.; Grau-Perez, M.; Kuo, C.C.; Best, L.G.; Yracheta, J.; Francesconi, K.; Goessler, W.; Mossavar-Rahmani, Y.; Hall, M.; et al. Arsenic metabolism and one-carbon metabolism at low-moderate arsenic exposure: Evidence from the strong heart study. *Food Chem. Toxicol.* **2017**, *105*, 387–397. [CrossRef] [PubMed]
20. Linares, M.E.; Bye, R. The under-utilized species of the milpa. *Rev. Digit. Univ.* **2015**, *16*, 22.
21. Santiago-Saenz, Y.O.; Hernández-Fuentes, A.D.; López-Palestina, C.U.; Garrido-Cauich, J.H.; Alatorre-Cruz, J.M.; Monroy-Torres, R. Nutritional importance and biological activity of bioactive compounds from quelites consumed in Mexico. *Rev. Chil. Nutr.* **2019**, *46*, 593–605. [CrossRef]
22. Santiago-Saenz, Y.O.; Hernández-Fuentes, A.D.; Monroy-Torres, R.; Cariño-Cortés, R.; Jiménez-Alvarado, R. Physicochemical, nutritional and antioxidant characterization of three vegetables (*Amaranthus hybridus*

L., *Chenopodium berlandieri* L., *Portulaca oleracea* L.) as potential sources of phytochemicals and bioactive compounds. *J. Food Meas. Charact.* **2018**, *12*, 2855–2864. [CrossRef]
23. Kokanova-Nedialkova, Z.; Nedialkov, P.; Kondeva-Burdina, M.; Simeonova, R.; Tzankova, V.; Aluani, D. *Chenopodium bonus-henricus* L.—A source of hepatoprotective flavonoids. *Fitoterapia* **2017**, *118*, 13–20. [CrossRef]
24. Gawlik-Dziki, U.; Swieca, M.; Sułkowski, M.; Dziki, D.; Baraniak, B.; Czyz, J. Antioxidant and anticancer activities of *Chenopodium quinoa* leaves extracts—In Vitro study. *Food Chem. Toxicol.* **2013**, *57*, 154–160. [CrossRef]
25. Wanyin, W.; Liwei, D.; Lin, J.; Hailiang, X.; Changquan, L.; Min, L. Ethanol extract of *Portulaca oleracea* L. protects against hypoxia-induced neurodamage through modulating endogenous erythropoietin expression. *J. Nutr. Biochem.* **2012**, *23*, 385–391. [CrossRef] [PubMed]
26. Liang, D.; Zhou, Q.; Gong, W.; Wang, Y.; Nie, Z.; He, H.; Li, J.; Wu, J.; Wu, C.; Zhang, J. Studies on the antioxidant and hepatoprotective activities of polysaccharides from *Talinum triangulare*. *J. Ethnopharmacol.* **2011**, *136*, 316–321. [CrossRef] [PubMed]
27. Al-Quraishy, S.; Dkhil, M.A.; Abdel-Moneim, A.E. Protective effects of *Portulaca oleracea* against rotenone mediated depletion of glutathione in the striatum of rats as an animal model of Parkinson's disease. *Pest. Biochem. Physiol.* **2012**, *103*, 108–114. [CrossRef]
28. Monroy-Torres, R.; Espinoza-Pérez, J.A.; Ramírez-Gómez, X.; Carrizalez-Yañez, L.; Linares-Segovia, B.; Mejía-Saavedra, J.J. Efecto de una suplementación multivitamínica de cuatro semanas sobre el estado nutricio y excreción urinaria de arsénico en adolescentes. *Nutr. Hosp.* **2018**, *35*, 894–902. [CrossRef] [PubMed]
29. Norma Oficial Mexicana (NOM-127-SSA1-1994). Salud ambiental. Agua para uso y consumo humano. Límites permisibles de calidad y tratamientos a que debe someterse el agua para su potabilización. Norma Oficial Mexicana NOM 1994; SSA, 2000. Available online: http://www.salud.gob.mx/unidades/cdi/nom/127ssa14.html (accessed on 17 September 2019).
30. Santiago-Saenz, Y.O.; López-Palestina, C.U.; Gutiérrez-Tlahque, J.; Monroy-Torres, R.; Pinedo-Espinoza, J.M.; Hernández-Fuentes, A.D. Nutritional and functional evaluation of three powder mixtures based on Mexican quelites: Alternative ingredients to formulate food supplements. *Food Sci. Technol. (Campinas)* **2020**, in press.
31. Grossman, C.M. The effect of amino acids on serum and urine creatine. *J. Clin. Investig.* **1945**, *24*, 380–383. [CrossRef]
32. Lohman, T.G.; Roche, A.F.; Martorell, R. *Anthropometric Standardization Reference Manual*; Human Kinetics Books: Champaign, IL, USA, 1988.
33. Organización Mundial de la Salud (OMS). Capacitación Sobre la Evaluación del Crecimiento del Niño. OMS, 2008. Available online: http://www.who.int/childgrowth/training/c_interpretando.pdf (accessed on 15 September 2019).
34. Shamah-Levy, T.; Villalpando-Hernández, S.; Rivera-Dommarco, J. *Manual de Procedimientos Para Proyectos de Nutrición*; Instituto Nacional de Salud Pública: Cuernavaca, México, 2006.
35. Cox, D.H. Arsine evolution-electrothermal atomic absorption method for the determination of nanogram levels of total arsenic in urine and water. *J. Anal. Toxicol.* **1980**, *4*, 207–211. [CrossRef]
36. National Academies (NAP). Dietary Reference Intakes Tables and Application. Dietary Reference Intakes: Macronutrients, Vitamins and Elements. NAP, 2019. Available online: http://nationalacademies.org/hmd/Activities/Nutrition/SummaryDRIs/DRI-Tables.aspx (accessed on 15 September 2019).
37. Meza-Lozano, B.; Ortíz-Pérez, M.D.; Ponce-Palomares, M.; Castillo-Gutiérrez, S.G.; Flores-Ramírez, R.; Cubillas-Tejeda, A.C. Implementación y evaluación de un programa de comunicación de riesgos por exposición a flúor en la comunidad de el fuerte, Santa María del Río, San Luís Potosí, México. *Rev. Int. Contam. Ambie.* **2016**, *32*, 87–100.
38. Organización Mundial de la Salud (OMS). Concentraciones de Hemoglobina Para Diagnosticar la Anemia y Evaluar su Gravedad. OMS, 2011. Available online: https://www.who.int/vmnis/indicators/haemoglobin_es.pdf (accessed on 15 September 2019).
39. Egbi, G.; Gbogbo, S.; Mensah, G.; Glover-Amengor, M.; Steiner-Asiedu, M. Effect of green leafy vegetables powder on anaemia and vitamin-A status of Ghanaian school children. *BMC Nutr.* **2018**, *4*, 27. [CrossRef]
40. You, C.S.; Parker, R.S.; Swanson, J.E. Bioavailability and vitamin A value of carotenes from red palm oil assessed by an intrinsic isotope reference method. *Asia Pac. J. Clin. Nutr.* **2002**, *11*, S438–S442. [CrossRef]

41. Wang, J.P.; Maddalena, R.; Zheng, B.; Zai, C.; Liu, F.; Ng, J.C. Arsenicosis status and urinary malondialdehyde (MDA) in people exposed to arsenic contaminated-coal in China. *Environ. Int.* **2009**, *35*, 502–506. [CrossRef] [PubMed]
42. Flora, S.J.S.; Bhadauria, S.; Kannan, G.M.; Singh, N. Arsenic induced oxidative stress and the role of antioxidant supplementation during chelation: A review. *J. Environ. Biol.* **2007**, *28*, 333–347. [PubMed]
43. Khuda-Bukhsh, A.R.; Pathak, S.; Guha, B.; Karmakar, S.R.; Das, J.K.; Banerjee, P.; Biswas, S.J.; Mukherjee, P.; Bhattacharjee, N.; Choudhury, S.C.; et al. Can homeopathic arsenic remedy combat arsenic poisoning in humans exposed to groundwater arsenic contamination? A preliminary report on first human trial. *eCAM* **2005**, *2*, 537–548. [CrossRef]
44. Pace, C.; Dagda, R.; Angermann, J. Antioxidants protect against arsenic induced mitochondrial cardio toxicity. *Toxics* **2017**, *5*, 38. [CrossRef] [PubMed]
45. Reddy, M.K.; Alexander-Lindo, R.L.; Nair, M.G. Relative inhibition of lipid peroxidation, cyclooxygenase enzymes, and human tumor cell proliferation by natural food colors. *J. Agric. Food Chem.* **2005**, *53*, 9268–9273. [CrossRef] [PubMed]
46. Centers for Disease Control and Prevention (CDC). Emergency Preparedness and Response: Arsenic. CDC, 2018. Available online: https://emergency.cdc.gov/agent/arsenic/casedef.asp (accessed on 15 September 2019).
47. Calderon, R.L.; Hudgens, E.; Le, X.C.; Schreinemachers, D.; Thomas, D.J. Excretion of arsenic in urine as a function of exposure to arsenic in drinking water. *Environ. Health Perspect.* **1999**, *107*, 663–667. [CrossRef] [PubMed]
48. Skröder, H.L.; Kippler, M.; Lu, Y.; Ahmed, S.; Kuehnelt, D.; Raqib, R.; Vahter, M. Arsenic metabolism in children differs from that in adults. *Toxicol. Sci.* **2016**, *152*, 29–39. [CrossRef]
49. Vahter, M.E. Interactions between arsenic-induced toxicity and nutrition in early life. *J. Nutr.* **2007**, *137*, 2798–2804. [CrossRef]
50. Queen-Samour, P.; King-Helm, K. *Handbook of Pediatric Nutrition*; Jones & Bartlett: Sudbury, MA, USA, 2005.
51. Kumar, U.C.; Mahmudur, M.R.; Kumar, M.S.; Lodh, D.; Ranjan, C.C.; Roy, S.; Quamruzzaman, Q.; Tokunaga, H.; Ando, M.; Chakraborti1, D. Pattern of excretion of arsenic compounds [Arsenite, Arsenate, MMA (V), DMA (V)] in urine of children compared to adults from an arsenic exposed area in Bangladesh. *J. Environ. Sci. Health Part A* **2003**, *38*, 87–113. [CrossRef]
52. Kile, M.; Hoffman, E.; Hsueh, Y.M.; Afroz, S.; Quamruzzaman, Q.; Rahman, M.; Mahiuddin, G.; Ryan, L.; Christiani, D. Variability in biomarkers of arsenic exposure and metabolism in adults over time. *Environ. Health Perspect.* **2009**, *117*, 455–460. [CrossRef]
53. Kurzius-Spencer, M.; da Silva, V.; Thomson, C.A.; Hartz, V.; Hsu, C.H.; Burgess, J.L.; O'Rourke, M.K.; Harris, R.B. Nutrients in one-carbon metabolism and urinary arsenic methylation in the National Health and Nutrition Examination Survey (NHANES) 2003–2004. *Sci Total Environ.* **2017**, *607*, 381–390. [CrossRef] [PubMed]
54. Monroy-Torres, R.; Espinoza-Pérez, J.A.; Pérez-González, R.M. Evaluación de las prácticas de alimentación y nutrición en una población expuesta a arsénico: Una propuesta para integrar indicadores de exposición nutricional. *Nutrición Clínica y Dietética Hospitalaria* **2016**, *36*, 140–149. [CrossRef]
55. Hervert-Hernández, D.; García, O.P.; Rosado, J.L.; Goñi, I. The contribution of fruits and vegetables to dietary intake of polyphenols and antioxidant capacity in a Mexican rural diet: Importance of fruit and vegetable variety. *Food Res. Int.* **2011**, *44*, 1182–1189. [CrossRef]
56. López-Carrillo, L.; Gamboa-Loira, B.; Becerra, W.; Hernández-Alcaraz, C.; Hernández-Ramírez, R.U.; Jay-Gandolfi, A.; Franco-Marina, F.; Cebrián, M.E. Dietary micronutrient intake and its relationship with arsenic metabolism in Mexican women. *Environ. Res.* **2016**, *151*, 445–450. [CrossRef]
57. Mitra, S.R.; Guha-Mazumder, D.N.; Basu, A.; Block, G.; Haque, R.; Samanta, S.; Ghosh, N.; Hira-Smith, M.M.; Von Ehrenstein, O.S.; Smith, A.H. Nutritional factors and susceptibility to arsenic-caused skin lesions in west Bengal, India. *Environ. Health Perspect.* **2004**, *112*, 1104–1109. [CrossRef]
58. Misbahuddin, M.; Islam, A.Z.; Khandker, S.; Al-Mahmud, I.; Islam, N.; Anjumanara. Efficacy of spirulina extract plus zinc in patients of chronic arsenic poisoning: A randomized placebo-controlled study. *Clin. Toxicol. (Phila)* **2006**, *44*, 135–141. [CrossRef]
59. Pilsner, J.R.; Hall, M.N.; Liu, X.; Ahsan, H.; Ilievski, V.; Slavkovich, V.; Levy, D.; Factor-Litvak, P.; Graziano, J.H.; Gamble, M.V. Associations of plasma selenium with arsenic and genomic methylation of leukocyte DNA in Bangladesh. *Environ. Health Perspect.* **2011**, *119*, 113–118. [CrossRef]

60. Berry, J.P.; Galle, P. Selenium-arsenic interaction in renal cells: Role of lysosomes. Electron microprobe study. *J. Submicrosc. Cytol. Pathol.* **1994**, *26*, 203–210.
61. Clemente, M.J.; Devesa, V.; Velez, D. In vitro reduction of arsenic bioavailability using dietary strategies. *J. Agric. Food Chem.* **2017**, *65*, 3956–3964. [CrossRef]
62. Sun, G.X.; Van de Wiele, T.; Alava, P.; Tack, F.; Du Laing, G. Arsenic in cooked rice: Effect of chemical, enzymatic and microbial processes on bioaccessibility and speciation in the human gastrointestinal tract. *Environ. Pollut.* **2012**, *162*, 241–246. [CrossRef]

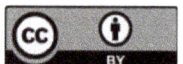

© 2019 by the authors. Licensee MDPI, Basel, Switzerland. This article is an open access article distributed under the terms and conditions of the Creative Commons Attribution (CC BY) license (http://creativecommons.org/licenses/by/4.0/).

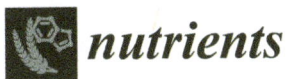 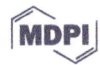

Article

Development of Dietary Supplement Label Database in Italy: Focus of FoodEx2 Coding

Alessandra Durazzo [1,*], Emanuela Camilli [1], Laura D'Addezio [1], Raffaela Piccinelli [1], Angelika Mantur-Vierendeel [2], Luisa Marletta [1], Paul Finglas [3], Aida Turrini [1] and Stefania Sette [1]

1. CREA-Research Centre for Food and Nutrition, Via Ardeatina 546, 00178 Rome, Italy; emanuela.camilli@crea.gov.it (E.C.); laura.daddezio@crea.gov.it (L.D.); raffaela.piccinelli@crea.gov.it (R.P.); luisa.marletta@crea.gov.it (L.M.); aida.turrini@crea.gov.it (A.T.); stefania.sette@crea.gov.it (S.S.)
2. EuroFIR AISBL, 40 Rue Washington, 1050 Brussels, Belgium; am@eurofir.org
3. Quadram Institute Bioscience, Norwich, Norfolk NR4 7UQ, UK; paul.finglas@quadram.ac.uk
* Correspondence: alessandra.durazzo@crea.gov.it; Tel.: +39-065-149-4430

Received: 20 November 2019; Accepted: 23 December 2019; Published: 27 December 2019

Abstract: The sector of food supplements is certainly varied and growing: an ever wider offer of new products is launched on the market every year. This is reflected in new reorganization of drug companies and new marketing strategies, in the adoption of new production technologies with resulting changes in dietary supplements regulation. In this context, information on composition reported in labels of selected dietary supplements was collected and updated for the development of a Dietary Supplement Label Database according to products' availability on the Italian market and also including items consumed in the last Italian Dietary Survey. For each item, a code was assigned following the food classification and description system FoodEx2, revision 2. A total of 558 products have been entered into the database at present, trying to give a uniform image and representation of the major classes of food supplements, and 82 descriptors have been compiled. Various suggestions on how the number of FoodEx2 system descriptors could be expanded were noted during the compilation of the database and the coding procedure, which are presented in this article. Limits encountered in compiling the database are represented by the changes in the formulation of products on the market and therefore by the need for a constant database update. The database here presented can be a useful tool in clinical trials, dietary plans, and pharmacological programs.

Keywords: Dietary Supplement Label Database; dietary supplements; food description; food classification; FoodEx2

---

1. Introduction

The sector of food supplements is certainly varied and growing: a wider and wider selection of new products is launched on the market every year. This is reflected in new reorganization of drug companies, in new marketing strategies, and in the adoption of new production technologies with resulting changes in the dietary supplements regulation. The growth of this sector is encouraged by growing interest of consumers in improving their health and physical and mental wellbeing, often to compensate for an incorrect lifestyle [1].

Dietary supplements are considered in epidemiological studies and in the analysis of food consumption patterns [2]. There are several implications in dietary adequacy assessment especially with regard to the issue of upper limits in daily intake of certain nutrients. Moreover, several factors may influence the use of dietary supplements, such as gender, age, socio-economic status, educational level, dietary habits, etc. A first attempt to harmonize information on food supplements between European countries was performed by EFSA [3] with the purpose of producing a food composition database including both foods and food supplements to estimate nutrient intakes in European Countries. In this regard, it is worth mentioning some ongoing initiatives such as Global Dietary Database (GDD) (https://globaldietarydatabase.org/) and FAO/WHO Global Individual Food consumption data Tool (FAO/WHO GIFT) (http://www.fao.org/gift-individual-food-consumption/en/) aimed at the harmonization of dietary datasets worldwide for global diet monitoring using a common food classification and description system [4,5]. Considering the importance of dietary supplements in the evaluation of dietary intake, it is worth mentioning in particular the Dietary Supplement Label Database (DSLD) (https://dsld.nlm.nih.gov/dsld/) by the National Institutes of Health [6,7]; at present, it contains label information (brand name, ingredients, amount per serving, and manufacturer contact information) of more than 71,000 dietary supplements present and consumed in the U.S. marketplace [8,9]. The DSLD can be used to track changes in product composition and capture new products entering the market. Browsing options were developed and organized to search by product, ingredient, or contact of manufacturer, representing a unique resource that policymakers, researchers, clinicians, and consumers may find valuable for multiple applications [8,9].

In this context, information on composition reported on the product labels of selected dietary supplements has been collected and updated for the development of a Dietary Supplement Label Database for Italy, according to products' availability on the Italian market and also including items from both the third Italian National Food Consumption Survey, INRAN-SCAI 2005-06 database [2] and the ongoing Italian national dietary survey IV SCAI. The design and construction of a food database requires above all identifying foods through an adequate food nomenclature and a precise description. The FoodEx2 system has been used for the classification and description of dietary supplements in the aforementioned database. FoodEx2 is a standardized food classification and description system developed by EFSA to better describe characteristics of foods and dietary supplements in exposure assessment studies; this system, nowadays at revised version 2, consists of flexible combinations of classifications and descriptions based on a hierarchical system for different food safety-related domains (i.e., food consumption, chemical contaminants, pesticide residues, zoonoses and food composition) [10–14]. This system is characterized by a compromise between comprehensiveness (sufficiently detailed description) and feasibility in different areas of food data collection. In fact, it consists of a fixed and sufficiently large set of food categories or groups (food classification—organization of terms identifying/assigning different food items into groups) defined at high level of detail that constitute the "core list" and represent the minimum recommended level for coding during data collection [15]. More detailed terms can be found on the "extended list"; terms present in the core and extended lists may be aggregated in a hierarchical parent–child relationship in several ways according to different food safety domains. Descriptors, defined "facets", are aimed at registering all relevant food items characteristics and can be used to add details to create new categories responding to particular study requirements.

This work has been undertaken to study the application of FoodEx2 system starting from FoodEx2 categories (or terms) belonging to the FoodEx2 group "Products for non-standard diets, food imitates and food supplements" (A03RQ) for classifying the items that make up the Italian Dietary Supplement Label Database here presented.

2. Materials and Methods

The starting set of supplements has been drawn from the nationwide dietary surveys including the third Italian National Food Consumption Survey, INRAN-SCAI 2005-06 database [2] and items from preliminary results of the ongoing Italian national dietary survey IV SCAI. National food consumption surveys were designed with the aim of representativeness of the total population at national level and in the four main geographical areas, taking energy intake as the referring parameter.

Subsequently, products' labels had been searched on the internet using the following keywords in Italian: dietary supplements, botanical, herbal formulations, vitamin-based supplements, mineral-based supplements, protein-based supplement, carnitine-based supplements, prebiotic formulations, probiotic formulations, algae-based formulations, enzyme-based formulations, yeast-based formulations, common supplements.

Afterwards, label surveys visiting retail points to directly observe products on shelves were carried out.

The official register of supplements authorized by the Italian Ministry of Health (http://www.salute.gov.it/imgs/C_17_pagineAree_3668_listaFile_itemName_1_file.pdf) was consulted.

The coding procedure was carried out by a qualified compiler who constantly follows the FoodEx2 system updates, taking part in training courses organized by system developers [14]. Another qualified compiler double-checked the codes.

Procedurally, information on composition of dietary supplements was taken from labels, and a code was assigned to each item following the food classification and description system FoodEx2, revision 2; the exposure hierarchy was used for coding [10–14]. The FoodEx2 categories (terms) belonging to the FoodEx2 group "Products for non-standard diets, food imitates and food supplements" (A03RQ) were considered for classification of the items.

FoodEx2 system consists of 21 clearly defined food groups. Detailed food groups represent the basis of the systems; a food only fits in one group and a parent–child structure is present within the food groups. Facets descriptors, of which there are 28 in total, can be viewed as characteristics of foods from different points of view; the facets give additional information for a peculiar aspect of food, i.e., part nature, ingredient, packaging material, production method, qualitative information, process, target consumer. Peculiarity of FoodEx2 is that each food group lists term with included implicit facet descriptors, to which further descriptors of different characteristics can be added; during compilation procedure, in FoodEx2 for each food item, the terms may be aggregated in different ways according to the needs [16]. "Implicit facets" means facets proper of the base term chosen for classification, and therefore, implicitly assigned to it, whereas "added facets" means the facet descriptors that are added by the coder to the chosen base term while coding a food item. The procedure consists of organizing them to reduce the coding time and prevent general imprecision.

For each food item, the terms may be aggregated in different ways according to the needs, without following a general scheme; a typical case is given by a base term, followed (optionally) by a hashtag "#" and a sequence of facet descriptors separated by dollar character "$".

During this practical experience of compiling the Dietary Supplement Label Database, feedbacks and suggestions for possible enhancement of FoodEx2 were formulated and forwarded to system developers. These suggestions can be grouped as "Additional items", "Clarifications", and "Typing suggestions".

3. Results and Discussion

A total of 558 products have been entered into the database at present, as an attempt to provide an adequate representation of the major categories of food supplements, and 82 descriptors have been compiled. Particular attention has been given to supplements/formulations based on medical herbs and plant extracts, one of the classes currently emerging [17,18].

3.1. Database Description

Items in the Dietary Supplements Label Database are organized in groups defined by base terms and additional facets.

Table S1 (Supplementary Material) reports ingredients and nutritional composition of the 558 products and Table S2 (Supplementary Material) reports the FoodEx2 codes of the 558 products.

3.1.1. Base Terms

The base terms reported for describing the 558 products are distributed in the subgroups as follows: 73 Mixed supplements/formulations [A03TC], 28 Vitamin only supplements [A03SL], 27 Mineral only supplements [A03SM], 49 Combination of Vitamin and mineral only supplements [A03SN],

6 Bee-produced formulations [A03SQ], 7 Fiber supplements [A03SR], 283 Herbal formulations and plant extracts [A03SS], 14 Algae-based formulations (e.g., spirulina, chlorella) [A03ST], 8 Probiotic or prebiotic formulations [A0F3Y], 15 Formulations containing special fatty acids (e.g., Omega-3, essential fatty acids) [A03SX], 10 Protein and amino acids supplements [A03SY], 2 Coenzyme Q10 formulations [A03SZ], 1 Enzyme-based formulations [A03TA], 4 Yeast-based formulations [A03TB], 10 Other common supplements [A03SV], 3 Protein and protein components for sports people [A03SA], 6 Micronutrients supplement for sports people [A03SB], 7 Carnitine or creatine-based supplement for sports people [A03SC], 2 Nutritionally complete formulae [A03SE], 3 Imitation yoghurt, non-soy [A03TZ].

3.1.2. Facets

Additional facets used for describing the dietary supplements are: FACET F03 "PHYSICAL STATE", FACET F04 "INGREDIENT", FACET F23 "TARGET CONSUMER", FACET F33 "LEGISLATIVE CLASSES". FACET F03 defines the physical state of a product such as: Tablets [A06JH], Powder [A06JD], Liquid [A06JL].

FACET F04 defines the characterizing ingredients. Common terms used are aggregation term Chemical elements [A0EVF], including core terms Calcium [A0EXH], Magnesium [A0EXF], Iron [A0EXD], Potassium [A0EXJ], Zinc [A0EXE], Fluorine [A0F3A]; aggregation term Vitamins [A0EVG], including core terms Vitamin C (Ascorbic acid) [A0EXN], Vitamin D (Cholecalciferol) [A0EXM], Vitamin E (Tocopherols, tocotrienols) [A0EXL, Vitamin A (retinol, carotenoids) [A0EXZ], Vitamin B9 (Folic acid, folinic acid) [A0EXQ], etc.; aggregation term Special fatty acids [A0EVS], including core terms Omega-3 fatty acids [A0EVV] and Omega-6 fatty acids [A0EVT]; aggregation term Phytochemicals [A0EVM], including core terms Phytosterols [A0EVQ], Polyphenols [A0EVP], Carotenoids [A0EVN]; the core term Dietary fiber [(A0EVR]; the extended terms Carnitine [A0F4N] and Creatine-creatinine [A0F4P]; the aggregation term Bee-produced fortifying agents [A0EVH], including the core term Royal jelly [A0CVG]; the aggregation term Live microorganisms for food production [A048X] including core terms Yeast cultures [A048Z]; the core term Caffeine [A0EVK]; the core term Algae-based fortifying agents (e.g., spirulina, chlorella) [A0EVL].

It is worth mentioning that the most used terms to indicate the ingredients present in the food supplements from the category Herbal formulations and plant extracts [A03SS] are Powdered extract of plant origin [A0ETZ], Liquid extract of plant origin [A0EVA], Extracts of plant origin [A0ETY], Dried herbs [A016T], Dried vegetables [A00ZQ], Dried fruit [A01MA], Dehydrated/powdered fruit juice [A03CG], Dehydrated/powdered vegetable juice [A03DA].

Examples of descriptors for FACET 23, used to indicate the target consumers for whom the product is intended are Children's food [A07TL], including the Children's food 4–8 years [A07TM] and Children's food 9–15 years [A07TN]; Infant or toddler's food [A07TF].

Within FACET F33, defining the legislative class, descriptors from the classification defined in the food additives legislation (Regulation (EC) No. 1333/2008) are used for dietary supplements as follows: FA-17.1 Food supplements supplied in a solid form including capsules and tablets and similar forms excluding chewable forms [A0C16], FA-17.2 Food supplements supplied in a liquid form [A0C15], FA-17.3 Food supplements supplied in a syrup-type or chewable form [A0C14].

3.1.3. Groups' Description

Examples of group Vitamin only supplements [A03SL] are dietary supplements containing vitamin D such as the product coded by [A03SL#F03.A06JH$F04.A0EXM$F33.A0C16] (Re-coded: Vitamin only supplements, STATE = Tablets, INGRED = Vitamin D (cholecalciferol), LEGIS = FA-17.1 Food supplements supplied in a solid form including capsules and tablets and similar forms, excluding chewable forms) or the one by [A03SL#F03.A06JL$F04.A0EXM$F33.A0C15] (Re-coded: Vitamin only supplements, STATE = Liquid, INGRED = Vitamin D (cholecalciferol), LEGIS = FA-17.2 Food supplements supplied in a liquid form); dietary supplements containing vitamin C such as the product coded by [A03SL#F04.A0EXN$F33.A0C14] (Re-coded: Vitamin only supplements, INGRED = Vitamin C (ascorbic acid), LEGIS = FA-17.3 Food supplements supplied in a syrup-type or chewable form); dietary supplements containing vitamin B9 such as the product coded by [A03SL#F03.A06JH$F04.A0EXQ$F33.A0C16], (Re-coded: Vitamin only supplements, STATE = Tablets, INGRED = Vitamin B9 (folic acid, folinic acid), LEGIS = FA-17.1 Food supplements supplied in a solid form including capsules and tablets and similar forms, excluding chewable forms); etc.

For group Mineral only supplements [A03SM], including all supplements based only on minerals, examples are dietary supplements containing, i.e., iron, potassium, magnesium, zinc, or combination such as potassium and magnesium widespread used. An example of FoodEx2 code of a product containing potassium and magnesium is as follows: FoodEx2 code [A03SM#F03.A06JH$F04.A0EXJ$F04.A0EXF$F33.A0C16], Re-coded: Mineral only supplements, STATE = Tablets, INGRED = Potassium, INGRED = Magnesium, LEGIS = FA-17.1 Food supplements supplied in a solid form including capsules and tablets and similar forms, excluding chewable forms.

Examples for group Combination of vitamin and mineral only supplements [A03SN] that comprises all supplements based only on formulations including both minerals and vitamins are dietary supplements containing vitamin D and Calcium, i.e., FoodEx2 Code: [A03SN#F04.A0EXM$F04.A0EXH], Re-coded: Combination of vitamin and mineral only supplements, INGRED = Vitamin D (cholecalciferol), INGRED = Calcium; dietary supplements containing vitamin C and iron, i.e., FoodEx2 Code: [A03SN#F03.A06JH$F04.A0EXN$F04.A0EXD$F33.A0C16], Re-coded: Combination of vitamin and mineral only supplements, STATE = Tablets, INGRED = Vitamin C (ascorbic acid), INGRED = Iron, LEGIS = FA-17.1 Food supplements supplied in a solid form including capsules and tablets and similar forms, excluding chewable forms.

The Herbal formulations and plant extracts [A03SS] include any type of supplement based on herbal formulations and/or plant extracts. Typical ingredients are ginkgo biloba, dog rose, star anise, tamarind, aloe, rhubarb, acacia, dandelion, astragalus, psyllium, holy basil, sage and others; these occur as dried products or liquid or powdered extracts. In addition to the classic medical herbs just mentioned, there are also foods with functional components such as artichoke, garlic, pineapple, black currant, whose use has become frequent. An example of coding of artichoke- based product is FoodEx2 Code: [A03SS#F03.A06JL$F04.A0EVA$F33.A0C15], (Re-coded: Herbal formulations and plant extracts, STATE = Liquid, INGRED = Liquid extract of plant origin, LEGIS = FA-17.2 Food supplements supplied in a liquid form), and in the Remark is noted: "The ingredient indicated as Liquid extract of plant origin is hydroalcoholic extract of artichoke leaves". For a garlic-based product, FoodEx2 Code is [A03SS#F04.A0ETZ$F33.A0C16] (Re-coded: Herbal formulations and plant extracts, INGRED = Powdered extract of plant origin, LEGIS = FA-17.1 Food supplements supplied in a solid form including capsules and tablets and similar forms, excluding chewable forms) and in the Remark is noted: "The ingredient indicated as Powdered extract of plant origin is garlic bulb dry extract".

The group Other Common Supplements [A03SV], referring to any type of other common supplements, includes formulations containing, as the main ingredient, compounds such as alpha lipoic acid, beta glucans, lactoferrin, melatonin, etc. An example of product containing lipoic acid is given by the code [A03SV#F03.A06JH$F04.A0F4M$F33.A0C16], (Re-coded: Other common supplements, STATE = Tablets, INGRED = Co-factors to metabolism, LEGIS = FA-17.1 Food supplements supplied in a solid form including capsules and tablets and similar forms, excluding chewable forms) and in the Remark is noted "The ingredient indicated as Co-factors of metabolism is α-lipoic acid".

Another example is given by a product containing melatonin coded as [A03SV#F03.A06JH$F04.A0EVM$F33.A0C16] (Re-coded: Other common supplements, STATE = Tablets, INGRED = Phytochemicals, LEGIS = FA-17.1 Food supplements supplied in a solid form including capsules and tablets and similar forms, excluding chewable forms) and in the Remark is noted "The ingredient indicated as phytochemicals is melatonin".

The group Mixed supplements/formulations [A03TC] includes any type of supplements combining different principles without a strong prevalence of one. Moreover, various products belonging to this group present bioactive molecules among the ingredients, such as rutin, quercetin, coenzyme Q10. An example is given by product containing powdered extract of plant origin and fish oil, quercetin, vitamin C, vitamin B5, and Methylsulfonylmethane; it is coded as [A03TC#F03.A06JH$F04.A0ETZ$F04.A0EVP$F04.A0EXN$F04.A0EXT$F04.A038M$F04.A0EVV$F33. A0C16] (Re-coded by Mixed supplements/formulations, STATE = Tablets, INGRED = Powdered extract of plant origin, INGRED = Polyphenols, INGRED = Vitamin C (ascorbic acid), INGRED = Vitamin B5 (pantothenic acid), INGRED = Fish oil, INGRED = Omega-3 fatty acids, LEGIS = FA-17.1 Food supplements supplied in a solid form including capsules and tablets and similar forms, excluding chewable forms) and in the Remark is noted "The ingredients indicated as licorice root dry extract, plantain leaves dry extract, chamomile flowers dry extracts, nettle aerial parts. The ingredient indicated as Polyphenols is quercetin. Methylsulfonylmethane is also contained".

3.2. Feedback and Suggestions for FoodEx2 Revision 2 Implementation: Focus on Dietary Supplements

Here we report the feedback and suggestions for implementation of FoodEx2 formulated during the development and updating of Dietary Supplement Label Database in Italy. Concerning additional items, supplementary aggregation terms for proteins and amino acids should be added, including core terms for main amino acids used in dietary supplements as well as within "Special fatty acids", extended terms for "Omega-3 fatty acids" and "Omega-6 fatty acids". Considering the widespread growth in the consumption of herbal remedies, additional items, such as powdered dried fruit, powdered dried vegetables and powdered dried herbs would be very useful. At the same time, attention should be given to additional terms linked to description of bioactive compounds; in this order, within the aggregation term "Phytochemicals", several core terms, i.e., alkaloids, nitrogen-containing compounds, organosulfur compounds, should be added, including their corresponding extended terms. Moreover, extended terms should be associated to the core terms just present in FoodEx2 System, "Carotenoids" and "Polyphenols".

In line with technological progress, facet descriptors, i.e., capsules, softgels, opercula, chewable tablets, and gastro-resistant tablets should be considered.

Details on additional items proposed were reported in Table 1.

"Clarification" about "scope notes" (textual information helping describing the selected term) of "protein and amino acids supplements" and "protein and protein components for sports people" should be underlined; differences in "protein and amino acids supplements [A03SY]" and "protein and protein components for sports people [A03SA]" should be clarified as well as if dietary supplements containing fiber with a marked prebiotic activity should be included in "Fiber supplements [A03SR]" or "Probiotic or prebiotic formulations [A0F3Y]". Moreover, several typing suggestions were indicated, i.e., "Chemical elements" should be replaced by "Minerals" and "Fiber" by "Fibre".

Table 1. Proposed descriptors for implementation of FoodEx2 distinguished by type of term in FoodEx2 hierarchical structure *.

Aggregation Terms	Core Terms	Extended Terms
AMINO ACIDS	ARGININE ASPARTIC ACID GLUTAMINE VALINE GLYCINE LEUCINE ISOLEUCINE LYSINE METHIONINE THREONINE TRYPTOPHAN TYROSINE BETA-ALANINE PHENYLALANINE CYSTEINE HISTIDINE	
PROTEINS		
Chemical elements [A0EVF]	SODIUM CHLORINE BORON CHROME TIN NICKEL SILICON	
Special fatty acids [A0EVS]	Omega-3 fatty acids [A0EVV]	DOCOSAHEXAENOIC ACID (DHA) EICOSAPENTAENOIC ACID (EPA) ALPHA LINOLENIC ACID (ALA)
	Omega-6 fatty acids [A0EVT]	LINOLEIC ACID ARACHIDONIC ACID GAMMA LINOLENIC ACID (GLA)
	OLEIC ACID	
Phytochemicals [A0EVM]	Carotenoids [A0EVN]	BETA-CAROTENE LUTEIN ASTAXANTHIN
	Polyphenols [A0EVP]	PHENOLIC ACIDS FLAVONOIDS STILBENES LIGNANS
	ALKALOIDS ORGANOSULFUR COMPOUNDS NITROGEN-CONTAINING COMPOUNDS	
Other plant oils [A037L]	BORAGE OIL ROSEMARY OIL EVENING PRIMROSE OIL	
	Brown algae [A00VK]	FUCUS ASCOPHYLLUM NODOSUM
	Green algae [A00VB]	CHLORELLA
	Dried fruit [A01MA]	POWDERED DRIED FRUIT
	Dried vegetables [A00ZQ]	POWDERED DRIED VEGETABLES
	Dried herbs [A016T]	POWDERED DRIED HERBS

* Proposed FoodEx2 descriptors are in upper case and bold.

4. Conclusions

A total of 558 products have been entered into the database at present, with the aim of providing an adequate representation of the major classes of food supplements, and 82 descriptors have been compiled.

This paper represents one of first works describing the procedure of coding dietary supplements through the FoodEx2 classification system and could be a useful tool/guide for other compilers and users.

The Dietary Supplement Label Database here presented is intended to be a first example of building a database of information on marketed dietary supplements and provides several suggestions for improving the adopted classification coding system. This database is intended as a basis for a dynamic database that can be expanded as new products are offered on the market. The main feature of a database dedicated to food supplements is its intrinsic dynamism linked to the frequent changes in the formulation of food supplements, with the consequent need to monitor the market and update the database regularly, both by inserting new formulations and expanding the number of descriptors. A precise and available description of the dietary supplements through coding is essential to recognize the type, the main ingredients, and the target consumers by users from different countries.

This database will help consumers to make healthy choices and will represent a valid tool for dietary intake calculations. This database can be useful in different contexts, such as, for example, in clinical trials, dietary plans and pharmacological programs, but also to expand the food composition databases for the purpose of daily nutrient intake estimations.

Considering the integrity of the labels of dietary supplements and whether they reflect the actual amount of each ingredient contained in the product or not, as properly pointed by Betz et al. [19], a new challenge is given by the development of analytically validated laboratory-derived dietary supplement databases. A valid, rapid, and environmental friendly tool in this direction could be represented by the use of infrared spectroscopy joined with chemometrics in the perspective of integrated research approach; as for instance, the development of a "fingerprint spectra database" of dietary supplements could be useful for further researches and applications in the assessment of quality and safety, i.e., monitoring production and/or shelf life of a product, identifying contaminants, and confirming an incoming product.

Supplementary Materials: The following are available online at http://www.mdpi.com/2072-6643/12/1/89/s1, Table S1: Ingredients and nutritional composition of the 558 products; Table S2: FoodEx2 codes of the 558 products.

Author Contributions: Conceptualization, A.D., A.T. and S.S.; Investigation, A.D., L.M., P.F. and A.T.; Data curation, A.D., L.D., E.C. and S.S.; Validation, A.D., L.D. and S.S.; Writing, Review & Editing, A.D., E.C., L.D., R.P., A.M.-V., L.M., P.F., A.T. and S.S. All authors have read and agreed to the published version of the manuscript.

Funding: The present work has been performed within the sub-contract agreement 'ITALIAN AND GREEK FOOD, RECIPES AND DIETARY SUPPLEMENTS COMPOSITION DATABASES AND DAILY REFERENCE VALUES FOR ITALY AND GREECE' (PD_Manager) awarded by EuroFIR and within the Service Contracts OC/EFSA/DATA/2014/02-LOT1-CT03 ("The children's survey") and OC/EFSA/DATA/2014/02-LOT2-CT05 ("The adults' survey"); "Support to National Dietary Surveys in Compliance with the EU-Menu methodology (fourth support)" call.

Conflicts of Interest: The authors declare no conflict of interest.

References

1. Giammarioli, S.; Boniglia, C.; Carratù, B.; Ciarrocchi, M.; Chiarotti, F.; Mosca, M.; Sanzini, E. Use of food supplements and determinants of usage in a sample Italian adult population. *Public Health Nutr.* **2013**, *16*, 1768–1781. [CrossRef] [PubMed]
2. Sette, S.; Le Donne, C.; Piccinelli, R.; Arcella, D.; Turrini, A.; Leclercq, C.; on behalf of the INRAN-SCAI 2005-06 Study Group. The third Italian National Food Consumption Survey, INRAN-SCAI 2005e06 e Part 1: Nutrient intakes in Italy. *Nutr. Metab. Cardiovasc. Dis.* **2011**, *21*, 922–932. [CrossRef] [PubMed]

3. Roe, M.A.; Bell, S.; Oseredczuk, M.; Christensen, T.; Westenbrink, S.; Pakkala, H.; Presser, K.; Finglas, P.M.; on behalf of EUROFIR Consortium. Updated food composition database for nutrient intake. *EFSA Support. Publ.* **2013**, *10*, 355E. [CrossRef]
4. Leclercq, C.; Allemand, P.; Balcerzak, A.; Branca, F.; Sousa, R.F.; Lartey, A.; Lipp, M.; Quadros, V.P.; Verger, P. FAO/WHO GIFT (Global Individual Food consumption data Tool): A global repository for harmonised individual quantitative food consumption studies. Africa Nutritional Epidemiology Conference (ANEC) VIII was held at Addis Ababa, Ethiopia on 1–5 October 2018. *Proc. Nutr. Soc.* **2019**, *78*, 484–495. [CrossRef] [PubMed]
5. Karageorgou, D.; Lara-Castor, L.; Leclercq, C.; Padula de Quadros, V.; Ioannidou, S.; Mozaffarian, D.; Micha, R. *Harmonizing Dietary Datasets around the World for Global Diet Monitoring: Methods from the Global Dietary Database and the Global Individual food Consumption Data Tool (or06-06-19)*; ASN Nutrition: Baltimore, MD, USA, 2019.
6. DSLD—Dietary Supplement Label Database. Available online: https://dsld.nlm.nih.gov/dsld/ (accessed on 8 June 2018).
7. Dwyer, J.T.; Saldanha, L.G.; Bailen, R.A.; Bailey, R.L.; Costello, R.B.; Betz, J.M.; Chang, F.F.; Goshorn, J.; Andrews, K.W.; Pehrsson, P.R.; et al. A free new dietary supplement label database for registered dietitiannutritionists. *J. Acad. Nutr. Diet.* **2014**, *114*, 1512–1517. [CrossRef] [PubMed]
8. Potischman, N.; Salazar, S.; Susser, J.; Saldanha, L.S.J.; Dwyer, J.; Kuzak, A.; Betz, J.; Bailen, R. Testingusability of the Dietary Supplement Label Database (DSLD): A resource for consumers, professionals, andresearchers. *J. Nutr. Educ. Behav.* **2017**, *49*, S99. [CrossRef]
9. Dwyer, J.T.; Bailen, R.A.; Saldanha, L.G.; Gahche, J.J.; Costello, R.B.; Betz, J.M.; Davis, C.D.; Bailey, R.L.; Potischman, N.; Ershow, A.G.; et al. The Dietary Supplement Label Database: Recent developments and applications. *J. Nutr.* **2018**, *148*, 1428S–1435S. [CrossRef] [PubMed]
10. European Food Safety Authority. The food classification and description system FoodEx2 (revision 2). *EFSA Support. Publ.* **2015**, *12*, 804E.
11. European Food Safety Authority; Vernazza, F.; Avon, V. FoodEx2 Browser—User's guide. *EFSA Support. Publ.* **2017**, *14*, 1291E.
12. European Food Safety Authority; Vernazza, F.; Avon, V. FoodEx2 Browser enhancement. *EFSA Support. Publ.* **2017**, *14*, 1292E.
13. European Food Safety Authority (EFSA); Ioannidou, S.; Nikolic, M.; Gibin, D. FoodEx2 maintenance 2016-2018. *EFSA Support. Publ.* **2018**, *16*, 1584E.
14. European Food Safety Authority (EFSA). Training on FoodEx2. *EFSA Support. Publ.* **2018**. [CrossRef]
15. Durazzo, A.; Camilli, E.; D'Addezio, L.; Sette, S.; Marconi, S.; Piccinelli, R.; Le Donne, C.; Turrini, A.; Marletta, L. Italian composite dishes: Description and classification by LanguaL™ and FoodEx2. *Eur. Food Res. Technol.* **2019**, 1–9. [CrossRef]
16. Durazzo, A.; Camilli, E.; D'Addezio, L.; Le Donne, C.; Ferrari, M.; Marconi, S.; Marletta, L.; Mistura, L.; Piccinelli, R.; Scalvedi, M.L.; et al. Food Groups and Individual Foods: Nutritional Attributes and Dietary Importance. *Ref. Mod. Food Sci.* **2018**. [CrossRef]
17. Restani, P. *Food Supplements Containing Botanicals: Benefits, Side Effects and Regulatory Aspects*; The Scientific Inheritance of the EU Project PlantLIBRA; Food Science & Nutrition; Springer International Publishing: Cham, Switzerland, 2018.
18. Durazzo, A.; D'Addezio, L.; Camilli, E.; Piccinelli, R.; Turrini, A.; Marletta, L.; Marconi, S.; Lucarini, M.; Lisciani, S.; Gabrielli, P.; et al. From plant compounds to botanicals and back: A current snapshot. *Molecules* **2018**, *23*, 1844. [CrossRef] [PubMed]
19. Betz, J.M.; Rimmer, C.A.; Saldanha, L.G.; Phillips, M.M.; Andrews, K.W.; Wise, S.A.; Wood, L.J.; Kuszak, A.J.; Gusev, P.A.; Pehrsson, P.R. Challenges in Developing Analytically Validated Laboratory-Derived Dietary Supplement Databases. *J. Nutr.* **2018**, *148*, 1406S–1412S. [CrossRef] [PubMed]

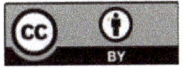

© 2019 by the authors. Licensee MDPI, Basel, Switzerland. This article is an open access article distributed under the terms and conditions of the Creative Commons Attribution (CC BY) license (http://creativecommons.org/licenses/by/4.0/).

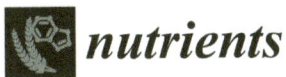

Article

Bioactivity Evaluation of a Novel Formulated Curcumin

Se-Chun Liao [1], Wei-Hsiang Hsu [2], Zi-Yi Huang [2], Kun-Lin Chuang [2], Kuan-Ting Lin [3], Chia-Ling Tseng [4], Tung-Hu Tsai [5], Anh-Hoang Dao [6], Chun-Li Su [4,7,*] and Chi-Ying F. Huang [1,2,8,*]

1. Institute of Clinical Medicine, National Yang-Ming University, Taipei 112, Taiwan; susanliao@everestpharm.com
2. Institute of Biopharmaceutical Sciences, National Yang-Ming University, Taipei 112, Taiwan; rabbitjim5@hotmail.com (W.-H.H.); laduree120@ym.edu.tw (Z.-Y.H.); jason101024004@gmail.com (K.-L.C.)
3. Cold Spring Harbor Laboratory, Cold Spring Harbor, NY 11724, USA; woodydon777@gmail.com
4. Department of Human Development and Family Studies, National Taiwan Normal University, Taipei 106, Taiwan; piiq2005@hotmail.com
5. Institute of Traditional Medicine, School of Medicine, National Yang-Ming University, Taipei 112, Taiwan; thtsai@ym.edu.tw
6. Department of Formulation and Processing, National Institute of Medicinal Materials, Hanoi 100000, Vietnam; bccb@nimm.org.vn
7. Graduate Program of Nutrition Science, School of Life Science, National Taiwan Normal University, Taipei 106, Taiwan
8. Department of Biochemistry, College of Medicine, Kaohsiung Medical University, Kaohsiung 807, Taiwan
* Correspondence: chunlisu@ntnu.edu.tw (C.-L.S.); cyhuang5@ym.edu.tw (C.-Y.F.H.);
Tel.: +886-277341436 (C.-L.S.); +886-228267904 (C.-Y.F.H.);
Fax: +886-223639635 (C.-L.S.); +886-228224045 (C.-Y.F.H.)

Received: 9 October 2019; Accepted: 19 November 2019; Published: 6 December 2019

Abstract: Curcumin has been used as a traditional medicine and/or functional food in several cultures because of its health benefits including anticancer properties. However, poor oral bioavailability of curcumin has limited its oral usage as a food supplement and medical food. Here we formulated curcumin pellets using a solid dispersion technique. The pellets had the advantages of reduced particle size, improved water solubility, and particle porosity. This pellet form led to an improvement in curcumin's oral bioavailability. Additionally, we used the C-Map and Library of Integrated Network-Based Cellular Signatures (LINCS) Unified Environment (CLUE) gene expression database to determine the potential biological functions of formulated curcumin. The results indicated that, similar to conventional curcumin, the formulated curcumin acted as an NF-κB pathway inhibitor. Moreover, ConsensusPathDB database analysis was used to predict possible targets and it revealed that both forms of curcumin exhibit similar biological functions, including apoptosis. Biochemical characterization revealed that both the forms indeed induced apoptosis of hepatocellular carcinoma (HCC) cell lines. We concluded that the formulated curcumin increases the oral bioavailability in animals, and, as expected, retains characteristics similar to conventional curcumin at the cellular level. Our screening platform using big data not only confirms that both the forms of curcumin have similar mechanisms but also predicts the novel mechanism of the formulated curcumin.

Keywords: curcumin; formulated curcumin; pharmacokinetics; aurora kinase A; hepatocellular carcinoma

1. Introduction

The use of nutraceutical or functional and medical foods as alternative medicine, in addition to supplementary foods, has been on the rise in recent years [1,2]. The delivery of active ingredients is important in order to obtain beneficial effects for the human body.

Curcumin has been used for many years as a naturally occurring alternative medicine and functional food for the treatment of many diseases. Curcumin is a polyphenol extracted from the rhizome of *Curcuma longa* L., which has phenolic groups and conjugated double bonds [3]. It has strong anti-oxidant, anti-inflammatory, anti-septic, anti-proliferative, and wound-healing properties [4–8]. In addition, curcumin can reverse multidrug resistance of cancer cells, suggesting that it can also serve as a supplement to traditional chemotherapy [9,10]. Several lines of evidence show that curcumin exerts potent anticancer effects against a broad range of human cancer cells, including prostate, colon, breast, ovarian, lung, and liver cancers, and can induce cancer cell apoptosis, for example, in liver cancer cell lines, including but not limited to HepG2, SK-Hep-1, Hep3B, SUN449, and Huh7 cells, with low cytotoxic effects on normal cells [11–16].

Despite curcumin's beneficial effects, its low oral bioavailability (due to its low absorption in the gut because of low solubility in water, fast metabolism by the liver, and rapid systemic elimination) has limited its applications [17–19]. Various methods have been developed to improve the oral bioavailability of curcumin, such as the use of a natural enhancer, a curcumin-phospholipid complex, cyclodextrin and microemulsions, and the development of curcumin analogs [20–22]. In this study, we selected the pellet form, a multiple-unit dosage form, as a vehicle for compound delivery. Pellets disperse freely in the gastrointestinal tract, so they invariably maximize drug absorption [23]. In addition, to improve the solubility of curcumin, we used a solid dispersion technique to formulate pellets. In solid dispersions, the particle size of poorly soluble drugs is reduced and their wettability and dispersibility enhanced, thereby improving their dissolution and absorption rate [24].

The Connectivity Map (C-Map) is a systematic database that establishes the relationship between diseases, genes, and compounds [25]. Recently, the database has been expanded and renamed C-Map and Library of Integrated Network-Based Cellular Signatures (LINCS) Unified Environment (CLUE) (https://clue.io/) [26]. Briefly, C-Map and CLUE use gene expression profiles to describe the biological states of cultured human cancer or normal cells to determine their chemical or genetic constructs (short hairpin RNA [shRNA] constructs). The new, low-cost, high-throughput generic solution for gene expression profiles is termed "L1000." CLUE not only expands the 1309 compounds listed in C-Map to 19,811 small molecules but also includes 5075 shRNA and overexpression genes. In addition, users find CLUE relatively convenient to quickly search for a drug class with a similar mechanism of action (MOA) as a target drug or the same gene family of genetic perturbagens, they codify the class-level annotation required considerable effort, perturbagen classes (PCLs). For example, users can compare their target, such as a disease gene signature or a novel compound, with C-Map and CLUE through pattern-matching algorithms and predict dissimilarities (search for a drug to reverse a disease) or similarities (search for a similar MOA via known compounds). They could upload gene expression profiles to C-Map and CLUE to calculate the connectivity score of each profile. A positive connectivity score would indicate a degree of similar mechanism, while a negative connectivity score would denote the reverse.

HCC is the fifth-most common malignancy worldwide. More than 75% of HCC cases occur in the Asia-Pacific region. The high mortality rate because of HCC is due to the difficulty in diagnosis and poor prognosis. Chemotherapy is a traditional choice for inoperable HCC, but drug resistance limits the therapeutic effect [27,28]. Sorafenib is a multi-kinase inhibitor that targets Raf kinases as well as vascular endothelial growth factor receptor (VEGFR)-2/VEGFR-3, platelet-derived growth factor receptor beta (PDGFR-β), Flt-3, and c-Kit. Because of its potential in providing a survival advantage of two to three months, as per results of two-phase III clinical studies, sorafenib is a Food and Drug Administration (FDA)-approved, first-line targeted therapy agent for treating advanced HCC patients [29,30]. However, the low tumor response rate and side effects of sorafenib indicate the need for investigating other new potential drugs or supplementary foods for HCC [31,32]. In this study, we investigated the anticancer activity of conventional and formulated curcumin and their combination with sorafenib in order to determine whether this combination can induce HCC cell apoptosis and autophagy and inhibit HCC cell proliferation. Formulated curcumin can be used as a functional food and alternative medicine in cancer therapy as it not only causes mitotic defects and cell cycle arrest in cancer cells but also alters chemosensitivity toward anticancer drugs by inducing Aurora-A suppression.

2. Materials and Methods

2.1. Materials and Methods Used in Manufacturing Formulated Curcumin

2.1.1. Preparation of Curcumin Solid Dispersion Loaded Pellet

A curcumin standard with a purity > 95.6% was purchased from Sigma-Aldrich.

We used a solid dispersion technique to enhance the solubility and dissolution rate of curcumin [24]. Briefly, the process of making formulated curcumin included dispersing curcumin powder into a solid dispersion solution and spraying it onto sugar spheres. Tumeric extract powder contained 95% curcumin in 80 g (as the active drug). The excipients used in the preparation process of solid dispersion curcumin were Polyvinylpyrrolidone #k30 800 g (PVP K30, as the non-volatile polymer solvent for curcumin) and alcohol 3200 g (as the volatile solvent for curcumin). The turmeric extract powder was mixed with the excipients. The drug-polymer interaction evenly dispersed curcumin in the solvent. Next, the solvent containing solid dispersion curcumin was loaded onto sugar spheres by spray-drying to make solid dispersion pellets; the solvent evaporated during fluid-bed granulation (Figure 1).

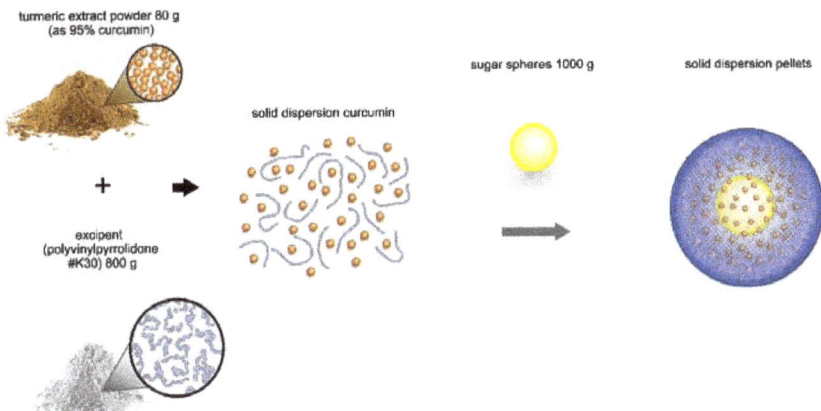

Figure 1. Preparation of solid dispersion curcumin. Turmeric extract powder, containing 80 g of 95% curcumin (as the active drug), was mixed with excipients (800 g PVP as the nonvolatile polymer solvent in the presence of alcohol as the volatile solvent for curcumin). The drug-polymer interaction evenly dispersed curcumin in the solvent. Then, the solvent containing solid dispersion curcumin was loaded onto sugar spheres by fluid-bed granulation to make solid dispersion curcumin pellets. PVP, polyvinylpyrrolidone.

2.1.2. Measurements of Particle Size and Zeta Potential

Particle size (Z-average, nm), polydispersity index (PDI), and ζ-potential (ZP, mV) of curcumin particles after re-dispersion in water were determined at 25 °C by dynamic light scattering (DLS) using a Zetasizer Nano ZS90 (Malvern Instruments, Malvern, UK). Measurements were performed with a detector at a fixed angle of 90°, in triplicate, and results were shown as mean ± SD. About 60 mg of pellets were dispersed into 2 mL water and centrifuged at 2000 × g for 1 minute to remove starch particles originated from sugar spheres. Supernatant was aspirated to measure size and ZP.

2.1.3. Dissolution Test

A dissolution test was conducted by the US Pharmacopeia 41 basket method (apparatus 1) using a dissolution tester (708-DS Dissolution apparatus, Agilent, USA). The samples of 89 mg conventional curcumin (equivalent to 72 mg curcumin) and 2180 mg formulated curcumin (equivalent to 72 mg curcumin) were placed into 900 mL of dissolution medium containing 1% sodium dodecyl sulfate (SDS) at 37 °C ± 0.5 °C, under a stirring speed of 100 ± 2 rpm. A 5 mL sample was withdrawn at each time interval (5, 10, 15, 20, 30, 45, and 60 minutes) and was mixed and filtered through a 0.45-μm pore membrane. Then, 2 mL of filtrate was diluted with mobile phase so that the total volume became 10 mL and subjected to HPLC analysis (Agilent 1260, USA). The HPLC program consisted of a mobile phase of tetrahydrofuran: 0.1% citric acid solution (4:6). The column used was 4.6 mm × 20 cm with 5-μm packing L1. The flow rate was 1 mL/minute, and the injection volume was 20 μL using a 420 nm wavelength detector. The percentages of curcumin dissolved from the conventional curcumin and pellets (formulated curcumin) into the medium were calculated and compared.

2.2. Pharmacokinetic Study

2.2.1. Animal Model

All animal treatment procedures followed the Guide for the Care and Use of Laboratory Animals (National Institutes of Health (NIH) publication, 85–23, revised 1996) as well as the Animal research: Reporting *in vivo* experiments (ARRIVE) guidelines, and were approved by the Animal Research Committee at National Yang-Ming University, Taipei, Taiwan, under Institutional Animal Care and Use Committees (IACUC) approval no: 990103. All surgeries and experimental procedure were carried out under anesthesia with all efforts to minimize animal suffering.

Twelve male Sprague Dawley (SD) rats (270 ± 15 g body weight) were obtained from Bio-Lasco, Taipei, Taiwan. Water was provided *ad libitum*, regardless of administration route. All animals were acclimatized and quarantined in quarantine room of the Rosetta animal facility for about 1 week, and then transferred to feeding room. The humidity and temperature were well controlled as 30%–70% and 19–25 °C. The light and dark cycle was set as 12 h: 12 h. Food and drinking water were allowed *ad libitum* during housing.

Rats were randomly divided into two groups treated with curcumin and formulated curcumin. Curcumin (conventional; 500 mg/kg, $n = 6$) and 500 mg/kg formulated curcumin (equal to curcumin 60 mg/kg, $n = 6$) were administered by gavage to the freely moving rats, respectively. A 300 μL blood sample was collected from the tail vein into a tube rinsed with heparin at 0, 0.25, 0.5, 1, 1.5, 2, 4, 6 h after oral administration.

2.2.2. Sample Pretreatment

Plasma was obtained by centrifuging the blood sample at 4000 rpm for 10 minutes at 4 °C. The 10 μL plasma was mixed with 50 μL of the internal standard solution containing 0.1 ng/μL of agomelatine. The samples were vortexed and centrifuged at 13,000 rpm for 5 minutes. The 50 μL of supernatant was transferred to the 1.5 mL tube contained 50 μL solution of 25% acetonitrile and 0.1% acetic acid. After that, 50 μL of the solution was injected onto LC-MS system.

2.2.3. LC/MS/MS Conditions and Data Analysis

Curcumin concentrations in the samples were determined by positive ion electrospray tandem mass spectrometry using multiple reaction monitoring (MRM). Separation of curcumin was conducted on a Cosmosil column (5C18-MS-IIPacked column, 120 Å, 5 μm, 4.6 mm I.D. x 150 mm; NACALAI TESQUE, Inc., Japan) with a mobile phase of acetonitrile-water-formic acid. MS/MS conditions consisted of a declustering potential of 50 V, desolvation temperature of 550 °C, spray needle of 5500 V, and collision energy of 30 V.

Pharmacokinetic analysis was calculated using a non-compartmental model with the Phoenix WinNonlin®(Version 8.0) software. The area under the drug concentration-time curve (AUC) was used to measure the total amount of curcumin reaching the systemic circulation. The relative oral bioavailability (BA) of curcumin was calculated according to the following equation: BA (%) = 100 × [(AUC$_{\text{formulated curcumin}}$/dose$_{\text{formulated curcumin}}$]/[(AUC$_{\text{curcumin}}$/dose$_{\text{curcumin}}$)]. The pharmacokinetic results were represented as the mean ± SD. Statistical analysis was performed by t test (SPSS version 10.0) to compare the differences between groups. The level of significance was set at $p < 0.05$.

2.3. Cell Lines and Cell Culture

The Huh7 and PLC5 cell lines were obtained from National Taiwan University Hospital, Taiwan. The Mahlavu cell lines were provided by Dr. Muh-Hwa Yang (Institute of Clinical Medicine, National Yang-Ming University, Taiwan). Hep3B cells were obtained from American Type Culture Collection (ATCC), Rockville, MD, USA.

HCC cell lines were cultured in Dulbecco's modified Eagle's medium (DMEM, GIBCO) supplemented with 10% (v/v) fetal bovine serum (FBS, GIBCO), non-essential amino acids (NEAA, GIBCO), L-glutamine (GlutaMAX™-I Supplement, GIBCO) and 10% penicillin-streptomycin (GIBCO). These cells were maintained in a humidified incubator with 5% CO_2 at 37 °C and were regularly subcultured every 2–3 days.

2.4. Drug Preparation and Cell Exposure

The conventional curcumin was prepared as a 30 mM stock solution in dimethyl sulfoxide (DMSO; Sigma) and stored at -20 °C. Final curcumin concentrations of 1–90 µM were obtained by dilution in culture medium so that the final concentration of DMSO was less than 1%. Controls contained 0.1% DMSO in all experiments.

The formulated curcumin was prepared as a 30 mM stock solution (based on the weight of curcumin) in double distilled water and stored at -20 °C. The formulated curcumin was diluted with cell culture medium to obtain the concentration indicated.

2.5. Proliferation and Viability Assays

Cells were seeded into a 96-well plate (1500–2000 cells/well) overnight and then treated with curcumin and the formulated curcumin respectively for 0, 24, 48, 72, 96 and 120 h. After treatment, 0.5 µg/mL 3-(4,5-cimethylthiazol-2-yl)-2,5-diphenyl tetrazolium bromide (MTT) was added to each well and cultured for 2 h at 37 °C. After incubation, the media were removed from the wells. The formazan crystals formed were then solubilized in DMSO at room temperature for 10 minutes, and then the absorbance was measured in a multimode microplate reader at 570 nm.

2.6. Mitochondrial Membrane Potential Assay

We employed 5, 5′, 6, 6′-tetrachloro-l, 1′, 3, 3′-tetraethylbenzimidazolcarbocyanine iodide (JC-1), which was obtained from Cayman Chemical Co., to analyze the mitochondrial membrane potential. The cells were seeded in 96-well black plates at a density of 7000 cells/well and cultured overnight. After treatment, JC-1 staining solution was added to each well and incubated at 37 °C for 15–30 minutes in the dark. The plates were obtained by centrifuged at 400 × g at room temperature for 5 minutes, and the supernatant was discarded. Then, JC-1 assay buffer was added to each well, followed by centrifugation at 400 × g at room temperature for 5 minutes, after which the supernatant was discarded. Finally, JC-1 assay buffer was added again to each well for fluorescent analysis using a fluorescent plate reader.

2.7. Annexin V and Propidium Iodide (PI) Double Staining by Flow Cytometry

The Huh7 were incubated with various concentrations of conventional and formulated curcumin for 24 h. Annexin V/PI staining was performed to quantify cell apoptosis using an Annexin V-fluorescein isothiocyanate (FITC) Apoptosis Detection Kit (BioVision, Inc., Milpitas, CA, USA) according to the manufacturer's protocol. Annexin V-FITC was then added followed by incubation for 15 minutes in the dark in a 100 µL cell suspension. PI was then spiked into 400 µL Annexin V binding buffer and added immediately to the cell suspension, and subsequently analyzed on a FACScan flow cytometer (BD Biosciences, USA).

2.8. Western Blot

The cells were incubated with various treatment (conventional and formulated curcumin or combination of sorafenib and conventional and formulated curcumin), and then collected for western blot. Aliquots of cell lysates containing 20–50 µg of protein were separated by SDS-polyacrylamide gel electrophoresis (SDS-PAGE), transferred onto a polyvinylidene difluoride (PVDF) membrane and detected using specific primary and secondary antibodies. The protein bands were visualized by an enhanced chemiluminescence (ECL) detection kit (Immobilon^{TM} western, Millipore). The membranes were reprobed for β-actin as a loading control. All western blots were carried out at least three times for each experiment. The data were normalized to β-actin. The following primary antibodies were used: anti-extracellular regulated protein kinases (ERK), anti-caspase-3, anti-poly (ADP-ribose) polymerase (PARP) (all from Cell Signaling Technology) and anti-aurora kinase A (AURKA) (BD Biosciences). All antibodies were used at a 1:1000 dilution.

2.9. Cell Cycle Analysis

After treatment, the cells were collected by trypsinization and fixed in precooled 70% ethanol overnight. The cells were then incubated with PI in the presence of RNase A. The DNA content was analyzed by a FACSCalibur, and the data were analyzed by Flowjo software. The percentage of cells in the sub-G1 was used to indicate the apoptosis rate.

2.10. Analysis the Similar Mechanism of Gene Expression Profiles of Conventional and Formulated Curcumin Using the L1000 Microarray

Human HCC (HepG2) and human colorectal cancer (HT29) cell lines (ATCC) were treated in triplicate with 20 µM of conventional curcumin or 2 µM of formulated curcumin. Briefly, for experiments using formulated curcumin, 2 µM of curcumin formulation and curcumin excipient were dissolved in DMSO and incubated with HepG2 and HT29 cell lines. The samples were submitted to Genometry, Inc. (Cambridge, MA, USA) for L1000 microarray analysis and to obtain the gene expression profiles of formulated curcumin in HepG2 and HT29. Each set of gene expression profiles consisted of up- and down-regulated gene signatures. Subsequently, CLUE was used to decipher the gene signatures in order to uncover potential mechanisms via mapping to compounds with known MOAs. To filter output data, we used a score > 90 for compounds and a score > 70 for PCLs.

2.11. Statistical Analysis

All values were expressed as the mean ± SD. The data were analyzed using a two-tailed student's t test. A $p < 0.05$ was considered as statistically significant.

3. Result

3.1. Preparation and Evaluation Formulated Curcumin

First, we prepared the formulated curcumin from powder to pellets with a solid dispersion technique as described in detail in the Materials and Methods section. The pellet size of formulated curcumin estimated by sieving was distributed in the range of 830–1000 µm. Curcumin content quantified by HPLC was 3.3%. Z-average (nm), PDI, and ZP (mV) of curcumin particles after re-dispersion in water were 141.9 ± 5.1, 0.308 ± 0.029 and −2.49 ± 0.39, respectively (Table 1). The dissolution rates of conventional curcumin were 0.00%, 9.80%, 13.60%, 14.05%, 17.28%, 19.41%, 24.06%, and 26.28%, while those of the formulated curcumin were 0.00%, 59.03%, 87.50%, 98.78%, 100.22%, 101.20%, 102.29%, and 103.65% at 0, 5, 10, 15, 20, 30, 45, and 60 minutes, respectively (Supplementary Figure S1). In the 1% SDS medium, more than 85% of curcumin was almost immediately released from the pellets after 10 minutes. Additionally, when compared to the US Pharmacopeia specifications for dissolution of curcuminoid capsules or curcuminoid tablets, the dissolution of the formulated curcumin was not lower than 75% after 60 minutes, suggesting that the formulation greatly increased curcumin's solubility.

Table 1. Properties of formulated curcumin.

Properties of Formulated Curcumin	Value
Pellet size (µm)	830–1000
Curcumin level (%)	3.3
Z-average (nm)	141.9 ± 5.1
Polydispersity index (PDI)	0.308 ± 0.029
Zeta potential (mV)	−2.49 ± 0.39

3.2. Oral Administration of Formulated Curcumin Shows an Increase in Bioavailability over Conventional Curcumin via Pharmacokinetic Analysis

To determine the actual amount of curcumin that was released and existed in the formulated curcumin, a high-performance liquid chromatography assay and LC-MS method was adopted for the quantification of curcumin. To investigate whether the bioavailability of curcumin was increased after formulation, 60 mg/kg of formulated curcumin was orally administered in a rat model and the plasma samples were subjected to chromatography. To confirm the reliability of the method for analyzing curcumin in plasma samples, a method validation was performed. The retention times of curcumin were about 5.14 minutes, with no visible interference peak in the blank plasma chromatogram (data not shown). To perform a pharmacokinetic analysis, the curcumin concentrations in rat plasma at different time points following oral administration of 500 mg/kg of curcumin and 60 mg/kg of formulated curcumin were compared (Figure 2). However, administration of 500 mg/kg of curcumin had very low amount of curcumin in rat plasma and resulted to a huge increase of bioavailability. Therefore, the pharmacokinetic parameters of curcumin represented an estimated number and will be compared with others from literatures (see later in discussion). AUC represents the total drug exposure over time. Based on the pharmacokinetic parameters (Table 2), the AUC represents the total drug exposure over time. The AUC normalized by dose of curcumin was increased from 0.0021 to 1.864, which is an 887.6-fold increase after formulation. Overall, this result showed that oral administration of formulated curcumin significantly increased the oral bioavailability of curcumin compared with conventional curcumin.

3.3. Gene Expression Analysis of Formulated Curcumin and Prediction of Highly Correlated Pathways

We queried CLUE with regard to the analyzed group of genes in order to identify potential biological functions of formulated curcumin. The top 30 compounds (Figure 3C) and PCLs (Figure 3A) with the highest scores were obtained from CLUE. Intersection of results from both cell lines revealed that seven compounds (e.g., menadione and angiogenesis inhibitor; Figure 3D) and two PCLs (e.g., NF-κB pathway inhibitors; Figure 3B) shared common functions with conventional curcumin. In summary, formulated curcumin was similar to conventional curcumin, and both functioned as, for example, NF-κB pathway inhibitors, which is consistent with previous studies [33]. We intersected two sample groups to identify common PCL/compound classes between formulated curcumin treatment of HT29 cells and formulated curcumin treatment of HepG2 cells. Consequently, we identified two PCLs (including NF-κB pathway inhibitors and vesicular transport loss of function (LOF; Figure 3B), and seven compounds belonging to the NF-κB pathway inhibitor PCL class were common among all groups.

In fact, CLUE revealed that only the MOA of compounds or shRNAs was similar to that of formulated curcumin; CLUE did not indicate the target of formulated curcumin. Therefore, to obtain more information about formulated curcumin, we used another database for assistance pathway analysis, ConsensusPathDB (CPDB). CPDB comprises interactions among different types of various intracellular information, such as genes, RNA, proteins, and metabolites, to predict a relatively comprehensive and unbiased cellular biology signal result. We used the Venny website to intersect our two sets of PCL results (Figure 3B) and selected their targets and members genes to predict potential pathways of formulated curcumin (Figure 4). According to $q < 0.001$, we listed the top 20 pathways at the bottom of Figure 4, and the details are in Supplementary Figure S2. In addition, we showed similar effects in L1000 microarray profiles between conventional and formulated curcumin in heatmaps (Figure 5). These data suggested that formulated curcumin exhibits similar biological functions as conventional curcumin.

Table 2. Pharmacokinetic parameters of curcumin in rat plasma following oral administration.

Parameters	Oral	
	Conventional Curcumin* ($n = 5$)	Formulated Curcumin ($n = 6$)
	500 mg/kg	60 mg/kg
C_{max} (ng/mL)	0.704 ± 0.272	109.200 ± 41.651
AUC_{0-t} (h × ng/mL)	1.1 ± 1.2	111.8 ± 16.4
AUC_{0-t}/Dose	0.0022 ± 0.0024	1.863 ± 0.273
T_{max}(h)	1.25 ± 0.83	0.38 ± 0.14

The data are expressed as the mean ± SD. C_{max}: the maximum plasma concentration; T_{max}: the time at which C_{max} is observed; AUC_{0-t}: area under the concentration-time curve from the time of drug administration to the last quantifiable concentration. *: Conventional curcumin in some rat plasma samples was very low and was assigned to 0 for calculations. We were unable to detect curcumin from the plasma of one rat during the experimental periods, and thus data from five rats were used for calculations.

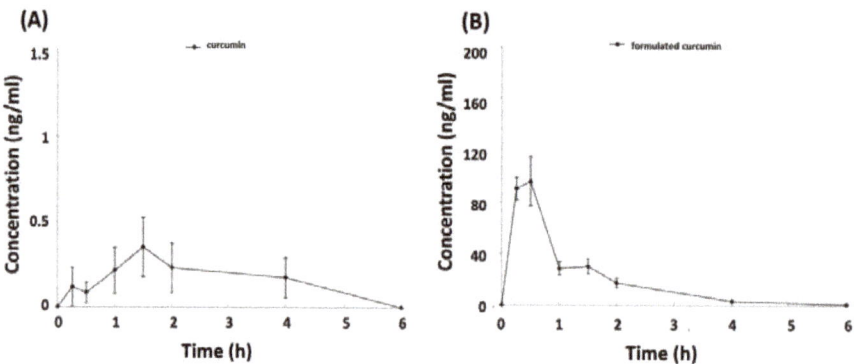

Figure 2. Mean plasma concentration-time profiles of curcumin in male SD rats following 500 mg/kg conventional curcumin (A) and 60 mg/kg formulated curcumin (B) after single dose oral gavage (P.O.) linear ordinate. The data are expressed as mean ± SD, $n = 5$ for curcumin and $n = 6$ for formulated curcumin.

(A)

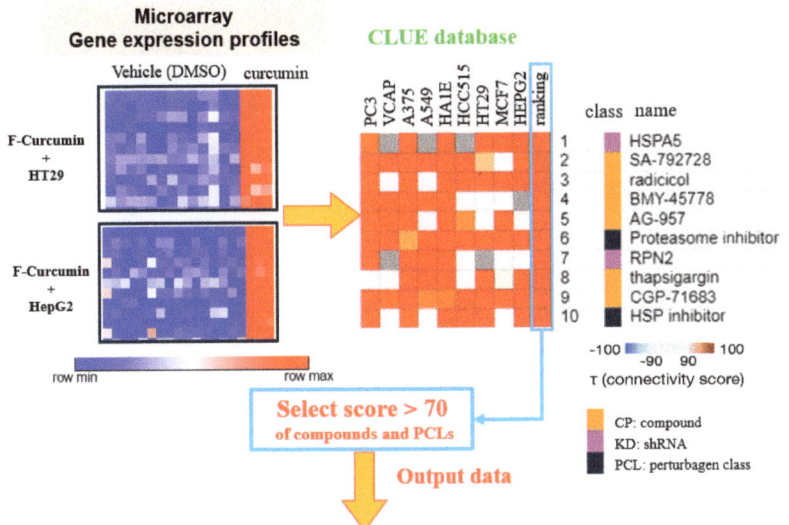

(B)

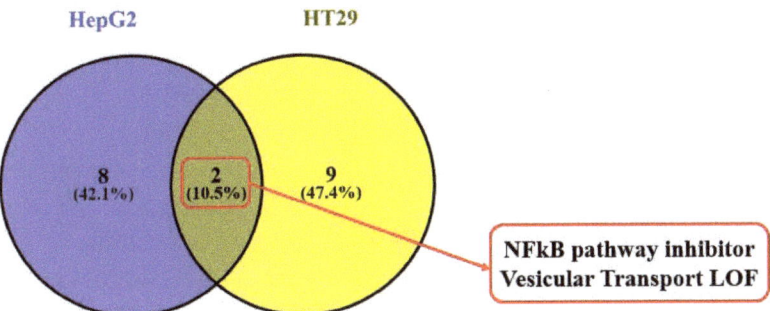

Figure 3. Cont.

(C)

	HepG2			HT29	
rank	Drug name	score	rank	Drug name	score
1	iodoacetic-acid	99.4	1	celastrol	99.93
2	tretinoin	98.84	2	erythrosine	99.93
3	Ala-Ala-Phe-CMK	98.73	3	RO-90-7501	99.72
4	WR-216174	98.7	4	clopidogrel	99.58
5	sappanone-a	98.41	5	W-7	99.34
6	caffeic-acid	98.17	6	PPT	99.33
7	AG-957	97.77	7	gatifloxacin	99.26
8	capsazepine	97.42	8	carbidopa	99.19
9	4-hydroxy-2-nonenal	97.4	9	SU-11652	99.19
10	pifithrin-mu	97.36	10	dipropyl-dopamine	99.08
11	tosyl-phenylalanyl-chloromethyl-ketone	97.32	11	n-formylmethionylalanine	98.73
12	SA-792709	97.26	12	metformin	98.73
13	SSR-69071	97.22	13	oxindole-I	98.44
14	15-delta-prostaglandin-j2	96.97	14	dichloroacetic-acid	98.34
15	BCL2-inhibitor	96.95	15	acyclovir	98.14
16	quinidine	96.88	16	rifampicin	98.13
17	isoliquiritigenin	96.72	17	thiothixene	98.06
18	parthenolide	96.69	18	AKT-inhibitor-1-2	97.83
19	SA-792728	96.62	19	methyl-angolensate	97.46
20	NSC-3852	96.62	20	LDN-193189	97.32
21	SCH-58261	96.59	21	BRD-A81377415	97.29
22	LDN-193189	96.58	22	auranofin	97.29
23	menadione	96.58	23	cefoxitin	97.25
24	rhamnetin	96.52	24	propranolol	96.86
25	atracurium	96.39	25	methylene-blue	96.85
26	flavokavain-b	96.34	26	rimcazole	96.61
27	MDM2-inhibitor	96.2	27	doxazosin	96.61
28	pyrrolidine-dithiocarbamate	96.17	28	temsirolimus	96.41
29	sulforaphane	96.02	29	maprotiline	96.33
30	tyrphostin-47	95.92	30	tivozanib	96.3

(D)

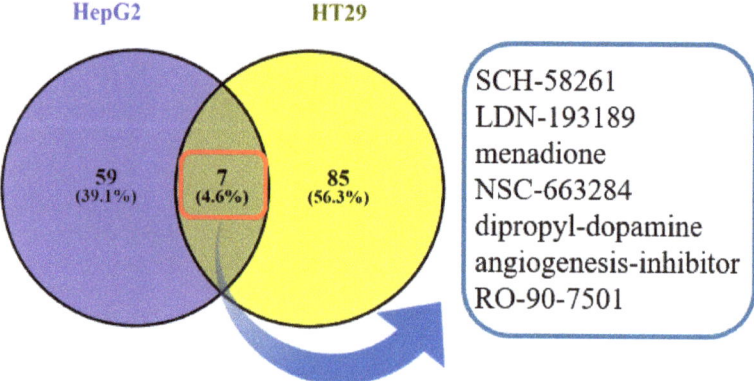

Figure 3. Gene analysis data of formulated curcumin. (**A**) The L1000 gene expression profiles of HT29 and HepG2 cells treated with formulated curcumin were analyzed by CLUE. The output data of PCLs

in both HT29 and HepG2 are shown at the bottom (score > 70). (**B**) PCLs list a score > 70 and are intersected by Venny website. Two common PLCs, NF-κB pathway inhibitor and vesicular transport LOF, are shown in the diagram. To avoid missing possible predicted functions of formulated curcumin, we used an intersection-driven approach to broadly cover these PCLs (score > 70). (**C**) The top 30 compounds (CP) are representative, while the complete list is provided in the Supplementary Information (score > 90). Details are in Supplementary Figure S3. (**D**) Intersection compounds using L1000 array analysis of formulated curcumin by CLUE. The connectivity score is based on the Kolmogorov–Smirnov enrichment statistical evaluation of each gene expression profile. The results provided from CLUE are expressed as a comprehensive connectivity score, showing that the same drug has a similar MOA on different cancer cells in CLUE, Connectivity Map and Library of Integrated Network-Based Cellular Signatures (LINCS) unified environment; PCL, perturbagen class; MOA, mechanism of action.

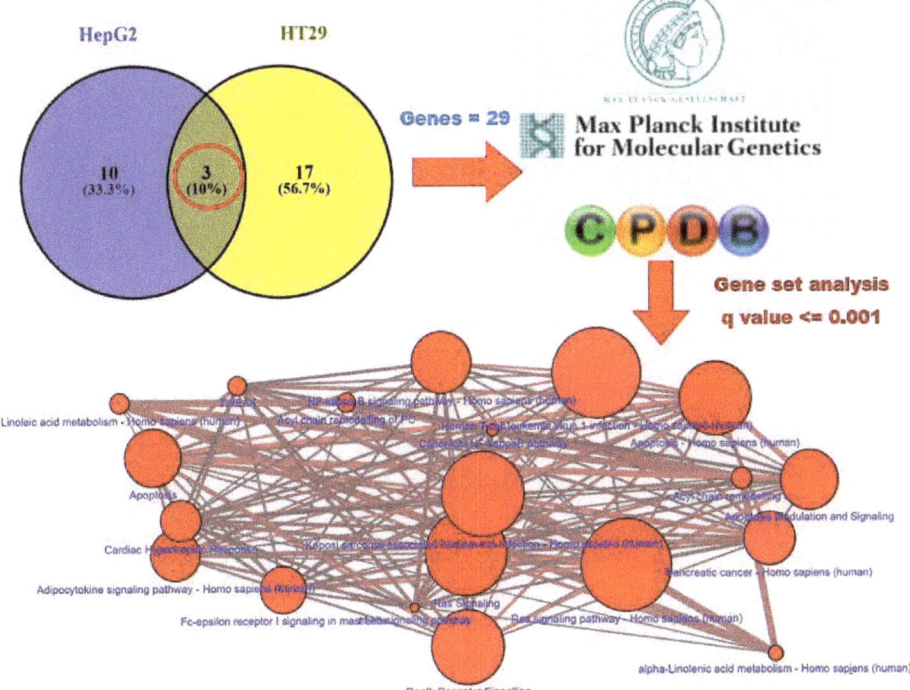

Figure 4. Possible pathways of formulated curcumin predicted by CPDB. Genes in two datasets were used to query CPDB in order to predict the pathways in which these genes were likely participating. The Venn diagram shows the intersecting PCLs (top, right). We focused on intersection results indicated by red circles. The results contained two PCLs, NF-κB pathway inhibitors and vesicular transport LOF and used their targets and member gene lists (total 22 genes) to query CPDB in order to analyze interaction network modules, biochemical pathways, and functional information. Top 50 prediction pathways are listed in Supplementary Figure S2, and top 20 pathways identified by CPDB analysis ($q < 0.001$) are shown at the bottom of the figure. The size of each dot denotes the entity number of genes in the pathway. The line between two dots was calculated by the function of these two pathways to indicate the number of genes overlapping said pathways. The breadth of the line denotes the strength of the correlation between two dots. The apoptosis was analyzed in this study (highlighted in yellow, Supplementary Figure S2). CPDB, ConsensusPathDB; PCL, perturbagen class; shRNA, short hairpin RNA.

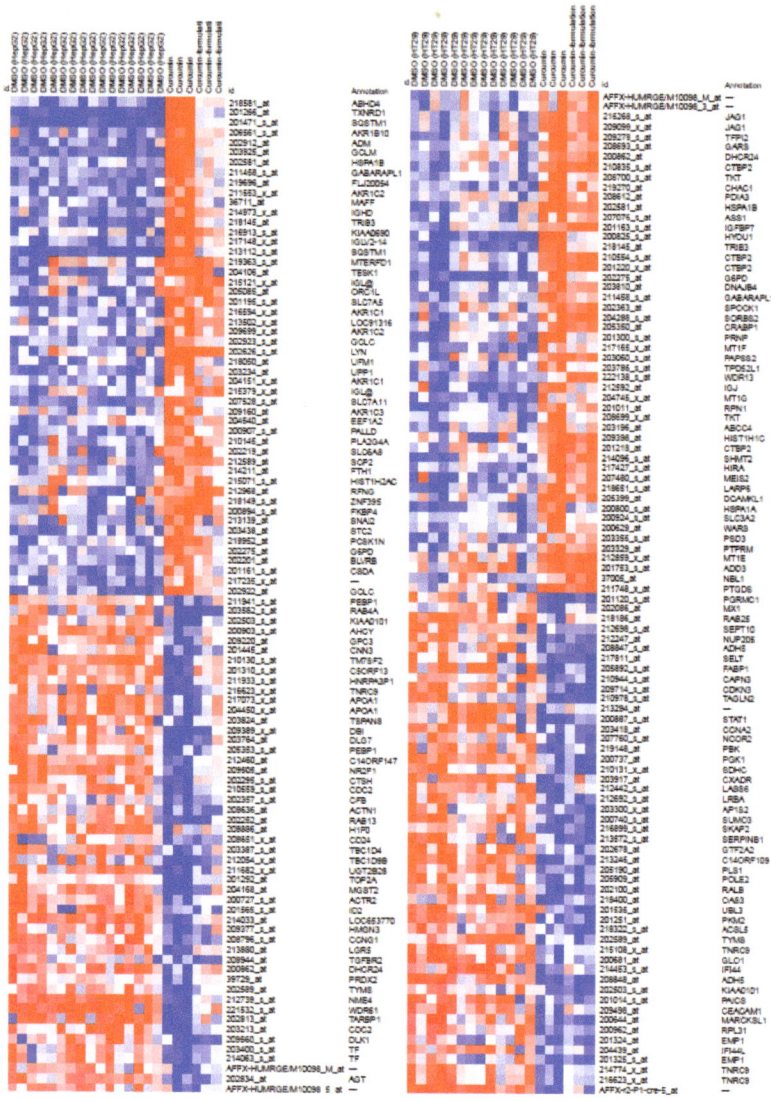

Figure 5. Heatmaps showing the top 50 up/down L1000 probes with similar expression patterns between conventional and formulated curcumin in HepG2 and HT29 cells, respectively. The horizontal axis denotes the treatments in three groups: (1) DMSO, (2) conventional curcumin, and (3) formulated curcumin. The vertical axis denotes the L1000 probe IDs and their corresponding gene names.

3.4. Formulated Curcumin Displays Stronger Inhibition on Population Growth of Huh7 Cells

To determine whether formulated curcumin retains the biological functions of conventional curcumin, we performed MTT assay to assess the cell proliferation and cell viability of conventional curcumin and formulated curcumin-treated Huh7 cells. As shown in Supplementary Figure S4, when the concentration of conventional or formulated curcumin increased, cell viability decreased after treatment with curcumin for 24–120 h. We also observed cytotoxicity of curcumin in Huh7 cells. The 50% inhibitory concentration (IC_{50}) value for conventional curcumin at 24, 48, 72, 96, and 120 h was around 90, 90, 60, 45, and 30 µM, respectively, while the IC_{50} value for formulated curcumin was around 60, 60, 30, 10, and 10 µM, respectively.

3.5. Cytotoxic Effect of Curcumin on Other HCC Cell Lines

To determine whether conventional and formulated curcumin could mediate the survival of other HCC cell lines, we first examined the effect of conventional and formulated curcumin on the viability of Huh7, Mahlavu, and PLC5 cells using MTT assay. While Huh7 cells are well differentiated, Mahlavu and PLC5 cells are poorly differentiated and carry *p53* mutations. To explore the cytotoxic activity of conventional and formulated curcumin against these HCC cell lines, we initiated an *in vitro* study by treating Huh7, Mahlavu, and PLC5 cells each with increasing dosages of conventional and formulated curcumin (0, 1, 3, 10, 30, 60, and 90 µM) for 72 h. MTT assay results indicated that both conventional and formulated curcumin significantly inhibit the viability of Huh7 (Figure 6A), Mahlavu (Figure 6B), and PLC5 (Figure 6C) cells. After 72 h post-treatment, formulated curcumin caused cytotoxicity in Huh7, Mahlavu, and PLC5 cells with an IC_{50} value of 38.1, 10.1, and 60.9 µM, respectively, while the IC_{50} values of conventional curcumin were 53.3, 35.4, and 82.5 µM, respectively (Figure 6A–C). Taken together, the results showed that both conventional and formulated curcumin inhibited the survival and proliferation of HCC cell lines in a dose-dependent manner. In addition, formulated curcumin was more effective than conventional curcumin.

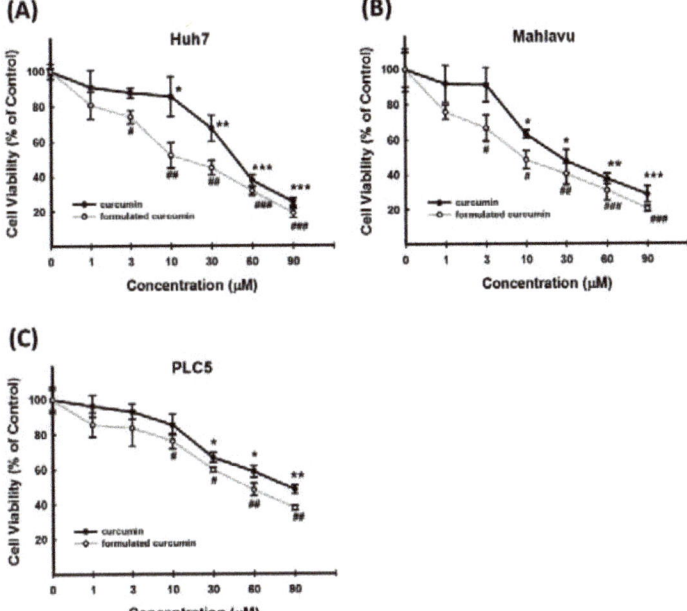

Figure 6. Cytotoxic effect of curcumin and formulated curcumin on other HCC cell lines (Huh7, Mahlavu, and PLC5). After separate treatment with 1, 3, 10, 30, 60, and 90 µM of conventional and formulated curcumin for 72 h, cell viability was determined by MTT assay and expressed as a percentage relative to the control group. Formulated curcumin was more effective than conventional curcumin on the basis of cell viability in the three cell lines tested. Formulated curcumin has higher cytotoxicity in (**A**) Huh7, (**B**) Mahlavu, and (**C**) PLC5 compared to conventional curcumin. #$p < 0.05$; ##$p < 0.01$; ###$p < 0.005$ compared to the control group (formulated curcumin). *$p < 0.05$; **$p < 0.01$; ***$p < 0.005$ compared to the control group (conventional curcumin). MTT, 3-(4,5-cimethylthiazol-2-yl)-2,5-diphenyl tetrazolium bromide.

3.6. Effects of Curcumin on Apoptosis-Related Protein Expression

MTT assay indicated that both conventional and formulated curcumin suppress cell viability. To determine whether cell viability inhibition is due to apoptosis, we examined the degree of apoptosis by PI and annexin V staining using flow cytometry. The results clearly demonstrated that 24 h post-treatment with 10–60 μM of conventional and formulated curcumin, the percentage of cells undergoing early apoptosis (annexin V$^+$/PI$^-$) and late apoptosis (annexin V$^+$/PI$^+$) increased, while the percentage of viable cells decreased (annexin V$^-$/PI$^-$) in a dose-dependent manner (Figure 7A). Comparison of effectiveness between conventional and formulated curcumin showed no significant statistical difference.

Caspase-3 activation is crucial for mitochondrial-dependent and mitochondrial-independent apoptotic pathways. Therefore, we examined the activity of caspase-3 by observing its active form (cleaved form) by western blotting in Huh7 cells (Figure 7B). Both conventional and formulated curcumin increased caspase-3 activity in Huh7 cells in a dose-dependent manner (Figure 7B). Caspase-3 activation led to cleavage of several substrates, including PARP. PARP cleavage was also determined by western blotting (Figure 7B). Therefore, conventional and formulated curcumin separately induced apoptosis by activating caspase-3 (Figure 7B).

Many antineoplastic drugs induce apoptosis of cancer cells via mitochondrial apoptotic pathways [34–36]. A hallmark of apoptosis induction via these pathways is a rapid, early breakdown of the mitochondrial membrane potential. Therefore, in this study, we also analyzed the mitochondrial function integrity posttreatment with conventional and formulated curcumin. Both conventional and formulated curcumin significantly induced mitochondrial membrane potential breakdown ($\Delta\Psi m$) in a concentration-dependent manner (Figure 7C), as determined by ELISA using the potential-sensitive dye JC-1.

Previous studies have shown that curcumin inhibits cancer cell proliferation via suppression of the ERK signaling pathway [37–39]. To investigate whether the ERK signaling pathway is involved in curcumin-induced apoptosis, ERK activation was evaluated by detecting ERK phosphorylation. Huh7 cells were exposed to 10–60 μM of conventional curcumin and formulated curcumin separately for 48 h, and ERK activation was determined by western blotting. As shown in Figure 7D, both conventional and formulated curcumin-induced phosphor-ERK down-regulation but with little change in the total ERK protein in Huh7 cells.

Recent studies have suggested that a curcumin-induced mitotic spindle defect and cell cycle arrest in human cancer cells occur through Aurora kinase inhibition [40–42]. To determine whether conventional and formulated curcumin inhibit Huh7 cell proliferation via down-regulation of Aurora-A expression, Huh7 cells were incubated with 0–60 μM of conventional and formulated curcumin separately for 48 h. We observed a significant decrease in the level of Aurora-A by western blotting (Figure 7D). These data suggested that the biological function of both conventional and formulated curcumin involves caspase-3 activation and ERK and Aurora-A down-regulation.

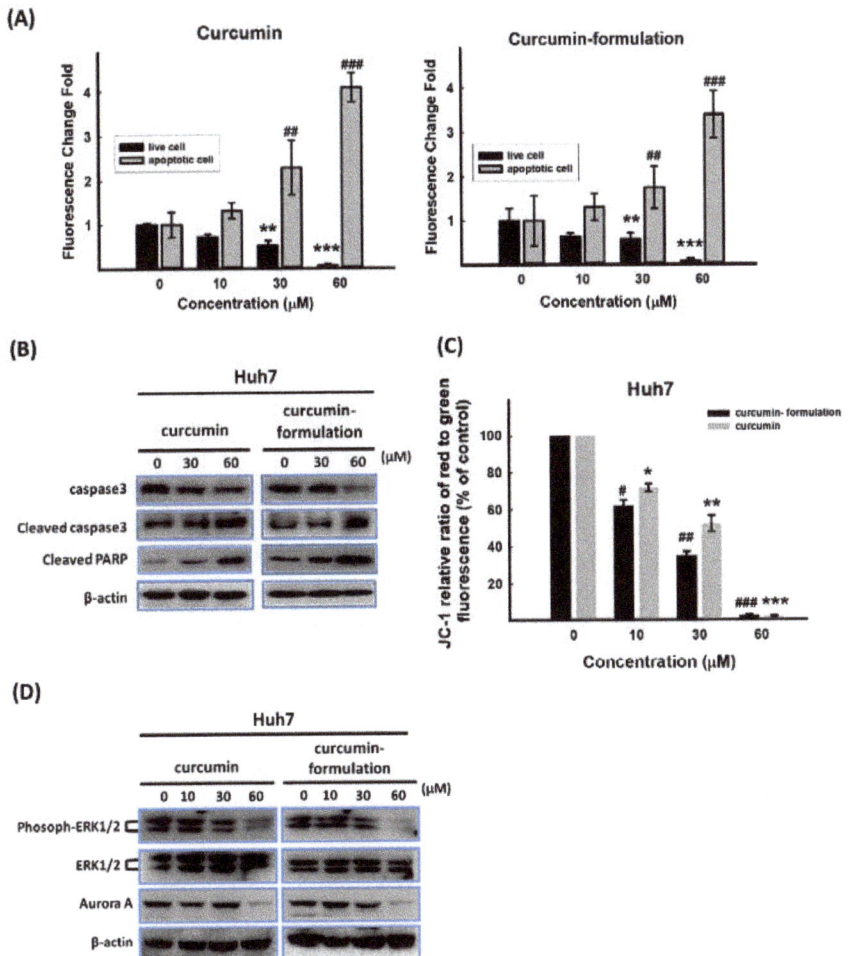

Figure 7. Both conventional and formulated curcumin caused apoptosis of Huh7 cells. (**A**) The cells were incubated and treated with conventional and formulated curcumin. After 24 h, the cells were subjected to annexin V/PI staining and analyzed by flow cytometry. Quantitative analysis of PI- or annexin V-positive cells is shown ($n = 3$). **$p < 0.01$ and ***$p < 0.005$ compared to the live-cell group without treatment. #$p < 0.01$ and ###$p < 0.005$ compared to the apoptotic cell group without treatment. (**B**) Huh7 cell lysates treated with conventional and formulated curcumin separately were subjected to immunoblot analysis. The expression levels of cleaved caspase-3, caspase-9, and PARP increased, demonstrating that the cells had undergone apoptosis. (**C**) The mitochondrial membrane potential ($\Delta\Psi m$) in Huh7 cells was analyzed using the JC-1 mitochondrial membrane potential assay. $\Delta\Psi m$ was lower in HCC cell lines treated with different concentrations (10, 30, and 60 µM) of conventional or formulated curcumin compared to control HCC cell lines (n = 3). *$p < 0.05$; **$p < 0.01$; and ***$p < 0.005$ compared to the group without conventional curcumin treatment. #$p < 0.05$; ##$p < 0.01$; and ###$p < 0.005$ compared to the group without formulated curcumin treatment. (**D**) P-ERK and AURKA expression was down-regulated by conventional and formulated curcumin in a concentration-dependent manner, as shown by immunoblot analysis results with anti-ERK, anti-P-ERK, and anti-AURKA antibodies. PI, propidium iodide; PARP, poly (ADP-ribose) polymerase; ERK, extracellular regulated protein kinase; AURKA, aurora kinase A.

3.7. Effects of Combination of Curcumin and Sorafenib

Sorafenib and curcumin both inhibited cell viability of two HCC cell lines (Huh7 and Hep3B) in a dose-dependent manner (Supplementary Figures S5 and S6). Therefore, we explored the potential effects of sorafenib in combination with conventional or formulated curcumin on Huh7, Mahlavu, and Hep3B cell proliferation. The cells were treated with various concentrations of sorafenib in combination with conventional or formulated curcumin for 48 h (Supplementary Figures S5A and S6). The results indicated that the combination of conventional or formulated curcumin with sorafenib has a stronger inhibitory effect on the population growth of HCC cell lines.

In this study, we demonstrated that both conventional and formulated curcumin inhibit Aurora kinase, preferentially suppress proliferation, and induce apoptosis of HCC cell lines. A previous study also indicated that curcumin induces apoptosis-associated autophagy [43,44]. Therefore, we investigated whether the combination of sorafenib and conventional or formulated curcumin can increase apoptosis of HCC cell lines. Cell cycle analysis revealed that adding conventional curcumin for 48 h leads to an apoptosis rate of 13.5% (sub-G1 population), similar to the 10.9% rate induced by sorafenib. We further examined whether conventional curcumin induces apoptosis of Hep3B cells. We found that the levels of cleaved caspase-3 proteins increased in conventional curcumin-treated, sorafenib-treated, and combination-treated cells (Supplementary Figure S5C). There was no notable difference between the three groups. Conventional curcumin and its combination with sorafenib both significantly induced accumulation of LC3-II (Supplementary Figure S5D), a lipidated form of LC3 that is considered an autophagosomal marker in mammals. Similar results were found with formulated curcumin treatment (data not shown). These results suggested that the combination of conventional curcumin and formulated curcumin separately with sorafenib induces apoptosis-associated autophagy in HCC cell lines.

4. Discussion

In this study, we reported that (i) both conventional and formulated curcumin induce apoptosis of HCC cell lines and down-regulate Aurora-A and (ii) a combination of conventional or formulated curcumin with sorafenib has a stronger inhibitory effect on HCC cell viability, demonstrating a possible prevention and therapeutic application for formulated curcumin to be used as a food supplement and medical food.

HCC most often develops and progresses with a lot of oxidative stress and inflammation. Phytochemicals, such as dietary polyphenols, endowed with potent antioxidant and anti-inflammatory properties, provide a suitable alternative for alleviation of HCC. Previous studies have reported that systemic bioavailability of curcumin in humans is very poor [45,46]. Solid dispersion manufacturing of poorly soluble drugs by spray-drying is a practical commercialization strategy to improve solubility and dissolution rates because of the reasonable cost of required materials and ease of scale-up [47].

Several methods have been developed to solve issue of low oral bioavailability of curcumin. One method is the use of a natural enhancer, such as alkaloid piperine. When 20 mg of piperine was given concomitantly with 2 g of curcumin, the serum curcumin increased by 20 times in humans and 1.56 times in rats. However, because piperine is a relatively selective CYP3A inhibitor [14], drug and food interactions with piperine are a concern. Some studies have used phospholipids as a delivery vehicle for curcumin. The oral bioavailability of curcumin-silica-coated flexible liposomes (curcumin-SLs) and curcumin-flexible liposomes (curcumin-FLs) was found to be 7.76- and 2.35-fold higher, respectively, compared to curcumin suspensions [20]. However, large-scale manufacturing will incur a substantial cost.

In the pharmaceutical industry, solid dispersion pellets are one of the drug delivery solutions for poorly soluble drugs. Solid dispersion pellets increase the solubility and release rate of a drug. For example, itraconazole is a triazole antifungal agent with low solubility. In some itraconazole solid dispersion pellets, the formulated itraconazole showed around 30- and 70-fold increase in the dissolution rate compared to pure drug [48]. Tanshinone IIA (TA), one of the liposoluble bioactive constituents extracted from the root of *Salvia miltiorrhiza* Bunge, has positive cardiovascular functions such as vasorelaxation and cardioprotective effects. The oral bioavailability of TA tSD pellets (a solid dispersion of a combination of PVP and poloxamer 188) in rabbit increased by 5.4 times compared to TA [49]. In this study, the oral bioavailability of formulated curcumin (solid dispersion pellets) increased significantly compared to conventional curcumin. Except for curcumin itself, all the materials used are inert and safe. In addition, because of the simple manufacturing process, solid dispersion pellets are also suitable for continuous and large-scale manufacturing, and the formulated curcumin can be used as a food supplement and medical food.

As mentioned in Section 3.1, 830–1000 μm is the size distribution of the pellets (formulated curcumin) determined by the sieving method. These pellets were formed by spraying ethanol solution of curcumin and PVP-K30 onto sugar spheres in a fluid-bed granulator machine. After re-dispersion in water, they were disintegrated to release free curcumin into the water as nanoparticles. The size of the curcumin particles (Z-average) measured using Zetasizer Nano ZS90 was determined to be 141.9 ± 5.1 nm, which could be filtered by a 0.45-μm pore filter. The nano size of the curcumin particles made it possible for them to be dissolved quickly in the dissolution medium. This was compatible with the data of the dissolution test.

In addition, using 1% SDS solution as the media for the dissolution test is mentioned in the US Pharmacopeia for curcuminoid tablets or curcuminoid capsules. Therefore, we used SDS in the medium to evaluate how well our newly formulated curcumin was improved in its dissolution by comparison with conventional curcumin. The results showed that dissolution of conventional curcumin in 1% SDS solution was only about 20% after 60 minutes, whereas that of the formulated curcumin was more than 85% after 10 minutes.

Supplementary Table S1 summarizes several studies that have reported techniques for enhancing curcumin oral bioavailability. While the formulated curcumin increases bioavailability over 800-fold, only approximately 5–100-fold increases have been achieved by other formulations. To clarify this difference, we investigated several pharmacokinetic parameters of conventional curcumin from these studies (supplementary Table S2) ([50–52]). In our study, administration of 500 mg/kg of curcumin resulted in a very low amount of curcumin in rat plasma: AUC_{0-t} (h × ng/mL) was 1.1, whereas in other studies the AUC_{0-t} (h × ng/mL) were 8.76, 80, and 60 after doses of 50, 340, and 500 mg/kg, respectively, were administered. If we used these AUC_{0-t} (h × ng/mL) from un-formulated curcumin to calculate the AUC for the formulated curcumin, an approximately 8–16-fold increase in bioavailability was obtained. In short, this study showed that oral administration of a novel solid dispersion of curcumin significantly increased its oral bioavailability compared with that of conventional curcumin. Although the C_{max} of the formulated curcumin is far below the effective concentrations of our cell culture experiments, administration of conventional curcumin (200 mg/kg) for days or weeks has been reported to exhibit significant biological activity against both chemically induced and xenograft hepatocarcinogenesis [53]. Because the formulated curcumin (single administration of 60 mg/kg) significantly increased the oral bioavailability compared with conventional curcumin (single administration of 500 mg/kg), repeating administration of the formulated curcumin at a higher dosage for a longer period of time can be expected to achieve a much higher C_{max}, and especially AUC, to display the biological effect of curcumin observed *in vitro*. It is noteworthy that the formulated curcumin, as expected, retains similar characteristics to conventional curcumin at the cellular level.

It is well known that the low oral bioavailability of curcumin is due to its poor solubility, poor intestinal permeability and extensive metabolism. In another study [52], authors have used phospholipid to formulate liposome of curcumin in order to enhance intestinal absorption of curcumin. In the fasted rat model (rats were fasted overnight to avoid interference by food), they proved that the AUC for liposome of curcumin increased about 5.5-fold compared with that for the conventional curcumin after administration of 340 mg/kg dose; the AUC 26.7 μg × min/mL is equivalent to 445 h × ng/mL. In our study, rats had free access to food and water. After administrating 60 mg/kg of the formulated curcumin, the AUC recorded was approximately 111 h × ng/mL. In addition, AUC/dose calculated in our study was higher than that in the previous study. Although we enhanced solubility of curcumin, we suggest that after administration of our formulation, curcumin was quickly released as nano particles then dissolved in gastric fluid or tiny oil droplet in food. Therefore, a part of curcumin was absorbed as free form and the rest was absorbed by pathway of oil absorption supported by bile salts. This was one of the advantages of the formulated curcumin which can be prepared easily and scaled up in industry. In future, we will conduct more experiments to verify this conclusion.

Both conventional and formulated curcumin were effective in decreasing proliferation and viability of HCC cell lines in a dose-dependent manner and induced apoptosis of HCC cell lines via mitochondria dysfunction *in vitro*. In the cell culture study, both forms of curcumin were dissolved completely before experiments, thus the benefits of formulated curcumin with improved solubility and dissolution rates could not be displayed. The *in vitro* study was carried out mainly to determine if the formulated curcumin retained similar characteristics of conventional curcumin at the cellular level. Mitochondrial hyperpolarization is a prerequisite for curcumin-induced apoptosis, and mitochondrial DNA (mtDNA) damage might be a probable mechanism for curcumin-induced apoptosis of HepG2 cells and might serve as the initial event triggering a chain of events leading to apoptosis [12]. Aurora kinases, such as Aurora-A, Aurora-B, and Aurora-C, comprise a family of centrosome-associated serine/threonine kinases that are overexpressed in various cancers and are potentially correlated with chemoresistance [54–56]. Curcumin administration [57] or Aurora-A inhibition by short interfering RNA (siRNA) [58] induces apoptosis. Curcumin has also been shown to down-regulate Notch1, the janus kinase (JAK)/signal transducer and activator of transcription (STAT) pathway, and multidrug resistance protein 1 (MDR1) expression and to inhibit histone deacetylase 1 (HDAC1) activity [12,13,42,59,60]. Sorafenib is the only chemotherapeutic drug that has been shown to be effective in prolonging the survival of HCC patients. However, the low rate of tolerance to sorafenib among HCC patients limits its use [31,32]. Recent preclinical studies have reported that combining sorafenib with other chemotherapeutic agents exerts synergistic effects [61,62], which could provide a promising strategy for the treatment of advanced HCC. In this study, conventional or formulated curcumin in combination with sorafenib inhibited the proliferation of HCC cell lines and exhibited a stronger inhibitory effect on HCC cell lines. Taken together, the formulated curcumin appeared to have properties similar to conventional curcumin, raising the possibility that our formulated curcumin could enhance cytotoxicity against HCC.

In addition, our bioinformatics screening platform effectively identified the molecular mechanisms of a phytochemical via gene expression profiles. C-Map can be queried to identify specific gene signatures from small molecules, including FDA-approved drugs. CLUE is similar to C-Map but considerably larger, with > 1.1 million L1000 profiles; therefore, similarity scores for compounds in CLUE can be obtained to identify their molecular actions. Similar results for conventional and formulated curcumin suggested that only solubility and oral bioavailability have been altered in formulated curcumin. Curcumin is known to exert strong anti-inflammatory effects by interrupting NF-κB signaling at multiple levels. Based on CLUE analysis, formulated curcumin can be predicted to have a similar action as NF-κB pathway inhibitors. Furthermore, analysis via CPDB suggests that curcumin can be linked to TNF related weak inducer of apoptosis as well as TNF mediated NF-κB pathway. Therefore, our screening platform not only confirms that the formulated curcumin has similar mechanism with unformulated curcumin, but it also predicts the novel mechanism of formulated curcumin, such as suppression of HMGB1 mediated inflammation by THBD (label in red in Supplementary Figure S2).

In conclusion, our curcumin was formulated in pellet form, which not only improved its oral bioavailability but also provided high flexibility of use. For example, it would be easy to adjust the dosage and combine the pellets with other ingredients. In addition, as a functional food and alternative medicine, it would be suitable for those who cannot swallow tablets or capsules.

Supplementary Materials: The following are available online: http://www.mdpi.com/2072-6643/11/12/2982/s1. Figure S1. The dissolution rates of conventional and formulated curcumin in 1% sodium dodecyl sulfate medium, Figure S2. Prediction of highly correlated pathways, Figure S3. The output data of compounds (CP, score ≥ 90) was analyzed via CLUE, and detected their similarity among these gene expression profiles, Figure S4. Curcumin and the formulated curcumin affect the cell viability of Huh7 cells, Figure S5. Inhibitory effect of the combination of sorafenib and conventional or formulated curcumin on HCC cell lines, Figure S6. Effect of sorafenib with or without curcumin/formulated curcumin on Mahlavu and Hep3B cell viability, Table S1. Comparison between our study and previous studies on the improvement of solubility/oral bioavailability of curcumin formulation, Table S2. Comparison of pharmacokinetic parameters of curcumin in rat plasma following oral administration.

Author Contributions: S.-C.L. and W.-H.H. initiated the studies, performed and analyzed the majority of the experiments. C.-L.S., T.-H.T., and C.-Y.F.H. conceived and designed the experiments. K.-T.L., Z.-Y.H., K.-L.C., C.-L.T., and A.-H.D. performed the experiments and analyzed data. All authors contributed his/her efforts to write the manuscript.

Funding: This work was supported by the grants from the Yang-Ming University collaboration project (YM106C024). This work was also supported by grants from the National Science Council, Taiwan (NSC 101-2313-B-003-002-MY3) and the Ministry of Science and Technology, Taiwan (MOST 106-2320-B-003-006-MY3, MOST 107-2320-B-003-002-MY2, and MOST 107-2320-B-010-040-MY3).

Acknowledgments: We thank the Everest Pharm. Industrial Co., LTD., Chiayi, Taiwan, for the experiment drug supply and Rosetta Pharmamate Co., Ltd. for helping with animal pharmacokinetic study.

Conflicts of Interest: No potential conflicts of interest were disclosed. Competing financial interests statement: The authors declare that there is no conflict of interest.

Abbreviations

Full Name	Abbreviations
area under curve	AUC
aurora kinase A	AURKA
bioavailability	BA
dimethyl sulfoxide	DMSO
Dulbecco's modified Eagle's medium	DMEM
enhanced chemiluminescence	ECL
extracellular regulated protein kinases	ERK
hepatocellular carcinoma	HCC
high performance liquid chromatography	HPLC
histone deacetylase 1	HDAC1
janus kinase	JAK
limit of quantification	LOQ
limits of detection	LOD
multidrug resistance protein 1	MDR1
platelet-derived growth factor receptor beta	PDGFR-β
poly (ADP-ribose) polymerase	PARP
polydispersity index	PDI
polyvinylidene difluoride	PVDF
propidium iodide	PI
signal transducer and activator of transcription	STAT
sodium dodecyl sulfate	SDS
Tanshinone IIA	TA
The Food and Drug Administration	FDA
vascular endothelial growth factor receptor	VEGFR

References

1. Sheikh, B.Y.; Sarker, M.M.R.; Kamarudin, M.N.A.; Ismail, A. Prophetic medicine as potential functional food elements in the intervention of cancer: A review. *Biomed. Pharm.* **2017**, *95*, 614–648. [CrossRef] [PubMed]
2. Shahidi, F. Nutraceuticals, Functional Foods and Dietary Supplements in Health and Disease. *J. Food Drug Anal.* **2012**, *20*, 226–230.

3. Sharma, R.A.; Gescher, A.J.; Steward, W.P. Curcumin: The story so far. *Eur. J. Cancer.* **2005**, *41*, 1955–1968. [CrossRef] [PubMed]
4. Oyama, Y.; Masuda, T.; Nakata, M.; Chikahisa, L.; Yamazaki, Y.; Miura, K.; Okagawa, M. Protective actions of 5′-n-alkylated curcumins on living cells suffering from oxidative stress. *Eur. J. Pharmacol.* **1998**, *360*, 65–71. [CrossRef]
5. Maheshwari, R.K.; Singh, A.K.; Gaddipati, J.; Srimal, R.C. Multiple biological activities of curcumin: A short review. *Life Sci.* **2006**, *78*, 2081–2087. [CrossRef]
6. Ono, K.; Hasegawa, K.; Naiki, H.; Yamada, M. Curcumin has potent anti-amyloidogenic effects for Alzheimer's beta-amyloid fibrils *in vitro*. *J. Neurosci. Res.* **2004**, *75*, 742–750. [CrossRef]
7. Pal, S.; Choudhuri, T.; Chattopadhyay, S.; Bhattacharya, A.; Datta, G.K.; Das, T.; Sa, G. Mechanisms of curcumin-induced apoptosis of Ehrlich's ascites carcinoma cells. *Biochem. Biophys. Res. Commun.* **2001**, *288*, 658–665. [CrossRef]
8. Pal, S.; Bhattacharyya, S.; Choudhuri, T.; Datta, G.K.; Das, T.; Sa, G. Amelioration of immune cell number depletion and potentiation of depressed detoxification system of tumor-bearing mice by curcumin. *Cancer Detect. Prev.* **2005**, *29*, 470–478. [CrossRef]
9. Nautiyal, J.; Banerjee, S.; Kanwar, S.S.; Yu, Y.; Patel, B.B.; Sarkar, F.H.; Majumdar, A.P. Curcumin enhances dasatinib-induced inhibition of growth and transformation of colon cancer cells. *Int. J. Cancer* **2011**, *128*, 951–961. [CrossRef]
10. Duvoix, A.; Blasius, R.; Delhalle, S.; Schnekenburger, M.; Morceau, F.; Henry, E.; Dicato, M.; Diederich, M. Chemopreventive and therapeutic effects of curcumin. *Cancer Lett.* **2005**, *223*, 181–190. [CrossRef]
11. Kunwar, A.; Barik, A.; Mishra, B.; Rathinasamy, K.; Pandey, R.; Priyadarsini, K.I. Quantitative cellular uptake, localization and cytotoxicity of curcumin in normal and tumor cells. *Biochim. Biophys. Acta* **2008**, *1780*, 673–679. [CrossRef]
12. Cao, J.; Liu, Y.; Jia, L.; Zhou, H.M.; Kong, Y.; Yang, G.; Jiang, L.P.; Li, Q.J.; Zhong, L.F. Curcumin induces apoptosis through mitochondrial hyperpolarization and mtDNA damage in human hepatoma G2 cells. *Free Radic. Biol. Med.* **2007**, *43*, 968–975. [CrossRef] [PubMed]
13. Wang, W.Z.; Zhang, B.Y.; Yuan, J.; Mao, J.W.; Mei, W.J. [Effect of curcumin on JAK-STAT signaling pathway in hepatoma cell lines]. *Yao Xue Xue Bao Acta Pharm. Sin.* **2009**, *44*, 1434–1439.
14. Deguchi, A. Curcumin targets in inflammation and cancer. *Endocr. Metab. Immune Disord. Drug Targets* **2015**, *15*, 88–96. [CrossRef] [PubMed]
15. Lin, L.I.; Ke, Y.F.; Ko, Y.C.; Lin, J.K. Curcumin inhibits SK-Hep-1 hepatocellular carcinoma cell invasion *in vitro* and suppresses matrix metalloproteinase-9 secretion. *Oncology* **1998**, *55*, 349–353. [CrossRef] [PubMed]
16. Magini, A.; Polchi, A.; Di Meo, D.; Mariucci, G.; Sagini, K.; De Marco, F.; Cassano, T.; Giovagnoli, S.; Dolcetta, D.; Emiliani, C. TFEB activation restores migration ability to Tsc1-deficient adult neural stem/progenitor cells. *Hum. Mol. Genet.* **2017**, *26*, 3303–3312. [CrossRef]
17. Pan, M.H.; Huang, T.M.; Lin, J.K. Biotransformation of curcumin through reduction and glucuronidation in mice. *Drug Metab. Dispos. Biol. Fate Chem.* **1999**, *27*, 486–494.
18. Vareed, S.K.; Kakarala, M.; Ruffin, M.T.; Crowell, J.A.; Normolle, D.P.; Djuric, Z.; Brenner, D.E. Pharmacokinetics of curcumin conjugate metabolites in healthy human subjects. *Cancer Epidemiol. Biomark. Prev.* **2008**, *17*, 1411–1417. [CrossRef]
19. Wahlstrom, B.; Blennow, G. A study on the fate of curcumin in the rat. *Acta Pharmacol. Toxicol.* **1978**, *43*, 86–92. [CrossRef]
20. Siviero, A.; Gallo, E.; Maggini, V.; Gori, L.; Mugelli, A.; Firenzuoli, F.; Vannacci, A. Curcumin, a golden spice with a low bioavailability. *J. Herb. Med.* **2015**, *5*, 57–70. [CrossRef]
21. Song, J.X.; Sun, Y.R.; Peluso, I.; Zeng, Y.; Yu, X.; Lu, J.H.; Xu, Z.; Wang, M.Z.; Liu, L.F.; Huang, Y.Y.; et al. A novel curcumin analog binds to and activates TFEB *in vitro* and *in vivo* independent of MTOR inhibition. *Autophagy* **2016**, *12*, 1372–1389. [CrossRef] [PubMed]
22. Magini, A.; Polchi, A.; Di Meo, D.; Buratta, S.; Chiaradia, E.; Germani, R.; Emiliani, C.; Tancini, B. Curcumin analogue C1 promotes hex and gal recruitment to the plasma membrane via mTORC1-independent TFEB activation. *Int. J. Mol. Sci.* **2019**, *20*, 1363. [CrossRef] [PubMed]
23. Vikash, K.; Kumar, M.S.; Amit, L.; Singh, R. Multiple unit dosage form-pellet and pelletization techniques: An overview. *Int. J. Res. Ayurveda Pharm.* **2011**, *2*, 121–125.
24. Dhirendra, K.; Lewis, S.; Udupa, N.; Atin, K. Solid dispersions: A review. *Pak. J. Pharm. Sci.* **2009**, *22*, 234–246.

25. Lamb, J.; Crawford, E.D.; Peck, D.; Modell, J.W.; Blat, I.C.; Wrobel, M.J.; Lerner, J.; Brunet, J.P.; Subramanian, A.; Ross, K.N.; et al. The Connectivity Map: Using gene-expression signatures to connect small molecules, genes, and disease. *Science* **2006**, *313*, 1929–1935. [CrossRef]
26. Subramanian, A.; Narayan, R.; Corsello, S.M.; Peck, D.D.; Natoli, T.E.; Lu, X.; Gould, J.; Davis, J.F.; Tubelli, A.A.; Asiedu, J.K.; et al. A Next Generation Connectivity Map: L1000 Platform and the First 1,000,000 Profiles. *Cell* **2017**, *171*, 1437–1452. [CrossRef]
27. Guo, J.; Li, L.; Guo, B.; Liu, D.; Shi, J.; Wu, C.; Chen, J.; Zhang, X.; Wu, J. Mechanisms of resistance to chemotherapy and radiotherapy in hepatocellular carcinoma. *Transl. Cancer Res.* **2018**, *7*, 765–781. [CrossRef]
28. Lohitesh, K.; Chowdhury, R.; Mukherjee, S. Resistance a major hindrance to chemotherapy in hepatocellular carcinoma: An insight. *Cancer Cell Int.* **2018**, *18*, 44. [CrossRef]
29. Llovet, J.M.; Ricci, S.; Mazzaferro, V.; Hilgard, P.; Gane, E.; Blanc, J.F.; de Oliveira, A.C.; Santoro, A.; Raoul, J.L.; Forner, A.; et al. Sorafenib in advanced hepatocellular carcinoma. *N. Eng. J. Med.* **2008**, *359*, 378–390. [CrossRef]
30. Reig, M.; Bruix, J. Sorafenib for hepatocellular carcinoma: Global validation. *Gastroenterology* **2009**, *137*, 1171–1173. [CrossRef]
31. Welker, M.W.; Lubomierski, N.; Gog, C.; Herrmann, E.; Engels, K.; Vogl, T.J.; Bechstein, W.O.; Zeuzem, S.; Trojan, J. Efficacy and safety of sorafenib in advanced hepatocellular carcinoma under daily practice conditions. *J. Chemother.* **2010**, *22*, 205–211. [CrossRef] [PubMed]
32. Morimoto, M.; Numata, K.; Kondo, M.; Hidaka, H.; Takada, J.; Shibuya, A.; Kobayashi, S.; Ohkawa, S.; Okuse, C.; Morita, S.; et al. Higher discontinuation and lower survival rates are likely in elderly Japanese patients with advanced hepatocellular carcinoma receiving sorafenib. *Hepatol. Res.* **2011**, *41*, 296–302. [CrossRef] [PubMed]
33. Liao, S.C.; Hsu, H.W.; Chuang, K.L.; Huang, Z.Y.; Lin, K.T.; Hsu, W.H.; Chang, K.H.; Huang, C.F.; Su, C.L. Using the Pleiotropic Characteristics of Curcumin to Validate the Potential Application of a Novel Gene Expression Screening Platform. *Nutrients* **2019**, *11*, 1397. [CrossRef]
34. Jendrossek, V.; Handrick, R.; Belka, C. Celecoxib activates a novel mitochondrial apoptosis signaling pathway. *FASEB J.* **2003**, *17*, 1547–1549. [CrossRef] [PubMed]
35. Wieder, T.; Essmann, F.; Prokop, A.; Schmelz, K.; Schulze-Osthoff, K.; Beyaert, R.; Dorken, B.; Daniel, P.T. Activation of caspase-8 in drug-induced apoptosis of B-lymphoid cells is independent of CD95/Fas receptor-ligand interaction and occurs downstream of caspase-3. *Blood* **2001**, *97*, 1378–1387. [CrossRef]
36. Engels, I.H.; Stepczynska, A.; Stroh, C.; Lauber, K.; Berg, C.; Schwenzer, R.; Wajant, H.; Janicke, R.U.; Porter, A.G.; Belka, C.; et al. Caspase-8/FLICE functions as an executioner caspase in anticancer drug-induced apoptosis. *Oncogene* **2000**, *19*, 4563–4573. [CrossRef]
37. Shin, H.K.; Kim, J.; Lee, E.J.; Kim, S.H. Inhibitory effect of curcumin on motility of human oral squamous carcinoma YD-10B cells via suppression of ERK and NF-kappaB activations. *Phytother. Res.* **2010**, *24*, 577–582. [CrossRef]
38. Xie, Y.Q.; Wu, X.B.; Tang, S.Q. Curcumin treatment alters ERK-1/2 signaling *in vitro* and inhibits nasopharyngeal carcinoma proliferation in mouse xenografts. *Int. J. Clin. Exp. Med.* **2014**, *7*, 108–114.
39. Guo, Y.; Shan, Q.; Gong, Y.; Lin, J.; Shi, F.; Shi, R.; Yang, X. Curcumin induces apoptosis via simultaneously targeting AKT/mTOR and RAF/MEK/ERK survival signaling pathways in human leukemia THP-1 cells. *Pharmazie* **2014**, *69*, 229–233.
40. Wolanin, K.; Magalska, A.; Mosieniak, G.; Klinger, R.; McKenna, S.; Vejda, S.; Sikora, E.; Piwocka, K. Curcumin affects components of the chromosomal passenger complex and induces mitotic catastrophe in apoptosis-resistant Bcr-Abl-expressing cells. *Mol. Cancer Res.* **2006**, *4*, 457–469. [CrossRef]
41. Liu, H.S.; Ke, C.S.; Cheng, H.C.; Huang, C.Y.; Su, C.L. Curcumin-induced mitotic spindle defect and cell cycle arrest in human bladder cancer cells occurs partly through inhibition of aurora A. *Mol. Pharmacol.* **2011**, *80*, 638–646. [CrossRef] [PubMed]
42. Ke, C.S.; Liu, H.S.; Yen, C.H.; Huang, G.C.; Cheng, H.C.; Huang, C.Y.; Su, C.L. Curcumin-induced Aurora-A suppression not only causes mitotic defect and cell cycle arrest but also alters chemosensitivity to anticancer drugs. *J. Nutr. Biochem.* **2014**, *25*, 526–539. [CrossRef] [PubMed]
43. Li, B.; Takeda, T.; Tsuiji, K.; Wong, T.F.; Tadakawa, M.; Kondo, A.; Nagase, S.; Yaegashi, N. Curcumin induces cross-regulation between autophagy and apoptosis in uterine leiomyosarcoma cells. *Int. J. Gynecol. Cancer* **2013**, *23*, 803–808. [CrossRef] [PubMed]

44. Zhou, T.; Ye, L.; Bai, Y.; Sun, A.; Cox, B.; Liu, D.; Li, Y.; Liotta, D.; Snyder, J.P.; Fu, H.; et al. Autophagy and apoptosis in hepatocellular carcinoma induced by EF25-(GSH)2: A novel curcumin analog. *PLoS ONE* **2014**, *9*. [CrossRef] [PubMed]
45. Lao, C.D.; Ruffin, M.T.T.; Normolle, D.; Heath, D.D.; Murray, S.I.; Bailey, J.M.; Boggs, M.E.; Crowell, J.; Rock, C.L.; Brenner, D.E. Dose escalation of a curcuminoid formulation. *BMC Complementary Altern. Med.* **2006**, *6*, 10. [CrossRef]
46. Sharma, R.A.; Euden, S.A.; Platton, S.L.; Cooke, D.N.; Shafayat, A.; Hewitt, H.R.; Marczylo, T.H.; Morgan, B.; Hemingway, D.; Plummer, S.M.; et al. Phase I clinical trial of oral curcumin: Biomarkers of systemic activity and compliance. *Clin. Cancer Res.* **2004**, *10*, 6847–6854. [CrossRef]
47. Vasconcelos, T.; Sarmento, B.; Costa, P. Solid dispersions as strategy to improve oral bioavailability of poor water soluble drugs. *Drug Discov. Today* **2007**, *12*, 1068–1075. [CrossRef]
48. Ye, G.; Wang, S.; Heng, P.W.; Chen, L.; Wang, C. Development and optimization of solid dispersion containing pellets of itraconazole prepared by high shear pelletization. *Int. J. Pharm.* **2007**, *337*, 80–87. [CrossRef]
49. Li, J.; Liu, P.; Liu, J.P.; Zhang, W.L.; Yang, J.K.; Fan, Y.Q. Novel Tanshinone II A ternary solid dispersion pellets prepared by a single-step technique: In vitro and in vivo evaluation. *Eur. J. Pharm. Biopharm.* **2012**, *80*, 426–432. [CrossRef]
50. Yang, K.Y.; Lin, L.C.; Tseng, T.Y.; Wang, S.C.; Tsai, T.H. Oral bioavailability of curcumin in rat and the herbal analysis from Curcuma longa by LC-MS/MS. *J. Chromatogr. B* **2007**, *853*, 183–189. [CrossRef]
51. Khalil, N.M.; do Nascimento, T.C.; Casa, D.M.; Dalmolin, L.F.; de Mattos, A.C.; Hoss, I.; Romano, M.A.; Mainardes, R.M. Pharmacokinetics of curcumin-loaded PLGA and PLGA-PEG blend nanoparticles after oral administration in rats. *Colloids Surf. B Biointerfaces* **2013**, *101*, 353–360. [CrossRef] [PubMed]
52. Marczylo, T.H.; Verschoyle, R.D.; Cooke, D.N.; Morazzoni, P.; Steward, W.P.; Gescher, A.J. Comparison of systemic availability of curcumin with that of curcumin formulated with phosphatidylcholine. *Cancer Chemother. Pharmacol.* **2007**, *60*, 171–177. [CrossRef] [PubMed]
53. Darvesh, A.S.; Aggarwal, B.B.; Bishayee, A. Curcumin and liver cancer: A review. *Curr. Pharm. Biotechnol.* **2012**, *13*, 218–228. [CrossRef] [PubMed]
54. Lin, Z.Z.; Jeng, Y.M.; Hu, F.C.; Pan, H.W.; Tsao, H.W.; Lai, P.L.; Lee, P.H.; Cheng, A.L.; Hsu, H.C. Significance of Aurora B overexpression in hepatocellular carcinoma. Aurora B Overexpression in HCC. *BMC Cancer* **2010**, *10*, 461. [CrossRef]
55. Carmena, M.; Earnshaw, W.C. The cellular geography of aurora kinases. *Nat. Rev. Mol. Cell Biol.* **2003**, *4*, 842–854. [CrossRef]
56. Jeng, Y.M.; Peng, S.Y.; Lin, C.Y.; Hsu, H.C. Overexpression and amplification of Aurora-A in hepatocellular carcinoma. *Clin. Cancer Res.* **2004**, *10*, 2065–2071. [CrossRef]
57. Woo, J.H.; Kim, Y.H.; Choi, Y.J.; Kim, D.G.; Lee, K.S.; Bae, J.H.; Min, D.S.; Chang, J.S.; Jeong, Y.J.; Lee, Y.H.; et al. Molecular mechanisms of curcumin-induced cytotoxicity: Induction of apoptosis through generation of reactive oxygen species, down-regulation of Bcl-XL and IAP, the release of cytochrome c and inhibition of Akt. *Carcinogenesis* **2003**, *24*, 1199–1208. [CrossRef]
58. Du, J.; Hannon, G.J. Suppression of p160ROCK bypasses cell cycle arrest after Aurora-A/STK15 depletion. *Proc. Natl. Acad. Sci. USA* **2004**, *101*, 8975–8980. [CrossRef]
59. Ning, L.; Wentworth, L.; Chen, H.; Weber, S.M. Down-regulation of Notch1 signaling inhibits tumor growth in human hepatocellular carcinoma. *Am. J. Transl. Res.* **2009**, *1*, 358–366.
60. Wang, W.; Zhang, B.; Chen, H.; Zhang, L. Anticancer activities of curcumin on human hepatocarcinoma cell line Sk-hep-1. *Zhongguo Zhong Yao Za Zhi* **2010**, *35*, 485–488.
61. Singh, S.; Singh, P.P.; Roberts, L.R.; Sanchez, W. Chemopreventive strategies in hepatocellular carcinoma. *Nat. Rev. Gastroenterol. Hepatol.* **2014**, *11*, 45–54. [CrossRef] [PubMed]
62. Abou-Alfa, G.K.; Johnson, P.; Knox, J.J.; Capanu, M.; Davidenko, I.; Lacava, J.; Leung, T.; Gansukh, B.; Saltz, L.B. Doxorubicin plus sorafenib vs doxorubicin alone in patients with advanced hepatocellular carcinoma: A randomized trial. *JAMA* **2010**, *304*, 2154–2160. [CrossRef] [PubMed]

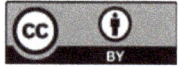

© 2019 by the authors. Licensee MDPI, Basel, Switzerland. This article is an open access article distributed under the terms and conditions of the Creative Commons Attribution (CC BY) license (http://creativecommons.org/licenses/by/4.0/).

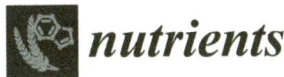 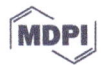

Article

Anti-Atherosclerotic Properties of Wild Rice in Low-Density Lipoprotein Receptor Knockout Mice: The Gut Microbiome, Cytokines, and Metabolomics Study

Mohammed H. Moghadasian [1,2,*], Ramandeep Kaur [1,2], Kayla Kostal [1,2], Akhila A. Joshi [1,2], Mahboubeh Molaei [2], Khuong Le [2], Gabor Fischer [3], Francesca Bonomini [4], Gaia Favero [4], Rita Rezzani [4], Branden S. J. Gregorchuk [5], Vanessa Leung-Shing [5], Michelle Wuzinski [5], Andy I. Seo [5] and Denice C. Bay [5]

1. Department of Human Nutritional Sciences, University of Manitoba, Winnipeg, MB R3T 2N2, Canada; kaurr27@myumanitoba.ca (R.K.); kkostal@sbrc.ca (K.K.); joshiaa@myumanitoba.ca (A.A.J.)
2. Canadian Center for Agri-food Research in Health and Medicine, St. Boniface Hospital Research Center, Winnipeg, MB R2H 2A6, Canada; mahbobe.molaei@gmail.com (M.M.); kle@sbrc.ca (K.L.)
3. Department of Pathology, University of Manitoba, Winnipeg, MB R3T 2N2, Canada; Gabor.Fischer@umanitoba.ca
4. Department of Clinical and Experimental Sciences, University of Brescia, 25121 Brescia, Italy; francesca.bonomini@unibs.it (F.B.); gaia.favero@unibs.it (G.F.); rita.rezzani@unibs.it (R.R.)
5. Department of Medical Microbiology & Infectious Diseases, University of Manitoba, Winnipeg, MB R3E 0J9, Canada; umgreg43@myumanitoba.ca (B.S.J.G.); V.LeungShing1@nuigalway.ie (V.L.-S.); wuzinskm@myumanitoba.ca (M.W.); seoi@myumanitoba.ca (A.I.S.); denice.bay@umanitoba.ca (D.C.B.)
* Correspondence: mmoghadasian@sbrc.ca; Tel.: +1-204-235-3934; Fax: +204-237-4018

Received: 22 October 2019; Accepted: 16 November 2019; Published: 28 November 2019

Abstract: Background and aim: We previously reported the anti-atherogenic properties of wild rice in low-density lipoprotein receptor knockout (LDL-r-KO) mice. The present study aimed to discover the mechanism of action for such effects. Materials: Fecal and plasma samples from the wild rice treated and control mice were used. Fecal bacterial population was estimated while using 16S rDNA technology. The plasma samples were used to estimate the levels of 35 inflammatory markers and metabolomics, while using Meso Scale multiplex assay and liquid chromatography-mass spectrometry (LC-MS/MS) techniques. Results: Many bacteria, particularly *Anaeroplasma sp.*, *Acetatifactor sp.*, and *Prophyromonadaceae sp.*, were found in higher quantities in the feces of wild rice fed mice as compared to the controls. Cytokine profiles were significantly different between the plasma of treated and control mice. Among them, an increase in the level of IL-10 and erythropoietin (EPO) could explain the anti-atherogenic properties of wild rice. Among many metabolites tested in plasma of these animals, surprisingly, we found an approximately 60% increase in the levels of glucose in the wild rice fed mice as compared to that in the control mice. Conclusion: Additional studies warrant further investigation of the interplay among gut microbiome, inflammatory status, and macronutrient metabolism.

Keywords: wild rice; microbiome; metabolomics; atherosclerosis; LDL-r-KO mice; cytokines; 16S rDNA; plasma; feces; proteins; carbohydrates; functional food

1. Introduction

Appropriate types of diets and levels of physical activities are believed to be major determinants of maintaining optimal health [1,2]. Many studies have reported that regular consumption of certain foods, particularly plant-based foods, such as whole grains, fruits, and vegetables, as well as fish, are associated with decreased prevalence of chronic diseases, specifically cardiovascular disease [3,4]. Phytochemicals that are contained within these foods are believed to mediate these health benefits and include phytosterols, dietary fiber, dietary antioxidants, oleic acid, and docosahexaenoic acid (DHA). On the other hand, food ingredients, such as saturated fat, heavy metals, and other contaminants, may increase the risk of cardiovascular disease [5,6]. One of the common chronic diseases with a significant negative impact on the quality of life is atherosclerotic vascular disease, which remains the main cause of global morbidity and mortality [7]. A fundamental contributor in the pathogenesis of atherosclerosis is the oxidation of low-density lipoprotein (LDL) particles, which are taken up by macrophages, initiating foam cell formation in the arterial wall [8]. Therefore, foods with an ability to lower LDL cholesterol and prevent LDL oxidation have been at the center of atherosclerosis prevention [3].

Wild rice has many health benefits when consumed, as noted in historical documents of the indigenous peoples of North America for centuries, as well as other nations, including Chinese and Europeans [9]. Although it is not a grain, wild rice is recognized as a 'whole grain' [10]. Unlike conventional rice, wild rice is usually consumed unprocessed, meaning that wild rice maintains its natural outer layers and contains significantly higher amounts of dietary fiber, micronutrients, and phytochemical compounds. Another important difference between wild rice and conventional white rice is the type of starch they produce [9]. Wild rice contains resistant starch, being often considered to act like a prebiotic; prebiotics are compounds within foods that beneficially affect gut bacterial population and diversity [11]. Gut bacteria produce many metabolites that can either benefit or harm the cardiovascular system [12].

We have previously reported cholesterol-lowering effects and anti-atherosclerotic properties of plant sterols in apolipoprotein E knockout (apo E-KO) mice [13,14]. Over the past few years, we also tested the potential anti-atherosclerotic effects of wild rice in LDL receptor knockout (LDL-r-KO) mice [15,16]. In these studies, we observed significant anti-atherogenic effects of wild rice; however, we were not able to identify a mechanism of action. Atherosclerosis is a multi-factorial disease, in which alterations in inflammatory pathways and oxidative stress, including LDL particle oxidation, play a major role [17]. Furthermore, recent studies reported an association between gut microbiome biology and atherogenesis [18]. Therefore, this study aimed to investigate the impact of wild rice on bacterial species abundance and diversity from 16S rDNA data analysis collected from mouse feces and monitor the metabolic products from the feces and plasma of LDL-r-KO mice.

2. Materials and Methods

2.1. Animals and Diets

Sixteen male, four week old LDL-r-KO mice were purchased from the Jackson Laboratory, USA. The animals were kept in pairs while using standard cages and fed regular mouse chow in a controlled environment for one week. After a week of chow adaptation, fasting blood samples were taken from the jugular vein under light anesthesia; body weight was also recorded. Plasma total cholesterol was estimated, and the animals were divided into two groups of treated ($n = 8$) and controls ($n = 8$), as previously reported [15]. The treated group was fed an atherogenic diet that contained 60% (w/w) wild rice powder, whereas the control group received the same atherogenic diet without wild rice powder, as previously reported [15]. Briefly, the mouse chow diet contained 9% fat that was purchased from Ren's Feed & Supplies Ltd. (Whitby, ON, Canada). This diet was supplemented with 0.06% (w/w) cholesterol to make it atherogenic; the atherogenic diet was further supplemented with or without 60% (w/w) wild rice powder and then used for this study. This supplementation was performed by replacing the atherogenic diet by the ground wild rice at 60%. Therefore, the amounts and types of dietary fiber in the control diet and the wild rice diet were not identical. The experiments lasted for 24 weeks.

2.2. Sample Collection

The blood samples were taken every four weeks. Fecal samples were collected and stored at −80°C until analysis. At autopsy, final blood samples were taken from the hearts and animals were euthanized while using CO_2 gas followed by cardiac puncture [15]. The hearts and aortae were collected for the assessment of atherosclerotic lesion development [15]. The Animal Care Committee approved the study at the University of Manitoba, Winnipeg, Canada; refer to Protocol number 18-048 [15].

2.3. Plasma Cytokine Levels

Plasma samples that were taken at week 16 of the experiments were used for the estimation of 35 inflammatory biomarkers, using Meso Scale Discovery U-PLEX multiplex assay kit for a mouse (Meso Scale Diagnostics, Rockville, MD 20850-3173, USA) [19]. These markers include interleukins (IL-2, IL-4, IL-9, IL-10, IL-13, IL-17A, IL-17E/IL 25, IL-17F, IL-21, IL-22), tumor necrosis factor-alpha (TNF-α)), TH1/TH2 Combo (IL-1β, IL-5, and IL-12p70A), TH17 Combo 1 (IL-17C, IL-23, and IL-33), TH17 Combo 2 (IL-6, erythropoietin (EPO), IL-27p28/IL-30, vascular endothelial growth factor A (VEGF-A), IL-15, IL-16, and IL-17A/F), interferon gamma-induced protein-10 (IP-10), growth regulated oncogenes (KC/GRO), monocyte chemo-attractant protein-1 (MCP-1), macrophage inflammatory proteins (MIP-1α, MIP-1β, MIP 2, and MIP-3α), granulocyte-macrophage colony-stimulating factor (GM-CSF), and interferon-gamma (IFN-γ). This cytokine analysis was performed on the pooled samples ($n = 4$). MSD SI2400 Imager device and MSD Workbench 3.0 software were used to detect and analyze the standard curves and intensity of the cytokines. The intensity for each biomarker was included in statistical analysis and then reported herein.

2.4. Fecal Microbiome Analysis

Microbial diversity and species changes in mice that were fed wild rice as compared to controls were estimated based on extracted 16S rDNA from fecal samples that were collected from pairs of mice at weeks, 0, 4, 16, and 24 during the study. Feces from four cages, where each cage contained two mice (eight mice total), were collected ($n = 4$) for each experimental diet group and stored at −80 °C. Microbial genomic DNA from each thawed fecal sample were extracted with a QIAamp Fast DNA Stool Mini kit (51604, QIAGEN Inc., Germantown, MD, USA), according to its recommended DNA extraction procedures. Fecal DNA was resuspended in nuclease-free water, where the DNA quantity and quality were assessed while using a Qubit™ dsDNA BR Assay Kit (Q32853, Life Technologies, Carlsbad, CA, USA). Fecal DNA samples were stored at −20 °C until they were shipped on dry ice to LC Sciences, LLC (Houston, TX, USA) for 16S rDNA sequencing services. The sequencing methodology that was used by this service and for this study was described previously [20]. Briefly, 16S rDNA sequencing with an Illumina MiSeq platform was carried out, using 338F/806R primers. Further amplification of V3 and V4 regions (around 469 bp in length) was performed by the polymerase chain reaction (PCR). Bioinformatics analysis of 16S rDNA sequence data was assisted by LC Sciences LLC (Houston, TX, USA). Briefly, QIIME software 1.9.1 was used to analyze paired-end reads that were merged into single tags, according to the overlapped region between pairs. The tags were filtered based on their Phred quality score (Q20 and Q30). Chimera sequences that were generated during PCR amplification of the 16S rDNA gene were also excluded, resulting in the final dataset for analysis. This 16S rDNA sequences in the dataset were mapped to the ribosome database project (RDP; http://rdp.cme.msu.edu/) and NCBI 16S rDNA Microbial databases (NT-16S; ftp://ftp.ncbi.nlm.nih.gov/blast/db/nt.gz; as of August 2018) to produce taxonomically annotated sequences, which are referred to as operational taxonomic units (OTUs), described herein. The sequence dataset was grouped using the UCLUST algorithm program. A minimum sequence identity of 99% was used to align the most abundant sequences within each OTU against the reference database sequences, and the hypervariable regions were removed and used to classify the OTUs.

2.5. Metabolomics Studies

Metabolites from fecal and plasma samples from week 18 of the study were analyzed by a previously described the liquid chromatography (LC)-mass spectrometry (MS/MS) analysis method [21]. This method combines derivatization and extraction of analytes from the samples, and the selective mass-spectrometric detection using multiple reaction monitoring pairs. The isotope-labeled internal standards were used for metabolite quantification. A total of 133 metabolites were included in the full panel. This analysis was performed through a service contract with The Metabolomics Innovation Centre (TMIC) at the University of Alberta, Edmonton, Canada. It is acknowledged that the use of fecal samples from two mice that were housed in one cage is a limitation for microbiome studies as each mouse can behave as a single ecosystem; however, the average changes among multiple mice were the objective of this study.

2.6. Atherosclerotic Lesion Assessment

Sections from the beginning of the aortae were cut and processed for morphological evaluation of the atherosclerotic lesions, as previously described [15]. The sections were stained with hematoxylin and eosin (H&E) and trichrome. Light microscopy techniques were used for semi-quantitative analysis of atherosclerotic lesions in the wild rice treated and control mice [15].

2.7. Statistical Analysis

Non-parametric Mann–Whitney tests (also known as the Wilcoxon rank-sum test) and Kruskal–Wallis rank-sum tests were used to calculate the p-values and identify significant differences between the two groups of wild rice fed and control mice with an $n = 4$. These statistical analyses were also used to identify significant differences between time course measurements for each animal group when appropriate. Statistical analyses of fecal microbial composition differences were assessed by non-parametric tests, as described by White et al. 2009 [22]. The Venn diagrams of OTUs determined from these analyses were generated while using 'R' statistics software (version 3.6.1, https://www.r-project.org/) 'Venn Diagram' package to show the number of common OTUs in feces of control and wild rice diet groups. Data are presented as means and standard deviations, where p-values ≤ 0.05 were deemed to be significantly different based on the degrees of freedom for each sample group. All of the statistical analyses were performed, while using either Microsoft Office Excel (365, Microsoft, Redmond, USA) or the comprehensive 'R' Archive Network (CRAN) statistics software (version 3.6.1, https://www.r-project.org/), with the 'PMCMR' analysis package, using 'kruskal.test' and 'wilcox.test' functions.

3. Results

3.1. Consumption of Wild Rice Was Associated with Changes in Fecal Bacterial Species Populations

Insights into microbial taxonomic alterations could only be confidently determined for high abundance OTUs due to the small number of fecal samples ($n = 4$) examined in this analysis. Microbial 16S rDNA analysis identified more than 200,000 bacterial species (OTUs) in the mouse fecal samples. Figure 1A shows a Venn diagram comparing similar OTUs that were observed between the control and wild rice fed fecal samples collected at various weeks 0, 4, 16, and 24. The majority of all OTUs (732 total) shown in the center of the Venn diagram were identical among all diet treatments, as would be expected in a study involving similar mouse breeds and housing conditions. The wild rice diet fecal samples showed a decrease in the number of unique OTUs over time, where 135 unique OTUs at week 0 reduced to 73 OTUs by week 24. The control samples showed no differences in unique OTUs over time, suggesting that the introduction of the wild rice diet reduced species diversity as compared to the control diets.

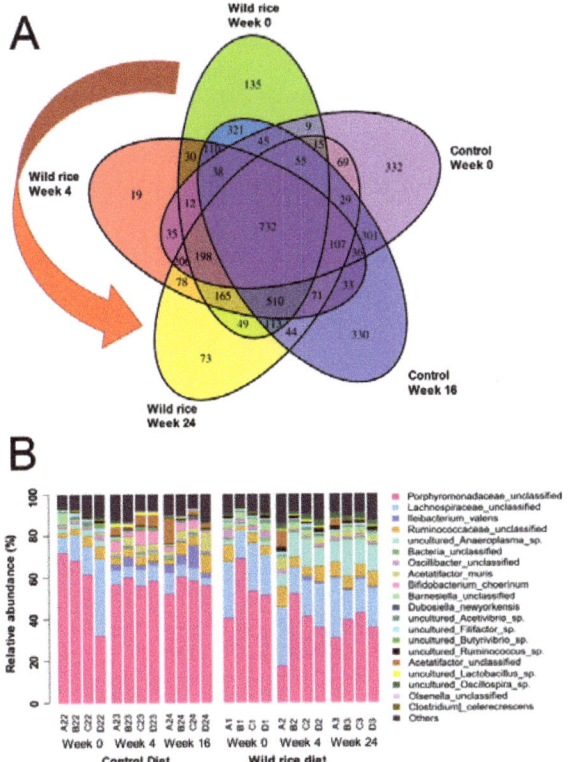

Figure 1. (**A**) Venn diagram comparing 16S rDNA operational taxonomic units (OTUs) from the feces of wild rice and control diet fed mice at weeks 0, 4, 16, and 24. The red curved arrow highlights the decrease in the unique total OTUs in the wild rice fed mice from week 0 to week 24 of the study. (**B**) The relative abundance of the top 20 most abundant bacterial OTUs identified from wild rice or control diet fecal samples at weeks 0 to 24. Identified OTUs are listed according to their order (bottom to top) and color within the bar chart.

Microbial composition changes were further investigated by performing 16S rDNA sequence clustering, where the top 20 most abundant OTUs determined from each fecal sample are shown as a stacked bar chart (Figure 1B). No significant differences were detected between the two major taxa, unclassified Porphyromonadales and Lachnospirales, over time (weeks 0–16 or weeks 0–24) between the control and wild rice diet fecal samples (Figure 1B). Wild rice diets significantly increased ($p < 0.05$) the proportion and appearance of a number of major OTUs when comparing week 0 to week 24 fecal samples; specifically, uncultured *Anaeroplasma sp.* (8.8-fold increase), *Acetatifactor muris* (4.4-fold increase), uncultured *Lactobacillus* sp. (3-fold increase), uncultured *Oscillospira* sp. (3-fold increase), and *Dubosiella newyorkensis* (0.07% appearance) increased (Figure 1B). Losses or significant reductions ($p < 0.05$) in OTUs within the fecal wild rice diet microbiomes after comparing them to the control diet microbiomes were also noted over time (weeks 4 and/or 24). Specifically, reductions in unclassified *Barnesiella* sp. (2-fold reduction), uncultured *Butyrivibrio* sp. (2-fold reduction), and unclassified *Oscillibacter* sp. (2-fold reduction;) were detected. *Bifidobacterium choerinium* was also undetectable in the wild rice diet samples at weeks 4 and 24 as compared to control diet (Figure 1B). Altered proportions of OTUs were also noted within the control diet fecal samples over time (weeks 0 to 16); significant ($p < 0.05$) reductions in uncultured *Anaeroplasma* sp. (undetectable at week 16), uncultured *Ruminococcus* sp. (2-fold reduction), and uncultured *Filifactor* sp. (undetectable at week 16) were noted, as well as significant increases ($p < 0.05$) in *Ileibacterium valens* (2–5% appearance) and *Bifidobacterium choerinum* (43-fold increase). It is noteworthy that the control diet OTUs, as mentioned above, were either low or completely absent in the wild rice diet fecal samples (Figure 1B). Overall, fecal microbiome analyses indicate that the wild rice diet significantly alters many high abundance bacterial species.

Figure 2 shows values for three OTUs that reached statistically significant differences ($p < 0.05$) between the treated and control animals. The abundance of unclassified *Prophyromonadaceae sp.* and uncultured *Anaeroplasma sp.* in wild rice fed mice were approximately 5000 and 1000, respectively, more than those in the control group.

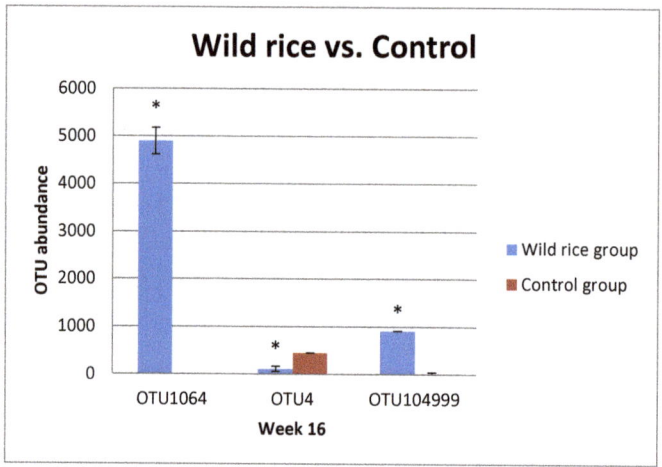

Figure 2. The abundance of OTUs for selected species identified from 16S rDNA analysis of wild rice fed and control fecal samples. All samples were collected at week 16 of the study with an $n = 4$ per group. OTU 4: *Acetatifactor sp.* unclassified; OTU 1064: *Porphyromonadaceae sp.* unclassified; OTU 104999: uncultured *Anaeroplasma sp.* *: $p < 0.05$ as compared with the controls.

3.2. Wild Rice Consumption Is Associated with Changes in Plasma Inflammatory Markers

Our analysis included an estimation of 35 different markers in inflammatory pathways. Statistical analyses between data from the wild rice fed and control groups only identified five markers with a significant change in their mean values (Table 1). The levels of EPO and interleukin 10 (IL-10) increased by approximately 109% and 130%, respectively, in the wild rice diet mice. In contrast, wild rice diet mice had reduced markers of approximately 18%, 18%, and 35% of tumor necrosis factor-alpha (TNF-α), vascular endothelial growth factor (VEGF), and interleukin-16 (IL-16), respectively, as compared with the control animals.

Table 1. Plasma cytokine intensity from the wild rice fed and control groups.

Plasma Cytokines (pg/mL)	Experimental Groups		% Change
	Control Group ($n = 4$)	Wild Rice Group ($n = 4$)	
EPO	6.69 ± 2.7	14.01 ± 4.7 *	↑109
TNF-α	6.77 ± 0.7	5.57 ± 0.5 *	↓18
VEGF	6.06 ± 0.6	5.0 ± 0.5 *	↓18
IL10	4.32 ± 1.77	9.94 ± 3.14 *	↑130
IL16	645.83 ± 14.4	422.07 ± 64.3 *	↓35

Data are presented as means ± standard deviation. Statistical analyses were performed using the Mann Whitney test; *: $p < 0.05$ as compared with the controls. EPO: erythropoietin, TNF-α: tumor necrosis factor-α, VEGF: vascular endothelial growth factor, IL-16: interleukin-16. ↓: Decrease. ↑: Increase

3.3. Wild Rice Diets Show Differences in Fecal and Plasma Metabolites

LC-MS/MS analysis of metabolites that were extracted from wild rice and control diet fecal and plasma samples identified a total of 133 metabolites. We performed a Mann-Whitney rank-sum test on metabolite values between the sample groups to improve the confidence in metabolite analyses due to our lower sampling numbers ($n = 4$). We focused our results on metabolites with significant differences from the control diet group ($p < 0.05$). Table 2 show significant changes in the levels of 11 plasma metabolites that were differentially detected. Glucose increased in wild rice fed mice by approximately 61%, whereas 10 metabolites, including short-chain fatty acids (C8, C10, and C12), medium-chain fatty acids (C14:1, and C16), and long-chain fatty acids (C18 and C18:1) decreased by 17–48% in the wild rice diet plasma samples as compared to those in the controls.

Table 2. Metabolomics data from plasma samples of mice fed wild rice and control diets.

Plasma Metabolomics		Control Group ($n = 4$) (µM)	Wild Rice Group (µM) ($n = 4$)	% Change from Control Diet
Nutrients	Metabolites			
Proteins	Putrescine	1.21 ± 0.19	0.83 ± 0.16 *	↓32%
Carbohydrates	Glucose	10,208.17 ± 2575.4	16,405.98 ± 2966.73 *	↑61%
Short Chain Fatty Acids	Caprylic acid	0.06 ± 0.009	0.05 ± 0.007 *	↓25%
	Capric acid	0.09 ± 0.009	0.06 ± 0.010 *	↓30%
	Lauric acid	0.08 ± 0.014	0.05 ± 0.0002 *	↓41%
Medium Chain Fatty Acids	Myristic acid (C14)	0.17 ± 0.026	0.10 ± 0.008 *	↓41%
	3-Hydroxytetradecenoyl-carnitine (C14:1-OH)	0.03 ± 0.0047	0.02 ± 0.0027 *	↓29%
	Palmitic acid (C:16)	0.51 ± 0.158	0.32 ± 0.032 *	↓38%
	Hydroxyhexadecadienyl-L-Dcarnitine (C16:2OH)	0.01 ± 0.0026	0.01 ± 0.002 *	↓35%
Long Chain Fatty Acids	Stearic (C18)	0.18 ± 0.0205	0.12 ± 0.012 *	↓31%
	Hydroxy-Oleyl-L-Carnitine (C18:1OH)	0.05 ± 0.011	0.03 ± 0.002 *	↓34%

Data are presented as means ± standard deviation. Statistical analyses were performed using the Mann-Whitney test; *, $p < 0.05$ as compared with controls. ↓: Decrease. ↑: Increase

Among 24 fecal metabolites listed in Table 3, only four metabolites, butyric acid and three phospholipids increased by 51–323%. The remaining metabolites, which included amino acids, short-chain fatty acids (except butyric acid), and long-chain fatty acids, showed a decrease of 30–70% by wild rice fed fecal samples as compared to those in the control group (Table 3).

Table 3. Fecal metabolomics data from the wild rice fed and control groups.

Fecal Metabolomics Assay		Control Group (n = 4)	Wild Rice Group (n = 4)	% Change
Nutrients	Metabolites (μM)			
Amino acids	Glycine	1.15 ± 0.529	0.34 ± 0.12 *	↓70%
	Alanine	2.79 ± 1.31	1.18 ± 0.32 *	↓58%
	Proline	0.52 ± 0.179	0.18 ± 0.07 *	↓66%
	Valine	0.81 ± 0.381	0.26 ± 0.13 *	↓67%
	Leucine	0.92 ± 0.497	0.32 ± 0.11 *	↓66%
	Isoleucine	0.91 ± 0.424	0.28 ± 0.11 *	↓69%
	Methionine-sulfoxide	0.16 ± 0.061	0.06 ± 0.04 *	↓60%
	Tryptophan	0.07 ± 0.034	0.03 ± 0.01 *	↓62%
Short-Chain Fatty acids	Butyric acid	0.11 ± 0.029	0.20 ± 0.05 *	↑81%
	Succinic acid	0.18 ± 0.088	0.08 ± 0.01 *	↓58%
	Isobutyric acid	0.07 ± 0.014	0.03 ± 0.01 *	↓60%
	Methylmalonic acid	0.003 ± 0.0003	0.0009 ± 0.004 *	↓72%
	Dodecanedioyl-L-Carnitine (C12DC)	$7.93 \times 10^{-5} \pm 8.72 \times 10^{-6}$	$4.44 \times 10^{-5} \pm 9.71 \times 10^{-6}$ *	↓44%
Long-Chain Fatty Acids	Vaccenic acid (C18:1)	$3.50 \times 10^{-5} \pm 1.33 \times 10^{-5}$	$1.63 \times 10^{-5} \pm 1.40 \times 10^{-6}$ *	↓53%
	Lenoleic acid (C18:2)	$6.01 \times 10^{-5} \pm 8.50 \times 10^{-6}$	$3.48 \times 10^{-5} \pm 3.21 \times 10^{-6}$ *	↓42%
Phospholipids	LYSOC16:1	$0.0002 \pm 4.98 \times 10^{-5}$	$0.0004 \pm 9.77 \times 10^{-5}$ *	↑72%
	LYSOC16:0	0.005 ± 0.0009	0.01 ± 0.002 *	↑93%
	LYSOC18:2	0.001 ± 0.0003	0.002 ± 0.001 *	↑157%
	LYSOC18:1	0.001 ± 0.0002	0.004 ± 0.001 *	↑226%
	16:1SM	$0.0001 \pm 3.57 \times 10^{-5}$	$4.91 \times 10^{-5} \pm 5.62 \times 10^{-6}$*	↓69%
	20:2SM	$1.43 \times 10^{-5} \pm 5.50 \times 10^{-7}$	$2.15 \times 10^{-5} \pm 5.64 \times 10^{-6}$*	↑51%
	PC36:6AA	$8.01 \times 10^{-5} \pm 3.10 \times 10^{-5}$	$0.0003 \pm 8.66 \times 10^{-5}$ *	↑323%
	PC38:0AA	$0.0004 \pm 9.23 \times 10^{-5}$	$0.0003 \pm 3.83 \times 10^{-5}$ *	↓30%
	PC40:2AA	$6.93 \times 10^{-5} \pm 1.39 \times 10^{-5}$	$4.33 \times 10^{-5} \pm 2.19 \times 10^{-6}$ *	↓37%

Data are presented as means ± standard deviation; each fecal sample represents feces from 2 caged mice, eight mice total and n = 4 fecal samples per experimental group. Statistical analyses were performed using the Kruskal Wallis test; *, $p < 0.05$ as compared to the controls. ↓: Decrease. ↑: Increase

3.4. Wild Rice Consumption Prevents Atherogenesis

In agreement with our previous findings [15,16], we report that the mice fed with wild rice had much smaller atherosclerotic lesions in their aortae as compared to that in the control animals. Figure 3 illustrates advanced atherosclerotic lesions at the beginning of aortae in the control animals (arrows), but similar lesions were absent or minimal in the similar anatomical region of aortae of the wild rice fed mice.

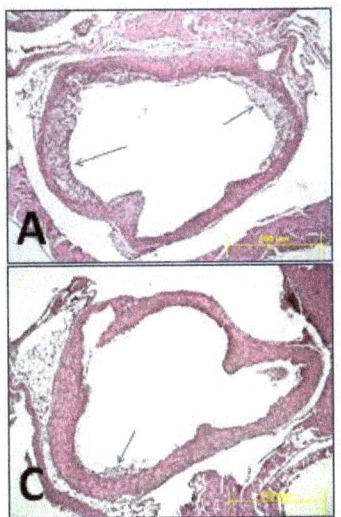
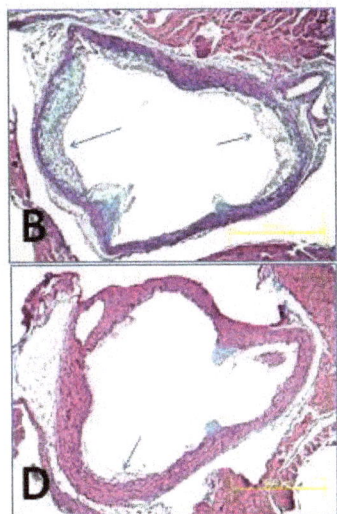

Figure 3. Representative photomicrographs were taken at the beginning of aorta from one control mouse (**A,B**) and one wild rice fed mouse (**C,D**) illustrating atherosclerotic lesions (arrows). As it is seen in (**A,B**), atherosclerotic lesions are large and well established in the control mouse (arrows), while such advanced lesions are missing in the wild rice fed mouse (**C,D**). H&E staining (**A,C**); trichrome staining (**B,D**).

4. Discussion

We have previously shown that wild rice consumption is associated with the prevention of atherosclerotic vascular disease in LDL-r-KO mice [15,16]. This effect could be related to reductions in plasma cholesterol levels. We have shown alterations in LDL-r-KO mice microbiomes may influence the detection of inflammatory markers, and alter concentrations of metabolites when fed a diet rich in wild rice based on the results of our study. LDL-r-KO mice exhibit atherosclerosis, which is known to be an inflammatory disease [23]. Therefore, treatment with agents that possess pro-inflammatory properties are expected to increase the risk for this disease and anti-inflammatory states should prevent atherosclerosis [24]. LDL-r-KO mice fed a wild rice diet had approximately 75% lower atherosclerotic lesions (0.46 ± 0.11 vs. 1.95 ± 0.16 mm^2) in their aortic roots as compared to the control diet mice [15].

The results from the current study have identified that wild rice feeding is associated with a 130% change increase in IL-10; IL-10 was shown in previous studies to possess anti-atherogenic activities [25]. Another interesting observation was a 109% increase in the levels of EPO in plasma of wild rice fed mice. Recent studies have shown the anti-atherogenic properties for EPO [26]. The mechanism by which IL-10 and EPO levels were increased in wild rice treated animals is not presently understood, but it may be associated with changes in gut microbiome composition. We have reported a beneficial change in the inflammatory pathways of mice that were fed either wild rice or Saskatoon berries [27,28]. Additionally, a recent study monitoring dietary changes in mice demonstrated that specific microbes can alter gut T-cell responses [29]. It is possible that the changes in cytokine concentrations that we observed in wild rice fed LDL-r-KO mice may indirectly influence plasma when phytochemicals produced by altered gut microbiome species reach the blood.

We also reported that starch from wild rice is different in nature from the starch found in conventional white rice; wild rice also contains a significant amount of dietary fiber [9,16]. These forms of carbohydrates may act as prebiotics, which thereby alters the diversity and population of the gut microbiome [11,12]. In the present study, we observed that unclassified Prophyromonadaceae decreased in the fecal samples of wild rice fed mice (Figure 1B). When we examined different OTUs associated with unclassified Prophyromonadaceae, we observed that many OTUs increased in wild rice group as compared to those in the control (Figure 2). This suggests that specific Prophyromonadaceae, such as unclassified *Barnesiella* sp., differ between control and wild rice fed mice (Figure 1B). Previous studies examining changes in mouse gut microbial species showed that mice that were fed with polysaccharides from the mushroom *Auricularia auricular* altered quantities of Prophyromonadaceae in their intestine as compared to control diet animals [30]. This study highlights the importance of carbohydrates on microbial species diversity. In the same mushroom study, the treated animals showed higher serum IgA and IgG, indicating changes in gut microbiome due to mushroom carbohydrate consumption also modulated the immune system of the mice [30]. Another noteworthy observation was the difference in *Anaeroplasma* sp. between the wild rice fed and control fecal samples. A study by Zeng et al. [31] reported an increased abundance of *Anaeroplasma* species in the intestines of wild type mice that were fed a high-fat diet. These authors concluded that high-fat diets promoted colonic aberrant crypt formation accompanied by an increase in the abundance of opportunistic pathogens, such as *Anaeroplasma* sp. in the colon of C57BL/6 mice [31]. *Acetatifactor* sp. was also identified in high abundance over time within the wild rice fed fecal samples. Although not much is known about *Acetatifactor* species' influence on murine microbiomes, Pfeiffer et al. [32] suggested the name *Acetatifactor muris* due to its isolation from the cecum of mice fed a high-fat diet, which we also observed in our study only among control diet LDL-r-KO mice (Figure 1B). *Acetatifactor* species are not known to metabolize glucose and they are associated with higher phenylalanine arylamidase activities. In our study, we identified that wild rice diets reduced the *Acetatifactor muris* levels, suggesting that this species, might indirectly influence atherosclerosis in an LDL-r-KO mouse model.

Analysis of fecal metabolic compounds revealed that wild rice consumption was associated with altered metabolite abundances, particularly metabolites that are associated with amino acids, carbohydrates, and fats. All amino acids that were detected in fecal samples were significantly reduced from mice fed wild rice diets. Wild rice diets may promote the growth and predominance of these amino acid utilizing species to catabolize more amino acids, since the most abundant bacterial species *Anaeroplasma* sp., *Acetatifactor* sp., and *Prophyromonadaceae* sp. significantly differed in wild rice as compared to the control group. For example, *Acetatifactor muris* may be a species promoting greater amino acid usage, as it possesses phenylalanine arylamidase, which breaks down L-phenylalanine from peptides [32]. This might suggest that a significant reduction in the concentrations of several amino acids could be associated with bacteria containing this and other relevant enzymes.

Among several short-chain fatty acids and their derivatives, butyric acid was found in the fecal materials from the wild rice fed mice 81% more than that in the control animals. This finding coincides with specific and significant increases in butyric acid-producing uncultured *Butyrivibrio* species identified from 16S rDNA wild rice fed fecal microbiomes (Figure 1B). *Butyrivibrio* sp. is commonly enriched in the guts of ruminant animals, where they produce butyrate from the breakdown of plant fibers and structural carbohydrates, specifically hemicellulose [33,34]. Many studies have reported the metabolic benefits of short-chain fatty acids [35,36]. Analysis of blood plasma samples did not correlate well to metabolic and microbiome changes despite increases in butyrate in the intestine of wild rice fed mice. Plasma concentrations of other short-chain fatty acids, such as caproic acid and caprylic acid, were significantly lower in the wild rice fed mice as compared to those in the controls. However, there was an association between the levels of long-chain fatty acids in the fecal and plasma samples, as these levels were increased in both samples from the wild rice fed mice as compared to those in the controls. Another observation was a significant increase in plasma glucose concentrations in the wild rice fed mice as compared to that in the control group. Increased plasma glucose levels are seen during diabetes or insulin resistance in animals as well as humans [37,38]. However, the consumption of high fiber diets is generally recommended to combat complications that are caused by diabetes [39,40]. Wild rice is a rich source of dietary fiber; therefore, this observation seems to be in contrast with our general knowledge and it certainly begs more investigation. To conclude, additional investigations examining the interplay between changes in intestinal microflora, inflammatory response, and metabolic biomarkers are warranted, as they may play a role in the pathogenesis of chronic diseases, like atherosclerosis. Overall, it should be mentioned that a low number of animals, pooled fecal, and plasma samples, as well as a lack of different doses of wild rice, could be viewed as limitations of the present study.

5. Conclusions

In conclusion, we hereby report that the long term consumption of wild rice at 60% (w/w) in LDL-r-KO mice is associated with the prevention of atherosclerosis. This effect was accompanied by significant alterations in the fecal bacterial population and diversity, as well as significant changes in several inflammatory and metabolic biomarkers. Of particular interest was an increase in the plasma glucose levels in the wild rice fed mice; currently, we have no explanation for this finding. Other findings that can support anti-atherogenic properties of wild rice are increases in the plasma levels of anti-inflammatory marker IL-10 and EPO. Altogether, this study provides preliminary evidence in support of additional studies on this animal model and others to improve our understanding of how gut bacterial species, plasma inflammatory markers, and metabolic biomarkers may prevent atherosclerosis. Furthermore, a dose-response study can help to establish whether lower doses of wild rice can result in similar findings in this animal model.

Author Contributions: M.H.M., R.K., K.K., M.M., and K.L. contributed to the preparation of manuscripts, A.A.J., B.S.J.G., V.L.-S., A.I.S., M.W., and D.C.B. contributed to microbiome study, D.C.B. and R.K. performed statistical analysis, G.F. (Gabor Fischer) contributed to atherosclerosis data, F.B., G.F. (Gaia Favero), and R.R. contributed to overall experimental design.

Funding: This study was supported by a grant from the Natural Sciences and Engineering Research Council (NSERC) of Canada to MHM (Grant number 298450). RK is a recipient of the University of Manitoba Graduate Fellowship.

Acknowledgments: Supports from St. Boniface Hospital Foundation for the provision of facilities needed to carry out this research are greatly appreciated.

Conflicts of Interest: Authors claim no conflict of interest.

References

1. Moghadasian, M.H.; Afqari, N.; Rideot, T.C.; Bonomini, F.; Favero, G.; Rezzani, R. The Mideterranean diet. An update. *Ann. Nutr. Food Sci.* **2018**, *2*, 1019.
2. Molendijk, I.; van der Marel, S.; Maljaars, P.W.J. Towards a Food Pharmacy: Immunologic Modulation through Diet. *Nutrients* **2019**, *11*, 1239. [CrossRef] [PubMed]
3. Moghadasian, M.H.; Frohlich, J.J. Effects of dietary phytosterols on cholesterol metabolism and atherosclerosis: Clinical and experimental evidence. *Am. J. Med.* **1999**, *107*, 588–594. [CrossRef]
4. Asgary, S.; Rastqar, A.; Keshvari, M. Functional Food and Cardiovascular Disease Prevention and Treatment: A Review. *J. Am. Coll. Nutr.* **2018**, *37*, 429–455. [CrossRef]
5. He, L.; Chen, Z.; Dai, B.; Li, G.; Zhu, G. Low-level lead exposure and cardiovascular disease: The roles of telomere shortening and lipid disturbance. *J. Toxicol. Sci.* **2018**, *43*, 623–630. [CrossRef]
6. Huang, L.; Lin, J.S.; Aris, I.M.; Yang, G.; Chen, W.Q.; Li, L.J. Circulating Saturated Fatty Acids and Incident Type 2 Diabetes: A Systematic Review and Meta-Analysis. *Nutrients* **2019**, *11*, 998. [CrossRef]
7. World Health Organization. Cardiovascular Disease Mortality and Morbidity. 2017. Available online: https://www.who.int/news-room/fact-sheets/detail/cardiovascular-diseases-(cvds) (accessed on 25 August 2019).

8. Zhong, S.; Li, L.; Shen, X.; Li, Q.; Xu, W.; Wang, X.; Tao, Y.; Yin, H. An update on lipid oxidation and inflammation in cardiovascular diseases. *Free Radic. Biol. Med.* **2019**, *144*, 266–278. [CrossRef]
9. Surendiran, G.; Alsaif, M.; Kapourchali, F.R.; Moghadasian, M.H. Nutritional constituents and health benefits of wild rice (Zizania spp). *Nutr. Rev.* **2014**, *72*, 227–236. [CrossRef]
10. Food and Drug Administration. Food Fact Sheet (April 2018). Available online: https://www.fda.gov/media/115280/download (accessed on 21 November 2019).
11. Slavin, J. Antioxidant, Fiber and prebiotics: Mechanisms and health benefits. *Nutrients* **2013**, *5*, 1417–1435. [CrossRef]
12. Marcelino, G.; Hiane, P.A.; Freitas, K.C.; Santana, L.F.; Pott, A.; Donadon, J.R.; Guimarães, R.C.A. Effects of Olive Oil and Its Minor Componentson Cardiovascular Diseases, Inflammation, and Gut Microbiota. *Nutrients* **2019**, *11*, 1826. [CrossRef]
13. Moghadasian, M.H.; McManus, B.M.; Nguyen, L.B.; Shefer, S.; Nadji, M.; Godin, D.V.; Green, T.J.; Hill, J.; Yang, Y.; Scudamore, C.H.; et al. Pathophysiology of apolipoprotein E deficiency in mice: Relevance to apo E-related disorders in humans. *FASEB J.* **2001**, *15*, 2623–2630. [CrossRef] [PubMed]
14. Moghadasian, M.H.; McManus, B.M.; Godin, D.V.; Rodrigues, B.; Frohlich, J.J. Proatherogenic and antiatherogenic effects of probucol and phytosterols in apolipoprotein E-deficient mice: Possible mechanisms of action. *Circulation* **1999**, *99*, 1733–1739. [CrossRef] [PubMed]
15. Moghadasian, M.H.; Alsaif, M.; Le, K.; Gangadaran, S.; Masisi, K.; Beta, T.; Shen, G.X. Combination effects of wild rice and phytosterols on prevention of atherosclerosis in LDL receptor knockout mice. *J. Nutr. Biochem.* **2016**, *33*, 128–135. [CrossRef] [PubMed]
16. Surendiran, G.; Goh, C.Y.; Le, K.; Zhao, Z.; Askarian, F.; Othman, R.; Nicholson, T.; Moghadasian, P.; Wang, Y.J.; Aliani, M.; et al. Wild rice prevents atherogenesis in LDL receptor knock-out mice. *Atherosclerosis* **2013**, *230*, 284–292. [CrossRef] [PubMed]
17. Herman, A.B.; Silva Afonso, M.; Kelemen, S.E.; Ray, M.; Vrakas, C.N.; Burke, A.C.; Scalia, R.G.; Moore, K.; Autieri, M.V. Regulation of Stress Granule Formation by Inflammation, Vascular Injury, and Atherosclerosis. *Arterioscler. Thromb. Vasc. Biol.* **2019**, *39*, 2014–2027. [CrossRef] [PubMed]
18. Jayachandran, M.; Chung, S.S.M.; Xu, B. A critical review on diet-induced microbiota changes and cardiovascular diseases. *Crit. Rev. Food Sci. Nutr.* **2019**, 1–12. [CrossRef]
19. Gupta, D.; Wen, J.C.; Huebner, J.L.; Stinnett, S.; Kraus, V.B.; Tseng, H.C.; Walsh, M. Cytokine biomarkers in tear film for primary open-angle glaucoma. *Clin. Ophthalmol.* **2017**, *11*, 411–416. [CrossRef]
20. Rintala, A.; Pietilä, S.; Munukka, E.; Eerola, E.; Pursiheimo, J.P.; Laiho, A.; Pekkala, S.; Huovinen, P. Gut microbiota analysis results are highly dependent on the 16S rRNA gene target region, whereas the impact of DNA extraction is minor. *J. Biomol. Tech.* **2017**, *28*, 19–30. [CrossRef]
21. Kervezee, L.; Cermakian, N.; Boivin, D.B. Individual metabolomic signatures of circadian misalignment during simulated night shifts in humans. *PLoS Biol.* **2019**, *17*, e3000303. [CrossRef]
22. White, J.R.; Nagarajan, N.; Pop, M. Statistical methods for detecting differentially abundant features in clinical metagenomic samples. *PLoS Comput. Biol.* **2009**, *5*, e1000352. [CrossRef]
23. Ross, R. Atherosclerosis is an inflammatory disease. *Am. Heart J.* **1999**, *138*, S419–S420. [CrossRef]
24. Ali, M.; Girgis, S.; Hassan, A.; Rudick, S.; Becker, R.C. Inflammation and coronary artery disease: From pathophysiology to Canakinumab Anti Inflammatory Thrombosis Outcomes Study (CANTOS). *Coron. Artery Dis.* **2018**, *29*, 429–437. [CrossRef] [PubMed]
25. Kusters, P.J.; Lutgens, E. Cytokines and Immune Responses in Murine Atherosclerosis. *Methods Mol. Biol.* **2015**, *1339*, 17–40.
26. Lu, K.Y.; Ching, L.C.; Su, K.H.; Yu, Y.B.; Kou, Y.R.; Hsiao, S.H.; Huang, Y.C.; Chen, C.Y.; Cheng, L.C.; Pan, C.C.; et al. Erythropoietin suppresses the formation of macrophage foam cells: Role of liver X receptor alpha. *Circulation* **2010**, *121*, 1828–1837. [CrossRef] [PubMed]
27. Moghadasian, M.H.; Zhao, R.; Ghazzawi, N.; Le, K.; Apea-Bah, F.B.; Beta, T.; Shen, G.X. Inhibitory effects of North American wild rice on monocyte adhesion and inflammatory modulators in low-density lipoprotein receptor-knockout mice. *J. Agric. Food Chem.* **2017**, *65*, 9054–9060. [CrossRef]
28. Zhao, R.; Le, K.; Li, W.; Ren, S.; Moghadasian, M.H.; Beta, T.; Shen, G.X. Effects of Saskatoon berry powder on monocyte adhesion to vascular wall of leptin receptor-deficient diabetic mice. *J. Nutr. Biochem.* **2014**, *25*, 851–857. [CrossRef]

29. Fuc, E.; Złotkowska, D.; Wróblewska, B. Milk and Meat Allergens from *Bos taurus* β-Lactoglobulin, α-Casein, and Bovine Serum Albumin: An In-Vivo Study of the Immune Response in Mice. *Nutrients* **2019**, *4*, 2095. [CrossRef]
30. Zhao, R.; Cheng, N.; Nakata, P.A.; Zhao, L.; Hu, Q. Consumption of polysaccharides from Aricularia auricular modulates the intestinal microbiota in mice. *Food Res. Int.* **2019**, *123*, 383–392. [CrossRef]
31. Zeng, H.; Ishaq, S.L.; Liu, Z.; Bukowski, M.R. Colonic aberrant crypt formation accompanies an increase of opportunistic pathogenic bacteria in C57BL/6 mice fed a high fat diets. *J. Nutr. Biochem.* **2018**, *54*, 18–27. [CrossRef]
32. Pfeiffer, N.; Desmarchelier, C.; Blaut, M.; Daniel, H.; Haller, D.; Clavel, T. Acetatifactor muris gen. nov., sp. nov., a novel bacterium isolated from the intestine of an obese mouse. *Arch. Microbiol.* **2012**, *194*, 901–907. [CrossRef]
33. Kock, S.G.; Kistner, A. Extent of Solubilization of a-Cellulose and Hemicellulose of Low-protein Teff Hay by Pure Cultures of Cellulolytic Rumen Bacteria. *J. Gen. Microbial.* **1969**, *55*, 459–462. [CrossRef] [PubMed]
34. Paillard, D. Relation between phylogenetic position, lipid metabolism and butyrate production by different Butyrivibrio-like bacteria from the rumen. *Antonie Van Leeuwenhoek* **2007**, *91*, 417–422. [CrossRef] [PubMed]
35. Bartolomaeus, H.; Balogh, A.; Yakoub, M.; Homann, S.; Markó, L.; Höges, S.; Tsvetkov, D.; Krannich, A.; Wundersitz, S.; Avery, E.G.; et al. Short-Chain Fatty Acid Propionate Protects From Hypertensive Cardiovascular Damage. *Circulation* **2019**, *139*, 1407–1421. [CrossRef] [PubMed]
36. Bultman, S.J. Bacterial butyrate prevents atherosclerosis. *Nat. Microbiol.* **2018**, *3*, 1332–1333. [CrossRef] [PubMed]
37. Zhang, X.; Jiang, H.; Ma, X.; Wu, H. Increased serum level and impaired response to glucose fluctuation of asprosin is associated with type 2 diabetes mellitus. *J. Diabetes Investig.* **2019**. [CrossRef]
38. Azizi, F.; Hadaegh, F.; Hosseinpanah, F.; Mirmiran, P.; Amouzegar, A.; Abdi, H.; Asghari, G.; Parizadeh, D.; Montazeri, S.A.; Lotfaliany, M.; et al. Metabolic health in the Middle East and north Africa. *Lancet Diabetes Endocrinol.* **2019**. [CrossRef]
39. Dreher, M.L. Whole Fruits and Fruit Fiber Emerging Health Effects. *Nutrients* **2018**, *10*, 1833. [CrossRef]
40. Kyrø, C.; Tjønneland, A.; Overvad, K.; Olsen, A.; Landberg, R. Higher Whole-Grain Intake Is Associated with Lower Risk of Type 2 Diabetes among Middle-Aged Men and Women: The Danish Diet, Cancer, and Health Cohort. *J. Nutr.* **2018**, *148*, 1434–1444. [CrossRef]

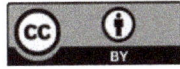

© 2019 by the authors. Licensee MDPI, Basel, Switzerland. This article is an open access article distributed under the terms and conditions of the Creative Commons Attribution (CC BY) license (http://creativecommons.org/licenses/by/4.0/).

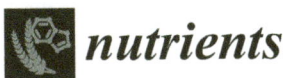

Article

Intervention Study on the Efficacy and Safety of *Platycodon grandiflorus* Ethanol Extract in Overweight or Moderately Obese Adults: A Single-Center, Randomized, Double-Blind, Placebo-Controlled Trial

Ye Jin Kim [1], Eun-Young Kwon [2,3], Ji-Won Kim [2,3], Youngmi Lee [2,3], Ri Ryu [4], Jongbok Yun [5], Manheun Kim [5] and Myung-Sook Choi [2,3,*]

[1] Division of Endocrinology and Metabolism, Department of Internal Medicine, Kyungpook National University, Daegu 41566, Korea; freewilly59@hanmail.net
[2] Center for Food and Nutritional Genomics Research, Kyungpook National University, 1370 San-Kyuk DongPuk-Ku, Daegu 41566, Korea; savage20@naver.com (E.-Y.K.); budy9497@naver.com (J.-W.K.); 6k5rsg@hanmail.net (Y.L.)
[3] Department of Food Science and Nutrition, Kyungpook National University, 1370 San-Kyuk Dong Puk-Ku, Daegu 41566, Korea
[4] Research Institute of Applied Animal Science, Institute of Green-Bio Science and Technology, Seoul National University, Pyeongchang 25354, Korea; riryu@anu.ac.kr
[5] Business Deveopment Division, GC WellBeing Corporation, Gyeonggi-do, Seongnam 13595, Korea; jb@greencross.com (J.Y.); caciclup@greencross.com (M.K.)
* Correspondence: mschoi@knu.ac.kr; Tel.: +82-53-950-6232

Received: 9 September 2019; Accepted: 5 October 2019; Published: 14 October 2019

Abstract: *Platycodon grandiflorus* root extract (PGE) has shown various properties, such as anti-hyperlipidemia, anti-diabetic, and anti-obesity, but mostly in animal studies. Therefore, we conducted a preliminary study on the anti-obesity effect of PGE in 108 Korean adults (aged 20–60 years, 30 kg/m² ≥ body mass index ≥ 23 kg/m²). The participants were randomly assigned to four groups and were administered the placebo, PGE571 (571 mg as PGE), PGE1142 (1142 mg as PGE), and PGE2855 (2855 mg as PGE), independently, for 12 weeks. Body composition, nutrient intake, computed tomography scan, and plasma adipokines, as well as hepatic/renal function markers, were assessed. The PGE571 group revealed a significant decrease in body fat mass and body fat percentage when compared with the placebo group. Moreover, the total abdominal and subcutaneous fat areas were significantly decreased following PGE (PGE2855 group) supplementation. These results provide useful information on the anti-obesity effect of PGE for overweight and obese adult humans.

Keywords: *Platycodon grandiflorus* root; BMI; body fat mass; abdominal fat area

1. Introduction

Obesity is associated with the morbidity and mortality of diabetes and cardiovascular disease, and it is a major public health problem that is increasing in prevalence worldwide [1]. Obesity increases the risk of metabolic abnormalities, associated insulin resistance, hyperglycemia, type 2 diabetes, and dyslipidemia, which generate high medical costs [2,3]. Obesity leads to the accumulation of body fat mass, as well as the loss of skeletal muscle mass. Recently, a new concept of sarcopenic obesity has emerged, reflecting a combination of sarcopenia and obesity, which describes the process of muscle loss combined with increased body fat as people age—a condition associated with the loss of muscle strength and function, reduced quality of life, and even mortality [4,5].

Platycodon grandiflorus (PG) root is widely used in traditional Chinese medicine. It contains many active constituents, such as steroidal saponins, flavonoids, phenolic acids, and sterols, among which, the saponins are regarded as the major active compounds [6]. Numerous studies have proven that the saponins of *P. grandiflorus* exhibit diverse pharmacological activities, such as antioxidant [7], anti-inflammatory [8], and anti-apoptosis effects [9]. These saponins are also believed to have protective effects against some chemically-induced hepatotoxic reactions. Indeed, platycodin D, the major triterpenoid saponin found in PG, was recently suggested for protecting against liver damage caused by ethanol and carbon tetrachloride [10]. In addition, PG is considered to be a legal medicine and dietary supplement; it is also frequently used as an ingredient in health foods and vegetable dishes [11].

Many studies have reported the effects of PG fractions or extracts on lipid metabolism regulation and insulin resistance improvement, but mostly in animal models [11–13]. Therefore, we conducted a preliminary study on the anti-obesity effect of PG extract (PGE) in overweight and obese adult humans. This is the first study to investigate the body fat loss effects of PGE in humans. In particular, this preliminary study provides information on the approximate daily dosage of PGE for the upcoming main study, which will be performed using dual-energy X-ray absorptiometry (DEXA) equipment for body fat measurement.

2. Materials and Methods

2.1. Participants

Volunteers (20–60 years old) were recruited from Daegu and among employees of Kyungpook National University in the Republic of Korea, in March 2017. After an initial screening, 108 participants with a body mass index (BMI) of 23–30 kg/m^2 were selected. The exclusion criteria were as follows: (1) taking diuretics for hypertension; (2) taking oral hypoglycemic agents or insulin injection; (3) serious cardiac, renal, hepatic, thyroid, or cerebrovascular disease; (4) serious cystic or gastrointestinal disease, gout, or porphyria; (5) psychiatric problems, such as depressive disorder, schizophrenia, alcoholism, and drug intoxication; (6) cancer diagnosis and treatment; (7) asthma or other allergies; (8) a history of surgery within the past 6 months; (9) pregnant or in lactation period. The study was approved by the Kyungpook National University Human Research Committee (KNU 2017-0113). All participants gave their written informed consent for inclusion before they participated in the study.

2.2. Sample Size

In order to eliminate the effects of gender differences, the gender of the participants was assigned by replicated randomized complete block design. The sample size was estimated using G* Power 3.1.9.2. Assuming a 95% statistical power, 0.05 significance level, and 0.40 effect size (Cohen's standard for a large effect), it was estimated that at least 120 participants were required to show a statistically significant difference in biomarkers of body fat among four groups.

2.3. Design

This single institution, randomized, double-blinded, and placebo-controlled study was conducted to confirm the effect of PGE supplementation on body fat loss in obese or overweight participants. The random assignment code was generated using the permed-block randomization method with the assistance of SAS Proc Plan (SAS Institute, Cary, NC, USA). All participants were randomly assigned in into four groups in a 1:1:1:1 ratio: placebo, PGE571 (571 mg as PGE), PGE1142 (1142 mg as PGE), and PGE2855 (2855 mg as PGE). The total content of test product for one tablet was 900 mg (including 571 mg of *Platycodon grandifloras* extract); all participants received two pouches per day of the placebo (including 666 mg of crystalline cellulose) and each PGE (PGE571, PGE1142, PGE2855), according to their assigned group, which were consumed from baseline (0 days) to the end of the 12-week experiment, at 30 min after breakfast and dinner. The placebo and PGEs were supplied by

GC WellBeing (Seongnam, Korea). All participants were instructed to maintain their routine food intake and physical activity during the study. Moreover, during the study period, we monitored the participants' compliance with the nutritional intervention and capsule consumption every week by telephone. At the end of the study, the participants were asked to return any pouches not consumed. The doses of PGE were selected by extrapolated calculations on the basis of a previous animal study [14].

2.4. Anthropometric and Biochemical Analyses

For anthropometric and physiological measurements at baseline and 4, 8, and 12 weeks post-test material supplementation, the participants visited the Science Research Center Laboratory at Kyungpook National University between 07:00 and 11:00 h after a 12 h overnight fast. The BMI, height, weight, and body composition were measured using an X-Scan Plus II body composition analyzer (Jawon Medical Co., Daejeon, Korea). Abdominal computed tomography (CT; Brivo CT385, GE Healthcare, Chicago, IL, USA) scans that included the lumbar spine were acquired at baseline and during follow-up [2,4]. The CT scans were taken at the Doctors Radiology Clinic, located in Daegu city (Korea). The waist and hip circumferences were measured with an anthropometric tape. The waist circumference was measured as the minimum circumference between the iliac crest and rib cage, and the hip circumference was measured as the maximum width over the greater trochanters. The waist-to-hip ratio was calculated by dividing the waist measurement by the hip measurement. Blood samples were collected in ethylenediaminetetraacetic acid-coated tubes and centrifuged at $1000 \times g$ for 15 min at 4 °C for plasma assays. To determine the dietary intake, 24 h dietary recalls were administered in face-to-face interviews at the participants' homes before and during the preliminary trial by dieticians. Three day dietary recalls were performed twice at baseline and during follow-up. We presented the mean of the 3 day dietary intake at each point. During the interview, the participants were asked what kinds of food they ate and drank on their dietary recall sheet. Food replicas were provided to help the participants estimate their dietary intakes and exact portions. Nutritional analysis was performed using CAN-Pro 3.0 software (The Korean Nutrition Society, Seoul, Korea), which provides a comprehensive database for the nutritional content of general foods and specific Korean foods.

2.5. Biochemical Analyses

Before and after the test, fasting blood was collected and analyzed by Seegene Co. Ltd. (Daegu, Korea). The levels of plasma adiponectin, leptin, interleukin-6, tumor necrosis factor-alpha, and monocyte chemoattractant protein-1 were determined using a Cobas 8000 analyzer (Roche Diagnostics, Mannheim, Germany). For the safety evaluation of the test material, the liver and renal function markers (albumin, blood urea nitrogen, total bilirubin, aspartate transaminase, alanine transaminase, and alkaline phosphatase (ALP)) were measured using a Hitachi LABOSPECT 008 AS (Hitachi, Tokyo, Japan).

2.6. Statistical Analysis

Data were analyzed using SPSS (IBM SPSS, version 21) and expressed as mean ± standard deviation. Statistical analysis was performed using the analysis of covariance (ANCOVA) test for comparison between the placebo control group (placebo) and the test groups. In the questionnaire, it was confirmed that there was a large difference in physical activity and drinking among the participants. Given that there is a high correlation between alcohol consumption and obesity rate [15], participants who frequently consumed alcohol (more than two bottles per week) and reported a very low physical activity (sedentary behavior) were excluded (Table 1). Paired t-test was used to verify the difference before and after ingestion at $p < 0.05$. Statistical analysis was also performed on all participants (23 kg/m^2 ≤ BMI ≤ 30 kg/m^2) without any discrimination of physical activity and alcohol consumption for safety assessment.

Table 1. Survey of physical activity and alcohol drinking status of subjects.

Score	Physical Activity	Drinking Behavior
1	Sedentary behavior	1–2 glasses/week
2	Light activity	Less than 1 bottle/week
3	Moderate activity	1–2 bottles/week
4	Vigorous activity	More than 2 bottles/week

3. Results

3.1. Study Flow

This study had an initial 130 candidates, and had 108 eligible individuals who were enrolled in this study through the eligibility tests. After 12 weeks, eight people dropped out for personal reasons. Participants with factors affecting obesity, very low physical activity, and frequent alcohol consumption were excluded. Physical activity and alcohol consumption were assessed through the questionnaire (Table 1). Thus, data from 72 participants were analyzed for evaluating the efficacy of PGE supplementation. Serious adverse effects were not reported by the participants consuming the PGEs or placebo supplements.

3.2. Baseline Clinical Characteristics and Nutrient Intake

The baseline characteristics of volunteers who completed the randomized controlled trial are shown in Table 2. There were no significant differences among all groups in terms of age, height, systolic blood pressure, diastolic blood pressure, and fasting blood glucose. Nutritional intake of the participants before and after the test food intake was measured six times (three times before the test, three times after the test) using the 24 h recall method. The energy and carbohydrate intake of the PGE1142 and PGE2855 groups were significantly higher than that of the placebo group. In other nutrients, no significant difference was found among all groups (Table 3).

Table 2. Baseline characteristics of 4 groups with overweight or obesity subjects who participated in efficacy test of *Platycodon grandiflorus* root extract (PGE).

	Placebo (M: 9, F: 7)	PGE571 (M: 6, F: 13)	PGE1142 (M: 5, F: 14)	PGE2855 (M: 6, F: 12)
Age (years)	40.89 ± 3.44	42.63 ± 2.52	44.95 ± 2.56	48.00 ± 2.03
Height (cm)	168.58 ± 2.79	163.59 ± 2.37	165.26 ± 1.73	162.49 ± 1.82
Body weight (kg)	74.07 ± 2.64	72.48 ± 2.40	70.14 ± 1.93	69.32 ± 1.75
BMI (kg/m^2)	25.98 ± 0.44	26.99 ± 0.44	25.62 ± 0.41	26.24 ± 0.48
Waist (cm)	93.34 ± 1.21	92.26 ± 1.12	91.76 ± 1.41	90.67 ± 0.84
Hip (cm)	103.00 ± 1.10	101.84 ± 1.00	101.16 ± 0.91	100.64 ± 0.97
WHR	0.91 ± 0.01	0.91 ± 0.01	0.91 ± 0.01	0.90 ± 0.01
Systolic BP (mmHg)	124.69 ± 3.68	133.95 ± 3.95	130.42 ± 3.50	139.11 ± 4.24
Diastolic BP (mmHg)	82.44 ± 2.97	90.21 ± 2.75	85.74 ± 2.27	87.83 ± 2.90

Values are the mean ± SD; PGE571: 571 mg administered as PGE, PGE1142: 1142 mg administered as PGE, PGE2855: 2855 mg administered as PGE, BMI: body mass index, WHR: waist hip ratio, BP: blood pressure, M: male, F: female.

Table 3. Comparison of physical activity and nutrients intake in four groups with overweight or obesity by 24 h dietary recall performed before and in a follow-up of the trial.

	Placebo (M: 9, F: 7)	PGE571 (M: 6, F: 13)	PGE1142 (M: 5, F: 14)	PGE2855 (M: 6, F: 12)
	Mean ± SD	Mean ± SD	Mean ± SD	Mean ± SD
Energy (kcal/day)				
Baseline	1571.86 ± 8.31	1680.07 ± 16.89	1520.09 ± 13.74	1747.36 ± 14.15
Follow-up	1384.56 ± 9.83 *	1545.68 ± 14.12	1706.26 ± 15.32	1757.60 ± 10.76
CFB	−187.30 ± 9.45	−134.4 ± 13.21	186.18 ± 12.04	10.24 ± 16.00
p-Value		0.437	0.013	0.045
Carbohydrate (d/day)				
Baseline	226.34 ± 1.32	222.70 ± 1.81	221.81 ± 1.85	244.70 ± 1.99
Follow-up	186.23 ± 1.82 **	211.71 ± 2.23	241.07 ± 1.71	245.17 ± 1.80
CFB	−40.12 ± 1.56	−10.99 ± 1.60	19.26 ± 1.89	0.46 ± 2.23
p-Value		0.185	0.007	0.021
Fat (g/day)				
Baseline	43.80 ± 0.46	53.95 ± 1.11	43.55 ± 0.68	51.61 ± 0.68
Follow-up	45.17 ± 0.53	48.84 ± 0.57	46.85 ± 0.64	52.97 ± 0.42
CFB	1.37 ± 0.58	−5.11 ± 1.13	3.30 ± 0.52	1.36 ± 0.80
p-Value		0.823	0.790	0.358
Protein (g/day)				
Baseline	64.13 ± 0.46	65.61 ± 0.81	57.33 ± 0.55	68.57 ± 0.63
Follow-up	58.72 ± 0.48	57.80 ± 0.55	65.03 ± 0.71	67.96 ± 0.43
CFB	−5.41 ± 0.63	−7.81 ± 0.61	7.70 ± 0.54	−0.61 ± 0.72
p-Value		0.804	0.145	0.242
Cholesterol (mg/day)				
Baseline	239.95 ± 3.79	213.90 ± 3.41	203.86 ± 3.40	274.73 ± 3.94
Follow-up	218.46 ± 3.32	234.29 ± 3.71	246.74 ± 3.44	244.84 ± 3.06
CFB	−21.48 ± 4.31	20.39 ± 3.10	42.87 ± 4.83	−29.89 ± 4.20
p-Value		0.564	0.341	0.692

p-Value: Analysis of covariance (ANCOVA) model with independent variable as baseline and treatment; * $p < 0.05$, ** $p < 0.01$ derived from paired t-tests performed for values obtained before and after the trial. CFB: changes from baseline.

3.3. Body Composition

Body composition, such as body weight, BMI, body fat mass, body fat percentage (BFP), and muscle weight, were analyzed by using data that considered drinking and exercise activities ($n = 72$) (Table 4). Body fat (ANCOVA, $p < 0.028$) and BFP (ANCOVA, $p < 0.001$) were significantly decreased in the PGE571 group compared with the placebo. Also, supplementation of PGE2855 led to a decrease in the body fat mass (ANCOVA, $p < 0.036$) and BPF (ANCOVA, $p < 0.035$). In contrast, muscle mass was significantly increased in the PGE571 (ANCOVA, $p < 0.002$)-supplemented group compared with the control (placebo) group (Table 4).

Moreover, we performed CT scans at baseline and after (follow-up) to observe the effects of PGE supplementation on the participants' abdominal fat area. The high-dose PGE group (PGE2855) was observed to have a significant effect when compared with the placebo group. In particular, the PGE2855 led to a significant decrease in the L4 total abdominal fat area (ANCOVA, $p = 0.029$) and subcutaneous fat area (ANCOVA, $p = 0.035$) (Table 5).

Table 4. Effect of PGE supplementation for 12 weeks on change of body composition measured by bioelectrical impedance analysis (BIA), WHR-related body measurements, and blood pressure in groups with overweight or obesity.

	Placebo (M: 9, F: 7)	PGE571 (M: 6, F: 13)	PGE1142 (M: 5, F: 14)	PGE2855 (M: 6, F: 12)
	Mean ± SD	Mean ± SD	Mean ± SD	Mean ± SD
Body weight (kg)				
Baseline	74.07 ± 2.64	72.48 ± 2.40	70.14 ± 1.93	69.32 ± 1.75
Follow-up	73.61 ± 2.70	72.12 ± 2.42	69.73 ± 1.95	68.03 ± 1.60 **
CFB	−0.46 ± 0.40	−0.36 ± 0.39	−0.42 ± 0.42	−1.28 ± 0.36
p-Value		0.901	0.969	0.128
BMI (kg/m^2)				
Baseline	25.98 ± 0.44	26.99 ± 0.44	25.62 ± 0.41	26.24 ± 0.48
Follow-up	25.71 ± 0.46 *	26.69 ± 0.42	25.39 ± 0.44	25.69 ± 0.46 ***
CFB	−0.27 ± 0.13	−0.30 ± 0.16	−0.23 ± 0.16	−0.54 ± 0.11
p-Value		0.933	0.924	0.213
Body fat mass (kg)				
Baseline	21.02 ± 0.95	22.76 ± 0.75	21.91 ± 0.85	22.11 ± 0.98
Follow-up	21.46 ± 0.93	22.12 ± 0.77	21.96 ± 0.91	21.54 ± 0.99 **
CFB	0.44 ± 0.30	−0.64 ± 0.38	0.05 ± 0.30	−0.57 ± 0.20
p-Value		0.028	0.432	0.036
BFP (%)				
Baseline	28.73 ± 1.45	31.95 ± 1.18	31.41 ± 1.12	31.97 ± 1.27
Follow-up	29.52 ± 1.42 *	31.11 ± 1.25 *	31.67 ± 1.17	31.73 ± 1.30
CFB	0.79 ± 0.30	−0.85 ± 0.41	0.26 ± 0.30	−0.24 ± 0.17
p-Value		0.001	0.273	0.035
Muscle weight (kg)				
Baseline	48.79 ± 2.41	45.61 ± 2.12	44.25 ± 1.68	43.24 ± 1.53
Follow-up	47.94 ± 2.42 **	45.91 ± 2.21	43.82 ± 1.67	42.62 ± 1.43 **
CFB	−0.85 ± 0.26	0.29 ± 0.25	−0.43 ± 0.26	−0.62 ± 0.19
p-Value		0.002	0.251	0.551

p-Value: ANCOVA model with independent variable as baseline and treatment; * $p < 0.05$, ** $p < 0.01$, *** $p < 0.001$ derived from paired t-tests performed for values obtained before and after the trial; CFB: changes from baseline; BFP: body fat percentage.

Table 5. Effect of PGE supplementation for 12 weeks on change of abdominal fat area assessed by computed tomography (CT) in subjects with overweight or obesity.

	Placebo (M: 9, F: 7)	PGE571 (M: 6, F: 13)	PGE1142 (M: 5, F: 14)	PGE2855 (M: 6, F: 12)
	Mean ± SD	Mean ± SD	Mean ± SD	Mean ± SD
L4 Total abdominal fat (cm^2)				
Baseline	305.72 ± 21.54	363.49 ± 15.51	331.80 ± 18.78	318.07 ± 14.08
Follow-up	316.84 ± 19.81	362.35 ± 15.12	331.36 ± 17.47	299.11 ± 11.53 *
CFB	11.12 ± 12.81	−1.13 ± 8.54	−0.44 ± 8.50	−18.95 ± 7.91
p-Value		0.959	0.651	0.029
L4 Subcutaneous fat (cm^2)				
Baseline	184.00 ± 20.17	215.13 ± 14.95	195.32 ± 13.65	179.18 ± 11.76
Follow-up	197.10 ± 18.16	222.43 ± 13.87	196.80 ± 12.28	171.04 ± 10.41
CFB	13.10 ± 11.17	7.30 ± 6.19	1.48 ± 7.15	−8.14 ± 6.73
p-Value		0.911	0.382	0.035
L4 Visceral fat (cm^2)				
Baseline	121.71 ± 7.32	148.35 ± 9.89	136.48 ± 10.37	138.88 ± 11.16
Follow-up	119.74 ± 8.96	139.92 ± 10.52	134.56 ± 10.88	128.07 ± 9.56 **
CFB	−1.97 ± 4.62	−8.43 ± 6.03	−1.92 ± 3.62	−10.81 ± 3.60
p-Value		0.561	0.828	0.245

p-Value: ANCOVA model with independent variable as baseline and treatment; * $p < 0.05$, ** $p < 0.01$ derived from paired t-tests performed for values obtained before and after the trial; CFB: changes from baseline.

3.4. Plasma Adipokines

Table 6 shows the levels of plasma adipokines. When ANCOVA was used, there were no significant differences in adipokine levels among the four groups. However, PGE571 supplementation significantly reduced leptin levels after 12 weeks from baseline. Also, the leptin:adiponectin (L:A) ratio was significantly lower after supplementation with PGE2855 compared with the baseline (before supplementation) measurement. In comparison to the baseline, PGE supplementation led to a significant decrease in leptin levels in the PGE571 (paired t-test, $p < 0.01$) and the L:A ratio in the PGE2855 (paired t-test, $p < 0.05$) after the 12 week experiment. In addition, when all participants were analyzed ($n = 100$), adiponectin levels (ANCOVA, $p < 0.059$) tended to decrease in the PGE571 group compared with the placebo (data not shown).

Table 6. Effect of supplementation of PGE for 12 weeks on changes of serum adipokine levels in subjects with overweight or obesity.

	Placebo (M: 9, F: 7)	PGE571 (M: 6, F: 13)	PGE1142 (M: 5, F: 14)	PGE2855 (M: 6, F: 12)
	Mean ± SD	Mean ± SD	Mean ± SD	Mean ± SD
Leptin (ng/mL)				
Baseline	3.58 ± 0.61	6.22 ± 0.96	4.15 ± 0.66	5.47 ± 0.84
Follow-up	3.11 ± 0.46	5.00 ± 0.78 **	4.24 ± 0.62	4.19 ± 0.67
CFB	−0.48 ± 0.42	−1.22 ± 0.35	0.09 ± 0.46	−1.16 ± 0.58
p-Value		0.776	0.133	0.888
Resistin (ng/mL)				
Baseline	31.66 ± 8.05	21.83 ± 1.84	19.16 ± 2.57	26.69 ± 4.51
Follow-up	23.65 ± 3.03	21.03 ± 2.79	17.74 ± 2.38	23.17 ± 2.80
CFB	−8.01 ± 6.22	−0.80 ± 2.07	−1.42 ± 2.39	−4.37 ± 2.91
p-Value		0.724	0.968	0.726
Adiponectin (ug/mL)				
Baseline	9.74 ± 1.28	8.44 ± 1.61	8.27 ± 1.28	13.53 ± 2.97
Follow-up	9.00 ± 1.37	13.38 ± 4.51	9.84 ± 1.64	11.95 ± 2.16
CFB	−0.74 ± 0.43	4.94 ± 4.60	1.58 ± 1.39	−0.70 ± 1.18
p-Value		0.174	0.633	0.792
L:A ratio				
Baseline	0.42 ± 0.07	1.14 ± 0.23	0.84 ± 0.22	0.75 ± 0.22
Follow-up	0.39 ± 0.05	0.74 ± 0.16	0.74 ± 0.20	0.53 ± 0.16 *
CFB	−0.02 ± 0.05	−0.40 ± 0.22	−0.10 ± 0.13	−0.24 ± 0.10
p-Value		0.789	0.466	0.758

p-Value: ANCOVA model with independent variable as baseline and treatment; * $p < 0.05$, ** $p < 0.01$ derived from paired t-tests performed for values obtained before and after the trial; CFB: changes from baseline, L:A: leptin:adiponectin.

3.5. Lipids Metabolism

Table 7 shows the changes in the indirect markers of lipids metabolism. There were no significant changes in lipids metabolism. When all participants were analyzed, there were no significant changes among the four groups in terms of cholesterol, triglyceride, high density lipoprotein cholesterol (HDL-C), low density lipoprotein cholesterol (LDL-C), and phospholipid. The changes were within the normal range and were considered to have no clinical implications in terms of the safety assessment.

Table 7. Effect of supplementation of PGE for 12 weeks on changes of lipids metabolism in subjects with overweight or obesity.

	Placebo (M: 9, F: 7)	PGE571 (M: 6, F: 13)	PGE1142 (M: 5, F: 14)	PGE2855 (M: 6, F: 12)
	Mean ± SD	Mean ± SD	Mean ± SD	Mean ± SD
Cholesterol (mg/dL): normal range 0~240 mg/dL				
Baseline	201.38 ± 10.42	210.25 ± 9.18	204.43 ± 7.70	198.84 ± 7.30
Follow-up	199.75 ± 10.56	204.55 ± 7.22	208.05 ± 9.69	195.72 ± 8.06
CFB	−1.63 ± 4.34	−5.70 ± 7.40	3.62 ± 5.46	−1.89 ± 5.65
p-Value		0.837	0.517	0.904
TG (mg/dL): normal range 36~150 mg/dL				
Baseline	96.00 ± 8.34	119.40 ± 10.81	116.38 ± 9.12	125.79 ± 25.42
Follow-up	119.38 ± 16.70	137.75 ± 15.98	112.00 ± 10.85	116.22 ± 17.78
CFB	23.38 ± 13.33	18.35 ± 11.36	−4.38 ± 8.13	−7.61 ± 21.67
p-Value		0.733	0.279	0.324
HDL-C (mg/dL): normal range 40~60 mg/dL				
Baseline	49.88 ± 2.50	53.80 ± 3.06	57.86 ± 2.95	50.11 ± 2.52
Follow-up	46.38 ± 2.49 *	50.95 ± 2.74	56.24 ± 2.23	45.56 ± 2.25 *
CFB	−3.5 ± 1.63	−2.85 ± 2.07	−1.62 ± 1.66	−4.39 ± 1.61
p-Value		0.299	0.088	0.704
LDL-C (mg/dL): normal range 0~130 mg/dL				
Baseline	131.69 ± 8.52	134.50 ± 8.47	123.38 ± 6.40	125.68 ± 7.12
Follow-up	130.25 ± 8.01	125.65 ± 6.42	128.38 ± 8.73	124.11 ± 6.50
CFB	−1.44 ± 3.77	−8.85 ± 7.87	5.00 ± 5.02	−0.39 ± 5.78
p-Value		0.427	0.563	0.877
Phospholipid (mmol/L): normal range 150~250 mg/dL				
Baseline	225.31 ± 8.88	242.40 ± 7.67	237.90 ± 6.50	229.74 ± 7.13
Follow-up	229.38 ± 8.56	241.85 ± 6.53	246.81 ± 6.78	226.17 ± 7.56
CFB	4.06 ± 5.87	−0.55 ± 6.92	8.9 ± 5.05	−2.11 ± 7.32
p-Value		0.812	0.333	0.560

p-Value: ANCOVA model with independent variable as baseline and treatment; * $p < 0.05$ derived from paired t-tests performed for values obtained before and after the trial; CFB: change from baseline; TG: triglyceride; HDL-C: high density lipoprotein cholesterol; LDL-C: low density lipoprotein cholesterol.

3.6. Safety Assessment and Indirect Markers of Hepatic and Renal Function Test

Hepatic and renal function markers in plasma were analyzed for safety assessment. When all participants were analyzed ($n = 100$), there were no significant changes in the safety-related markers of liver or renal function among the four groups. Table 8 shows the changes in the indirect markers of liver and renal function due to PGE supplementation. PGE1142 supplementation was observed to lower the glutamic-pyruvic transaminase (GPT) (ANCOVA, $p < 0.006$) levels more than the placebo. The changes were within the normal range and were considered to have no clinical implications.

Table 8. Effect of PGE supplementation for 12 weeks on plasma albumin, total bilirubin, alanine aminotransferase (ALP), glutamic oxalacetic transaminase (GOT), glutamic pyruvate transaminase (GPT), blood urea nitrogen (BUN), and creatinine levels in subjects with overweight or obesity ($n = 100$).

	Placebo (M: 15, F: 10)	PGE571 (M: 10, F: 16)	PGE1142 (M: 10, F: 15)	PGE2855 (M: 8, F: 16)
	Mean ± SD	Mean ± SD	Mean ± SD	Mean ± SD
ALB (g/dL): normal range 3.5~5.2 g/dL				
Baseline	4.45 ± 0.04	4.37 ± 0.06	4.37 ± 0.05	4.39 ± 0.04
Follow-up	4.51 ± 0.05 **	4.38 ± 0.05	4.46 ± 0.04 ***	4.42 ± 0.04
CFB	0.06 ± 0.03	0.02 ± 0.04	0.08 ± 0.02	0.03 ± 0.03
p-Value		0.080	0.991	0.205
Total bilirubin (mg/dL): normal range <1.3 mg/dL				
Baseline	0.82 ± 0.05	0.73 ± 0.06	0.74 ± 0.06	0.78 ± 0.07
Follow-up	0.84 ± 0.04	0.73 ± 0.06	0.67 ± 0.04	0.76 ± 0.07
CFB	0.01 ± 0.03	0 ± 0.06	−0.07 ± 0.04	−0.02 ± 0.05
p-Value		0.438	0.052	0.411
ALP (U/L): normal range 40~160 U/L				
Baseline	56.8 ± 3.20	56 ± 2.23	55.84 ± 2.74	61.08 ± 2.91
Follow-up	57.84 ± 2.99	55.04 ± 2.12	56.08 ± 2.94	59.5 ± 2.99
CFB	1.00 ± 1.37	−0.96 ± 1.80	0.23 ± 1.76	−1.52 ± 2.87
p-Value		0.412	0.696	0.608
GOT (AST) (U/L): normal range <40 U/L				
Baseline	32.88 ± 5.10	29.15 ± 3.46	26.68 ± 1.79	26.00 ± 1.87
Follow-up	30.24 ± 4.49	26.92 ± 2.88	23.16 ± 1.13 *	26.75 ± 2.40
CFB	−2.54 ± 3.35	−2.23 ± 4.30	−3.38 ± 1.44	0.72 ± 1.78
p-Value		0.668	0.258	0.959
GPT (ALT) (U/L): normal range <40 U/L				
Baseline	31.44 ± 8.21	26.54 ± 3.94	27.08 ± 3.38	24.21 ± 3.06
Follow-up	36.08 ± 9.47	26.46 ± 4.47	21.68 ± 2.25 *	23.17 ± 3.65
CFB	4.46 ± 2.07	−0.08 ± 2.80	−5.19 ± 2.08	−1 ± 2.84
p-Value		0.188	0.006	0.121
BUN (mg/dL): normal range 8~22 mg/dL				
Baseline	13.12 ± 0.58	13.31 ± 0.66	12.96 ± 0.49	15.04 ± 0.82
Follow-up	14.24 ± 0.79	12.85 ± 0.66	13.64 ± 0.55	14.08 ± 0.83
CFB	1.08 ± 0.55	−0.46 ± 0.61	0.65 ± 0.50	−0.92 ± 0.78
p-Value		0.070	0.550	0.118
Creatinine (mg/dL): normal range 0.5~1.30 mg/dL				
Baseline	0.74 ± 0.03	0.70 ± 0.04	0.70 ± 0.03	0.68 ± 0.03
Follow-up	0.79 ± 0.03 ***	0.74 ± 0.04 ***	0.77 ± 0.04 ***	0.71 ± 0.03
CFB	0.05 ± 0.01	0.04 ± 0.01	0.06 ± 0.02	0.04 ± 0.02
p-Value		0.540	0.630	0.365

p-Value: ANCOVA model with independent variable as baseline and treatment; * $p < 0.05$, ** $p < 0.01$, *** $p < 0.001$ derived from paired t-tests performed for values obtained before and after the trial; ALB: albumin, ALP: alanine aminotransferase, GOT: glutamic oxalacetic transaminase, GPT: glutamic pyruvate transaminase, BUN: blood urea nitrogen, CFB: changes from baseline.

4. Discussion

Many studies have reported on the health benefits of the extracts and saponin fractions of *P. grandiflorus*, such as anti-obesity and anti-lipid metabolism, but most of them have demonstrated efficacy in animal models. Our preliminary study also confirmed the weight loss and body fat loss efficacy of PGE in animal models of obesity. Indeed, PG extract increased thermogenic gene expression (such as SIRT1, PPARα, UCP1, PGC1α), thereby inducing the browning of white adipose tissue, resulting in an anti-obesity effect. Thus, this study was conducted to verify the effect of PGE in humans. Through the questionnaire, we found that there was a significant difference in the level of alcohol drinking and physical activity among the participants. Accordingly, the following statistics were used in this study: an analysis, excluding dropouts, but including the participants with very low physical activity and frequent drinking activities (more than two bottles per week).

This study was a small-scale experiment to set the effective dose of PGE in humans by confirming the anti-obesity effect. We conducted bioelectrical impedance analysis (BIA), which is generally highly correlated with body weight and body fat mass, although we did not measure body fat mass by DEXA.

In particular, we screened participants who frequently consumed alcohol and had a very low physical activity, two factors closely associated with obesity, to confirm the anti-obesity effect of PGE. Energy and carbohydrates were significantly higher in the PGE1142 and PGE2855 supplement groups compared with the placebo. Body composition changes induced by PGE revealed that supplementation of PGE571 and PGE2855 significantly reduced body fat mass and BFP, but also led to an increase in muscle mass in the PGE571 group. In our previous study [14], we found increased muscle mass associated with increased energy expenditure following supplementation of PGE in animal models of obesity. Similarly, in this study, PGE supplementation significantly increased the muscle mass of the participants. Therefore, this increase is considered to be an important candidate in obesity treatment or prevention. We performed abdominal CT, as well as BIA, to confirm the effect of PGE on body fat loss. Consistent with the BIA results, PGE2855 supplementation significantly lowered the subcutaneous fat and abdominal fat area of L4 when compared with the placebo, suggesting the association of BFP and fat mass reduction by PGE2855 supplementation. Although there was no change in the abdominal fat area in the PGE571 group, this may have been due to the relatively high baseline abdominal fat area, as the PGE571 group showed a high level of leptin in the blood, which is proportional to the amount of fat [16]. PGE571 not only significantly decreased body fat and BFP, but also significantly increased muscle mass when BIA was performed, regardless of the statistical method. This was similar to our previous studies that showed increased muscle mass by PGE, which is closely associated with increased energy expenditure [17]. When all participants were analyzed in terms of lipids metabolism and markers of hepatic and renal function test, there were no significant changes among the four groups in terms of cholesterol, triglyceride, HDL-C, LDL-C, phospholipid, and markers of liver and renal function. The changes were within the normal range and were considered to have no clinical implications for the safety assessment. In this context, it is considered that the increase of muscle mass can act as an important marker in obesity (or sarcopenic obesity) research. In this study, DEXA, which is highly correlated with BIA [18] and provides more accurate levels of body fat mass, was not measured. Therefore, it is presumed that DEXA measurement may be able to confirm the change of abdominal fat area due to PGE571 supplementation in future studies.

The limitations of this trial should be emphasized. Given that the participants of this study were restricted to volunteers, it was difficult to represent the general population with this small sample size. As the study was conducted on overweight or moderately obese adults who had BMI measurements ranging between 23 and 30, part of the results that we obtained via clinical trial were difficult to identify and generate statistically meaningful data. Hence, to have more statistical meaningful data, it would be prudent to conduct the trial in obese adults. This study was a clinical trial to determine whether PGE could improve obesity and estimate the appropriate daily dose of PGE for overweight or obese adult humans. In addition, we used CT scans to improve the accuracy of the body composition measurements, but this technique only measured the abdominal fat area. Therefore, a further experiment is underway to confirm the body fat reduction function of PGE571 using DEXA.

5. Conclusions

In conclusion, despite some limitations, we demonstrated that PGE is able to reduce body fat mass and body fat percentage, which is an anti-obesity marker, in overweight or obese adult humans. PGE supplementation significantly increased the muscle mass when compared with the placebo, indicating an excellent anti-obesity effect.

Author Contributions: Y.J.K. performed the experiments, analyzed the data, and wrote/edited the manuscript. E.-Y.K. performed the experiments and reviewed the manuscript. J.-W.K., Y.L., and R.R. performed the experiments. GC WellBeing (J.Y. and M.K.) contributed to the preparation of *Platycodon grandiflorus* ethanol extract for this experiment. M.-S.C. supervised this work and had full access to all the data and, therefore, takes full responsibility for the integrity of the results and accuracy of the data analysis.

Funding: This work was supported by the Support Research and Commercialization Project grant number (NRF-20170701C4048818) of the Ministry of Science, ICT, and Future Planning through the National Research Foundation of Korea.

Conflicts of Interest: The authors declare no conflict of interest.

References

1. Pi-Sunyer, X. The medical risks of obesity. *Postgrad. Med.* **2009**, *121*, 21–33. [CrossRef] [PubMed]
2. National Institutes of Health. Clinical Guidelines on the Identification, Evaluation, and Treatment of Overweight and Obesity in Adults—The Evidence Report. *Obes. Res.* **1998**, *6* (Suppl. 2), 51S–209S.
3. Grundy, S.M. Obesity, metabolic syndrome, and cardiovascular disease. *J. Clin. Endocrinol. Metab.* **2004**, *89*, 2595–2600. [CrossRef] [PubMed]
4. Batsis, J.A.; Mackenzie, T.A.; Jones, J.D.; Lopez-Jimenez, F.; Bartels, S.J. Sarcopenia, sarcopenic obesity and inflammation: Results from the 1999–2004 National Health and Nutrition Examination Survey. *Clin. Nutr.* **2016**, *35*, 1472–1483. [CrossRef] [PubMed]
5. Choi, K.M. Sarcopenia and sarcopenic obesity. *Korean J. Intern. Med.* **2016**, *31*, 1054–1060. [CrossRef] [PubMed]
6. Wang, C.; Zhang, N.; Wang, Z.; Qi, Z.; Zheng, B.; Li, P.; Liu, J. Rapid characterization of chemical constituents of Platycodon grandiflorum and its adulterant Adenophora stricta by UPLC-QTOF-MS/MS. *J. Mass Spectrom.* **2017**, *52*, 643–656. [CrossRef] [PubMed]
7. Ryu, C.S.; Kim, C.H.; Lee, S.Y.; Lee, K.S.; Choung, K.J.; Song, G.Y.; Kim, B.H.; Ryu, S.Y.; Lee, H.S.; Kim, S.K. Evaluation of the total oxidant scavenging capacity of saponins isolated from Platycodon grandiflorum. *Food Chem.* **2012**, *132*, 333–337. [CrossRef] [PubMed]
8. Wang, Y.; Zhang, X.; Wei, Z.; Wang, J.; Zhang, Y.; Shi, M.; Yang, Z.; Fu, Y. Platycodin D suppressed LPS-induced inflammatory response by activating LXRalpha in LPS-stimulated primary bovine mammary epithelial cells. *Eur. J. Pharmacol.* **2017**, *814*, 138–143. [CrossRef] [PubMed]
9. Lin, Y.C.; Lin, C.H.; Yao, H.T.; Kuo, W.W.; Shen, C.Y.; Yeh, Y.L.; Ho, T.J.; Padma, V.V.; Lin, Y.C.; Huang, C.Y.; et al. Platycodon grandiflorum (PG) reverses angiotensin II-induced apoptosis by repressing IGF-IIR expression. *J. Ethnopharmacol.* **2017**, *205*, 41–50. [CrossRef] [PubMed]
10. Fu, C.L.; Liu, Y.; Leng, J.; Zhang, J.; He, Y.F.; Chen, C.; Wang, Z.; Li, W. Platycodin D protects acetaminophen-induced hepatotoxicity by inhibiting hepatocyte MAPK pathway and apoptosis in C57BL/6J mice. *Biomed. Pharmacother.* **2018**, *107*, 867–877. [CrossRef] [PubMed]
11. Zhang, L.; Wang, Y.; Yang, D.; Zhang, C.; Zhang, N.; Li, M.; Liu, Y. Platycodon grandifloras—An ethnopharmacological, phytochemical and pharmacological review. *J. Ethnopharmacol.* **2015**, *164*, 147–161. [CrossRef] [PubMed]
12. Lee, J.S.; Choi, M.S.; Seo, K.I.; Lee, J.; Lee, H.I.; Lee, J.H.; Kim, M.J.; Lee, M.K. Platycodi radix saponin inhibits alpha-glucosidase in vitro and modulates hepatic glucose-regulating enzyme activities in C57BL/KsJ-db/db mice. *Arch. Pharm. Res.* **2014**, *37*, 773–782. [CrossRef] [PubMed]
13. Qin, H.; Du, X.; Zhang, Y.; Wang, R. Platycodin D, a triterpenoid saponin from Platycodon grandiflorum, induces G2/M arrest and apoptosis in human hepatoma HepG2 cells by modulating the PI3K/Akt pathway. *Tumor Biol.* **2014**, *35*, 1267–1274. [CrossRef] [PubMed]
14. Kim, Y.J.; Choi, J.Y.; Ryu, R.; Lee, J.; Cho, S.J.; Kwon, E.Y.; Lee, M.K.; Liu, K.H.; Rina, Y.; Sung, M.K.; et al. Platycodon grandiflorus Root Extract Attenuates Body Fat Mass, Hepatic Steatosis and Insulin Resistance through the Interplay between the Liver and Adipose Tissue. *Nutrients* **2016**, *8*, 532. [CrossRef] [PubMed]
15. Traversy, G.; Chaput, J.P. Alcohol Consumption and Obesity: An Update. *Curr. Obes. Rep.* **2015**, *4*, 122–130. [CrossRef] [PubMed]
16. Bravo, P.E.; Morse, S.; Borne, D.M.; Aguilar, E.A.; Reisin, E. Leptin and hypertension in obesity. *Vasc. Health Risk Manag.* **2006**, *2*, 163–169. [CrossRef] [PubMed]

17. August, G.P.; Caprio, S.; Fennoy, I.; Freemark, M.; Kaufman, F.R.; Lustig, R.H.; Silverstein, J.H.; Speiser, P.W.; Styne, D.M.; Montori, V.M.; et al. Prevention and treatment of pediatric obesity: An endocrine society clinical practice guideline based on expert opinion. *J. Clin. Endocrinol. Metab.* **2008**, *93*, 4576–4599. [CrossRef] [PubMed]
18. Tyrrell, V.J.; Richards, G.; Hofman, P.; Gillies, G.F.; Robinson, E.; Cutfield, W.S. Foot-to-foot bioelectrical impedance analysis: A valuable tool for the measurement of body composition in children. *Int. J. Obes. Relat. Metab. Disord.* **2001**, *25*, 273–278. [CrossRef] [PubMed]

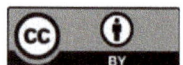

© 2019 by the authors. Licensee MDPI, Basel, Switzerland. This article is an open access article distributed under the terms and conditions of the Creative Commons Attribution (CC BY) license (http://creativecommons.org/licenses/by/4.0/).

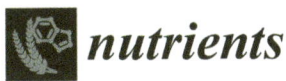

Article

Comparative Investigation of Frankincense Nutraceuticals: Correlation of Boswellic and Lupeolic Acid Contents with Cytokine Release Inhibition and Toxicity against Triple-Negative Breast Cancer Cells

Michael Schmiech [1], Sophia J. Lang [1], Judith Ulrich [1], Katharina Werner [1], Luay J. Rashan [2], Tatiana Syrovets [1,*] and Thomas Simmet [1,*]

[1] Institute of Pharmacology of Natural Products and Clinical Pharmacology, Ulm University, 89081 Ulm, Germany; michael.schmiech@uni-ulm.de (M.S.); sophia.lang@uni-ulm.de (S.J.L.); judith.ulrich@uni-ulm.de (J.U.); katharina.werner@uni-ulm.de (K.W.)
[2] Medicinal Plants Division, Research Center, Dhofar University, Salalah 211, Oman; lrashan@du.edu.om
* Correspondence: tatiana.syrovets@uni-ulm.de (T.S.); thomas.simmet@uni-ulm.de (T.S.); Tel.: +49-731-500-62604 (T.S.); +49-731-500-62600 (T.S.)

Received: 1 September 2019; Accepted: 26 September 2019; Published: 2 October 2019

Abstract: For centuries, frankincense extracts have been commonly used in traditional medicine, and more recently, in complementary medicine. Therefore, frankincense constituents such as boswellic and lupeolic acids are of considerable therapeutic interest. Sixteen frankincense nutraceuticals were characterized by high-performance liquid chromatography with tandem mass spectrometry (HPLC-MS/MS), revealing major differences in boswellic and lupeolic acid compositions and total contents, which varied from 0.4% to 35.7%. Frankincense nutraceuticals significantly inhibited the release of proinflammatory cytokines, such as TNF-α, IL-6, and IL-8, by LPS-stimulated peripheral blood mononuclear cells (PBMC) and whole blood. Moreover, boswellic and lupeolic acid contents correlated with TNF-α, IL-1β, IL-6, IL-8, and IL-10 inhibition. The nutraceuticals also exhibited toxicity against the human triple-negative breast cancer cell lines MDA-MB-231, MDA-MB-453, and CAL-51 in vitro. Nutraceuticals with total contents of boswellic and lupeolic acids >30% were the most active ones against MDA-MB-231 with a half maximal inhibitory concentration (IC$_{50}$) $\leq$ 7.0 µg/mL. Moreover, a frankincense nutraceutical inhibited tumor growth and induced apoptosis in vivo in breast cancer xenografts grown on the chick chorioallantoic membrane (CAM). Among eight different boswellic and lupeolic acids tested, β-ABA exhibited the highest cytotoxicity against MDA-MB-231 with an IC$_{50}$ = 5.9 µM, inhibited growth of cancer xenografts in vivo, and released proinflammatory cytokines. Its content in nutraceuticals correlated strongly with TNF-α, IL-6, and IL-8 release inhibition.

Keywords: frankincense; *Boswellia*; boswellic acid; lupeolic acid; AKBA; cytokine; breast cancer; pentacyclic triterpenic acid; triterpenoid; chorioallantoic membrane assay

1. Introduction

Frankincense is an oleogum resin from trees of the genus *Boswellia* Roxb. ex Colebr., which belong to the *Burseraceae* family. Herbal preparations from frankincense have been used for centuries in traditional Ayurvedic, African, Arab, and Chinese medicine for the treatment of skin ailments, infectious diseases, and other conditions, which today could be assigned to various chronic inflammatory diseases and cancer [1,2]. Likewise, modern medicine has rediscovered frankincense and its pain-relieving, sedative, anti-inflammatory, antimicrobial effects, and even potential anticancer properties [3–5].

Boswellia trees grow mainly in dry areas in India, the Arabian Peninsula, and the Horn of Africa and often have a shrubby appearance with an average high of 2–6 m [6,7], whereby the main representative species are *Boswellia sacra* (Oman and Yemen), *Boswellia carterii* (Somalia), and *Boswellia serrata* (India). However, there are about 25 *Boswellia* species reported, but it is still not clear whether this number contains some double-counted species [8]. Frankincense, the oleogum resin of *Boswellia* trees, which contains potential biologically-active compounds, emerges from cuts in trunks and branches as a sticky-milky liquid, which dries quickly in the air, yielding an oleogum resin containing 15–20% boswellic acids and lupeolic acids [9] (Figure 1). These pentacyclic triterpenic acids are believed to be effective in the prevention and treatment of chronic inflammatory diseases and cancer [3,5]. Previous studies have demonstrated that boswellic acids inhibit essential pathways of inflammatory responses by interaction with IκB kinases and therefore inhibition of proinflammatory gene expression or by inhibition of 5-lipoxygenase and leukotrienes biosynthesis [10,11]. Moreover, also recent clinical pilot studies claimed therapeutic efficacy of extracts containing boswellic acids in the treatment of chronic inflammatory diseases like asthma, rheumatoid arthritis, Crohn's disease, osteoarthritis, collagenous colitis, or colitis ulcerosa [12,13]. Furthermore, *Boswellia serrata* extracts as well as boswellic and lupeolic acids induce apoptosis in various cancer cell lines, such as leukemia, brain, and prostate [5,14–17]. There have also been reports indicating the efficacy of boswellic acids against breast cancer [18,19].

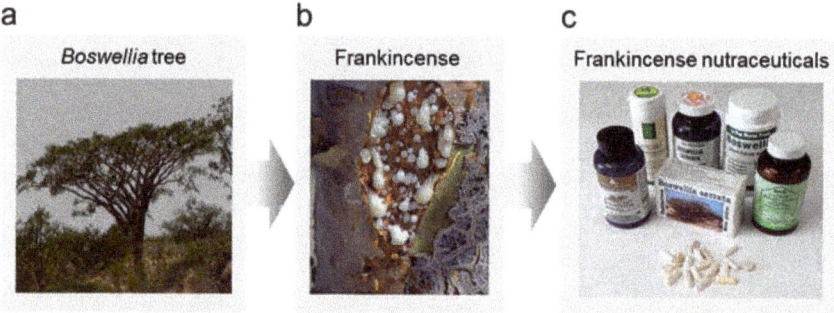

Figure 1. Production of frankincense nutraceuticals. *Boswellia* tree grown in Somalia (**a**), harvesting of the frankincense oleogum resin by bark incisions (**b**), commercial frankincense nutraceuticals (**c**). Pictures with permission from Georg Huber [20].

With 24.2%, breast cancer is the most common cancer of all female cancer cases, causing 15.0% of all female cancer deaths in 2018 [21]. Particularly, triple-negative breast cancer (TNBC) is an aggressive, highly metastatic breast cancer subtype affecting mainly younger women. TNBC is characterized by the lack of expression of hormone receptors (estrogen and progesterone) and the human epidermal growth factor receptor 2 (HER2), which countervails targeted therapy [22]. First, in 2011, Suhail et al. described the induction of apoptosis in human breast cancer cells in vitro by essential oil derived from *Boswellia sacra* [19]. In a later study, we demonstrated that mainly the acidic components of frankincense, i.e., boswellic and lupeolic acids, exhibit cytotoxic efficacy against the TNBC cell line MDA-MB-231 [18].

The global market size of dietary supplements and nutraceuticals was estimated to be worth USD 115 billion in 2018 with an expected compound annual growth rate (CAGR) of 7.8% till 2025 [23]. This demonstrates the strong aptness of the general public to use natural products to maintain good health and to prevent or treat diseases. However, due to insufficient regulation regarding quality and lack of standardization of dietary supplements and nutraceuticals, several questionable or even harmful products are on the market [24].

The aim of this study is to compare frankincense nutraceuticals (FNs) regarding their chemical composition, their efficacies in inhibiting production of inflammatory cytokines, and their cytotoxic efficacy against metastatic TNBC cells.

2. Materials and Methods

2.1. Materials

All solvents and chemicals were of analytical reagent grade. Dimethyl sulfoxide (DMSO) for sample preparation was purchased from Invitrogen (Thermo Fisher Scientific, Waltham, MA, USA). The solvents used for HPLC-MS/MS analysis were methanol, acetic acid (both HiPerSolv Chromanorm, VWR chemicals, Fontenay-sous-Bois, France) and ultrapure water (reverse-osmosis type water (pureAqua, Schnaitsee, Germany) coupled to a Milli-Q station (Millipore, Eschborn, Germany). The reference substances, acetyl-α-boswellic acid (α-ABA), acetyl-β-boswellic acid (β-ABA), α-boswellic acid (α-BA), β-boswellic acid (β-BA), acetyl-11-keto-β-boswellic acid (AKBA), and 11-keto-β-boswellic acid (KBA) were purchased from Extrasynthese (Genay Cedex, France). Acetyl-lupeolic acid (ALA) and lupeolic acid (LA) were isolated and characterized as previously published [9,25]. Samples of frankincense nutraceuticals (FNs) were purchased from the respective distributors (see Table A1). Stock solutions of FNs and pure boswellic (BAs) and lupeolic acids (LAs) were prepared in DMSO and further diluted in RPMI 1640 medium (Gibco, Thermo Fisher Scientific, Waltham, MA, USA). In all experiments, the final DMSO concentration did not exceed 0.5%.

2.2. Quantification of Boswellic and Lupeolic Acids by HPLC-MS/MS Analysis

The method development, chromatographic separation, mass spectrometry detection, and method validation for quantification of boswellic and lupeolic acids by HPLC-MS/MS have been previously published by us [18]. The quantification by HPLC-MS/MS analysis was performed on an Agilent 1260 Infinity system (Agilent, Santa Clara, CA, USA) coupled with an AB API 2000 triple quadrupole mass spectrometer (Applied Biosystems, Foster City, CA, USA). For chromatographic separation, an analytical reversed-phase HPLC column (Dr. Maisch ReproSil-Pur Basic-C18 HD, 3 µm, 125 × 3 mm; Dr. Maisch GmbH, Ammerbruch, Germany) with a precolumn (Dr. Maisch ReproSil Universal RP, 5 µm, 10 × 4 mm) were used. For sample preparation, contents were removed from the capsules, weighted, and dissolved in DMSO ($\beta = 1$ mg/mL, w/v), whereas pills were beforehand grounded. Samples were filtered through a 0.45 µm regenerated cellulose filter before injection. For quantification, three different capsules or pills were analyzed per product, each in duplicates.

2.3. Analysis of Cytokine Release

Whole human blood was collected from the antecubital vein of healthy male donors and incubated with FNs in concentrations of 30 µg/mL for 20 min followed by a stimulation with LPS (10 ng/mL) for 18 h. Plasma was separated by centrifugation and analyzed for IL-10 and TNF-α using ELISA Duo-Set Human from R&D Systems (Minneapolis, MN, USA). Peripheral blood mononuclear cells (PBMC) were isolated from whole venous blood from healthy male donors via density gradient centrifugation using Biocoll (Biochrom GmbH, Berlin, Germany). The collection and analysis of whole blood and peripheral blood mononuclear cells used in this study were approved by the Institutional Ethics Committee (# 177/18). The participating volunteers provided written informed consent to participate in this study. Cells were seeded into a 96-well plate (4×10^5 cells in 200 µL RPMI 1640 supplemented with 1% FCS and 100 U/mL penicillin, 100 µg/mL streptomycin (all from Gibco)). Cells were treated with FNs in concentrations of 10 µg/mL and pure BAs or LAs in final concentrations of 3 µg/mL for 20 min followed by a stimulation with LPS (10 ng/mL) and an 18 h incubation at 37 °C and in a 5% CO_2 atmosphere. After incubation, cells were centrifuged and supernatants were analyzed. The amounts of IL-12p70, TNF-α, IL-10, IL-6, IL-1β, and IL-8 were quantified by flow cytometry using Cytometric Bead Array (CBA) from Becton Dickinson (Franklin Lakes, NJ, USA) according to manufacturer's instructions.

2.4. Analysis of Antiproliferative and Cytotoxic Effects In Vitro

To verify that the concentrations of the FNs and pure BAs and LAs used, are not cytotoxic to PBMC but cytotoxic to cancer cells, analysis of lactate dehydrogenase (LDH) release (Roche,

Basel, Switzerland), XTT assay of cell viability and proliferation (Roche), and analysis of cell membrane integrity by propidium iodide staining [26] were carried out. Triple-negative human breast cancer cells MDA-MB-231 (ATCC, Rockville, MD, USA), CAL-51 and MDA-MB-453 (both from DSMZ, Braunschweig, Germany), and PBMC were analyzed. MDA-MB-231 cells were cultured in Dulbecco's Modified Eagle Medium (4.5 g/L glucose, GlutaMax; Life Technologies, Carlsbad, CA, USA) supplemented with 10% FCS, 0.1 mM MEM non-essential amino acids, 100 U/mL penicillin, and 100 mg/mL streptomycin. CAL-51 cells were cultured in Dulbecco's Modified Eagle Medium (4.5 g/L glucose; Life Technologies) supplemented with 10% FCS, 100 U/mL penicillin, and 100 mg/mL streptomycin. The MDA-MB-453 cells were cultured in Leibovitz's L-15 medium (Life Technologies) containing 10% FCS, 100 U/mL penicillin, and 100 mg/mL streptomycin and kept at atmospheric CO_2. When cancer cells reached 80% confluence, they were subcultured according to the supplier's recommendations. MDA-MB-231 and CAL-51 cells were treated 24 h after seeding. MDA-MB-453 cells were allowed to adhere for 72 h, because of slow adhesion. Subsequently, treatment with the respective compounds for 72 h followed. Different concentrations of the respective samples were applied using a Tecan D300e Digital Dispenser (Tecan, Männedorf, Switzerland). Absorbance was measured using an Infinite M1000 PRO Tecan plate reader. For analysis of viability, the blank values containing the respective compounds in the according concentration were subtracted and the percentage of viable cell was calculated by normalization to the vehicle control.

2.5. Human Tumor Xenografts on the Chick Chorioallantoic Membrane

TNBC xenografts were established by seeding 0.7×10^6 MDA-MB-231 cells in medium/matrigel (1:1) onto the chick chorioallantoic membrane (CAM) of fertilized chick eggs 7 days after fertilization. For the next 3 consecutive days, cells were treated topically with 20 µL of the respective FN or pure compounds dissolved in 0.9% NaCl (vehicle control: 0.5% DMSO). FN16 was used in concentrations of 5 and 10 µg/mL; AKBA and β-ABA were used in concentrations of 5 µg/mL (10 µM); and doxorubicin was used in a concentration of 1 µM. On day 4 after treatment initiation, tumors were collected, imaged, fixed, and embedded in paraffin for analysis by immunohistochemistry. Tumor volume (mm^3) was calculated with the formula length (mm) × width^2 (mm) × π/6. For immunohistochemical analysis, 5-µm slices of the collected tumors were stained using antibodies against the proliferation marker Ki-67. For analysis of apoptosis in vivo, DNA strand breaks were visualized by deoxynucleotidyl transferase dUTP nick end labeling (TUNEL) according to the manufacturer's recommendations (Roche). Images were recorded with an Axio Lab.A1 microscope (Carl Zeiss, Göttingen, Germany) and a Zeiss 2/3" CMOS camera using Progres Gryphax software (Carl Zeiss).

2.6. Statistical Analysis

Each experiment was repeated at least three times and the data are expressed as mean ± standard deviation (SD) or standard error of the mean (SEM) as indicated. Statistical analysis was performed using Minitab 18 software (Minitab, Munich, Germany) and SigmaPlot 14.0 (Systat Software Inc., San Jose, CA, USA). All data were tested for normal distribution by the Anderson-Darling test and equality of variances by Levene's test. Sample groups were compared by one-way analysis of variance (ANOVA) and post-hoc by Dunett's test for parametric data. Non-parametric data were either transformed prior to analysis by Box-Cox transformation or compared directly by Kruskal-Wallis one-way ANOVA on ranks and post-hoc by Dunn's test. Spearman's rank correlation was used to investigate correlations of non-parametric data. Cluster analysis was performed with hierarchical agglomerative clustering, complete-linkage, and Euclidean distances. Principal component analysis (PCA) was derived from a covariance matrix of the data.

3. Results

3.1. Compositions of Boswellic and Lupeolic Acids in Frankincense Nutraceuticals

Quantification of eight BAs and LAs including α-boswellic acid (α-BA), acetyl-α-boswellic acid (α-ABA), β-boswellic acid (β-BA), acetyl-β-boswellic acid (β-ABA), 11-keto-β-boswellic acid (KBA), acetyl-11-keto-β-boswellic acid (AKBA), lupeolic acid (LA), and acetyl-lupeolic acid (ALA), in 16 frankincense nutraceuticals (FNs) was performed by HPLC-MS/MS. The total contents (w/w) of BAs and LAs varied from 0.4% to 35.7% (Table 1). Related to the mass of a capsule or a pill, the total BA and LA contents varied from 3.5 to 157.3 mg/unit (Table S1). Many manufacturers and distributers promote their products as those with boswellic acids contents over 80%. Interestingly, these concentrations could not be confirmed. Manufacturers usually determine the boswellic acid content of their products by non-aqueous titration, for example, using 0.1 N potassium methoxide and 0.3% (w/v) thymol blue as the indicator [27]. These methods estimate unselectively all acidic compounds, not only boswellic acids. Here, a highly selective and accurate quantification method for analysis of BAs and LAs by HPLC-MS/MS was applied (Figure 2a,b). Consequently, the precise contents of the individual BAs and LAs in nutraceuticals could be determined (Table 1 and Table S1).

Table 1. Contents of boswellic and lupeolic acids in frankincense nutraceuticals (FN) quantified by HPLC-MS/MS analysis.

FN Sample	Concentrations of Boswellic and Lupeolic acids								Σ (%) (w/w)
	Deacetylated Compounds (µg/mg)				Acetylated Compounds (µg/mg)				
	KBA	LA	α-BA	β-BA	AKBA	ALA	α-ABA	β-ABA	
FN9	34.1	17.2	46.5	120.7	36.9	13.8	24.4	63.6	35.7
FN16	42.3	16.4	47.7	118.8	36.9	11.9	20.3	55.7	35.0
FN13	43.9	16.5	45.6	117.2	31.8	11.2	19.2	50.7	33.6
FN6	38.1	15.0	38.8	109.0	7.7	5.9	11.8	36.7	26.3
FN14	38.9	14.4	34.9	98.3	4.2	3.5	6.6	20.8	22.1
FN2	36.9	11.3	32.0	85.9	5.6	4.0	7.9	24.0	20.8
FN4	9.7	6.6	19.9	62.9	18.6	7.8	14.7	46.3	18.6
FN1	25.7	6.8	20.5	57.6	3.6	2.4	4.9	14.8	13.6
FN3	21.8	6.3	18.3	53.1	4.3	2.4	4.6	13.9	12.5
FN15	14.2	6.1	15.6	42.4	11.8	4.1	6.7	17.7	11.9
FN11	4.8	2.5	6.8	20.1	30.0	5.7	10.1	16.7	9.7
FN8	1.3	0.5	1.1	3.2	75.5	1.1	1.6	4.6	8.9
FN10	5.9	2.2	5.6	12.7	33.6	5.3	8.2	12.2	8.6
FN12	4.5	2.1	5.3	14.2	31.4	5.4	8.0	13.2	8.4
FN5	3.4	1.3	3.5	9.2	2.9	0.8	1.9	5.7	2.9
FN7	0.3	0.1	0.3	0.5	1.2	0.3	0.6	1.1	0.4

Samples are arranged by descending total contents of BAs and LAs (Σ in percent, w/w). KBA, 11-keto-β-boswellic acid; LA, lupeolic acid; α-BA, α-boswellic acid; β-BA, β-boswellic acid; AKBA, acetyl-11-keto-β-boswellic acid; ALA, acetyl-lupeolic acid; α-ABA, acetyl-α-boswellic acid; β-ABA, acetyl-β-boswellic acid.

In a previous study, we showed that oleogum resins of the species B. serrata are characterized by higher proportions of deacetylated compounds compared to acetylated compounds [18]. This pattern was also observed in the FN samples analyzed here, which contained mainly extracts from B. serrata. Unusually, particularly for B. serrata, sample FN8 exhibited an exceptionally high content of AKBA. Especially, the concurrence of the high content of AKBA and very low contents of the other BAs and LAs indicated a special enrichment procedure putting FN8 apart from the other samples. Meins et al. observed the same uncommon ratio between AKBA content and total BAs content in a product containing the same 5-Loxin® extract [28]. FN5 and FN7 showed the lowest contents of BAs and LAs of all investigated samples, with total BAs and LAs contents of 2.9% for FN5 and only 0.9% for FN7. In addition to the exceptionally low BAs and LAs contents, the large difference between the stated extract content of 400 mg for FN7 and the determined pill mass of 809.8 ± 5.0 mg points also to an oddly high amount of additives in FN7 (Table 1 and Table S1). According to the manufacturer, the AKBA content of FN7 is 52 mg per pill. However, analysis revealed an AKBA content <1 mg per pill. Hence, it can be assumed that either less *Boswellia* extract than stated was processed or other *Boswellia* oleogum resins containing little or no BAs and LAs were used like, for example, *B. frereana* [18,29].

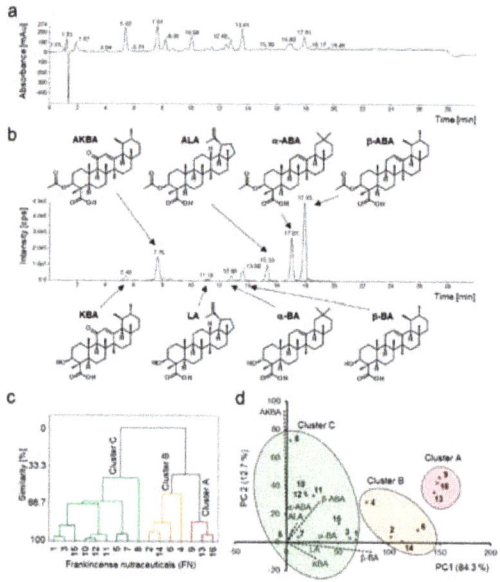

Figure 2. Chromatograms of HPLC-DAD-MS/MS analysis of sample FN9 and multivariate statistical analysis of BAs and LAs contents in different FNs. (**a**) Total wavelength chromatogram with detection at 210 nm, 254 nm, and 280 nm. (**b**) Multiple-reaction monitoring chromatogram and structures of BAs and LAs present in FNs. (**c**) The dendrogram shows FNs assigned to three different clusters according to their BAs and LAs composition: Cluster A >30%, Cluster B with 15–30%, and Cluster C <15% of total BAs and LAs. (**d**) Samples within clusters exhibit similarity in their individual BAs and LAs compositions. Biplot of principal component analysis is shown. Sample FN8 shows the highest deviation due to its unusually high AKBA content concomitantly with very low levels of all other BAs and LAs. Numbered scores visualize the individual FN1-16 in the biplot and dashed lines demonstrating the loadings of the individual BAs and LAs.

Multivariate statistical methods, cluster analysis and principal component analysis (PCA) were applied to the datasets to visualize the data and discover patterns of the BAs and LAs compositions in different FNs. Cluster analysis assigned the samples to three different clusters (Figure 2c). Cluster A contained samples FN9, FN13, and FN16 with the highest total BAs and LAs contents of over 30%. Furthermore, these FNs showed high similarity regarding the composition of the individual components (Figure 2d). Cluster B (samples FN2, FN4, FN6, and FN14) comprised samples with total BAs and LAs contents between 15% and 30%, and Cluster C (samples FN1, FN3, FN4, FN5, FN7, FN8, FN10, FN11, and FN12) contained less than 15% BAs and LAs. FN8 showed the lowest similarity to Cluster C (<50%) due to its unusual chemical composition with high AKBA concentration. Moreover, samples FN10, FN11, and FN12, which contained non-extracted oleogum resin, formed an additional subcluster, due to their similarity. Interestingly, these three samples contained oleogum resins of different *Boswellia* species. According to the manufacturers, sample FN10 was made of *B. sacra*, FN11 of *B. serrata*, and FN12 of *B. carterii*. Comparing with the BAs and LAs compositions determined in our previous studies [9,18], FN11 exhibited indeed general BAs and LAs patterns typical for *B. serrata* resins, with a higher proportion of deacetylated BAs and LAs than acetylated ones. However, FN10 and FN12 showed BAs and LAs patterns untypical for *B. sacra* or *B. carterii* resins, but more similar to *B. serrata*, too. Because these samples contain no extracts but untreated oleogum resin, these differences could not be caused by an extraction procedure. Therefore, it cannot be excluded that instead of *B. sacra* or *B. carterii*, possibly *B. serrata* oleogum resin might have been used for manufacturing of FN10 and FN12.

3.2. Inhibition of Proinflammatory Cytokine Release by Frankincense Nutraceuticals

For comparative investigation of the immunomodulatory activities of the FNs, whole blood of healthy donors was treated with lipopolysaccharide (LPS) to initiate an acute inflammatory response and to induce the release of proinflammatory cytokines. Pretreatment with FNs significantly decreased the expression of the proinflammatory cytokine TNF-α compared to the LPS-treated control group (Figure 3a). Interestingly, the production of the anti-inflammatory cytokine IL-10 was inhibited by the FNs, too. IL-10 acts to limit inflammatory responses by damping the uncontrolled production of proinflammatory cytokines including TNF-α [30]. However, also TNF-α regulates the production of IL-10. Thereby, the chronological sequence of cytokine expression during inflammation is essential. While high levels of proinflammatory cytokines IL-1, IL-6, IL-8, and TNF-α are released already 4–8 h after LPS stimulation, maximal levels of the anti-inflammatory IL-10 are observed only 24–48 h after stimulation [31]. Moreover, about 50–75% of IL-10 released by LPS-stimulated monocytes can be inhibited by anti-TNF-α [32], indicating that TNF-α is responsible for the majority of the released IL-10. Therefore, the decreased production of TNF-α by blood treated with FNs would decrease the later IL-10 release (Figure 3a).

The strong albumin-binding affinity of BAs complicates an accurate analysis of their immunomodulatory activity in whole blood [33]. In addition, blood contains varying amounts of different lipids aiding samples' solubility. Hence, analysis of variance (ANOVA) exhibited no significant differences between the samples or sample groups when analyzed in whole blood. As monocytes are the major producers of TNF-α and IL-10 in blood [34], for further analysis, peripheral blood mononuclear cells (PMBC) were used and the effects of the FNs on the production of a panel of cytokines including TNF-α, IL-1β, IL-6, IL-8, IL-10, and IL-12p70, were analyzed. Contents of IL-12p70 were too low for an adequate evaluation and are not presented. FNs were used at a concentration of 10 µg/mL, which did not affect cell viability as analyzed by XTT and lactate dehydrogenase release (LDH) assays and by propidium iodide staining.

FNs with BAs and LAs contents >30% (Cluster A: FN9, FN13, and FN16) exhibited a significant inhibition of TNF-α, IL-6, and IL-8 expression compared to the control LPS group (Figure 3b–f and Table S2). Moreover, FN4 and FN6 from Cluster B showed considerable inhibitory activity towards TNF-α, IL-6, and IL-8, too. The most potent five nutraceuticals, FN4, FN6, FN9, FN13, and FN16, decreased the release of proinflammatory cytokines to 20.7% for TNF-α, 9.2% for IL-6, and 16.8% for IL-8 (average values for all five FNs). Interestingly, these five samples also had the highest concentrations of ALA, α-ABA, and β-ABA. The proteasome inhibitor MG132 used as a positive control decreased cytokine release to 15.5% $\pm$ 7.2% for TNF-α, 18.5% $\pm$ 7.7% for IL-1β, 5.2% $\pm$ 3.5% for IL-6, 20.2 $\pm$ 7.2% for IL-8, and 37.5% $\pm$ 14.8% for IL-10 compared to the control group. Differently, samples FN5 and FN7, that were previously shown to contain the lowest BAs and LAs contents, exhibited no inhibitory effects on cytokine production at all but even enhanced the expression of the proinflammatory cytokines TNF-α, IL-6, and IL-8 with average values of 142.4% for FN5 and 210.7% for FN7 compared to the control group. The reason for the increased secretion of cytokines might be contamination of these FNs with bacterial products.

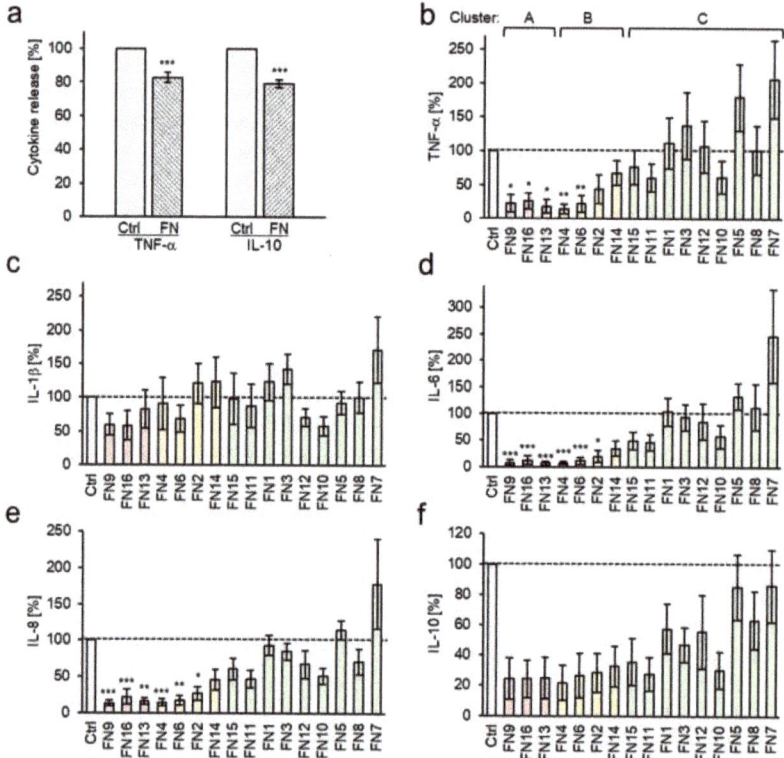

Figure 3. FNs inhibit cytokine production by LPS-stimulated blood and PBMC. (**a**) Inhibition of TNF-α and IL-10 expression by FNs (each at 30 µg/mL) in LPS-stimulated whole blood. Data are mean ± SEM of 16 FNs; each FN was analyzed in five independent experiments/donors, Wilcoxon test. (**b–f**) Inhibition of TNF-α, IL-1β, IL-6, IL-8, and IL-10 production by LPS-stimulated PBMC by the respective FN (each at 10 mg/mL). Samples are arranged according to β-ABA content in a descending order. Clusters are from cluster analysis of BAs and LAs compositions in Figure 2c,d: Cluster A (light red) >30%, Cluster B 30–15% (yellow), and Cluster C (green) <15% total contents of BAs and LAs. Box-Cox transformation followed by one-way ANOVA and post-hoc Dunnett's test. All data are mean ± SEM. $n = 7$ donors; * $p < 0.05$, ** $p < 0.01$, *** $p < 0.001$ compared to LPS-stimulated control groups (Ctrl).

Investigation of the correlation between the chemical composition and cytokine expression revealed that the total amount of BAs and LAs correlate positively with the inhibition of TNF-α, IL-6, IL-8, and IL-10 (Table 2 and Figure S1). Especially, the acetylated compounds ALA, α-ABA, and β-ABA exhibit the highest correlation coefficients, while the acetylated compound with keto group AKBA shows the lowest correlation. However, when FN8 with the extraordinarily high AKBA content was removed as an outlier (Grubbs test), AKBA contents in FNs exhibited significant correlation with all cytokines with $p = 0.007$ for TNF-α, $p < 0.001$ for IL-1β, $p = 0.011$ for IL-6, $p = 0.006$ for IL-8, and $p = 0.001$ for IL-10. Inhibition of IL-1β correlated only with AKBA, ALA, and α-ABA contents in FNs. Moreover, the inhibition of all five investigated cytokines correlated with each other. Whereby, IL-1β, the only cytokine in the panel activated by the NLRP3 inflammasome [35], showed the lowest correlation (Table 2 and Figure S1).

Table 2. Correlation between BAs and LAs contents and inhibition of cytokine production by LPS-stimulated PBMC.

Compound	TNF-α R	p	IL-1β R	p	IL-6 R	p	IL-8 R	p	IL-10 R	p
KBA	−0.621	*	−0.241	> 0.05	−0.744	***	−0.665	**	−0.656	**
LA	−0.721	**	−0.341	> 0.05	−0.832	***	−0.791	***	−0.765	***
α-BA	−0.709	**	−0.356	> 0.05	−0.815	***	−0.774	***	−0.774	***
β-BA	−0.735	***	−0.359	> 0.05	−0.850	***	−0.815	***	−0.794	***
AKBA	−0.537	*	−0.714	**	−0.430	> 0.05	−0.530	*	−0.511	*
ALA	−0.867	***	−0.784	***	−0.884	***	−0.890	***	−0.918	***
α-ABA	−0.879	***	−0.797	***	−0.891	***	−0.897	***	−0.932	***
β-ABA	−0.847	***	−0.447	> 0.05	−0.932	***	−0.903	***	−0.900	***
Σ BAs and LAs	−0.753	***	−0.318	> 0.05	−0.835	***	−0.818	***	−0.785	***
TNF-α			0.612	*	0.959	***	0.968	***	0.944	***
IL-1β					0.535	*	0.600	*	0.624	**
IL-6							0.976	***	0.947	***
IL-8									0.947	***

Spearman's rank correlation; R, correlation coefficient, * $p < 0.05$, ** $p < 0.01$, and *** $p < 0.001$, $n = 16$. PBMC, peripheral blood mononuclear cells.

3.3. Cytotoxic Efficacy of Frankincense Nutraceuticals Against Triple-Negative Breast Cancer Cells In Vitro

FN16, one of the most potent nutraceuticals with respect to cytokine release, concentration-dependently inhibited the viability of the highly metastatic, treatment-resistant breast cancer cell line MDA-MB-231 in vitro. Interestingly, cancer cells were more sensitive to FN16 compared to normal human PBMC, providing evidence for selectivity against cancer cells (Figure 4a). Also, FN1 with low contents of BAs and LAs, exhibited higher toxicity against MDA-MB-231 cells compared to PBMCs (Figure S2a), though the difference was not as strong as for FN16. Therefore, all FNs were investigated for their toxicity against MDA-MB-231 breast cancer cells and the half maximal inhibitory concentrations (IC_{50}) were determined (Table 3 and Figure 4b). The FNs exhibited cytotoxicity against MDA-MB-231 cells with an average IC_{50} of 15.9 µg/mL. The samples FN9, FN13, and FN16 (Cluster A) with the highest BAs and LAs contents exhibited also significantly higher cytotoxicity with IC_{50} values for FN9, FN13, and FN16 of 7.0 µg/mL, 6.6 µg/mL, and 6.0 µg/mL, respectively, compared to the average IC_{50} value of 15.9 µg/mL (Figure 4b). Samples FN5 and FN7 (Cluster C) demonstrated the lowest cytotoxicity against MDA-MB-231 with an $IC_{50} = 44.3$ µg/mL for FN5 and an $IC_{50} = 30.7$ µg/mL for FN7. Thus, FN5 and FN7 not only exhibited the lowest contents of BAs and LAs and the poorest cytokine modulatory properties, but also the cytotoxic efficacies against MDA-MB-231 were significantly below average. Hence, this points to a correlation between BAs and LAs compositions and cytotoxicity against breast cancer cells. A combination of principal component analysis (PCA) of the BAs and LAs concentrations with a contour plot that visualizes the IC_{50} values revealed correlation between the BAs and LAs contents and cytotoxic efficacy (Figure 4c). Interestingly, in addition to similar total BAs and LAs contents and similar effects on cytokine release, the compositions of the individual BAs and LAs in the most potent nutraceuticals FN9, FN13, and FN16 were highly alike. Spearman's rank correlation analysis revealed that contents of BAs and LAs without a keto group exhibit the highest correlation to FN cytotoxic efficacy (Figure S1). In this regard, the content of the boswellic acid β-ABA shows the highest correlation to cytotoxicity against MDA-MB-231.

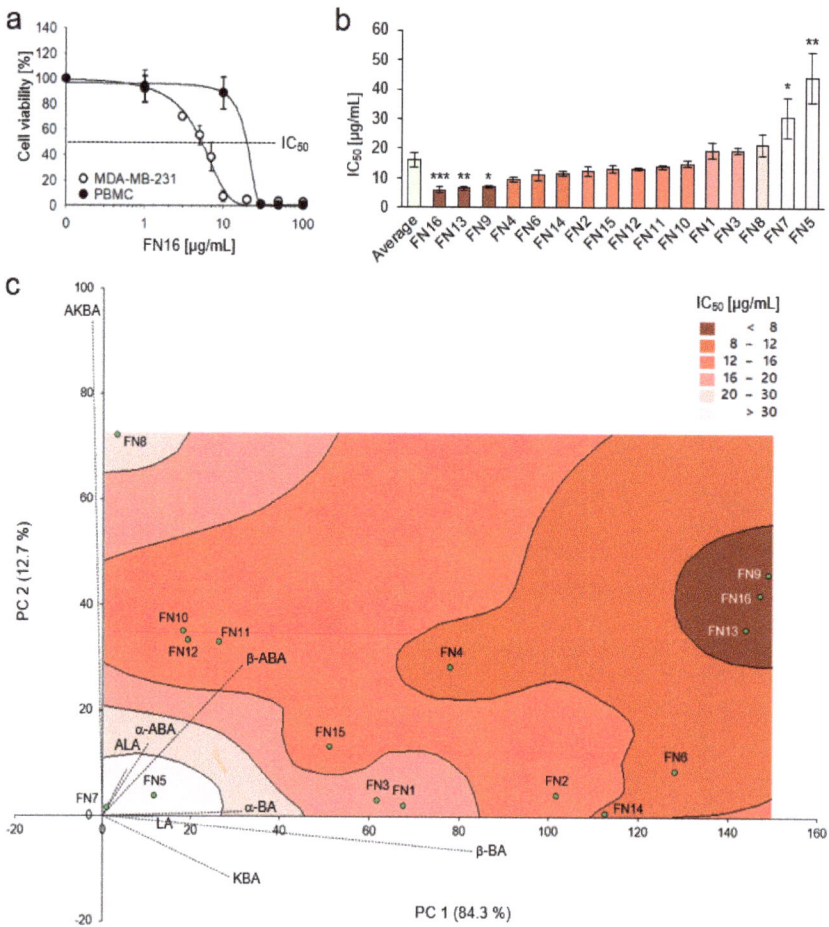

Figure 4. FNs are toxic to a TNBC cell line. (**a**) MDA-MB-231 cancer cells and peripheral blood mononuclear cells (PBMC) were treated for 72 h with FN16, and cell viability was analyzed by XTT assay (n = 3). (**b**) Half maximal inhibitory concentrations (IC$_{50}$) of FNs against MDA-MB-231 cell line. Comparison of IC$_{50}$ values of individual FNs with the average IC$_{50}$ value for all FNs (15.9 µg/mL) by Box-Cox transformation, one-way ANOVA, and post-hoc Dunnett's test. All data are mean ± SEM, n = 3 for the respective FN, n = 16 for the average value, * $p < 0.05$, ** $p < 0.01$, and *** $p < 0.001$. (**c**) Principal component analysis (PCA) and contour plot visualizing the correlation between toxicity of different FNs and their BAs and LAs contents.

Furthermore, a principal component regression analysis (PCR) based on known BAs and LAs contents in FNs was used, to avoid biases caused by multicollinearity. Sample FN5 was identified as an outlier by the Grubbs test and excluded from the regression analysis. The resulting regression model exhibited a R^2 of 96.5% and a significance of correlation of $p < 0.001$. The regression analysis yielded the following equations:

$$IC_{50}(\mu g/mL) = 31.6 - 0.223\, PC1 - 0.668\, PC2 + 0.000586\, PC1^2 + 0.00737\, PC2^2 + 0.00166\, PC1 \times PC2 \quad (1)$$

with

$$PC1 = 0.289\,[KBA] + 0.115\,[LA] + 0.316\,[\alpha\text{-}BA] + 0.830\,[\beta\text{-}BA] - 0.026\,[AKBA] + 0.056\,[ALA] \\ + 0.103\,[\alpha\text{-}ABA] + 0.316\,[\beta\text{-}ABA] \quad (2)$$

and

$$PC2 = -0.115\,[KBA] - 0.002\,[LA] + 0.008\,[\alpha\text{-}BA] - 0.064\,[\beta\text{-}BA] + 0.936\,[AKBA] + 0.088\,[ALA] \\ + 0.136\,[\alpha\text{-}ABA] + 0.285\,[\beta\text{-}ABA] \quad (3)$$

with concentrations of corresponding BA or LA in µg/mg FN given in square brackets.

The IC_{50} values calculated by the regression model exhibited an average absolute residue of only ± 1.0 µg/mL compared to the experimentally-derived values (Table 3). Hence, the regression equation could be used as a tool to predict cytotoxic efficacy of FNs and other frankincense herbal preparations with known BAs and LAs content. By expanding the data set, one could achieve an even more accurate prediction.

Table 3. Cytotoxic efficacy of FNs against MDA-MB-231 cell line.

FN Sample	XTT: IC_{50} (µg/mL)		Regression: IC_{50} (µg/mL)		Absolute Residue (µg/mL)
	Mean	SEM	Value	SE	
FN16	6.0	0.9	6.7	0.9	0.7
FN13	6.6	0.6	5.7	0.8	1.0
FN9	7.0	0.4	7.5	1.0	0.5
FN4	9.5	0.9	8.4	0.9	1.1
FN6	11.0	1.8	9.2	1.1	1.8
FN14	11.6	0.7	13.7	0.9	2.0
FN2	12.2	1.6	13.1	0.7	0.9
FN15	13.2	1.1	15.4	0.7	2.2
FN12	13.2	0.6	14.5	0.8	1.3
FN11	13.9	0.5	13.6	0.8	0.3
FN10	15.0	0.9	14.4	0.9	0.6
FN1	19.4	2.7	18.1	0.8	1.3
FN3	19.5	1.0	18.4	0.8	1.1
FN8	21.5	3.6	21.4	1.5	0.2
FN7	30.7	6.7	30.4	1.4	0.3
FN5	44.3	8.5	/	/	/

XTT, IC_{50} values were determined experimentally by XTT assay (72 h, $n = 3$). Regression, IC_{50} values were determined by principal component regression (PCR). Data are mean ± standard error of the mean (SEM) or standard error of the regression model (SE). Sample FN5 as an outlier (Grubbs test) was excluded from the regression analysis. Absolute residue is the difference between experimentally determined values and those determined by regression analysis. Samples are arranged by cytotoxicity (XTT) in a descending order.

Further, the three FNs, FN9, FN13, and FN16, showing the highest cytotoxicity against MDA-MB-231 cells, were investigated for their cytotoxic efficacy against two additional TNBC cell lines, MDA-MB-453 and Cal-51. Likewise, the investigated samples exhibited considerable cytotoxicity against MDA-MB-453 with IC_{50} values between 12.9 µg/mL and 17.3 µg/mL, and against Cal-51 with even lower IC_{50} values between 3.8 µg/mL and 4.0 µg/mL (Table 4). This indicates that FNs exhibit cytotoxic efficacy against different triple-negative treatment-resistant breast cancer cells.

The non-halogenated anthracycline doxorubicin, a chemotherapeutic agent used to treat patients with breast cancer, was analyzed as a positive control for FNs. Doxorubicin exhibited an $IC_{50} = 0.41 \pm 0.03$ µg/mL for MDA-MB-231, an $IC_{50} = 0.26 \pm 0.02$ µg/mL for MDA-MB-453, and an $IC_{50} = 0.033 \pm 0.004$ µg/mL for Cal-51. However, for doxorubicin, severe adverse effects including cardio- and nephrotoxicity have been reported [36,37]. Differently, for frankincense extracts, only mild adverse effects, like heartburn or nausea, have been described [38].

Table 4. Cytotoxic efficacy of FNs against triple-negative breast cancer cells (TNBC).

FN Sample	IC$_{50}$ (µg/mL)			
	MDA-MB-453		Cal-51	
	Mean	SEM	Mean	SEM
FN9	14.5	0.9	3.8	0.5
FN13	12.9	0.6	3.9	0.6
FN16	17.3	0.5	4.0	0.3

XTT assay, 72 h, $n = 3$.

3.4. Boswellic and Lupeolic Acids Inhibit Cytokine Release and Are Cytotoxic for TNBC Cells

Cytotoxicity of FNs against MDA-MB-231 cells correlated significantly to the total contents of BAs and LAs as well as to individual BAs and LAs contents, except for AKBA, in FNs (Spearman's rank correlation, $p < 0.001$) (Figure S1). The highest correlation coefficient exhibited β-ABA, whereas no significant correlation was detected for AKBA. The poor correlation of AKBA was caused mainly by the unusual chemical composition of the sample FN8 with unexpectedly high AKBA content concomitantly with very low contents of other BAs and LAs. After rejecting sample FN8 from the statistical analysis, the AKBA contents of the remaining samples correlated significantly with the cytotoxicity against MD-MB-231 cells ($p = 0.004$). Hence, we further investigated the cytotoxic efficacies of the pure individual BAs and LAs against MDA-MB-231 (Table 5). The acetylated forms of boswellic acids were more effective against MDA-MB-231 cells than their deacetylated forms; and the most cytotoxic compounds were AKBA with IC$_{50}$ = 6.6 µM, α-ABA with IC$_{50}$ = 7.2 µM, and β-ABA with IC$_{50}$ = 5.9 µM. Differently, for lupeolic acids, LA was more cytotoxic compared to ALA. We have previously shown that acetylated BAs, similar to anticancer drugs such as camptothecins and podophyllotoxins, inhibit activities of human topoisomerases [39]. Acetylated BAs also inhibit the activation of transcriptional factor NF-κB which regulates the synthesis of antiapoptotic proteins [11,17], whereas ALA is an inhibitor of the AKT kinase [16]. These molecular targets might explain the high cytotoxicity of BAs and LAs against proliferating cancer cells.

Table 5. Cytotoxic efficacies of the individual pure BAs and LAs against MDA-MB-231.

Compound	IC$_{50}$			
	µg/mL		µM	
	Mean	SEM	Mean	SEM
KBA	12.0	0.4	25.4	0.9
LA	5.6	0.1	12.3	0.2
α-BA	5.0	0.4	10.8	0.9
β-BA	4.2	0.1	9.3	0.2
AKBA	3.4	0.1	6.6	0.2
ALA	13.4	0.5	26.9	1.0
α-ABA	3.6	0.5	7.2	1.0
β-ABA	2.9	0.4	5.9	0.8

XTT assay, 72 h, $n = 3$. Acetylated boswellic acids (AKBA, α-ABA, and β-ABA) are more potent compared to their deacetylated forms (KBA, α-BA, and β-BA). Differently, LA is more potent than ALA.

Interestingly, similar to FN1 and FN16, AKBA, and in particular, β-ABA, showed higher toxicity against cancer cells compared to PBMC (Figure S2b,c), suggesting selectivity against cancer cells.

Moreover, toxicity against breast cancer cells strongly correlated with cytokine inhibition with $p = 0.023$ for IL-1β and $p < 0.001$ for TNF-α, IL-6, IL-8, and IL-10 (Figure S1). Cluster analysis of variables confirmed the correlation between toxicity against breast cancer cells and cytokine inhibition (Figure 5). In addition to the activation of genes coding for antiapoptotic proteins and for those necessary for continuous cell proliferation, NF-κB activation is central to the activation of cytokine and chemokine gene expression [40]. In previous studies, we have shown that acetylated boswellic acids AKBA and β-ABA specifically inhibited the activities of human IκB kinases (IKK) and the subsequent release of proinflammatory cytokines by human monocytes [11]. Moreover, intercepting the IKK activity by AKBA and β-ABA inhibited proliferation and promoted apoptosis in androgen-independent PC-3 prostate cancer cells in vitro and in vivo [17]. Hence, inhibition of NF-κB by boswellic acids might represent a clue as to why these compounds inhibit both inflammatory processes and cancer growth.

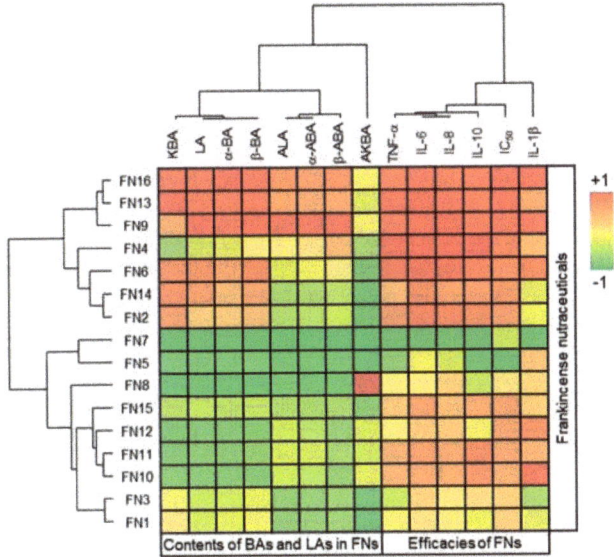

Figure 5. Heatmap visualizing correlations between BAs and LAs compositions in FNs and FN efficacies with respect to inhibition of cytokine release and cancer cell toxicity. Cluster analysis of variables (BAs, LAs, cytokines, IC_{50}) was performed with distances of correlation coefficients and complete linkage. Cluster analysis of objects (FN1-16) was performed with standardized variables, Euclidean distances, and complete linkage. All data were standardized and efficacy values were additionally inverted. +1 indicates high contents of BAs and LAs in FNs or high efficacies of FNs, −1 indicates low contents or efficacies. BAs and LAs contents were analyzed by HPLC-MS/MS; IC_{50} toxicity against MDA-MB-231 breast cancer cells was determined by XTT (72 h); and inhibition of cytokine release by PBMC was analyzed after 18 h by flow cytometry.

Interestingly, chronic inflammation is known to increase cancer risk. Particularly, activation of NF-κB and production of inflammatory cytokines by tumor-associated immune cells are important components aiding tumor initiation, growth, malignant transformation, invasion, and metastasis [41]. Hence, inhibition of inflammatory mediators prevents the development of experimental cancers, and treatment with anti-inflammatory drugs reduces cancer risks and progression [42]. Hence, inhibition of inflammation by frankincense constituents could benefit anticancer therapy.

Similar to FNs, pure BAs and LAs, in concentrations which do not affect PBMC viability, inhibited cytokine production by LPS-activated PBMC, but not as efficiently as FNs (Table S3). Although BAs and LAs are identified here as the active principle of FNs, frankincense extracts also contain a rather complex lipidome including a large number of different fatty acids [43]. The lipids are extracted from frankincense during extract preparation and are persistent components of FNs. Such lipids can act as a natural emulsifier for nonpolar compounds like BAs and LAs and increase their bioavailability [44]. Accordingly, the intake of a FN in combination with a high-fat meal improved the bioavailability of BAs in humans [45]. Hence, the intake of pure BAs and LAs in the absence of solubility enhancers might decrease their bioavailability and worsen the therapeutic response. This should be considered in the development of drugs based on BAs and LAs. Formulations with lecithin for oral administration and complexation with cyclodextrins or liposomes for injections can be beneficial [46,47].

3.5. Inhibition of Proliferation and Induction of Apoptosis in Breast Cancer Xenografts

The antitumor activity of FNs and BAs was further verified in vivo, in MDA-MB-231 breast cancer xenografts grown on the chorioallantoic membrane (CAM) of fertilized chick eggs. Xenografts were treated with FN16, because it contains high amounts of BAs and LAs and exhibited the highest cytotoxicity against MDA-MB-231 cells in vitro. Also, two acetylated BAs, AKBA and β-ABA, which exhibited the highest cytotoxic efficacy in vitro, were tested in an in vivo model.

Treatment of cancer xenografts with FN16 reduced dose-dependently and significantly the tumor volume compared to the control group (Figure 6a,b). Also, treatment with β-ABA significantly reduced the tumor volume. AKBA-treated xenografts were only non-significantly smaller than control. Immunohistochemical analysis of the tumors revealed that FN16 had a dose-dependent inhibitory effect on cancer cell proliferation (Figure 6c). Also, AKBA and β-ABA significantly inhibited cancer cell proliferation. FN16, AKBA, and β-ABA all induced apoptosis in TNBC xenografts as shown by analysis of apoptosis by using the TUNEL technique (Figure 6d). Whilst the chemotherapeutic drug doxorubicin exhibited eminent cytotoxicity against MDA-MB-231 cells in vitro, in vivo its efficacy was not sufficient to induce a significant reduction of tumor size or to induce apoptosis during the treatment period. Notably, no systemic toxicity of the FN16 or BAs on the chick embryos was observed.

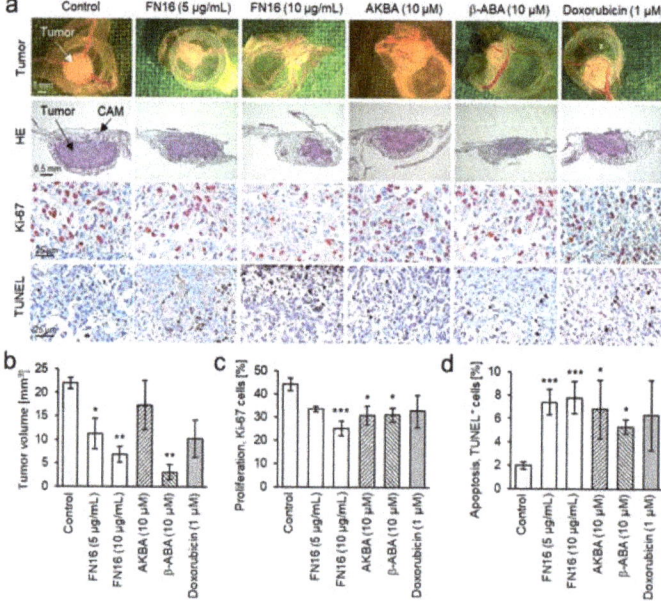

Figure 6. FNs and BAs inhibit growth and induce apoptosis in TNBC breast cancer xenografts in vivo. MDA-MB-231 cells were grafted on the chorioallantoic membrane (CAM) of fertilized chick eggs and treated for 3 consecutive days with either FN16 (5 mg/mL and 10 mg/mL), the boswellic acids AKBA or β-ABA (each 10 μM), doxorubicin (1 μM), or DMSO (0.5%) as control. (**a**) First row: tumor photographs immediately after extraction (original magnification 50×). Second row: hematoxylin and eosin staining. Third row: staining for proliferation marker Ki-67 (red-brown nuclear stain, original magnification 200×). Fourth row: staining for the apoptosis marker TUNEL (brown, original magnification 200×). (**b**) FN16 and β-ABA inhibit the tumor growth. (**c**) FN16, AKBA, and β-ABA inhibit cancer cell proliferation. (**d**) FN16, AKBA, and β-ABA induce apoptosis in cancer xenografts. All data are mean ± SEM, $n = 4$. Comparison with control by Kruskal-Wallis one-way ANOVA on ranks and post-hoc by Dunn's test with * $p < 0.05$, ** $p < 0.01$, and *** $p < 0.001$.

4. Conclusions

A comparative analysis of 16 frankincense nutraceuticals (FNs) revealed major differences in chemical compositions, cytokine modulatory properties, and cytotoxicities against triple-negative breast cancer cells. FNs with total boswellic and lupeolic acids (BAs and LAs) contents over 30% and/or β-ABA contents over 36 µg/mg significantly inhibited the expression of the proinflammatory cytokines TNF-α, IL-6, and IL-8. Moreover, FNs exhibited cytotoxic efficacy against triple-negative breast cancer cell lines MDA-MB-231, MDA-MB-453, and CAL-51 in vitro. In this regard, FNs with BAs and LAs contents over 30% and β-ABA contents over 50 µg/mg proved to be the most potent ones. A FN from this group and pure β-ABA inhibited growth and induced apoptosis in breast cancer xenografts in vivo. Moreover, a remarkable correlation between BAs and LAs contents, cytokine inhibition, and cytotoxicity against breast cancer cells could be observed. The contents of β-ABA exhibited the highest average correlation to inhibition of TNF-α, IL-6, and IL-8 cytokine release as well as cytotoxicity against breast cancer cells. Furthermore, pure β-ABA showed high cytotoxic efficacy against breast cancer cells in vitro and in vivo. Therefore, β-ABA should be considered as a compound for standardization of frankincense nutraceuticals and herbal preparations and it deserves further studies aiming at the development of new anticancer drugs.

Supplementary Materials: The following are available online at http://www.mdpi.com/2072-6643/11/10/2341/s1, Table S1: Frankincense nutraceutical (FN) capsule/pill contents and concentrations of boswellic and lupeolic acids per capsule/pill.; Table S2: Frankincense nutraceuticals (FNs) inhibit cytokine production by LPS-activated whole blood and isolated PBMC; Table S3: Boswellic and lupeolic acids inhibit cytokine production by LPS-activated PBMC; Figure S1: Correlations between contents of individual boswellic and lupeolic acids in frankincense nutraceuticals (FNs), FN cytokine inhibitory efficacies, and FN cytotoxicity against the MDA-MB-231 triple-negative breast cancer cell line (IC_{50}); Figure S2: Preferential toxicity of FN1, AKBA, and β-ABA against MDA-MB-231 cells compared to PBMC. (**a**) FN1, (**b**) AKBA, and (**c**) β-ABA. XTT assay, 72 h.

Author Contributions: M.S., T.S. (Tatiana Syrovets), T.S. (Thomas Simmet), and L.J.R. conceived and designed the experiments; M.S., S.J.L., J.U. and K.W. performed the experiments; M.S. analyzed the data; M.S. and S.J.L. wrote the original draft; T.S. (Thomas Simmet) and T.S. (Tatiana Syrovets) reviewed and edited the draft; T.S. (Thomas Simmet) and T.S. (Tatiana Syrovets) supervised and administrated the project.

Funding: This work was partially supported by the Academic Center for Complementary and Integrative Medicine (AZKIM), State Ministry of Baden-Württemberg for Science, Research, and Arts.

Acknowledgments: We thank Felicitas Genze and Eva Winkler for expert technical assistance and Georg Huber (https://weihrauch-blog.de/bilder) for providing photo material.

Conflicts of Interest: The authors declare no conflict of interest.

Appendix A

Table A1. Frankincense nutraceuticals (FNs) analyzed in the study.

FN Sample	Manufacturer/Distributor	Manufacturer's Specifications			RDA [1]
		Product	Batch	Stated Content	
FN1	Gall Pharma (Judenburg, Austria)	Boswellia serrata 200 mg GPH Kapseln	5260.53	200 mg B. serrata extract	2
FN2	Hecht Pharma (Bremervörde, Germany)	H15® Weihrauch Boswellia serrata 350 mg	2260.52	350 mg B. serrata extract	1 × 1
FN3	Hecht Pharma (Bremervörde, Germany)	H15® Weihrauch Kapseln 200 mg	5260.53	200 mg B. serrata extract	1 × 2
FN4	Heidelberg Pharmacy (Bisingen, Germany)	Weihrauch-Extrakt-Kapseln	HBMI07	300 mg B. serrata extract	3 × 1–2
FN5	The Nutri Store (Mauren, Liechtenstein)	Boswellia carterii Extrakt Kapseln	#7779529-1612	400 mg B. carterii extract	1 × 1

Table A1. Cont.

FN Sample	Manufacturer/Distributor	Manufacturer's Specifications			
		Product	Batch	Stated Content	RDA [1]
FN6	Wellnest Nutrazeutika (East Grinstead, England)	*Boswellia* Weihrauchextrakt	NB/BOS-1215189	400 mg *B. serrata* extract; 200 mg *B. carterii* extract	2
FN7	Vitabay (Masstricht, Netherlands)	Weihrauch Extrakt 400 mg	C17030104	400 mg *B. serrata* extract	2
FN8	Vitacost (Boca Raton, Florida)	Synergy 5-Loxin® *Boswellia serrata* Extract	#703657	150 mg *B. serrata* extract	2
FN9	Schloss Pharmacy (Koblenz, Germany)	Indische Weihrauchkapseln	611142B	400 mg *B. serrata* extract	
FN10	Heilsteine Methusalem (Neu-Ulm, Germany)	*Sacra* Weihrauch Gold	WS/102017/NT	430 mg *B. sacra* gum resin	2 × 2
FN11	Heilsteine Methusalem (Neu-Ulm, Germany)	Weihrauch *Boswellia serrata*	WBS/2425/12AS	500 mg *B. serrata* gum resin	2 × 1
FN12	Olibanum B.V. (Kerkrade, Netherlands)	Boscari®, original afrikanischer Weihrauch	B0417	400 mg *B. carterii* gum resin	3 × 1
FN13	Biotikon (Gorxheimertal, Germany)	85 Premium *Boswellia serrata*	BOSW-200917	400 mg *B. serrata* extract	1
FN14	Gall Pharma (Judenburg, Austria)	*Boswellia serrata* Tabletten 400 mg	261.29	400 mg *B. serrata* extract	3 × 1
FN15	Gufic Biosciences Ltd. (Mumbai, India)	Sallaki® Tablets 400 mg	AB17019	400 mg *B. serrata* extract	
FN16	Delphin Pharmacy (Langenau, Germany)	Weihrauch-Kapseln	BBD [2] 05.04.2018	400 mg *B. serrata* extract	

[1] Recommended daily allowance; [2] Best-before date.

References

1. Moussaieff, A.; Mechoulam, R. *Boswellia* resin: From religious ceremonies to medical uses; A review of in-vitro, in-vivo and clinical trials. *J. Pharm. Pharmacol.* **2009**, *61*, 1281–1293. [CrossRef]
2. Schrott, E. *Weihrauch*; Mosaik: Munich, Germany, 1998.
3. Ammon, H.P. Boswellic acids and their role in chronic inflammatory diseases. *Adv. Exp. Med. Biol.* **2016**, *928*, 291–327. [CrossRef]
4. Kluge, H.; Fernando, C.; Winking, M. *Weihrauch und Seine Heilende WIRKUNG*; Karl, F., Ed.; Haug Verlag: Heidelberg, Germany, 1998.
5. Roy, N.K.; Deka, A.; Bordoloi, D.; Mishra, S.; Kumar, A.P.; Sethi, G.; Kunnumakkara, A.B. The potential role of boswellic acids in cancer prevention and treatment. *Cancer Lett.* **2016**, *377*, 74–86. [CrossRef]
6. Bongers, F.; Groenendijk, P.; Bekele, T.; Birhane, E.; Damtew, A.; Decuyper, M.; Eshete, A.; Gezahgne, A.; Girma, A.; Khamis, M.A.; et al. Frankincense in peril. *Nat. Sustain.* **2019**, *2*, 602–610. [CrossRef]
7. Huber, G. *Weihrauch*; Ansata: Munich, Germany, 2018.
8. Martinetz, D.; Lohs, K.; Janzen, J. *Weihrauch und Myrrhe: Kulturgeschichte und wirtschaftliche Bedeutung, Botanik, Chemie, Medizin*; Wissenschaftliche Verlangsgesellschaft mbH Stuttgart: Stuttgart, Germany, 1988.
9. Belsner, K.; Büchele, B.; Werz, U.; Syrovets, T.; Simmet, T. Structural analysis of pentacyclic triterpenes from the gum resin of *Boswellia serrata* by NMR spectroscopy. *Magn. Reson. Chem.* **2003**, *41*, 115–122. [CrossRef]
10. Safayhi, H.; Mack, T.H.; Sabieraj, J.O.; Anazodo, M.I.; Subramanian, L.R.; Ammon, H.P. Boswellic acids: Novel, specific, nonredox inhibitors of 5-lipoxygenase. *J. Pharmacol. Exp. Ther.* **1992**, *261*, 1143–1146. [PubMed]
11. Syrovets, T.; Büchele, B.; Krauss, C.; Laumonnier, Y.; Simmet, T. Acetyl-boswellic acids inhibit lipopolysaccharide-mediated TNF-α induction in monocytes by direct interaction with IκB kinases. *J. Immunol.* **2005**, *174*, 498–506. [CrossRef] [PubMed]

12. Ernst, E. Frankincense: Systematic review. *BMJ* **2008**, *337*, a2813. [CrossRef] [PubMed]
13. Gupta, I.; Parihar, A.; Malhotra, P.; Singh, G.B.; Ludtke, R.; Safayhi, H.; Ammon, H.P. Effects of *Boswellia serrata* gum resin in patients with ulcerative colitis. *Eur. J. Med. Res.* **1997**, *2*, 37–43. [PubMed]
14. Glaser, T.; Winter, S.; Groscurth, P.; Safayhi, H.; Sailer, E.R.; Ammon, H.P.T.; Schabet, M.; Weller, M. Boswellic acids and malignant glioma: Induction of apoptosis but no modulation of drug sensitivity. *Br. J. Cancer* **1999**, *80*, 756–765. [CrossRef]
15. Hoernlein, R.F.; Orlikowsky, T.; Zehrer, C.; Niethammer, D.; Sailer, E.R.; Simmet, T.; Dannecker, G.E.; Ammon, H.P.T. Acetyl-11-keto-β-boswellic acid induces apoptosis in HL-60 and CCRF-CEM cells and inhibits topoisomerase I. *J. Pharmacol. Exp. Ther.* **1999**, *288*, 613–619. [PubMed]
16. Schmidt, C.; Loos, C.; Jin, L.; Schmiech, M.; Schmidt, C.Q.; El Gaafary, M.; Syrovets, T.; Simmet, T. Acetyl-lupeolic acid inhibits Akt signaling and induces apoptosis in chemoresistant prostate cancer cells in vitro and in vivo. *Oncotarget* **2017**, *8*, 55147–55161. [CrossRef] [PubMed]
17. Syrovets, T.; Gschwend, J.; Büchele, B.; Laumonnier, Y.; Zugmaier, W.; Genze, F.; Simmet, T. Inhibition of IκB kinase activity by acetyl-boswellic acids promotes apoptosis in androgen-independent PC-3 prostate cancer cells in vitro and in vivo. *J. Biol. Chem.* **2005**, *280*, 6170–6180. [CrossRef] [PubMed]
18. Schmiech, M.; Lang, S.J.; Werner, K.; Rashan, L.J.; Syrovets, T.; Simmet, T. Comparative analysis of pentacyclic triterpenic acid compositions in oleogum resins of different *Boswellia* species and their in vitro cytotoxicity against treatment-resistant human breast cancer cells. *Molecules* **2019**, *24*, 2153. [CrossRef]
19. Suhail, M.M.; Wu, W.; Cao, A.; Mondalek, F.G.; Fung, K.M.; Shih, P.T.; Fang, Y.T.; Woolley, C.; Young, G.; Lin, H.K. *Boswellia sacra* essential oil induces tumor cell-specific apoptosis and suppresses tumor aggressiveness in cultured human breast cancer cells. *BMC Complement. Altern. Med.* **2011**, *11*. [CrossRef]
20. Der Weihrauch Blog. Available online: https://weihrauch-blog.de/ (accessed on 29 May 2019).
21. Bray, F.; Ferlay, J.; Soerjomataram, I.; Siegel, R.L.; Torre, L.A.; Jemal, A. Global cancer statistics 2018: GLOBOCAN estimates of incidence and mortality worldwide for 36 cancers in 185 countries. *CA Cancer J. Clin.* **2018**, *68*, 394–424. [CrossRef]
22. Carey, L.; Winer, E.; Viale, G.; Cameron, D.; Gianni, L. Triple-negative breast cancer: Disease entity or title of convenience? *Nat. Rev. Clin. Oncol.* **2010**, *7*, 683. [CrossRef]
23. Grand View Research. *Dietary Supplements Market Size Analysis Report by Ingredient (Botanicals, Vitamins), by form, by Application (Immunity, Cardiac Health), by End User, by Distribution Channel, and Segment Forecasts, 2019–2025*; Grand View Research: San Francisco, CA, USA, 2019.
24. Yates, A.A.; Erdman, J.W., Jr.; Shao, A.; Dolan, L.C.; Griffiths, J.C. Bioactive nutrients–Time for tolerable upper intake levels to address safety. *Regul. Toxicol. Pharmacol.* **2017**, *84*, 94–101. [CrossRef]
25. Belsner, K.; Büchele, B.; Werz, U.; Simmet, T. Structural analysis of 3-α-acetyl-20(29)-lupene-24-oic acid, a novel pentacyclic triterpene isolated from the gum resin of *Boswellia serrata*, by NMR spectroscopy. *Magn. Reson. Chem.* **2003**, *41*, 629–632. [CrossRef]
26. Lang, S.J.; Schmiech, M.; Hafner, S.; Paetz, C.; Steinborn, C.; Huber, R.; Gaafary, M.E.; Werner, K.; Schmidt, C.Q.; Syrovets, T.; et al. Antitumor activity of an *Artemisia annua* herbal preparation and identification of active ingredients. *Phytomedicine* **2019**, *62*, 152962. [CrossRef]
27. Rajpal, V. *Standardization of Botanicals*, 2nd ed.; Business Horizons: New Delhi, India, 2011; Volume 1.
28. Meins, J.; Artaria, C.; Riva, A.; Morazzoni, P.; Schubert-Zsilavecz, M.; Abdel-Tawab, M. Survey on the quality of the top-selling european and american botanical dietary supplements containing boswellic acids. *Planta Med.* **2016**, *82*, 573–579. [CrossRef]
29. Mathe, C.; Culioli, G.; Archier, P.; Vieillescazese, C. High-performance liquid chromatographic analysis of triterpenoids in commercial frankincense. *Chromatographia* **2004**, *60*, 493–499. [CrossRef]
30. Iyer, S.S.; Ghaffari, A.A.; Cheng, G. Lipopolysaccharide-mediated IL-10 transcriptional regulation requires sequential induction of type I IFNs and IL-27 in macrophages. *J. Immunol.* **2010**, *185*, 6599–6607. [CrossRef] [PubMed]
31. De Waal Malefyt, R.; Abrams, J.; Bennett, B.; Figdor, C.G.; de Vries, J.E. Interleukin 10 (IL-10) inhibits cytokine synthesis by human monocytes: An autoregulatory role of IL-10 produced by monocytes. *J. Exp. Med.* **1991**, *174*, 1209–1220. [CrossRef] [PubMed]
32. Wanidworanun, C.; Strober, W. Predominant role of tumor necrosis factor-alpha in human monocyte IL-10 synthesis. *J. Immunol.* **1993**, *151*, 6853–6861.

33. Siemoneit, U.; Pergola, C.; Jazzar, B.; Northoff, H.; Skarke, C.; Jauch, J.; Werz, O. On the interference of boswellic acids with 5-lipoxygenase: Mechanistic studies in vitro and pharmacological relevance. *Eur. J. Pharmacol.* **2009**, *606*, 246–254. [CrossRef]
34. Belge, K.U.; Dayyani, F.; Horelt, A.; Siedlar, M.; Frankenberger, M.; Frankenberger, B.; Espevik, T.; Ziegler-Heitbrock, L. The proinflammatory $CD14^+CD16^+DR^{++}$ monocytes are a major source of TNF. *J. Immunol.* **2002**, *168*, 3536–3542. [CrossRef]
35. Swanson, K.V.; Deng, M.; Ting, J.P. The NLRP3 inflammasome: Molecular activation and regulation to therapeutics. *Nat. Rev. Immunol.* **2019**, *19*, 477–489. [CrossRef]
36. Ayla, S.; Seckin, I.; Tanriverdi, G.; Cengiz, M.; Eser, M.; Soner, B.C.; Oktem, G. Doxorubicin induced nephrotoxicity: Protective effect of nicotinamide. *Int. J. Cell Biol.* **2011**, *2011*, 390238. [CrossRef]
37. Swain, S.M.; Whaley, F.S.; Ewer, M.S. Congestive heart failure in patients treated with doxorubicin: A retrospective analysis of three trials. *Cancer* **2003**, *97*, 2869–2879. [CrossRef]
38. Gupta, I.; Parihar, A.; Malhotra, P.; Gupta, S.; Ludtke, R.; Safayhi, H.; Ammon, H.P. Effects of gum resin of *Boswellia serrata* in patients with chronic colitis. *Planta Med.* **2001**, *67*, 391–395. [CrossRef] [PubMed]
39. Syrovets, T.; Büchele, B.; Gedik, E.; Slupsky, J.R.; Simmet, T. Acetyl-boswellic acids are novel catalytic inhibitors of human topoisomerases I and IIa. *Mol. Pharmacol.* **2000**, *58*, 71–81. [CrossRef] [PubMed]
40. Karin, M.; Cao, Y.; Greten, F.R.; Li, Z.W. NF-κB in cancer: From innocent bystander to major culprit. *Nat. Rev. Cancer* **2002**, *2*, 301–310. [CrossRef] [PubMed]
41. Grivennikov, S.I.; Greten, F.R.; Karin, M. Immunity, Inflammation, and Cancer. *Cell* **2010**, *140*, 883–899. [CrossRef] [PubMed]
42. Balkwill, F.; Charles, K.A.; Mantovani, A. Smoldering and polarized inflammation in the initiation and promotion of malignant disease. *Cancer Cell* **2005**, *7*, 211–217. [CrossRef] [PubMed]
43. Ahmed, H.H.; Abd-Rabou, A.A.; Hassan, A.Z.; Kotob, S.E. Phytochemical analysis and anti-cancer investigation of *boswellia serrata* bioactive constituents in vitro. *Asian Pac. J. Cancer Prev.* **2015**, *16*, 7179–7188. [CrossRef] [PubMed]
44. Van Hoogevest, P.; Wendel, A. The use of natural and synthetic phospholipids as pharmaceutical excipients. *Eur. J. Lipid. Sci. Technol.* **2014**, *116*, 1088–1107. [CrossRef]
45. Sterk, V.; Buchele, B.; Simmet, T. Effect of food intake on the bioavailability of boswellic acids from a herbal preparation in healthy volunteers. *Planta Med.* **2004**, *70*, 1155–1160. [CrossRef]
46. Riva, A.; Morazzoni, P.; Artaria, C.; Allegrini, P.; Meins, J.; Savio, D.; Appendino, G.; Schubert-Zsilavecz, M.; Abdel-Tawab, M. A single-dose, randomized, cross-over, two-way, open-label study for comparing the absorption of boswellic acids and its lecithin formulation. *Phytomedicine* **2016**, *23*, 1375–1382. [CrossRef]
47. Wang, H.; Syrovets, T.; Kess, D.; Büchele, B.; Hainzl, H.; Lunov, O.; Weiss, J.M.; Scharffetter-Kochanek, K.; Simmet, T. Targeting NF-κB with a natural triterpenoid alleviates skin inflammation in a mouse model of psoriasis. *J. Immunol.* **2009**, *183*, 4755–4763. [CrossRef]

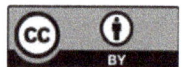

© 2019 by the authors. Licensee MDPI, Basel, Switzerland. This article is an open access article distributed under the terms and conditions of the Creative Commons Attribution (CC BY) license (http://creativecommons.org/licenses/by/4.0/).

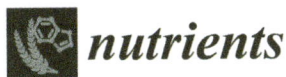

Article

Dietary and Supplement-Based Complementary and Alternative Medicine Use in Pediatric Autism Spectrum Disorder

Melanie S. Trudeau [1,*], Robyn F. Madden [1], Jill A. Parnell [2], W. Ben Gibbard [3] and Jane Shearer [1,3]

1. Department of Kinesiology, University of Calgary, 2500 University Dr NW, Calgary, AB T2N 1N4, Canada
2. Department of Health and Physical Education, Mount Royal University, Calgary, AB T3E 6K6, Canada
3. Department of Pediatrics, Cumming School of Medicine, University of Calgary, Alberta Children's Hospital, 28 Oki Drive NW, Calgary, AB T3B 6A8, Canada
* Correspondence: mstrudea@ucalgary.ca

Received: 3 July 2019; Accepted: 26 July 2019; Published: 1 August 2019

Abstract: Previous literature has shown that complementary and alternative medicine (CAM) is steadily increasing in autism spectrum disorder (ASD). However, little data is currently available regarding its use, safety, and efficacy in children with ASD. Thus, the purpose of this study is to describe the use of supplement-based CAM therapies in children between the ages of 4 to 17 years with ASD. This population-based, cross-sectional study evaluated children with ASD regarding supplement use. A total of 210 participants were recruited from a variety of sources including educational and physical activity programs, and social media to complete a questionnaire. Primary caregivers provided information on current supplement based CAM use. Data evaluated the proportion of children that used supplement therapies, the types of supplements used, reasons for use, perceived safety, and demographic factors associated with use (e.g., income, parental education, severity of disorder). Seventy-five percent of children with ASD consumed supplements with multivitamins (77.8%), vitamin D (44.9%), omega 3 (42.5%), probiotics (36.5%), and magnesium (28.1%) as the most prevalent. Several supplements, such as adrenal cortex extract, where product safety has not yet been demonstrated, were also reported. A gluten free diet was the most common specialty diet followed amongst those with restrictions (14.8%). Health care professionals were the most frequent information source regarding supplements; however, 33% of parents reported not disclosing all their child's supplements to their physician. In conclusion, the use of supplement therapies in children with ASD is endemic and highlights the need for further research concerning public health education surrounding safety and efficacy.

Keywords: Autism spectrum disorder; dietary supplements; pediatric; physician communication

1. Introduction

Autism spectrum disorder (ASD) is a group of heterogeneous chronic neurodevelopmental disorders characterized by qualitative impairments in social interaction, communication, and repetitive stereotyped patterns of behavior [1]. The etiology of these conditions is thought to be multifactorial, involving genetic, prenatal, and postnatal factors [2]. The Centre for Disease Control (CDC) reports that 1 in 59 children are diagnosed with ASD, with boys 4 times more likely to be diagnosed than girls. As such, ASD is the fastest growing developmental disorder in the United States [3].

Treatment for ASD focuses on educational and behavioral interventions such as applied behavioral analysis [4]. Psychotropic drugs are commonly prescribed to treat core behavioral symptoms, decrease maladaptive behavior, and support learning and development [5]. In addition to conventional treatment options, some parents of children with ASD seek out complementary and alternative medicine (CAM) to treat symptoms. The National Centre for Complementary and Integrative Health defines CAM as "a diverse group of medical and health care systems, practices, and products that are not generally considered part of conventional Western medicine" [6]. Complementary approaches fall broadly into 3 categories: Natural products such as dietary supplements and special diets, mind and body practices, and other complementary health approaches [7].

Evidence regarding the use of CAM in the general pediatric population is limited. Studies in the United States have shown that the prevalence of pediatric CAM use in populations with illness or disease can range up to 76% [8]. However, these studies are limited in several ways. First, while many employ sound methodologies, they often provide differing definitions of what constitutes a CAM therapy. For example, in their review of 136 studies on alternative medicines, Surette et al. [9] found 39 studies that included vitamins, 13 studies that excluded vitamins, and 41 studies that made no mention of their inclusion or exclusion criteria. Further, many of the pediatric CAM studies are characterized by wide variation in study populations and size, prevalence measurements, and research methodologies, all of which hinder the formulation of evidence-based recommendations.

Though limited in number, some studies have examined CAM effects in ASD. Levy et al. [10] found that greater than 9% of children with ASD used potentially harmful CAM, such as chelation, antibiotics, or excessive amounts of vitamins. These findings are consistent with anecdotal evidence of dangerous products used to "cure" ASD. For example, in 2014, the supplementation market saw an explosion of *Miracle Mineral Solution,* a solution of sodium chlorite and hydrochloric acid (i.e., bleach) as a treatment option for ASD. The US Food and Drug Administration has issued several warnings about the product and the treatment has been linked to 1 death and several serious injuries; however, *Miracle Mineral Solution* is still widely available, with 1000 + followers on social media promoting its use [11].

From a public health perspective, supplement-based therapies and specialty diets, a subcategory of CAM, requires further evaluation. While many supplements such as melatonin, vitamins, gluten-casein-free diet, and omega 3 fatty acids may have few adverse effects, their safety and effectiveness in reducing ASD symptomology have not been reliably established [2,12,13]. Research estimates that up to 74% of children with ASD have been provided with CAM and that supplement-based therapies make up approximately 50% of CAM therapies used by this population [14].

Despite its popularity, disclosure of CAM use to physicians is often poor, with rates as low as 23% [15]. Concurrent use of CAM and prescription medications is widespread and poses a possible risk to patients who may be unaware of the potential for interactions [16]. Further, research has documented that knowledge of CAM use is important for health care professionals, as it provides insight into patient values and health beliefs. Importantly, considering patient values may assist in providing optimum care, especially in the context of supplements that pose a safety risk to patients [15]. Given the rates of concurrent use, in conjunction with lack of disclosure, there is a pressing need to assess pediatric CAM use and parental perceptions of these therapies.

As the prevalence of supplements and specialty diets are high and many are unsupported by research, a better understanding of the use of supplementation in pediatric ASD could help provide better integrative care by (1) informing the public and health care professionals about the prevalence and types of supplement therapies and specialty diets used in children with ASD; (2) assessing patient-physician communication and interactions surrounding supplement and specialty diet use; and (3) highlighting priorities for evidence-based clinical trials for supplements in ASD. Therefore, this study seeks to describe the use of supplement-based CAM therapies in children with ASD.

2. Materials and Methods

2.1. Participants

This study was approved by the Conjoint Health Research Ethics Board at the University of Calgary (REB17-0970). Inclusion criteria for this population-based cross sectional study included (1) a physician-confirmed diagnosis of autism spectrum disorder (including previous diagnostic labels of Asperger's syndrome, pervasive developmental disorder—not otherwise specified, childhood disintegrative disorder, or Rett syndrome) and (2) between the ages of 4 and 17.99 years inclusive. A sample size calculation (margin of error 8% and 95% confidence interval) revealed 150 participants were required [17]. Many of the children were cognitively and/or developmentally delayed; therefore, the parents/legal guardians served as a proxy for describing their child's use of supplements, in order to maintain consistency between responses. The parents/legal guardians of children with ASD provided written informed consent and completed the questionnaire on their behalf.

2.2. Dietary Supplement Questionnaire

Data about supplement use with regards to ASD was collected via self-report online and paper form questionnaires. A validity and reliability tested supplement use questionnaire [18,19] was modified for children with ASD. Supplements were defined as a product that contains a vitamin, mineral, herb or botanical, amino acid, concentrate, metabolite, or other dietary ingredients intended to add further nutritional value to the diet. Supplements may be found in many forms such as tablets, capsules, soft gels, liquids, or powders. Examples include multivitamins, supplementary minerals, protein powders, energy drinks, meal replacements, etc. This definition was based on the definition provided by the National Centre for Complementary and Integrative Health [6]. Specialty diets such as the ketogenic diet, low-carb diet, and gluten free diet were also evaluated. The response format for the survey contained several closed-ended questions, short answer, and 5 item Likert scale questions. Several questions provided participants with answers to select from as well as short answer boxes to provide their answers. A pilot-test was conducted on a small sample of parents ($n = 34$) to ensure clarity of content. A sample of the questionnaire can be found in Supplementary Data File S1, Table S1.

2.3. Measures

The key outcomes were the demographic variables of the child (i.e., age, sex, ethnicity, medical characteristics) and parent (i.e., income, education level), and the types of therapies (i.e., gluten free diet, omega 3 fatty acids, probiotics) used. Secondary outcomes included reasons why parents have or have not used supplement therapies for their children, the information sources consulted by parents regarding therapies, and the proportion of parents who perceive the therapies used as being safe. In addition, parent perceived satisfaction with their child's family physician or pediatrician, comfort level in discussing nutrition and supplements, number of supplements/dietary patterns disclosed to the physician (if applicable), and reasons why they might have chosen not to disclose supplements were quantified.

2.4. Procedures

Children were recruited from clinics at the Alberta Children's Hospital, Autism Calgary, and physical literacy programs around the city. Researchers also utilized schools that focus on inclusive and accessibility programs to recruit eligible participants. Recruitment posters were displayed throughout the facilities to describe the study, explain eligibility criteria, and provide contact information should parents of children with ASD want to participate. Researchers also contacted program organizers and asked permission to approach parents directly during recreation and instructional sessions and enroll them in the study. Many of these organizations promoted the study on their social media platforms, which provided an online consent form and a link to complete the survey.

2.5. Statistical Analysis

Data from the question 'has your child previously taken or currently taking any dietary supplements' was categorized as yes or no. Dietary supplement use data were categorized into groups based on sex, age (4 to 8 years, 9 to 13 years, and 14 to 17 years), and abilities. The age groups were based on dietary reference intake (DRI) values [20]. Ability groups were based on 4 ability categories (verbal, intellectual, social, and physical) in which parents ranked their child as "very weak/weak," "neutral," or "strong/very strong. Differences between sex, age, and ability groups were determined by a Fisher's exact test. All analyses were performed using SPSS statistics version 25 (IBM Corporation, Armonk, NW, USA).

3. Results

3.1. Participant Characteristics

A total of 210 parents agreed to participate in the study on behalf of their child(ren) and completed the questionnaire. Descriptive characteristics and demographic characteristics of the participants are outlined in Tables 1 and 2, respectively.

Table 1. Descriptive characteristics.

Descriptive Characteristics	All	Males	Females
Participants	210	157 (74.8%)	53 (25.2%)
Age, years	9.2 (3.6)	9.0 (3.6)	9.5 (3.7)
Year of Diagnosis			
2003–2007	16 (7.8%)	14 (6.8%)	2 (1.0%)
2008–2012	42 (20.5%)	28 (13.7%)	14 (6.8%)
2013–2018	147 (71.7%)	113 (55.1%)	34 (16.6%)

Participants and year of diagnosis are listed as a count (percentage of total); age is listed as a mean (standard deviation).

Table 2. Demographic characteristics.

Characteristic	All n (%)	Males n (%)	Females n (%)
Ethnicity			
Caucasian	170 (81.3)	124 (59.3)	46 (22.0)
Asian/Pacific Islander	13 (6.2)	11 (5.3)	2 (1.0)
Hispanic or Latino	2 (1.0)	2 (1.0)	0 (0.0)
Black or African American	5 (2.4)	2 (1.0)	3 (1.4)
First Nations or Metis or Inuit	6 (2.9)	5 (2.4)	1 (0.5)
Multiracial	13 (6.2)	12 (5.7)	1 (0.5)
Household Income			
>$20,000	10 (4.8)	7 (3.3)	3 (1.4)
$20,000–40,000	23 (11.0)	18 (8.6)	5 (2.4)
$40,000–60,000	23 (11.0)	17 (8.1)	6 (2.9)
$60,000–80,000	33 (15.7)	25 (11.9)	8 (3.8)
$80,000–$100,000	35 (16.7)	23 (11.0)	12 (5.7)
$100,000+	75 (35.7)	60 (28.6)	15 (7.1)
Not Applicable	11 (5.2)	7 (3.3)	4 (1.9)
Parent Level of Education			
High School Diploma	17 (8.2)	13 (6.3)	4 (1.9)
Trade School Diploma	4 (1.9)	3 (1.4)	1 (0.5)
Some College	17 (8.2)	13 (6.3)	4 (1.9)
College Diploma	51 (24.5)	41 (19.7)	10 (4.8)
Some University	19 (9.1)	17 (8.2)	2 (1.0)
University Degree	52 (25.0)	40 (19.2)	12 (5.8)
Master's Degree	30 (14.4)	21 (10.1)	9 (4.3)
Professional Degree	11 (5.3)	5 (2.4)	6 (2.9)
Ph.D.	7 (3.4)	3 (1.4)	4 (1.9)

The category "Multiracial" was created as a result of multiple parents indicating this option in the "other" category to reflect the demographic of our sample. Data is presented as a count (percentage of total).

3.2. Dietary Supplement Use

A total of 167 parents (79.5%) indicated that their child had previously taken or was currently taking at least 1 supplement (males 77.1%; females 86.8%, $p = 0.168$). Eighty-three percent (83%) of parents reported thinking supplements were safe, 3.8% reported that they did not consider them safe, and 13.3% were undecided or perceived supplements as safe under certain conditions (i.e., evidence-based, supervised by a health care professional, etc.). There were no statistical differences between sexes in perceived safety of dietary supplement use ($p = 234$).

The top 10 previous and current pediatric supplement use is summarized in Figure 1. A more extensive list of the supplements listed by the questionnaire can be found in Supplementary Data, Table S2. The 5 most common supplements were multivitamins (77.8%), vitamin D (44.9%), omega 3 (42.5%), probiotics (36.5%), and magnesium (28.1%). Other supplements such as alpha lipoic acid, sodium butyrate, N-Acetyl Cysteine, 5HTP, fluoride, methylfolate, adrenal cortex extract, selenium, milk thistle, liposomal curcumin, cannabidiol, and melatonin were also mentioned. Differences between sexes were found in calcium (male = 9.1%, female = 21.7%, $p = 0.037$) and vitamin K (male = 1.7%, female = 10.9%, $p = 0.018$). When analyzed by age group, significant differences were found in calcium ($p = 0.049$), vitamin B ($p = 0.010$), and energy drinks ($p = 0.027$). The percentage of children who have/are taking more than 1 supplement was 88.6%. In addition, a Pearson's correlation determined that there was no relationship between number of supplements used and years since diagnosis ($p = 240$). The average number of supplements per child was 4.49 and the mean year of diagnosis was 2013.

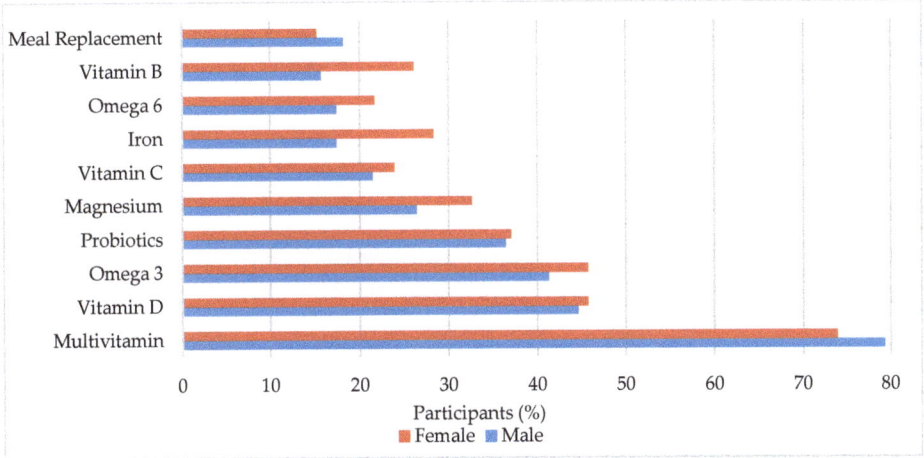

Figure 1. Dietary supplements commonly used in pediatric autism spectrum disorder (ASD). Male and female is percent within sex.

Of the 167 parents who indicated their child has or is currently taking supplements, 126 rated the perceived degree of change on their child's overall well-being between neutral and positive (69.1 ± 15.9) on a scale of 1 (negative impact) to 100 (positive impact). The most common supplements cited to have the largest impact on the child's health were melatonin, multivitamins, omega fatty acids, and magnesium.

3.3. Dietary Supplement Reasons for Use

Parental reasons for providing their children with supplements are outlined in Table 3. The top 3 reasons for consuming supplements were to enhance the child's diet, promote immune system function, and increase quality/duration of sleep. Improvement in gut health was listed 7 times under the "other" section. Parents also indicated several reasons for omitting supplements including: Inadequate knowledge/information (n = 14), too expensive (n = 8), and may be considered harmful (n = 5). Six parents indicated that supplements were not necessary, as their child eats a balanced diet.

Table 3. Reasons for and against dietary supplement use.

	All n (%)	Males n (%)	Females n (%)	p
Reasons for Use				
Enhance diet	127 (76.0)	94 (56.3)	33 (19.8)	0.424
Promote immune system function	88 (52.7)	66 (39.5)	22 (13.2)	0.490
Increase quality/duration of sleep	76 (45.5)	53 (31.7)	23 (13.8)	0.602
Improve cognitive ability	54 (32.3)	34 (20.4)	20 (12.0)	0.066
Decrease repetitive or restrictive behavior	21 (12.6)	16 (9.6)	5 (3.0)	0.798
Promote sociability	18 (10.8)	12 (7.2)	6 (3.6)	0.581
Increase interactions with others	13 (7.8)	8 (4.8)	5 (3.0)	0.349
Enhance motor skills	12 (7.2)	9 (5.4)	3 (1.8)	1.000
Reasons Against Use				
Inadequate knowledge/information	14 (32.6)	12 (27.9)	2 (4.7)	1.000
Too expensive	8 (18.6)	7 (16.3)	1 (2.3)	1.000
May be considered harmful	5 (11.6)	5 (11.6)	0 (0.0)	0.574
Based on suggestion from close family/friends	4 (9.3)	4 (9.3)	0 (0.0)	1.000
Read in scholarly article	4 (9.3)	4 (9.3)	0 (0.0)	1.000

Reasons for use are listed for the parents who indicated that their child had taken supplements (n = 167). Reasons against use are listed for the parents who indicated that their child had not taken supplements (n = 43). Data is presented as a count (percentage of total).

3.4. Special Diets and Information Sources

Current diet information is summarized in Table 4. The top 4 diets followed in our sample included no restrictions, gluten free, high carbohydrate, and lactose free, with a significant difference between sex in diets with no restrictions (male = 72.0%, female = 54.7%, p = 0.027), gluten free (male = 5.1%, female = 24.5%, p < 0.001), and lactose free (male = 4.5%, female = 17.0%, p = 0.006). Other diets such as the paleo diet, nut-free, dye-free, and low sugar diets were also mentioned. In addition, 6 parents also stated that their children were picky eaters and had "very limited diets."

Table 4. Special diet use in pediatric autism.

	All n (%)	Males n (%)	Females n (%)	p
No restrictions	142 (67.6)	113 (72.0)	29 (54.7)	**0.027**
Gluten free	21 (10.0)	8 (5.1)	13 (24.5)	**<0.001**
High carb	17 (8.1)	14 (8.9)	3 (5.7)	0.570
Lactose free	16 (7.6)	7 (4.5)	9 (17.0)	**0.006**
Casein free	12 (5.7)	8 (5.1)	4 (7.5)	0.734
High protein	8 (3.8)	4 (2.5)	4 (7.5)	0.206
Ketogenic diet (i.e., high fat, low card)	7 (3.3)	6 (3.8)	1 (1.9)	0.682
Vegetarian	4 (1.9)	2 (1.3)	2 (3.8)	0.574
Vegan	0 (0.0)	0 (0.0)	0 (0.0)	n/a

Diet data is presented as a count (percentage within sex) who follow each diet. Differences between sex were determined using a Fisher's exact test. p < 0.05 was considered significant. Significant differences are bolded. n/a, not applicable.

The primary information sources regarding dietary supplements used by parents are shown in Figure 2. Sixty-five percent (65%) of parents indicated that health care professionals (e.g., physician, nurse, nutritionist) were their primary source of information regarding dietary supplements. Published literature and media (e.g., news, magazines, journals) were listed as the second and third most popular sources of information. Social media was the least utilized source, with only 5.8% of parents indicating use. Two participants did not indicate a primary information source and two other participants indicated "knowledge over the years," and "myself (pharmacist)" in the "other" section.

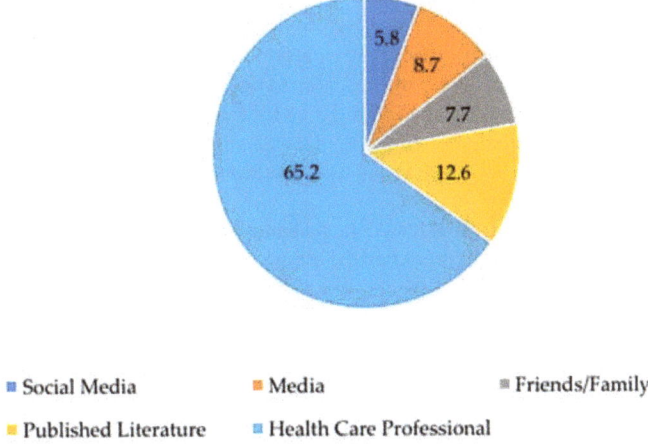

- Social Media
- Media
- Friends/Family
- Published Literature
- Health Care Professional

Figure 2. Primary information sources about dietary supplements. Data is presented as % of respondents. Participants could only choose one source or answer in the "other" section. One participant indicated in the "other" section that they use a combination of social media and health care professionals, so a "yes" was put into each category.

3.5. Physician Communication

Nearly all families (98.1%) indicated that they have a family doctor and/or a pediatrician. Eleven percent (11%) of families ($n = 21$) rated their overall level of satisfaction with the primary care physician as not satisfied or partially unsatisfied on a scale of 1 (not satisfied) to 5 (very satisfied), whereas 87% of parents ($n = 169$) rated their level of comfort in discussing supplements with physicians as comfortable or very comfortable. A large majority (72.4%; $n = 152$) had never met with a dietician. The frequency of disclosure of supplement use to a physician is summarized in Table 5. Results revealed that 33.5% of parents did not disclose all supplements to their physician. Several reasons were reported for omitting disclosure of supplementation use to primary care physicians including perceived "physician lack of knowledge", "no benefit", "too time consuming", and "scared of judgment".

Table 5. Disclosure of supplement use to physician.

Disclosure of Number of Supplements (%)	Frequency n (%)
None (0)	11 (6.6)
Some (1–49)	14 (8.4)
Half (50)	8 (4.8)
Most (51–99)	23 (13.8)
All (100)	111 (66.5)

Frequency data is presented as a count (percentage of total).

4. Discussion

The use of complementary and alternative medicine (CAM) is increasing among children and is common in those with chronic illness or disorders, such as ASD [13]. Critically, however, a complete profile of dietary supplement use in children with ASD is lacking; making it difficult to develop educational strategies. The present study is impactful, as it provides a fully powered assessment of supplement-based CAM therapies in children with ASD.

4.1. Dietary Supplement Patterns and Special Diet Use

In this study, 75.9% of the children sampled have consumed dietary supplements, supporting the upper end of the prevalence range of supplement use in pediatric ASD cited in previous literature [14]. As the most recent studies evaluating supplement use in children with ASD were conducted several years ago, it is possible that the high prevalence reported here reflects a continued increase in supplement use. Additionally, this study utilized a broad definition of supplements when compared to other studies, therefore, it is likely we captured a wider variety of supplements used by children with autism. Nevertheless, the reported high rates of dietary and supplement use in this study would indicate these products continue to be of interest as a complementary approach to standard treatment of care.

Multivitamins, vitamin D, omega 3 fatty acids, probiotics, and magnesium were the most common supplement therapies used. Research regarding the efficacy of these supplements in ASD populations requires further evaluation [21]. Multivitamins, for example, are considered a popular CAM therapy in ASD [22]. The rationale for this treatment is based on the frequently observed dietary deficiency of vitamins and micronutrients in children with ASD. Children with ASD are often deficient in calcium, vitamin D, vitamin K, vitamin A, vitamin E, zinc, vitamin B6, and tetrahydrobiopterin [21]. These deficiencies could be the result of food selectivity or altered gastrointestinal absorption. Adams et al. [23] conducted a double-blind randomized control trial to examine the effect of a common commercial vitamin supplement on observed improvements in parent-rated pre and post autism symptomatology. They found significant improvements in hyperactivity, tantrumming, overall, and receptive language, suggesting it as a reasonable adjunct therapy for children with ASD. However, no other study has evaluated or been able to replicate the effectiveness or safety of this biological therapy. Similarly, preliminary studies on probiotics have shown improvement in core symptomatology in ASD [21], but they have been minimally replicated and several other studies have denounced their effects. It is also possible that there are responders and non-responders to individual treatments, further complicating interpretation.

Recently, vitamin D has been proposed as a potential treatment for ASD [24]. In 2015, an open trial demonstrated significant improvements in autism rating scales following 3 month vitamin D3 supplementation [25]. However, this small sample study has been the only experimental study to demonstrate the potential efficacy of vitamin D in children with ASD, highlighting the need for more wide-scale studies to critically validate the efficacy of vitamin D before drawing any definite conclusions.

Collectively, these supplements require more systematic and rigorous research. As a result, there is little evidence to support the use of any nutritional supplement or dietary therapy for children with ASD [26]. Furthermore, some of the other supplements reported in this study confirm anecdotal reports regarding the consumption of dangerous biological therapies. The Food and Drug Administration has issued several health warnings about adrenal cortex extract, for example, and has deemed it "unsafe and ineffective for labeled indications for human use" [27–29]. Evidently, there are gaps in the transmission of scholarly literature to quality educational materials for families, as many children continue to consume dietary supplements that are unsupported by research. In addition, several parents indicated that they were undecided about the safety of supplements and listed inadequate knowledge about supplements as the number one factor barring use.

Research evaluating specialty diets (e.g., gluten free casein free, lactose free, etc.) shows similar ambiguity. More specifically, there are few studies that demonstrate conclusive results in the gluten free and casein (or lactose) free diets reported in this study [30]. Many are small in size and lack strict dietary controls, both common problems in conducting dietary research in children, which limits the ability of researchers to drawn firm conclusions. Consequently, many studies regarding specialty diets point to the need for further research and illustrate how clinicians often find themselves unable to offer the most up-to-date and scientifically credible information to their patients. Of note, the ketogenic diet has emerged as a leader in specialty diets for ASD in the past several years and has offered promising, though preliminary, results in both animal and human studies [31–33]. Seven participants reported utilizing this diet.

4.2. Physician-Patient Communication

Sixty-five percent (65%) of parents disclosed that their primary source of information regarding supplements were health care providers. In addition, 72% of families indicated that they had never met a dietician, signifying that many are relying on their physician for quality information regarding supplements and special diets. However, 33% admitted to not disclosing all supplements to their physician due to perceived physician lack of knowledge, no apparent benefit, the time commitment, and fear of judgment. Alarmingly, as 36.7% reported taking prescribed medication, a lack of disclosure may pose a risk to patients who may be unaware of the potential for interactions with concurrent CAM use. An open, patient-centered, non-judgmental approach is recommended for physicians when discussing supplement therapies [34]. This study highlights that patients would like to receive information about CAM from their conventional health care team, underscoring the importance of clinician knowledge about CAM and emerging research findings.

4.3. Limitations

There are a couple areas to consider when examining the limitations of this study. While the study provides novel information about the use of supplement therapies and special diet use in children with ASD, the study is limited as the majority of its participants are from Canada, therefore, may not be generalizable to other geographic regions. Further, as this is a descriptive study, it does not provide causal information regarding the effect of individual supplement therapies (e.g., omega 3 fatty acids causing relief of gastroenteritis symptoms). Finally, social desirability, a common bias where respondents answer in a way viewed favorably by others, may have influenced the data.

5. Conclusions

Supplement use continues to be a prevalent form of CAM used in ASD. While a variety of supplements and dietary interventions are utilized, the scientific consensus remains that there is currently little evidence to support the use of any nutritional supplement or dietary therapy for children with ASD. Future investigation into the effects of individual supplements on physiological and psychological functioning to determine optimal supplementation strategies in ASD is required.

Supplementary Materials: The following are available online at http://www.mdpi.com/2072-6643/11/8/1783/s1, File S1: Dietary Patterns and Supplement Use in Pediatric Autism, Table S1. All Supplement Use in Children with ASD, Table S2. Supplements listed in the "Other" Category by Parents.

Author Contributions: Conceptualization, M.S.T., R.F.M. and J.S.; Data curation, R.F.M.; Formal analysis, R.F.M. and J.A.P.; Funding acquisition, M.S.T.; Investigation, M.S.T.; Methodology, M.S.T.; Project administration, M.S.T.; Supervision, J.A.P., W.B.G. and J.S.; Validation, W.B.G.; Writing—original draft, M.S.T.; Writing—review & editing, M.S.T., R.F.M., J.A.P., W.B.G. and J.S.

Funding: This research was funded by Alberta Innovates Health Solutions, Alberta. (M.S.T. Alberta Innovates Research Studentship).

Acknowledgments: The authors would like to acknowledge Jodi Siever for her assistance with the statistical analysis, and Sarah Tabler, Yegor Korchemagin, and Madeleine Brulotte for their assistance with data collection and distribution. The authors would like to acknowledge Taking Strides for its continued support and promotion of participation.

Conflicts of Interest: The authors declare no conflict of interest. The funders had no role in the design of the study; in the collection, analyses, or interpretation of data; in the writing of the manuscript, or in the decision to publish the results.

References

1. American Psychiatric Association. *Diagnostic and Statistical Manual of Mental Disorders*, 5th ed.; American Psychiatric Pub.: Philadelphia, PA, USA, 2013; Volume 21, ISBN 9780890425541.

2. Lai, M.-C.; Lombardo, M.V.; Baron-Cohen, S. Autism. *Lancet* **2014**, *383*, 896–910. [CrossRef]
3. Redfield, R.R.; Kent, C.K.; Leahy, M.A.; Martinroe, J.C.; Spriggs, S.R.; Yang, T.; Doan, Q.M.; King, P.H.; Maitland, P.D.; Starr, T.M.; et al. Prevalence of Autism Spectrum Disorder Among Children Aged 8 Years-Autism and Developmental Disabilities Monitoring Network, 11 Sites, United States, 2014 Surveillance Summaries Centers for Disease Control and Prevention MMWR Editorial and Production Staf. *MMWR Surveill Summ.* **2018**, *67*, 2.
4. Klein, N.; Kemper, K.J. Integrative approaches to caring for children with autism. *Curr. Probl. Pediatr. Adolesc. Health Care* **2016**, *46*, 195–201. [CrossRef] [PubMed]
5. Bryson, S.E.; Rogers, S.J.; Fombonne, E. Autism spectrum disorders: Early detection, intervention, education, and psychopharmacological management. *Can. J. Psychiatry* **2003**, *48*, 506–516. [CrossRef] [PubMed]
6. National Centre for Complementary and Integrative Health. The Use of Complementary and Alternative Medicine in the United States. Available online: https://nccih.nih.gov/research/statistics/2007/camsurvey_fs1.htm (accessed on 14 May 2019).
7. National Centre for Complementary and Integrative Health. Complementary, Alternative, or Integrative Health: What's In a Name? Available online: https://nccih.nih.gov/health/integrative-health (accessed on 14 June 2019).
8. Sanders, H.; Davis, M.F.; Duncan, B.; Meaney, F.J.; Haynes, J.; Barton, L.L. Use of complementary and alternative medical therapies among children with special health care needs in southern Arizona. *Pediatrics* **2003**, *111*, 584–587. [CrossRef] [PubMed]
9. Surette, S.; Vanderjagt, L.; Vohra, S. Surveys of complementary and alternative medicine usage: A scoping study of the paediatric literature. *Complement. Ther. Med.* **2013**, *21*, S48–S53. [CrossRef] [PubMed]
10. Levy, S.E.; Mandell, D.S.; Merhar, S.; Ittenbach, R.F.; Pinto-Martin, J. A Use of complementary and alternative medicine among children recently diagnosed with autistic spectrum disorder. *J. Dev. Behav. Pediatr.* **2003**, *24*, 418–423. [CrossRef]
11. Connett, D. Autism: Potentially lethal bleach "cure" feared to have spread to Britain. Available online: https://www.independent.co.uk/life-style/health-and-families/health-news/autism-potentially-lethal-bleach-cure-feared-to-have-spread-to-britain-a6744291.html (accessed on 1 May 2019).
12. Anagnostou, E.; Hansen, R. Medical treatment overview: Traditional and novel psycho-pharmacological and complementary and alternative medications. *Curr. Opin. Pediatr.* **2011**, *23*, 621–627. [CrossRef]
13. Huffman, L.C.; Sutcliffe, T.L.; Tanner, I.S.D.; Feldman, H.M. Management of symptoms in children with autism spectrum disorders: A comprehensive review of pharmacologic and complementary-alternative medicine treatments. *J. Dev. Behav. Pediatr.* **2011**, *32*, 56–68. [CrossRef]
14. Hanson, E.; Kalish, L.A.; Bunce, E.; Curtis, C.; McDaniel, S.; Ware, J.; Petry, J. Use of complementary and alternative medicine among children diagnosed with autism spectrum disorder. *J. Autism Dev. Disord.* **2007**, *37*, 628–636. [CrossRef]
15. Robinson, A.; McGrail, M.R. Disclosure of CAM use to medical practitioners: A review of qualitative and quantitative studies. *Complement. Ther. Med.* **2004**, *12*, 90–98. [CrossRef] [PubMed]
16. Izzo, A.; Ernst, E. Interactions Between Herbal Medicines and Prescribed Drugs. *Drugs* **2009**, *69*, 1777–1798. [CrossRef] [PubMed]
17. Lenth, R. Java Applets for Power and Sample Size. Available online: https://homepage.divms.uiowa.edu/~{}rlenth/Power/ (accessed on 17 May 2019).
18. Wiens, K.; Erdman, K.A.; Stadnyk, M.; Parnell, J.A. Dietary supplement usage, motivation, and education in young Canadian athletes. *Int. J. Sport Nutr. Exerc. Metab.* **2014**, *24*, 613–622. [CrossRef] [PubMed]
19. Parnell, J.A.; Wiens, K.P.; Erdman, K.A. Dietary intakes and supplement use in pre-adolescent and adolescent Canadian athletes. *Nutrients* **2016**, *8*, 526. [CrossRef] [PubMed]
20. The National Academies of Science and Medicine Dietary Reference Intakes Tables and Application. Available online: http://nationalacademies.org/hmd/Activities/Nutrition/SummaryDRIs/DRI-Tables.aspx (accessed on 13 June 2019).
21. Brondino, N.; Fusar-Poli, L.; Rocchetti, M.; Provenzani, U.; Barale, F.; Politi, P. Complementary and alternative therapies for autism spectrum disorder. *Evidence-Based Complement. Altern. Med.* **2015**, *2015*. [CrossRef] [PubMed]

22. Stewart, P.A.; Hyman, S.L.; Schmidt, B.L.; Macklin, E.A.; Reynolds, A.; Johnson, C.R.; James, S.J.; Manning-Courtney, P. Dietary Supplementation in Children with Autism Spectrum Disorders: Common, Insufficient, and Excessive. *J. Acad. Nutr. Diet.* **2015**, *115*, 1237–1248. [CrossRef] [PubMed]
23. Adams, J.B.; Audhya, T.; McDonough-Means, S.; Rubin, R.A.; Quig, D.; Geis, E.; Gehn, E.; Loresto, M.; Mitchell, J.; Atwood, S. Effect of a vitamin/mineral supplement on children and adults with autism. *BMC Pediatr.* **2011**, *11*, 111. [CrossRef]
24. Cannell, J.J. Vitamin D and autism, what's new? *Rev. Endocr. Metab. Disord.* **2017**, *18*, 183–193. [CrossRef]
25. Saad, K.; Abdel-rahman, A.A.; Elserogy, Y.M.; Al-Atram, A.A.; Cannell, J.J.; Bjørklund, G.; Abdel-Reheim, M.K.; Othman, H.A.K.; El-Houfey, A.A.; Abd El-Aziz, N.H.R.; et al. Vitamin D status in autism spectrum disorders and the efficacy of vitamin D supplementation in autistic children. *Nutr. Neurosci.* **2015**, *19*, 346–351. [CrossRef]
26. Sathe, N.; Andrews, J.C.; McPheeters, M.L.; Warren, Z.E. Nutritional and Dietary Interventions for Autism Spectrum Disorder: A Systematic Review. *Pediatrics* **2017**, *139*. [CrossRef]
27. Food and Drug Administration. Report to the Honorable Barry M. Goldwater Jr. House of Representatives—Adrenal Cortex Extract Taken Off the Market. Available online: http://archive.gao.gov/f0102/115802.pdf (accessed on 25 July 2019).
28. Hurt, R.T.; Mundi, M.S. Over-the-Counter Adrenal Supplements: More than Meets the Eye. *Mayo Clin. Proc.* **2018**, *93*, 276–277. [CrossRef] [PubMed]
29. Food and Drug Administration. Important Alert Adrenal Cortext Extract. Available online: https://www.accessdata.fda.gov/cms_ia/importalert_172.html (accessed on 14 September 2018).
30. Piwowarczyk, A.; Horvath, A.; Łukasik, J.; Pisula, E.; Szajewska, H. Gluten- and casein-free diet and autism spectrum disorders in children: A systematic review. *Eur. J. Nutr.* **2018**, *57*, 433–440. [CrossRef] [PubMed]
31. Castro, K.; Faccioli, L.S.; Baronio, D.; Gottfried, C.; Perry, I.S.; Dos Santos Riesgo, R. Effect of a ketogenic diet on autism spectrum disorder: A systematic review. *Res. Autism Spectr. Disord.* **2015**, *20*, 31–38. [CrossRef]
32. El-Rashidy, O.; El-Baz, F.; El-Gendy, Y.; Khalaf, R.; Reda, D.; Saad, K. Ketogenic diet versus gluten free casein free diet in autistic children: A case-control study. *Metab. Brain Dis.* **2017**, *32*, 1935–1941. [CrossRef] [PubMed]
33. Newell, C.; Bomhof, M.R.; Reimer, R.A.; Hittel, D.S.; Rho, J.M.; Shearer, J. Ketogenic diet modifies the gut microbiota in a murine model of autism spectrum disorder. *Mol. Autism* **2016**, *7*, 1–6. [CrossRef] [PubMed]
34. Kemper, K.J.; Vohra, S.; Walls, R. The Use of Complementary and Alternative Medicine in Pediatrics. *Pediatrics* **2008**, *122*, 1374–1386. [CrossRef] [PubMed]

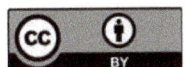

© 2019 by the authors. Licensee MDPI, Basel, Switzerland. This article is an open access article distributed under the terms and conditions of the Creative Commons Attribution (CC BY) license (http://creativecommons.org/licenses/by/4.0/).

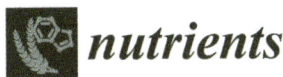

Review

Exploring the Science behind *Bifidobacterium breve* M-16V in Infant Health

Chyn Boon Wong [1], Noriyuki Iwabuchi [2] and Jin-zhong Xiao [1,*]

1. Next Generation Science Institute, Morinaga Milk Industry Co., Ltd., Zama, Kanagawa 252-8583, Japan
2. Food Ingredients and Technology Institute, Morinaga Milk Industry Co., Ltd., Zama, Kanagawa 252-8583, Japan
* Correspondence: j_xiao@morinagamilk.co.jp; Tel.: +81-46(252)3064

Received: 9 July 2019; Accepted: 24 July 2019; Published: 25 July 2019

Abstract: Probiotics intervention has been proposed as a feasible preventative approach against adverse health-related complications in infants. Nevertheless, the umbrella concept of probiotics has led to a massive application of probiotics in a range of products for promoting infant health, for which the strain-specificity, safety and efficacy findings associated with a specific probiotics strain are not clearly defined. *Bifidobacterium breve* M-16V is a commonly used probiotic strain in infants. M-16V has been demonstrated to offer potential in protecting infants from developing the devastating necrotising enterocolitis (NEC) and allergic diseases. This review comprehends the potential beneficial effects of M-16V on infant health particularly in the prevention and treatment of premature birth complications and immune-mediated disorders in infants. Mechanistic studies supporting the use of M-16V implicated that M-16V is capable of promoting early gut microbial colonisation and may be involved in the regulation of immune balance and inflammatory response to protect high-risk infants from NEC and allergies. Summarised information on M-16V has provided conceptual proof of the use of M-16V as a potential probiotics candidate aimed at promoting infant health, particularly in the vulnerable preterm population.

Keywords: *Bifidobacterium breve* M-16V; infant health; clinical efficacy; probiotics; gut microbiota

---

1. Introduction

Gut microbiota has become an important aspect of human health. Gut microbes regulate host intestinal, immunological and metabolic activities through their wide array of modulatory capabilities and enzymatic armoury [1]. Recent advances in microbial research have revealed the importance of early gut microbiome for neonatal health development and disease pathologies [2]. Aberrations of infant gut microbiota—a state of altered microbial composition and functionality—are associated with adverse health-related consequences including asthma [3], necrotising enterocolitis (NEC) [4], eczema [5] and inflammatory bowel disease [6] in neonatal stage or later in life.

Microbial ecosystem is established during the first three years of life for which a host–microbe symbiotic interaction that mutually benefits both is initiated [7]. It has been implicated that a number of extrinsic factors, such as gestational age, delivery mode and feeding types, are affecting the process of microbial colonisation in newborns [7,8]. Initial neonatal gut microbial colonisation represents a crucial window of opportunity for shaping a healthy gastrointestinal tract and immune system [9], and positive modulation of gut microbiota during this critical period could be an effective preventative approach against immune-mediated and microbiome-related disease pathologies. Consequently, probiotics intervention is receiving significant attention as a non-invasive attempt to optimize the infant microbiota as a means to improve health or prevent disease.

Probiotics are defined as "live microorganisms, which when administered in adequate amounts, confer a health benefit on the host" [10]. Studies over the last decade have demonstrated that probiotics supplementation could promote gut microbial colonisation and prevent or treat diseases in infants [11,12]. These reports have led to a massive application of probiotics in a range of products including foods, infant formula, dietary supplements, and pharmaceutical products for promoting infant health. Nevertheless, many of the marketed probiotic products encompass limited well-consolidated regulatory oversight and a lack of human substantiation of efficacy [13]. Moreover, the safety and effects of probiotics in the vulnerable preterm population remain relatively limited and inconsistent [14,15]. Therefore, a detailed review of the scientific basis of a specific probiotic strain has emerged as an important aspect for an optimised selection of suitable probiotic candidates for use in infants.

Bifidobacterium breve M-16V (designated as M-16V) is a commonly used probiotic strain in infants for modulation of gut microbiota as a means to support healthy growth and promote health. Some evidence suggests that M-16V can stimulate bifidobacterial colonisation, alleviate allergic disorders and protect premature infants against NEC. Nevertheless, despite its nutritional and medicinal benefits, a comprehensive review of its specific clinical effects for infant health is still lacking. In this review, we discuss the effects of probiotic administration on infant health, with specific attention to the probiotic strain M-16V. We conducted a systematic survey for publications related to M-16V using the databases including MEDLINE [16], EMBase [17], medical journal web [18] and JDreamIII [19] from inception to 12 May 2019. Search terms were: M-16V OR M16V and the languages used were English and Japanese. A total of 60 articles including in vitro, preclinical and clinical studies were extracted (two review and 58 original articles). Among them, 31 were on the single strain of M-16V, five were on the probiotics mixture with other strains, and 24 were on synbiotics (Supplementary Tables S1 and S2). Herein, we summarise the significant effects of M-16V on premature birth complications and allergic disorders from the most relevant in vitro, animal and clinical studies. We believed that improved understanding of the role of M-16V in governing development of healthy gut microbiota during early life would inform rational therapeutic application of probiotics aimed at promoting infant health, especially in the vulnerable preterm population, and ultimately preventing chronic diseases later in life.

2. Probiotics for Infant Health

Probiotics intervention has gained overwhelming popularity over the last two decades as a potential nutritional supplementation approach to promote and maintain a healthy gut milieu and protect against dysbiosis in early life [20]. Accumulating evidence suggests that manipulation of the microbiota with the use of probiotics at an early stage may lead to an appropriate microbial colonisation and could have long-lasting impacts on child and adult health [21]. Probiotics that have been commonly given to neonates and infants include species of *Bifidobacterium* and *Lactobacillus*. Among them, *Bifidobacterium* is thought to be a keystone taxon in infant gut microbiota that plays a vital role in regulating immunological and physiological functions [22].

Bifidobacterial species have been isolated from the gastrointestinal tract of humans and animals as well as a few that have been isolated from human vagina, oral cavity, breast milk, sewage and foods, and could be categorised into two major groups; bifidobacterial species of human origins as human-residential bifidobacteria (HRB), whereas other species which are the natural inhabitants of animals or environment as non-HRB [23]. It has been demonstrated that bifidobacterial species of different residential origins display different levels of adaptability and functionality in the infant gut [23]. Of note, *B. longum* subsp. *infantis* (*B. infantis*), *B. longum* subsp. *longum* (*B. longum*), *B. bifidum*, and *B. breve*, which are frequently isolated from infant intestines and are referred to as infant-type HRB [23,24], have a large repertoire of genes for the utilisation of human milk oligosaccharides (HMOs) [25,26]. Studies have reported that infant-type HRB are capable of utilising HMOs with different metabolic pathways and degrees of degradation, highly compatible with human breast milk and tolerant to lysozyme [25,27], demonstrating how well adapted they are to the transmission routes and growth conditions in the infant gut. In fact, infant-type HRB have been shown to be the exclusive members of healthy breastfed infants [28,29], while formula-fed infants are also colonised with species that are commonly isolated from adult intestines (adult-type HRB) such as B. adolescentis and B. pseudocatenulatum [30], implying the strains of infant-type HRB could be better probiotic candidates for infant use.

Several studies have demonstrated the use of infant-type HRB, including the strains of B. breve [31], B. longum [32], B. infantis [33] and B. bifidum [34], as probiotics for therapeutic purposes in neonates and infants. Administration of infant-type HRB probiotic strains in the first stage of life may result in the prevention of NEC and reduction in the risk as well as treatment of infectious and atopic disease [11,12]. Despite the promise, questions and concerns have been raised about the safety and clinical efficacy of probiotics administration, especially if the product is destined for use in infants. It is increasingly apparent that not all probiotics are equally safe, and the effects demonstrated with one strain cannot be extrapolated to another strain, even if they belong to the same species [35]. Of note, among many infant-type HRB probiotic strains that have been studied, M-16V possesses a proven track record of safety and a number of beneficial attributes that make it an attractive probiotic candidate for infant use. The following paragraphs will review the safety and specific health benefits of M-16V in infants within the field that seek to provide rigorous preclinical characterisation and substantial clinical evidence of M-16V for successful probiotics selection.

3. *Bifidobacterium breve* M-16V as Infant Probiotic

3.1. Origin and Characteristics

M-16V was originated from the gut of an infant in 1963 and was first commercially available in Japan in 1976 with the launch of Vinelac dietary supplement. In 1982, M-16V was added to a growing-up powdered formula called Yochien-Jidai in Japan and has since been incorporated in several other products including term and preterm infant formula.

M-16V is a non-motile, non-spore forming, rod-shaped anaerobic Gram-positive bacterium. It was identified as *B. breve* based on morphological, physiological and genetic characteristics. M-16V is highly accessible to human gastrointestinal tract with strong adherence activity [36]. In addition, lyophilised powder of M-16V manufactured by Morinaga Milk Industry Co., Ltd. possesses excellent stability during storage and high survivability in finished products such as powdered formula until consumption [37].

3.2. Safety

M-16V is well-evaluated for safety and has met the safety standards regulated by the Food and Agriculture Organization of the United Nations/World Health Organization (FAO/WHO) guidelines for the evaluation of microbes for probiotics use in foods [38]. In 2013, M-16V attained not only FDA-Notified Generally Recognized as Safe (GRAS) status for food uses (GRN No., 453) [39], but also GRAS status for infants (GRN No., 454) [40]. In addition, in 2016, M-16V has been included in the list of authorised probiotic strains for infant's food in China, in which M-16V is the only infant-type HRB strain among the nine strains in the list [41]. To date, there has been broad use of M-16V in low birth weight infants to reduce the risk of preterm birth complications in more than 120 neonatal intensive care units (NICU) in affiliated hospitals in Japan, Australia, New Zealand and Singapore [42–44].

Comprehensive safety evaluation of M-16V, which includes functional, genomic, and in vivo analyses, demonstrated that M-16V is a non-pathogenic, non-toxigenic, non-haemolytic and non-antibiotic resistant probiotic bacterium that does not contain any plasmids and does not display harmful metabolic activities [36,40,45,46]. M-16V produces L-lactic acid but no D-lactic acid. In addition, M-16V was reported to possess conjugated bile salt hydrolytic activity [36]. M-16V was able to hydrolyse conjugated bile acids taurocholic and glycocholic acid to the primary bile acid (cholic acid) and glycochenodeoxycholic and taurochenodeoxycholic acid to chenodeoxycholic acid, while the production of hepatotoxic and carcinogenic secondary bile acids (deoxycholic and lithocholic acid) was not detected upon complete biotransformation of bile salts [47]. These results resolve the concern about the safety of administering a secondary bile acids-producing bacterium.

Studies on acute and chronic toxicological features of M-16V revealed that both single and repeated oral administration of M-16V did not cause death and any toxic symptoms in a rat model [45]. For instance, groups of 10 male and 10 female three-week-old Crj:CD (SD) rats were orally administered with a single dose of M-16V at 6000 mg/kg (1.4×10^{12} CFU/kg) or 3000 mg/kg (6.9×10^{11} CFU/kg) and examined for acute toxic symptoms for 14 days. There were no gross abnormalities or histopathological findings attributable to the treatment in all organs throughout the test period, although slightly lower body weight was observed in male rats administered a high dose of M-16V as compared to the control on days 8 and 10. Furthermore, oral administration of M-16V with a 90-day repeated dose (2.3×10^{11} CFU/kg/day) to five-week-old Crj:CD (SD) IGS rats revealed no adverse effects attributed to M-16V during the study period. M-16V induced no significant histopathological changes in all organs examined. These findings demonstrate the absence of acute and chronic toxicity by consumption of M-16V. Additional in vitro tests showed that M-16V did not possess mucin degradation ability [48]. Taken together, these studies support that M-16V is safe for use as a probiotic in humans.

4. Effects of M-16V on Premature Birth Complications

Prematurity, prolonged hospitalisation, immunodeficiency, antibiotics use and delayed enteral feeding are challenging ways to begin life for preterm infants [49]. Premature infants are at elevated risk to develop multiple health comorbidities; one of which is the devastating necrotising enterocolitis (NEC) [50]. It is a major cause of morbidity and mortality in extremely preterm infants that is associated with severe sepsis and intestinal perforation [51]. Although the exact aetiology and pathogenesis of NEC remain elusive, perturbation of the gut microbiota, leading to a hyperinflammatory response, appears to be a key factor that predisposes neonates to NEC [52]. Premature infants often present with an immature gut and exhibit delayed gut colonisation with beneficial commensal bacteria such as *Bifidobacterium* and *Bacteroides*, where instead they are more susceptible to colonisation by *Enterobacteriaceae* and *Enterococcus* [53,54]. Moreover, the use of antibiotics in premature and low birth weight infants disturbs the colonisation patterns of *Bifidobacterium* and shifts the gut microbial composition toward a high abundance of Proteobacteria, with a decreased in the overall diversity of the infant's gut microbiota [55–57]. To this end, the neonatal period has; therefore, emerged as an opportune time for preventive M-16V probiotics intervention to promote bifidobacterial colonisation, facilitate the development of gut mucosal immune system and improve infant health.

4.1. Preclinical Studies

Several animal studies have demonstrated the potential role of M-16V in improving the maturation of intestinal immune system and promoting bifidobacterial colonisation during early infancy. In a neonatal Lewis rat model, oral supplementation with M-16V (4.5×10^8 CFU/100 g of body weight/day; $n = 8$) during suckling period (days 6 to 18) showed potential in enhancing the homing process of naïve T cells to the mesenteric lymph nodes (MLN) and the retention of activated T cells in the intraepithelial (IEL) compartment [58]. The control group ($n = 8$) was administered with a matched volume of mineral water. Administration of M-16V increased the proportion of cells bearing toll-like receptor 4 (TLR4) in the MLN and IEL compartments, and enhanced the percentage of the integrin $\alpha E\beta 7+$ and CD62L+ cells in the MLN and that of the integrin $\alpha E\beta 7+$ cells in the IEL, as compared to the control. However, M-16V did not exert a systemic immune-enhancing effect in which the proportions of the main lymphocyte subset in spleen were not significantly affected by M-16V. In addition, M-16V induced no harmful effects on the rats wherein no significant differences were observed in the growth curve of the control and M-16V groups. Administration of M-16V significantly increased the levels of intestinal immunoglobulin A (IgA) as compared to the control, indicating M-16V could also strengthen the humoral intestinal immune response.

Furthermore, M-16V has also been reported to be able to regulate immune responses and appear to exert anti-inflammatory effects in rats at different developmental periods [59,60]. Oral administration of M-16V (5×10^8 CFU/day) to F344/Du rats significantly reduced the expression of inflammatory molecules during the newborn period (days 1 to 14) and regulated the expression of co-stimulatory molecules during the weaning period (days 21 to 34) [60]. In addition, the numbers of *Bifidobacterium* were also significantly increased in both the caecum and colon during the newborn period but not during weaning, as compared to the control groups [60].

Similarly, significant improvements in inflammatory conditions were also observed in DSS-induced colitis F344/N rats administered with M-16V (2.5×10^9 CFU/day) during weaning period (from postnatal days 21 to 34), as compared to the control rats. M-16V showed potential in altering systemic T-cell immune functions and suppressing inflammatory responses in colitis rats during the weaning period [59]. Taken together, these preclinical studies imply that supplementation with M-16V may aid in the development of intestinal immunity and prevention of intestinal inflammation during early infancy.

4.2. Clinical Studies

Multiple implementation cohort studies have demonstrated the potential effect of early administration of M-16V in improving bifidobacterial colonisation in preterm infants (gestation < 33 weeks) [42,61] and low birth weight infants (<2250 g) [32,42,62,63]. Earlier detection and longer maintenance of a bifidobacteria-dominant gut microbiome were observed in M-16V-supplemented infants. For instance, in a randomised, double-blind, placebo-controlled trial involving 159 preterm neonates (gestation < 33 weeks) ready to commence or on feeds for <12 h, supplementation of M-16V (3×10^9 CFU/day) for three weeks significantly increased the levels of faecal *B. breve* as compared to placebo control where the *B. breve* counts were below detection level [42]. M-16V supplement was well-tolerated by all enrolled preterm neonates with no adverse effects including probiotic sepsis and deaths. These findings suggest that M-16V is a suitable probiotic strain for routine use in preterm neonates to promote the acquisition of beneficial commensal bacteria.

Another randomised, placebo-controlled trial involving 30 preterm low birth weight infants, with mean gestation 32.8 weeks and birth weight 1486 g, also revealed a positive effect of M-16V on early gut colonisation with commensal *Bifidobacterium* spp. [63]. The subjects were randomly divided into three groups; (A) subjects received M-16V supplementation within several hours (mean: 7.2 h) of birth, (B) subjects received M-16V supplementation >24 h (mean: 36.5 h) after birth, and (C) subjects who were fed normally without M-16V supplementation as control group. Intragastrical administration of M-16V (1.6×10^8 CFU in 0.5 mL of 5% glucose sterile distilled water, twice daily) until the subjects were discharged from the hospital remedied the delayed bifidobacterial colonisation in both groups A and B, while no *Bifidobacterium* was detected in eight out of ten infants in group C during the observation period of seven weeks [63]. Notably, a significant earlier detection of bifidobacteria and a significant decrease in the cell numbers of *Enterobacteriaceae* were observed at two weeks after birth in infants administered with M-16V within several hours of birth (group A), indicating timing of administration of M-16V is highly important for which the earlier the administration of M-16V to preterm low birth weight infants, the better the effects of M-16V in promoting the colonisation of bifidobacteria and reducing the susceptibility to colonisation by potentially harmful bacteria.

A comparative, non-randomised controlled, prospective trial involving 44 low birth weight infants (body weight 1000–2000 g), who were ready for feeds within seven days of birth, administered with either single strain of M-16V (5×10^8 CFU/day) or probiotics mixture containing three bifidobacterial strains, M-16V, *B. infantis* M-63, and *B. longum* BB536 (5×10^8 CFU/day of each strain), for six weeks has also revealed a significant increase in the detection rates and cell numbers of bifidobacteria in the faeces [32]. Notably, administration of the three-species probiotics mixture resulted in an earlier formation of a bifidobacteria-dominant microbiota and a significantly lower level of *Enterobacteriaceae* than those administered with M-16V alone [32]. It was noted that not only the total cell numbers of bifidobacteria but also the cell numbers of M-16V was higher in infants administered with the three-strain probiotics mixture than those administered with M-16V alone. This study suggests that M-16V may act synergistically and cooperatively with other *Bifidobacterium* strains to confer a more remarkable beneficial effect in premature infants. Nevertheless, the comparison between probiotics and control groups from the different timeline in this trial may introduce bias that tends to compromise the efficacy of M-16V and is likely to result in unfair comparisons. Additionally, two comparable pilot studies involving ten very low birth weight premature infants (<1250 g) administered with either M-16V or *B. longum* at a dose of 5×10^8 CFU/day for eight weeks have also suggested a potential capability of M-16V to colonise in the premature gut [62,64]. Supplementation with M-16V had a longer colonisation rate than those with *B. longum*, for which, while M-16V was found to colonise the premature gut as early as week two after birth and remain dominant, the administered strain of *B. longum* was not detected from week six after birth [62,64]. Collectively, these data have exemplified that M-16V is potentially beneficial at promoting early colonisation of bifidobacteria and may; therefore, support healthy growth in premature infants.

Furthermore, M-16V has also been evaluated for the preventive effects on NEC, death and late-onset sepsis in premature infants; however, the clinical findings are not conclusive [43,44,65]. The first evidence of the potential preventive effects of M-16V on NEC came from a non-randomised clinical trial involving 338 infants (220 extremely low birth weight (ELBW) and 118 very low birth weight (VLBW) infants) receiving M-16V supplementation (1×10^9 CFU/day in raw breast milk or formula milk) started within several hours (mean 7.2 h) after birth and continued until discharged from NICU, and 226 infants (101 ELBW and 125 VLBW infants) as a historical control [44]. The study revealed that administration of M-16V was potentially effective at reducing the incidence of NEC in ELBW and VLBW infants as compared to that in the historical control group. A significant reduction in morbidity and mortality rate, as well as the mortality due to infection, was also observed in ELBW and VLBW infants receiving M-16V supplementation [44]. These encouraging results have suggested a potential role of M-16V in protecting premature infants from NEC and infection. However, the use of historical control from another timeline in this trial may introduce bias that tends to compromise the efficacy of M-16V and is likely to result in unfair comparisons.

More recently, M-16V was reported to be associated with decreased incidence of "NEC ≥ Stage II" and "NEC ≥ Stage II or all-cause mortality" in preterm neonates <34 weeks [43]. The study was a retrospective cohort study involving 835 preterm neonates as historical control and 920 preterm neonates receiving M-16V routine probiotics supplementation (3×10^9 CFU/day in 1.5 mL breast milk or sterile water) started when the infants were ready for enteral feeds and continued until the corrected age of 37 weeks. The initial daily dose for neonates <28 weeks was 1.5×10^9 CFU/day until reaching feeds of 50 mL/kg/day. It was noted that M-16V significantly lowered the incidence of NEC in preterm VLBW neonates born <34 weeks, while the incidence of NEC was lower but not statistically significant in those born <28 weeks, although the small sample size used [43]. Despite the encouraging results, the trial may introduce potential bias in comparisons with the historical control drawn from another timeline.

In addition, a recent strain-specific systematic review revealed that the significant efficacy of M-16V to reduce the risk of NEC remains controversial [65]. It was concluded that current evidence is limited regarding the potential of M-16V as a probiotic for preterm neonates, albeit the meta-analysis of non-randomised controlled trials showed a significant effect of M-16V intervention in NEC [65]. No significant benefits on stage ≥2 NEC, late-onset sepsis, mortality and postnatal age at full feeds were reported in the meta-analysis of randomised controlled trials. Well-designed and adequately-powered randomised controlled trials are needed for definite confirmation. Nonetheless, all clinical studies included in the systematic review have concluded that M-16V supplementation was not associated with probiotic-associated sepsis in this vulnerable population [65], suggesting the risk of developing sepsis related to M-16V administration in the setting of severe illness to be relatively low. In fact, issues on *B. breve* sepsis in immunocompromised infants [66,67] and meningitis caused by other strain of *B. breve* in preterm infants [68] have been reported. Another systematic review using a network meta-analysis approach showed that only few probiotic strains have statistically significant effects in reducing mortality, NEC, late-onset sepsis, and time until full enteral feeding [69]. M-16V was one of the many studied probiotic strains that did not show significant efficacy in preterm birth complications, reflecting a lack of adequately-powered randomised controlled trials to precisely define the clinical efficacy [69]. Further large and well-powered trials are needed to evaluate the effectiveness of M-16V in preventing NEC.

Taken together, these clinical studies underscore the potential roles of M-16V as a promising infant probiotic that could potentially impact the incidence, morbidity and mortality associated with NEC (Table 1).

Table 1. Summary from clinical studies of the effects of M-16V on premature birth complications.

Reference	Study Design	Study Characteristics
Effect of M-16V on bifidobacterial colonisation		
Patole et al., 2014 [42]	Randomised, double-blinded, placebo-controlled	Study population: Preterm infants (<33 weeks; BW < 1500 g)
		Country: Australia
		Sample size: $n = 159$ (Probiotics: 79; Placebo: 80)
		Intervention and dose: 3×10^9 CFU/day in 1.5 mL of sterile water or breast milk.
		Duration of supplementation: Supplementation started when infants were on enteral feeds for <12 h, continued till 37 weeks of corrected gestational age.
		Main outcomes: (1) Significant increase in *B. breve* faecal counts three weeks after M-16V supplementation. (2) No probiotic sepsis and death in M-16V-supplemented infants.
		Study limitations: Nil
Patole et al., 2016 [61]	Non-RCT comparative analytical study	Study population: Preterm infants (<33 weeks; BW < 1500 g)
		Country: Australia
		Sample size: $n = 159$; subjects were divided into two groups based on their gestational age: (1) SGA due to IUGR (Probiotics: 22; Placebo: 20). (2) Non-SGA (Probiotics: 55; Placebo: 56)
		Intervention and dose: 3×10^9 CFU/day in 1.5 mL of sterile water or breast milk.
		Duration of supplementation: Supplementation started when infants were on enteral feeds for <12 h, continued till 37 weeks of gestational age.
		Main outcomes: (1) *B. breve* faecal counts did not differ between SGA and non-SGA infants. (2) M-16V-treated SGA infants reached full feeds earlier than SGA controls, after adjustment for age at starting feeds and gestation <28 weeks.
		Study limitations: (1) This was a comparative analytical study that relies on the results obtained from the previous study [42]. (2) Assessment of outcome could not be blinded; however, that was not expected to introduce a major bias because of the objectivity of the outcome.
Li et al., 2004 [63]	Randomised controlled trial	Study population: Preterm VLBW infants (BW < 1250 g)
		Country: Japan
		Sample size: $n = 30$ (A) M-16V given several hours (mean: 7.2 h) after birth; $n = 10$ (B) M-16V given >24 h (mean: 36.5 h) after birth; $n = 10$ (C) Control fed normally without probiotic supplement; $n = 10$
		Intervention and dose: 1.6×10^8 CFU twice daily in 0.5 mL of 5% glucose sterile water.
		Duration of supplementation: Continued until discharged.
		Main outcomes: (1) Significant increase in bifidobacterial colonisation in both groups A and B. (2) Significant earlier detection of bifidobacteria and a significant decrease in the cell numbers of *Enterobacteriaceae* were observed in group A.
		Study limitations: (1) This was a non-double-blinded randomised controlled trial which may introduce potential bias. (2) The sample size was relatively small. (3) Assessment of outcome could not be blinded; however, that was not expected to introduce a major bias because of the objectivity of some of the outcomes.

Table 1. Cont.

Reference	Study Design	Study Characteristics
Ishizeki et al., 2013 [32]	Non-RCT prospective study	Study population: Low birth weight infants (<33 weeks; BW 1000–2000 g) who were ready for feeds within seven days of birth in three cohorts: (1) Control group: October 1999 to June 2000; $n = 16$ (2) Single-strain M-16V group: December 2000 to June 2001; $n = 15$ (3) Three-strain probiotics mixture group: April 2002 to April 2003; $n = 13$
		Country: Japan
		Sample size: 44
		Intervention and dose: (1) Control group: No probiotics (2) Single strain M-16V group: 5×10^8 CFU/day in 1.5 mL sterile water (3) Three-strain probiotics mixture group: *B. longum* BB536, *B. breve* M-16V and *B. infantis* M-63; 5×10^8 CFU/day of each strain in 1.5 mL sterile water
		Duration of supplementation: Six weeks.
		Main outcomes: (1) Both single-strain M-16V and three-strain probiotics mixture groups significantly increased the detection rates and cell numbers of *Bifidobacterium* in the faeces as compared to the control group. (2) Bifidobacteria proportion was significantly higher in the single-strain M-16V group at weeks one to four and in the three-strain probiotics mixture group at weeks one to six as compared to the control group. (3) The proportion of bifidobacteria in the three-strain probiotics mixture group was significantly higher than that in the single-strain M-16V group at weeks one and six. (4) The detection rates of *Clostridium* and proportions of *Enterobacteriaceae* were significantly lower in both probiotic groups.
		Study limitations: (1) This was a retrospective study that relies on the quality of record keeping. (2) The study was conducted at three different timelines which may introduce potential bias. (3) Outcome evaluation could not be blinded; however, that was not expected to introduce a major bias because of the objective of some of the outcomes.
Akiyama et al., 1994 [62]	Non-RCT	Study population: Preterm LBW infants with mean gestation (range) 32.8 weeks (27.8–37.6 weeks) and BW 1486 g (780–2250 g)
		Country: Japan
		Sample size: $n = 10$ (Probiotics: 5; Control: 5)
		Intervention and dose: 5×10^8 CFU/day of M-16V in 1.0 mL of sterile water
		Duration of supplementation: Continued until eight weeks of age
		Main outcomes: (1) Significant increase in bifidobacterial colonisation in M-16V-supplemented infants.
		Study limitations: (1) This was a non-randomised controlled trial which may introduce potential bias. (2) The sample size was very small. (3) Assessment of outcome could not be blinded; however, that was not expected to introduce a major bias because of the objectivity of the outcome.
Akiyama et al., 1994 [64]	Non-RCT	Study population: Preterm LBW infants with mean gestation (range) 32.8 weeks (27.8–37.6 weeks) and BW 1486 g (780–2250 g)
		Country: Japan
		Sample size: $n = 10$ (Probiotics: 5; Control: 5)
		Intervention and dose: 5×10^8 CFU/day of *B. longum* BB536 in 1.0 mL of sterile water
		Duration of supplementation: Continued until eight weeks of age
		Main outcomes: (1) Significant increase in bifidobacterial colonisation in *B. longum* BB536-supplemented infants. (2) This study compared the results obtained in the previous study using M-16V and revealed that while M-16V colonised the premature gut as early as week two after birth and remain dominant, the administered strain of *B. longum* was not detected from week six after birth.
		Study limitations: (1) This was a non-randomised controlled trial comparing the results from the previous study which may introduce potential bias. (2) The sample size was very small. (3) Assessment of outcome could not be blinded; however, that was not expected to introduce a major bias because of the objectivity of the outcome.

Table 1. Cont.

Reference	Study Design	Study Characteristics
Effect of M-16V on prevention of NEC		
Satoh et al., 2007 [44]	Non-RCT retrospective study	Study population: Preterm VLBW and ELBW infants in two cohorts: (1) Control group: January 1994 to December 1998; n = 226 (ELBW: 101, VLBW: 125) (2) M-16V group: January 1999 to December 2003; n = 338 (ELBW: 220, VLBW: 118)
		Country: Japan
		Sample size: n = 564
		Intervention and dose: 1×10^9 CFU/day in milk or mixed with formula
		Duration of supplementation: Commenced within several hours after birth (mean: 7.2 h) and continued till discharge at 37 weeks
		Main outcomes: (1) Significant reduction in the incidence of Stage 1 NEC and infection. (2) Significant reduction in mortality due to infection. (3) Increased survival to discharge: 64.2% (301–600 g), 94% (601–1000 g), and 97.8% (1001–1500 g)
		Study limitations: (1) This was a retrospective study that relies on the quality of record keeping. (2) The study was conducted at two different timelines which may introduce potential bias. (3) Outcome evaluation could not be blinded; however, that was not expected to introduce a major bias because of the objective of some of the outcomes.
Patole et al., 2016 [43]	Non-RCT retrospective study	Study population: Preterm neonates <34 weeks over two epochs: (1) Before probiotic supplementation: December 2008 to November 2010 (2) After probiotic supplementation: June 2012 to May 2014
		Country: Australia
		Sample size: n = 1755 (Epoch 1: 835; Epoch 2: 920)
		Intervention and dose: 3×10^9 CFU/day in 1.5 mL of sterile water or breast milk
		Duration of supplementation: Started when the infant was ready for feeds and continued till 37 weeks corrected gestational age
		Main outcomes: (1) Significant reduction in the incidence of NEC ≥ Stage II in infants supplemented with M-16V. (2) Significant reduction in "NEC ≥ Stage II or all-cause mortality", late-onset sepsis, and age at full feeds in M-16V group. (3) For the subgroup of neonates <28 weeks, the beneficial effects of M-16V did not reach statistical significance.
		Study limitations: (1) This was a retrospective study that relies on the quality of record keeping. (2) The study was conducted at two different timelines which may introduce potential bias.
Clinical studies related to the potential mechanisms of action of M-16V		
Fuji et al., 2006 [70]	Randomised controlled trial	Study population: Preterm infants with mean gestation and mean BW of (1) Probiotics group: 31.3 ± 3.16 weeks and 1378 ± 365 g (2) Control group: 31.2 ± 1.98 weeks and 1496 ± 245 g
		Country: Japan
		Sample size: n = 19 (Probiotics: 11; Control: 8)
		Intervention and dose: 1×10^9 CFU/day twice daily in 0.5 mL of 5% glucose solution
		Duration of supplementation: Commenced within several hours after birth and continued till discharge.
		Main outcomes: (1) Significant increase in the expression of serum TGF-β1 level and expression of TGF-β signalling molecule (Smad3) on day 28 in M-16V group. (2) Serum cytokine levels were not different in the two groups.
		Study limitations: (1) The sample size was small. (2) Assessment of outcome could not be blinded; however, that was not expected to introduce a major bias because of the objectivity of the outcome.

Table 1. Cont.

Reference	Study Design	Study Characteristics
Wang et al., 2007 [71]	Randomised controlled trial	Study population: Preterm LBW, VLBW, and ELBW infants (gestation: 23–36 weeks, BW: 414–2124 g)
		Country: Japan
		Sample size: n = 66 (ELBW, <1000 g: n =22; VLBW, <1500 g: n = 22; LBW, <2500 g: n = 22). The infants were divided into two groups: Probiotics and Control, 11 each).
		Intervention and dose: 1.6×10^8 CFU/day twice daily in 0.5 mL of 5% glucose sterile distilled water.
		Duration of supplementation: From birth till discharge
		Main outcomes: (1) Significant increase in the ratio of acetate to total SCFAs in all M-16V-supplemented infants. (2) Significant reduction in faecal butyrate levels in ELBW and VLBW infants supplemented with M-16V.
		Study limitations: (1) The sample size was small. (2) Assessment of outcome could not be blinded; however, that was not expected to introduce a major bias because of the objectivity of the outcome.

BW, birth weight; CFU, colony-forming units; Non-RCT, non-randomised controlled trial; B. breve, Bifidobacterium breve; B. infantis, Bifidobacterium infantis; B. longum, Bifidobacterium longum; SGA, small for gestational age; IUGR, intrauterine growth retardation; LBW, low birth weight; VLBW, very low birth weight; ELBW, extremely low birth weight; NEC, necrotising enterocolitis; SCFAs, short-chain fatty acids; TGF-β, transforming growth factor-beta.

4.3. Potential Mechanisms of Action

Colonisation by commensal bifidobacteria during early life is indispensable for the normal development and growth of the gastrointestinal tract, particularly for epithelial barrier function and mucosal immunity [72,73]. A high abundance of bifidobacteria may contribute to improved health status and protect premature infants from diseases [74]. In fact, instability of the microbiome and a lack of bifidobacteria have been reported to be associated with NEC [74]. Towards this end, it seems likely that M-16V may potentially reduce the risk of developing NEC in premature infants by promoting the colonisation of bifidobacteria. Additional studies have been deployed to understand the mechanisms by which M-16V potentially reduces the risk of developing NEC [60,75]. In an experimental rat model of NEC, oral administration of M-16V was found to be effective at reducing the pathological scores of NEC and promoting survivability via modulation of TLR expressions and suppression of inflammatory responses [75]. Multiple reports have suggested that functional expression of TLRs is critical in the dynamic interaction between the host epithelium and the microbiota that enables normal intestinal epithelial development and immune homeostasis [76–78]. Differences in the expression of TLRs may; therefore, alter a host's response to a commensal or pathogenic microorganism [79]. Specifically, TLR4, which recognises the lipopolysaccharides of Gram-negative bacteria, was demonstrated as the key mediator in NEC development [76]. Increasing evidence suggests that NEC develops in response to an exaggerated pro-inflammatory signalling upon activation of TLR4 in the mucosa of the premature gut, leading to increased enterocyte apoptosis, mucosal injury, intestinal ischemia, and bacterial translocation [76,77,79,80]. It has indeed been demonstrated that TLR4 is expressed at higher levels in the premature infant gut than the full-term intestine [76,81]. Importantly, oral administration of M-16V to the experimental NEC rats significantly normalised the expression of TLR4, enhanced the expression of TLR2, and rectified the increased expression of pro-inflammatory cytokines, including interleukin-1β (IL-1β), IL-6 and tumour necrosis factor alpha (TNF-α) that resulted from NEC induction [75]. The superior anti-inflammatory effects of M-16V in colonic inflammation have also been demonstrated in an in vivo study using F344/Du rat pups models, wherein the expression of inflammation-related genes, including lipoprotein lipase (Lpl), glutathione peroxidase 2 (Gpx2) and lipopolysaccharide-binding protein (Lbp), was significantly reduced in the colon during the newborn period [60].

Furthermore, M-16V was also able to restore the tight junction barrier function by stimulating TLR2 expression and consequently protect the host against the development of NEC [75]. It has been reported that enhanced TLR2 expression by probiotics treatment could contribute to the down-regulation of TLR4 signalling that is activated by NEC [82,83]. Of note, aberrant TLR4 signalling was found to have a direct role in the breakdown of the gut barrier in NEC. Enhanced TLR4 signalling impairs mucosal repair and weakens the integrity of the gut, allowing for bacterial translocation and the downstream inflammatory response, which in aggregate lead to NEC [77]. Remarkably, M-16V showed potential in protecting the experimental NEC rats from intestinal barrier dysfunction via suppression of the NEC-induced elevated expressions of tight junction-related proteins, including ZO-1, claudin-1 and occludin [75].

Studies have also shown that daily M-16V supplementation may potentially facilitate the development of gut immune function and attenuate inflammation in preterm infants [58,59,70]. Administration of M-16V (1×10^9 CFU in 0.5 mL of 5% glucose solution), starting several hours after birth, twice daily, was shown to be capable of significantly elevating the levels of serum transforming growth factor beta-1 (TGF-β1) and enhancing the expression of TGF-β signalling molecule Smad3, while suppressing the levels of Smad antagonist, Smad7 in 19 preterm infants (mean birth weight of 1,378 ± 365 g and mean gestational age of 31.3 ± 3.16 weeks) as compared to the control on day 28 [70]. TGF-β1 is an important immune regulatory cytokine that prevents adverse immunologic reactions in infants. It exerts potent anti-proliferative and anti-inflammatory effects by activating Smad signalling pathway that mediates cell cycle arrest and induction of apoptosis [84]. Deficiency in TGF-β1 or its receptor has been implicated in fulminant inflammatory disease that proves lethal in the first week of life [85]. The encouraging result obtained in the clinical study has; therefore, implied that M-16V may assist the development of mucosal immunity and attenuate inflammatory reactions in preterm infants through upregulation of TGF-β signalling.

In addition to interacting with the immune system, M-16V may also potentially protect premature infants against gut mucosal injury and NEC through the production of short chain fatty acids (SCFAs) that can affect the health and integrity of the intestinal epithelial and immune cells [71]. In a randomised controlled trial involving 66 premature infants (birth weight ranged from 414 to 2124 g and gestation age ranged from 23 to 36 weeks), the effects of oral administration of M-16V on faecal SCFAs were evaluated. Based on birth weight, the infants were divided into three groups: 22 extremely low birth weight infants (ELBW; <1000 g), 22 very low birth weight infants (VLBW; <1500 g), and 22 low birth weight infants (LBW; <2500 g) and within each group, the subjects were further randomly divided into M-16V-supplemented or control groups. Administration of M-16V (1.6×10^8 CFU in 0.5 mL of 5% glucose sterile distilled water) at time of normal feeding, twice daily for four weeks led to an intestinal environment where the levels of butyrate was significantly decreased in ELBW and VLBW infants, while the ratio of acetate to total SCFAs was significantly increased in ELBW, VLBW, and LBW infants as compared with those of the control groups [71]. The exact significant contribution of such changes in the levels of SCFAs to premature infant health upon M-16V administration remains unclear. Although evidence is limited, higher acetate level in infants, which is often associated with a high abundance of bifidobacteria, has been reported to potentially improve intestinal immunity and promote epithelial cell barrier function [86,87]. Nevertheless, the healthy composition of an infant faecal metabolome remains understudied.

The premature gut is known to have structural and biochemical deficiencies which predispose infants to NEC. Although bacterial production of SCFAs plays an important role in the intestinal maturation and functions, it has been reported that overproduction of certain SCFA could be associated with an increased risk of NEC in premature infants [88]. Study has suggested that *Clostridium* spp., for which the abundance was higher in premature infants, may be implicated in NEC through excessive production of butyrate as a result of colonic lactose fermentation [89]. Overproduction of butyrate may cause gut mucosal injury and lead to intestinal inflammation in premature infants [90,91]. However, numerous studies have also demonstrated the importance of butyrate for colon health and its beneficial effects on intestinal inflammation and barrier integrity [92–94]. Further studies are warranted to resolve the contradictory roles of butyrate and to investigate the association between reduction of butyrate production by M-16V and protection against NEC.

Taken together, the findings from both animal and clinical studies have shed lights into the potential protective mechanisms of M-16V against NEC in premature infants. It is evident that M-16V may potentially reduce the risk of developing NEC in premature infants by promoting bifidobacterial colonisation, modulating the expressions of TLRs and inflammatory responses, and aiding in the development of mucosal immunity (Figure 1).

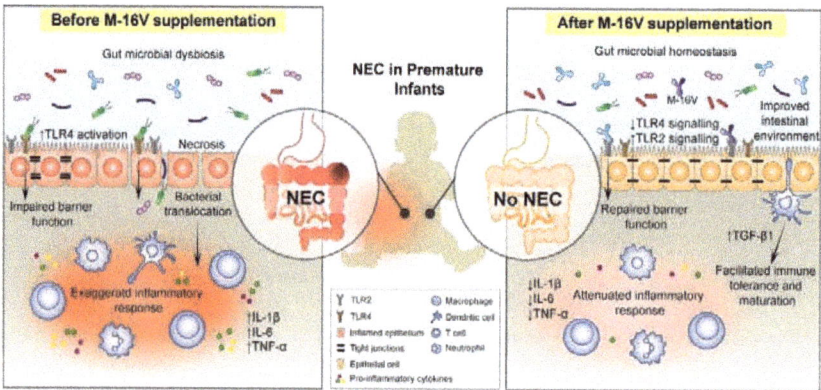

Figure 1. Administration of *Bifidobacterium breve* M-16V showed potential in reducing the risk of developing necrotising enterocolitis (NEC) in premature infants. M-16V stimulates the colonisation of bifidobacteria and could potentially improve the intestinal environment and gut barrier function. Additional mechanistic studies revealed that M-16V may assist the development of mucosal immunity through up-regulation of transforming growth factor-beta (TGF-β) signalling in premature infants and attenuate inflammatory reactions by modulating the expressions of toll-like receptor 2 (TLR2) and TLR4. IL-1β, interleukin-1β; IL-6, interleukin-6; TNF- α, tumour necrosis factor alpha; ↑, increased; ↓, decreased.

5. Effects of M-16V on Allergic Disorders

The prevalence of allergic diseases in infants has increased strikingly worldwide in the past few decades [95]. While the pathogenesis of allergic diseases is likely to be multifactorial, deviations in gut colonisation during early life are possible major factors promoting abnormal postnatal immune maturation [96]. The hygiene hypothesis suggests that insufficient or aberrant microbial stimulation during the critical neonatal period may lead to an exaggerated adaptive immune response and reduced tolerance [97]. Although compelling evidence for microbiota associations with allergic disease and related conditions is emerging, a causal relation between specific bacterial taxa and the development of allergy remains unclear. Several studies have reported differences in gut microbiota composition and lower abundance of bifidobacteria and lactobacilli in the infant's gut precede the onset of allergic manifestations [98,99]. In addition, multiple cohort studies suggested that high abundance of *Escherichia coli* or *Clostridium difficile* was associated with the development of eczema or atopy [100,101], while a low gut microbial diversity and an elevated *Enterobacteriaceae* to *Bacteroidaceae* (E/B ratio) in early infancy may contribute to the development of food allergy [102]. In this instance, a notable higher abundance of Firmicutes particularly *Clostridium* spp., *Blautia* spp., and a lower abundance of Actinobacteria in the early gut microbiota has also been described to contribute to the development of allergic diseases such as food allergy in infants [103], and type 1 diabetes in children [104]. On this basis, modulation of gut microbiota during early life through M-16V intervention has emerged as a potential measure to prevent allergic disorders in infants.

5.1. Preclinical Studies

The anti-allergic capability of M-16V in allergic airways disease, food allergy, and chronic asthma has been consolidated in a number of in vitro and animal studies [105–110]. In a bacterial strains comparative study assessing the capability of a panel of six bacterial strains (M-16V, *B. infantis* NumRes251, *B. animalis* NumRes252 and NumREs253, *Lactobacillus plantarum* NumRes8 and *L. rhamnosus* NumRes6) to alleviate allergic symptoms in ovalbumin (OVA)-sensitized BALB/c mice, M-16V was identified as the most effective strain in reducing allergic response [105]. Remarkably, in contrast to the other tested bifidobacteria, only the oral treatment with M-16V significantly inhibited the airway reactivity to methacholine and reduced acute allergic skin reactions to OVA. These discrepancies emphasise that the immuno-modulatory activity of probiotic strains is highly strain-specific.

Numerous studies have also shown that a synbiotic intervention, comprising M-16V and a galacto–fructooligosaccharide (GOS/FOS) mixture, was protective against the development of symptoms of oral sensitization with whey in mice model [110]. The promising effect was confirmed in an in vivo study demonstrating the partial prevention of skin reaction due to cow's milk allergy, following the probiotic administration in combination with specific β-lactoglobulin-derived peptides and a specific blend of short and long-chain fructo-oligosaccharides in mice [106]. Particularly, besides increasing the caecal content of propionic and butyric acid, the treatment with M-16V synbiotic formulation increased the expression of IL-22, which plays an antimicrobial role in the innate immune response and on the anti-inflammatory cytokine IL-10 in the Peyer's patches [106].

Additional preclinical studies revealed that administration of M-16V alone (10^9 CFU) [108], or in combination with non-digestible oligosaccharides (scFOS, lcFOS and pectin-derived acidic-oligosaccharides (AOS)) [109], could suppress pulmonary airway inflammation in murine OVA-induced chronic asthma model. M-16V treatments (both single-strain and synbiotic interventions) reduced T cell activation and mast cell degranulation, modulated expression of pattern recognition receptors, cytokines and transcription factors, and reduced airway remodelling [108,109]. More specifically, the treatments induced regulatory T cell responses in the airways by increasing IL-10 and Foxp3 transcription in lung tissue and systemically. These studies suggest that M-16V intervention, either as a single organism or as synbiotic, could be beneficial in the treatment of chronic inflammation in allergic asthma. Altogether, these findings laid the ground for the preventive and therapeutic effects of M-16V on allergic disorders.

5.2. Clinical Studies

Several interventional studies suggest that M-16V could promote bifidobacterial colonisation and prevent or reduce the severity of allergic diseases, including atopic dermatitis (eczema), food allergy, allergic rhinitis and asthma [111–113]. In a randomised controlled trial, oral administration of M-16V significantly improved the symptoms of atopic dermatitis in infants as compared to the control group [112]. The study randomly allocated 15 infants (aged 8.6 ± 4.5 months) with atopic dermatitis who had a *Bifidobacterium*-deficit gut microbiota to receive either lyophilised powder of M-16V ($n = 8$; 5×10^9 CFU/day) for one month or no M-16V supplementation as a control. It was noted that administration of M-16V was not only effective at alleviating the severity of allergic symptoms but also significantly increased the proportion of *Bifidobacterium* and decreased the levels of total aerobes in the gut microbiota of infants with atopic dermatitis [112]. Nevertheless, a significant correlation between alleviation of allergic symptoms and changes of the gut microbiota was not detected; suggesting M-16V may possess a direct immuno-modulatory effect on intestinal epithelial cells and not necessarily through the interaction with the gut microbiota.

Another clinical study involving 17 infants with cow's milk hypersensitivity with atopic dermatitis (aged 3.1–18.5 months) has also revealed the capability of M-16V supplementation (5×10^9 CFU/day for three months) to ameliorate allergic symptoms and improve gut microbiota composition [113]. The preventive effects of M-16V on allergic disorders have further been exemplified in a remarkable placebo-controlled, double-blinded and randomised trial involving 40 Italian children (mean age

9 ± 2.2 years) treated with a probiotics mixture containing M-16V (1×10^9 CFU), *B. longum* BB536 (3×10^9 CFU) and *B. infantis* M-63 (1×10^9 CFU), for four weeks [111]. Administration of probiotics mixture protected the children against pollen-induced IgE-mediated allergic rhinitis and intermittent asthma and improved their quality of life, for which these parameters were worsened in the placebo group. This study implies that, in addition to its effectiveness as a single organism, as aforementioned, M-16V could also dampen allergic disorders when combined with other *Bifidobacterium* strains.

More interestingly, in an open trial, administration of a probiotics mixture including M-16V during pregnancy as well as in postnatal period tied to lower the risk of developing allergic disorders in infants [114]. The study involved 130 mothers who were provided with a daily powder formulation (two sachets daily, 1 g/sachet) containing M-16V and *B. longum* BB536 (5×10^9 CFU/g of each strain) one month before the expected date of delivery and postnatally to their infants (one sachet daily) for six months. Another 36 mother–infant pairs who did not receive the bifidobacterial supplementation were served as the control. Prenatal and postnatal supplementation with the bifidobacteria mixture significantly reduced the risk of developing eczema and atopic dermatitis in infants during the first 18 months of life as compared to the control group [114]. Additionally, the probiotics intervention (M-16V and *B. longum* BB536) resulted in slight changes in the gut microbial composition, wherein a significantly higher proportion of *Bacteroidetes* was observed in the microbiota of infants receiving the bifidobacteria mixture than in that of the control group at four months of age. The relative abundance of Proteobacteria was also significantly lower in mothers receiving the bifidobacteria mixture at the time of delivery than those in the control group, and was positively correlated with that of infants at four months of age. These findings implicate that supplementation with bifidobacteria mixture of M-16V and *B. longum* BB536 during pregnancy may modulate both the maternal and neonatal gut microbiota for prevention of allergies upset in infants later in life. Further studies are needed to elucidate the association between the probiotics-modulated gut microbiota and allergy development in infants. Collectively, these findings are cautiously promising with respect to the use of probiotics for the primary prevention of eczema in pregnant mothers of infants at high risk for developing allergy and in high-risk infants, as recommended in recent guidelines from the World Allergy Organization [115].

Furthermore, synbiotic intervention of M-16V has also been reported to be effective in preventing asthma-like symptoms in infants with atopic dermatitis [116]. The study was a double-blind, placebo-controlled, multicentre trial involving 90 infants with atopic dermatitis (aged <7 months) who received either an extensively hydrolysed formula containing M-16V (1.3×10^9 CFU/100 mL and a GOS/FOS mixture (90%/10%; 0.8 g/100 mL) or the same formula without synbiotics for 12 weeks. The follow-up period for this trial was one year. It was noted that the synbiotic intervention significantly reduced the prevalence of frequent wheezing and/or noisy breathing apart from colds as well as the usage of asthma medication as compared to the placebo group [116]. As a result, it seems to be likely that combining M-16V with prebiotics—synbiotic intervention—could result in stronger immunomodulatory effects for prevention against allergic disorders. Collectively, these findings serve as a basis to incorporate M-16V in prebiotics-supplemented infant formula as a means to promote infant health.

Taken together, these clinical findings support the notion that administration of M-16V can be a potential prophylaxis approach to improve immune tolerance and consequently protect high-risk infants from allergic diseases (Table 2), although larger clinical trials are needed for definite confirmation.

Table 2. Summary from clinical studies of the effects of M-16V on allergic disorders.

Reference	Type of Allergy	Study Design	Study Characteristics
Hattori et al., 2003 [112]	Atopic dermatitis (eczema)	Randomised controlled trial	Study population: Infants aged 8.6 ± 4.5 months
			Country: Japan
			Sample size: $n = 15$ (Probiotics: 8; Control: 7)
			Intervention and dose: 5×10^9 CFU/day
			Duration of supplementation: One month
			Main outcomes: (1) Significant increase in the proportion of *Bifidobacterium* in the faecal microflora in M-16V group. (2) Significant reduction in the proportion of total aerobes in M-16V group. (3) Significant improvement in the allergic symptoms (cutaneous symptom score and total allergic score) in M-16V group. (4) No significant correlation between the changes in allergic symptoms and changes in intestinal microflora.
			Study limitations: (1) The sample size was small. (2) Assessment of outcome could not be blinded; however, that was not expected to introduce a major bias because of the objectivity of some of the outcomes.
Taniuchi et al., 2005 [113]	Food allergy	Randomised controlled trial	Study population: Infants aged 3.1–18.5 months with cow's milk hypersensitivity and atopic dermatitis
			Country: Japan
			Sample size: $n = 17$ (Probiotics: 10; Control: 7)
			Intervention and dose: 5×10^9 CFU/day
			Duration of supplementation: Three months
			Main outcomes: (1) Significant increase in the proportion of *Bifidobacterium* in the faecal microflora in M-16V group. (2) Significant reduction in the proportion of total aerobic bacteria in M-16V group. (3) Significant improvement in the allergic symptoms in M-16V group as compared to the beginning of the study. (4) In the control group, no changes to the overall faecal microflora and total allergic score during the entire study period.
			Study limitations: (1) The sample size was small. (2) Assessment of outcome could not be blinded; however, that was not expected to introduce a major bias because of the objectivity of some of the outcomes. (3) Outcomes were compared with the baseline but not the control group.
Del Giudice et al., 2017 [111]	Allergic rhinitis	Randomised, double-blinded, placebo-controlled	Study population: Children aged 9 ± 2.2 years with pollen-induced IgE-mediated allergic rhinitis and intermittent asthma
			Country: Italy
			Sample size: $n = 40$ (Probiotics: 20; Placebo: 20)
			Intervention and dose: one sachet/day *B. breve* M-16V: 1×10^9 CFU *B. longum* BB536: 3×10^9 CFU *B. infantis* M-63: 1×10^9 CFU
			Duration of supplementation: Four weeks
			Main outcomes: (1) Significant improvement of allergic symptoms and quality of life in children treated with the probiotics mixture. (2) The intergroup analysis showed that probiotics mixture was significantly more superior to the placebo for all parameters.
			Study limitations: The sample size was relatively small.

Table 2. Cont.

Reference	Type of Allergy	Study Design	Study Characteristics
Enomoto et al., 2014 [114]	Atopic dermatitis (eczema)	Non-RCT open trial	Study population: Mother–infant pairs; maternal age: (1) Probiotics group: 22–41 years; (2) Control group: 21–38 years.
			Country: Japan
			Sample size: $n = 166$ (Probiotics: 130; Control: 36)
			Intervention and dose: Pregnant women: 2 sachets/day; infants: 1 sachet/day *B. breve* M-16V: 5×10^9 CFU *B. longum* BB536: 5×10^9 CFU
			Duration of supplementation: One month before the expected date of delivery and postnatally to the infants for six months.
			Main outcomes: (1) Significant reduction in the risk of developing eczema/atopic dermatitis during the first 18 months of life in the probiotics group. (2) The proportion of Proteobacteria was significantly lower in mothers at the time of delivery who received probiotics supplementation when compared with the control group and was positively correlated with that of infants at four months of age. (3) No adverse effects were related to the use of probiotics.
			Study limitations: (1) This was a non-randomised trial which may introduce potential bias. (2) Assessment of outcome could not be blinded; however, that was not expected to introduce a major bias because of the objectivity of some of the outcomes.
Van der Aa et al., 2011 [116]	Atopic dermatitis (eczema)	Double-blinded, placebo-controlled multicentre trial	Study population: Full-term infants aged <7 months with atopic dermatitis.
			Country: Netherlands
			Sample size: $n = 90$ (Synbiotics: 46; Placebo: 44)
			Intervention and dose: Synbiotics consisted of *B. breve* M-16V at a dose of 1.3×10^9 CFU/100 mL and a mixture of 90% scGOS and 10% lcFOS (Immunofortis®), 0.8 g/100 mL.
			Duration of supplementation: 12 weeks
			Main outcomes: (1) Of the 75 children (mean age 17.3 months) completed the one-year follow-up evaluation, the prevalence of "frequent wheezing" and "wheezing and/or noisy breathing apart from colds" was significantly lower in the synbiotic than in the placebo. (2) Significantly fewer children in the synbiotic than in the placebo group had started to use asthma medication after baseline. (3) Total IgE levels did not differ between the two groups.
			Study limitations: The study tested the effect of M-16V in a synbiotic formulation.

CFU, colony-forming units; IgE, immunoglobulin E; Non-RCT, non-randomised controlled trial; *B. breve*, *Bifidobacterium breve*; *B. infantis*, *Bifidobacterium infantis*; *B. longum*, *Bifidobacterium longum*; scGOS, short-chain galactooligosaccharides; lcFOS, long-chain fructooligosaccharides.

5.3. Potential Mechanisms of Action

The mechanisms through which M-16V acts to protect infants against allergic disorders are not fully understood but clearly involve the contributions from M-16V to promote bifidobacterial colonisation, modulate Th2-skewed immune response and attenuate inflammatory reactions (Figure 2). M-16V has been shown to exert immuno-regulatory effect and anti-inflammatory capability in vitro, albeit the effect on allergic reaction has not been specifically demonstrated. M-16V was reported to interact with TLR2, upregulate the expression of ubiquitin-editing enzyme A20 in porcine intestinal epithelial cells challenged with heat-killed enterotoxigenic *Escherichia coli*, and beneficially modulate the subsequent TLR4 activation by reducing the activation of MAPK and NF-κB pathways and the production of pro-inflammatory cytokines (IL-8, monocyte chemotactic protein (MCP)-1, and IL-6) [83]. Furthermore, in an experimental OVA-immunised mice model, oral administration of M-16V (5×10^8 CFU/0.5 mL/day/animal) for 21 days significantly reduced the serum levels of total IgE, OVA-specific IgE and OVA-specific IgG1 and ex vivo production of IL-4 by the splenocytes, as compared to control [117]. In addition, M-16V could potentially modulate the systemic Th1/Th2 balance in vitro wherein the production of OVA-induced total IgE and IL-4 was suppressed and the secretion of IFN-γ and IL-10 was induced by M-16V in a dose-dependent manner. Nonetheless, M-16V did not induce IL-12 production. It is; therefore, suggested that M-16V may have the potential to restore Th2 skewed immune response, which was at least partially independent of the Th1 cytokine induction [117].

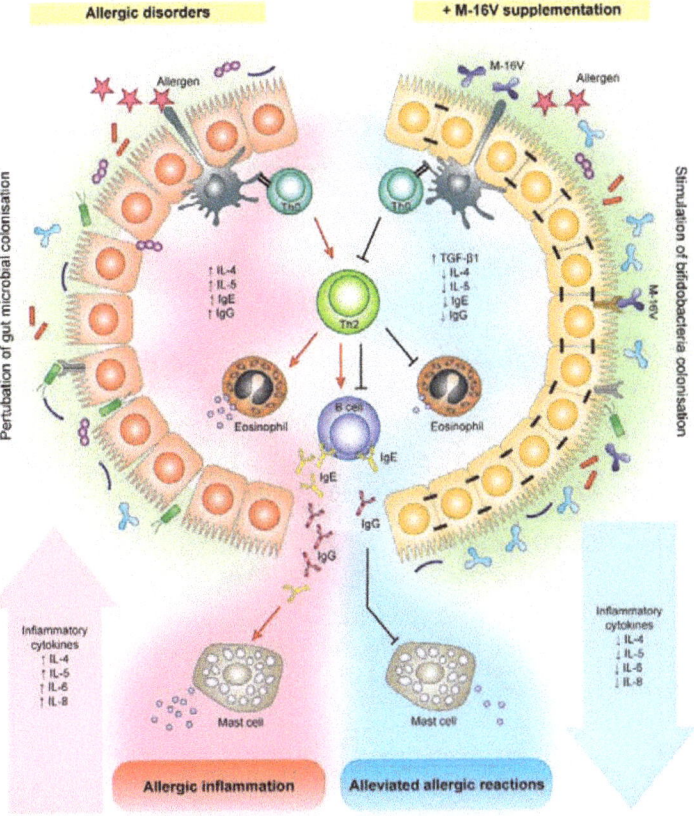

Figure 2. *Bifidobacterium breve* M-16V could potentially promote bifidobacterial colonisation and may prevent or reduce the severity of allergic diseases in infants. Specifically, M-16V may suppress the differentiation naïve T-helper cells (Th0) into T-helper (Th) 2 cells and the production of Th2 cytokines such as interleukin-4 (IL-4) and IL-5, and subsequently attenuate allergic inflammation by reducing the production of immunoglobulin E (IgE) and IgG1 in B cells and the release of pro-inflammatory mediators including IL-6 and IL-8. In addition, M-16V could also potentially assist immune tolerance and attenuate allergic reactions in infants through modulation of TGF-β signalling. ↓, decreased; ↑, increased.

It has been suggested that the pathology of allergic disease is driven by the allergen-specific Th2 cytokines such as IL-4 and IL-5, which play a triggering role in the activation/recruitment of IgE antibody-producing B cells, mast cells and eosinophils [118–120]. Notably, in an OVA-allergic asthma mouse model, oral administration of M-16V (10^9 CFU/0.4 mL/day/animal) for 17 days prevalently reduced the number of eosinophils in the bronchoalveolar lavage fluid and reduced the levels of OVA-specific IgE and IgG1 and Th2 cytokines (IL-4 and IL-5) [105]. In addition, M-16V has also been shown to potentially assist immune tolerance and attenuate allergic reactions in premature infants through modulation of TGF-β signalling [70]. Altogether, these findings provide proof of the potential of M-16V in modulating Th2 skewed allergic immune response. Further in-depth studies are required to elucidate the exact mechanisms by which M-16V prevents and ameliorates allergic disorders in infants.

6. Conclusions

Bifidobacterium breve M-16V has emerged as a probiotic strain that exerts positive effects on infant health. With the data from in vitro animal and clinical studies, M-16V holds promise to treat adverse health-related conditions in infants, particularly the vulnerable premature populations, and possesses a proven track record of safety. Mounting evidence favours the use of M-16V as a worthy and suitable infant probiotic in early life for promoting a healthy gut microbial colonisation and maturation in premature infants and preventing the development of NEC and allergic diseases. Although the mechanistic insights supporting the use of M-16V are not robust, it has become clear that M-16V may modulate the gut microbiota, interact with TLRs and regulate inflammatory responses to reduce the risk of developing life-threatening diseases and immune-mediated disorders. Despite the promising results, many studies summarised here have multiple limitations such as potential bias in non-randomised controlled trials and small sample size. Therefore, additional well-designed randomised controlled trials with larger sample size are needed to serve as the basis for developing conclusive evidence on M-16V intervention in vulnerable preterm populations. In addition, further investigations are required for an increased understanding of the protective mechanisms of M-16V and to releasing the full potential of M-16V as a human probiotic in paediatrics.

Supplementary Materials: The following are available online at http://www.mdpi.com/2072-6643/11/8/1724/s1, Table S1. Summary of publications related to *Bifidobacterium breve* M-16V; Table S2. Articles related to *Bifidobacterium breve* M-16V.

Author Contributions: Conceptualization, C.B.W. and J.-z.X.; resources, C.B.W.; data curation, C.B.W.; writing—original draft preparation, C.B.W.; writing—review and editing, C.B.W., N.I. and J.-z.X.; visualization, C.B.W.; supervision, J.-z.X.

Funding: This research received no external funding. Our work was funded by Morinaga Milk Industry Co., LTD. Employees of Morinaga Milk Industry Co., LTD., C.B.W., N.I., and J.-z.X. received a salary from the company. The specific roles of these authors are articulated in the "author contributions" section. The funders had no role in study design, data collection and analysis, decision to publish, or preparation of the manuscript.

Acknowledgments: The authors are grateful to all the researchers whom we cited in this review for their significant and valuable research.

Conflicts of Interest: The authors, C.B.W., N.I., and J.-z.X. are employees of Morinaga Milk Industry Co., Ltd., which has several probiotic products marketed worldwide. This does not alter our adherence to Nutrients policies on sharing data and materials.

References

1. Jandhyala, S.M.; Talukdar, R.; Subramanyam, C.; Vuyyuru, H.; Sasikala, M.; Reddy, D.N. Role of the normal gut microbiota. *World J. Gastroenterol.* **2015**, *21*, 8787. [CrossRef] [PubMed]
2. Arrieta, M.-C.; Stiemsma, L.T.; Amenyogbe, N.; Brown, E.M.; Finlay, B. The intestinal microbiome in early life: Health and disease. *Front. Immunol.* **2014**, *5*, 427. [CrossRef]

3. Abrahamsson, T.R.; Jakobsson, H.E.; Andersson, A.F.; Björkstén, B.; Engstrand, L.; Jenmalm, M.C. Low gut microbiota diversity in early infancy precedes asthma at school age. *Clin. Exp. Allergy* **2014**, *44*, 842–850. [CrossRef]
4. Cassir, N.; Benamar, S.; Khalil, J.B.; Croce, O.; Saint-Faust, M.; Jacquot, A.; Million, M.; Azza, S.; Armstrong, N.; Henry, M. Clostridium butyricum strains and dysbiosis linked to necrotizing enterocolitis in preterm neonates. *Clin. Infect. Dis.* **2015**, *61*, 1107–1115. [CrossRef] [PubMed]
5. Fujimura, K.E.; Sitarik, A.R.; Havstad, S.; Lin, D.L.; Levan, S.; Fadrosh, D.; Panzer, A.R.; LaMere, B.; Rackaityte, E.; Lukacs, N.W. Neonatal gut microbiota associates with childhood multisensitized atopy and T cell differentiation. *Nat. Med.* **2016**, *22*, 1187. [CrossRef] [PubMed]
6. Gevers, D.; Kugathasan, S.; Denson, L.A.; Vázquez-Baeza, Y.; Van Treuren, W.; Ren, B.; Schwager, E.; Knights, D.; Song, S.J.; Yassour, M. The treatment-naive microbiome in new-onset Crohn's disease. *Cell Host Microbe* **2014**, *15*, 382–392. [CrossRef]
7. Rodríguez, J.M.; Murphy, K.; Stanton, C.; Ross, R.P.; Kober, O.I.; Juge, N.; Avershina, E.; Rudi, K.; Narbad, A.; Jenmalm, M.C. The composition of the gut microbiota throughout life, with an emphasis on early life. *Microb. Ecol. Health Dis.* **2015**, *26*, 26050. [CrossRef] [PubMed]
8. Chong, C.; Bloomfield, F.; O'Sullivan, J. Factors affecting gastrointestinal microbiome development in neonates. *Nutrients* **2018**, *10*, 274. [CrossRef]
9. Cox, L.M.; Yamanishi, S.; Sohn, J.; Alekseyenko, A.V.; Leung, J.M.; Cho, I.; Kim, S.G.; Li, H.; Gao, Z.; Mahana, D. Altering the intestinal microbiota during a critical developmental window has lasting metabolic consequences. *Cell* **2014**, *158*, 705–721. [CrossRef]
10. Hill, C.; Guarner, F.; Reid, G.; Gibson, G.R.; Merenstein, D.J.; Pot, B.; Morelli, L.; Canani, R.B.; Flint, H.J.; Salminen, S. Expert consensus document: The International Scientific Association for Probiotics and Prebiotics consensus statement on the scope and appropriate use of the term probiotic. *Nat. Rev. Gastroenterol. Hepatol.* **2014**, *11*, 506. [CrossRef]
11. Chang, H.-Y.; Chen, J.-H.; Chang, J.-H.; Lin, H.-C.; Lin, C.-Y.; Peng, C.-C. Multiple strains probiotics appear to be the most effective probiotics in the prevention of necrotizing enterocolitis and mortality: An updated meta-analysis. *PLoS ONE* **2017**, *12*, e0171579. [CrossRef] [PubMed]
12. Cuello-Garcia, C.A.; Brożek, J.L.; Fiocchi, A.; Pawankar, R.; Yepes-Nuñez, J.J.; Terracciano, L.; Gandhi, S.; Agarwal, A.; Zhang, Y.; Schünemann, H.J. Probiotics for the prevention of allergy: A systematic review and meta-analysis of randomized controlled trials. *J. Allergy Clin. Immunol.* **2015**, *136*, 952–961. [CrossRef] [PubMed]
13. de Simone, C. The Unregulated Probiotic Market. *Clin. Gastroenterol. Hepatol.* **2018**, *17*, 809–817. [CrossRef] [PubMed]
14. Quin, C.; Estaki, M.; Vollman, D.M.; Barnett, J.A.; Gill, S.K.; Gibson, D.L. Probiotic supplementation and associated infant gut microbiome and health: A cautionary retrospective clinical comparison. *Sci. Rep.* **2018**, *8*, 8283. [CrossRef] [PubMed]
15. Rees, C.M.; Hall, N.J.; Fleming, P.; Eaton, S. Probiotics for the prevention of surgical necrotising enterocolitis: Systematic review and meta-analysis. *BMJ Paediatr. Open* **2017**, *1*. [CrossRef] [PubMed]
16. MEDLINE. Available online: https://www.nlm.nih.gov/bsd/medline.html (accessed on 14 June 2019).
17. EMBase. Available online: https://www.elsevier.com/solutions/embase-biomedical-research (accessed on 14 June 2019).
18. Medical Journal web. Available online: https://www.jamas.or.jp/english/ (accessed on 14 June 2019).
19. JDreamIII. Available online: https://jdream3.com/service/search/ (accessed on 14 June 2019). (In Japanese)
20. Gritz, E.C.; Bhandari, V. The human neonatal gut microbiome: A brief review. *Front. Pediatr.* **2015**, *3*, 17. [CrossRef] [PubMed]
21. Chassard, C.; de Wouters, T.; Lacroix, C. Probiotics tailored to the infant: A window of opportunity. *Curr. Opin. Biotechnol.* **2014**, *26*, 141–147. [CrossRef] [PubMed]
22. Laforest-Lapointe, I.; Arrieta, M.-C. Patterns of early-life gut microbial colonization during human immune development: An ecological perspective. *Front. Immunol.* **2017**, *8*, 788. [CrossRef] [PubMed]
23. Wong, C.B.; Sugahara, H.; Odamaki, T.; Xiao, J.-Z. Different physiological properties of human-residential and non-human-residential bifidobacteria in human health. *Benef. Microbes* **2018**, *9*, 111–122. [CrossRef] [PubMed]

24. Turroni, F.; Van Sinderen, D.; Ventura, M. Genomics and ecological overview of the genus Bifidobacterium. *Int. J. Food Microbiol.* **2011**, *149*, 37–44. [CrossRef]
25. Katayama, T. Host-derived glycans serve as selected nutrients for the gut microbe: Human milk oligosaccharides and bifidobacteria. *Biosci. Biotechnol. Biochem.* **2016**, *80*, 621–632. [CrossRef] [PubMed]
26. Odamaki, T.; Horigome, A.; Sugahara, H.; Hashikura, N.; Minami, J.; Xiao, J.-Z.; Abe, F. Comparative genomics revealed genetic diversity and species/strain-level differences in carbohydrate metabolism of three probiotic bifidobacterial species. *Int. J. Genom.* **2015**, *2015*. [CrossRef] [PubMed]
27. Minami, J.; Odamaki, T.; Hashikura, N.; Abe, F.; Xiao, J.Z. Lysozyme in breast milk is a selection factor for bifidobacterial colonisation in the infant intestine. *Benef. Microbes* **2016**, *7*, 53–60. [CrossRef] [PubMed]
28. Roger, L.C.; Costabile, A.; Holland, D.T.; Hoyles, L.; McCartney, A.L. Examination of faecal Bifidobacterium populations in breast-and formula-fed infants during the first 18 months of life. *Microbiology* **2010**, *156*, 3329–3341. [CrossRef] [PubMed]
29. Sakata, S.; Tonooka, T.; Ishizeki, S.; Takada, M.; Sakamoto, M.; Fukuyama, M.; Benno, Y. Culture-independent analysis of fecal microbiota in infants, with special reference to Bifidobacterium species. *FEMS Microbiol. Lett.* **2005**, *243*, 417–423. [CrossRef] [PubMed]
30. Turroni, F.; Foroni, E.; Pizzetti, P.; Giubellini, V.; Ribbera, A.; Merusi, P.; Cagnasso, P.; Bizzarri, B.; de'Angelis, G.L.; Shanahan, F. Exploring the diversity of the bifidobacterial population in the human intestinal tract. *Appl. Environ. Microbiol.* **2009**, *75*, 1534–1545. [CrossRef] [PubMed]
31. Bozzi Cionci, N.; Baffoni, L.; Gaggìa, F.; Di Gioia, D. Therapeutic Microbiology: The Role of Bifidobacterium breve as Food Supplement for the Prevention/Treatment of Paediatric Diseases. *Nutrients* **2018**, *10*, 1723. [CrossRef] [PubMed]
32. Ishizeki, S.; Sugita, M.; Takata, M.; Yaeshima, T. Effect of administration of bifidobacteria on intestinal microbiota in low-birth-weight infants and transition of administered bifidobacteria: A comparison between one-species and three-species administration. *Anaerobe* **2013**, *23*, 38–44. [CrossRef] [PubMed]
33. Liu, M.-Y.; Yang, Z.-Y.; Dai, W.-K.; Huang, J.-Q.; Li, Y.-H.; Zhang, J.; Qiu, C.-Z.; Wei, C.; Zhou, Q.; Sun, X. Protective effect of Bifidobacterium infantis CGMCC313-2 on ovalbumin-induced airway asthma and β-lactoglobulin-induced intestinal food allergy mouse models. *World J. Gastroenterol.* **2017**, *23*, 2149. [CrossRef]
34. Yeşilova, Y.; Çalka, Ö.; Akdeniz, N.; Berktaş, M. Effect of probiotics on the treatment of children with atopic dermatitis. *Ann. Dermatol.* **2012**, *24*, 189–193. [CrossRef]
35. McFarland, L.V.; Evans, C.T.; Goldstein, E.J. Strain-specificity and disease-specificity of probiotic efficacy: A systematic review and meta-analysis. *Front. Med.* **2018**, *5*. [CrossRef] [PubMed]
36. Toscano, M.; De Vecchi, E.; Gabrieli, A.; Zuccotti, G.V.; Drago, L. Probiotic characteristics and in vitro compatibility of a combination of Bifidobacterium breve M-16 V, Bifidobacterium longum subsp. infantis M-63 and Bifidobacterium longum subsp. longum BB536. *Ann. Microbiol.* **2015**, *65*, 1079–1086. [CrossRef]
37. Abe, F.; Miyauchi, H.; Uchijima, A.; Yaeshima, T.; Iwatsuki, K. Stability of bifidobacteria in powdered formula. *Int. J. Food Sci. Technol.* **2009**, *44*, 718–724. [CrossRef]
38. Guidelines for the Evaluation of Probiotics in Food. Available online: https://www.who.int/foodsafety/fs_management/en/probiotic_guidelines.pdf (accessed on 24 April 2019).
39. GRAS Notice (GRN) No. 453. Available online: http://wayback.archive-it.org/7993/20171031043458/https://www.fda.gov/downloads/Food/IngredientsPackagingLabeling/GRAS/NoticeInventory/UCM346877.pdf (accessed on 24 April 2019).
40. GRAS Notice (GRN) No. 454. Available online: http://wayback.archive-it.org/7993/20171031043455/https://www.fda.gov/downloads/Food/IngredientsPackagingLabeling/GRAS/NoticeInventory/UCM346879.pdf (accessed on 24 April 2019).
41. List of Authorised Probiotic Strains for Infant's Food in China. Available online: http://law.foodmate.net/show-188701.html (accessed on 24 April 2019).
42. Patole, S.; Keil, A.D.; Chang, A.; Nathan, E.; Doherty, D.; Simmer, K.; Esvaran, M.; Conway, P. Effect of Bifidobacterium breve M-16V supplementation on fecal bifidobacteria in preterm neonates-a randomised double blind placebo controlled trial. *PLoS ONE* **2014**, *9*, e89511. [CrossRef]
43. Patole, S.K.; Rao, S.C.; Keil, A.D.; Nathan, E.A.; Doherty, D.A.; Simmer, K.N. Benefits of Bifidobacterium breve M-16V supplementation in preterm neonates-a retrospective cohort study. *PLoS ONE* **2016**, *11*, e0150775. [CrossRef] [PubMed]

44. Satoh, Y.; Shinohara, K.; Umezaki, H.; Shoji, H.; Satoh, H.; Ohtsuka, Y.; Shiga, S.; Nagata, S.; Shimizu, T.; Yamashiro, Y. Bifidobacteria prevents necrotizing enterocolitis and infection in preterm infants. *Int. J. Probiotics Prebiotics* **2007**, *2*, 49.
45. Abe, F.; Yaeshima, T.; Iwatsuki, K. Safety evaluation of two probiotic bifidobacterial strains, Bifidobacterium breve M-16V and Bifidobacterium infantis M-63, by oral toxicity tests using rats. *Biosci. Microflora* **2009**, *28*, 7–15. [CrossRef]
46. Xiao, J.-Z.; Takahashi, S.; Odamaki, T.; Yaeshima, T.; Iwatsuki, K. Antibiotic susceptibility of bifidobacterial strains distributed in the Japanese market. *Biosci. Biotechnol. Biochem.* **2010**, *74*, 336–342. [CrossRef]
47. Grill, J.P.; Manginot-Dürr, C.; Schneider, F.; Ballongue, J. Bifidobacteria and probiotic effects: Action of *Bifidobacterium* species on conjugated bile salts. *Curr. Microbiol.* **1995**, *31*, 23–27. [CrossRef]
48. Abe, F.; Muto, M.; Yaeshima, T.; Iwatsuki, K.; Aihara, H.; Ohashi, Y.; Fujisawa, T. Safety evaluation of probiotic bifidobacteria by analysis of mucin degradation activity and translocation ability. *Anaerobe* **2010**, *16*, 131–136. [CrossRef]
49. Shane, A.L.; Deshpande, G.C.; Merenstein, D. Improved neonatal outcomes with probiotics. *JAMA Pediatr.* **2013**, *167*, 885–886. [CrossRef] [PubMed]
50. Berdon, W.E.; Grossman, H.; Baker, D.H.; Mizrahi, A.; Barlow, O.; Blanc, W.A. Necrotizing enterocolitis in the premature infant. *Radiology* **1964**, *83*, 879–887. [CrossRef] [PubMed]
51. Linder, N.; Hammel, N.; Hernandez, A.; Fridman, E.; Dlugy, E.; Herscovici, T.; Klinger, G. Intestinal perforation in very-low-birth-weight infants with necrotizing enterocolitis. *J. Pediatr. Surg.* **2013**, *48*, 562–567. [CrossRef] [PubMed]
52. Groer, M.W.; Luciano, A.A.; Dishaw, L.J.; Ashmeade, T.L.; Miller, E.; Gilbert, J.A. Development of the preterm infant gut microbiome: A research priority. *Microbiome* **2014**, *2*, 38. [CrossRef] [PubMed]
53. Arboleya, S.; Binetti, A.; Salazar, N.; Fernández, N.; Solís, G.; Hernandez-Barranco, A.; Margolles, A.; de los Reyes-Gavilan, C.G.; Gueimonde, M. Establishment and development of intestinal microbiota in preterm neonates. *FEMS Microbiol. Ecol.* **2012**, *79*, 763–772. [CrossRef] [PubMed]
54. Arboleya, S.; Sánchez, B.; Milani, C.; Duranti, S.; Solís, G.; Fernández, N.; Clara, G.; Ventura, M.; Margolles, A.; Gueimonde, M. Intestinal microbiota development in preterm neonates and effect of perinatal antibiotics. *J. Pediatr.* **2015**, *166*, 538–544. [CrossRef]
55. Fricke, W.F. The more the merrier? Reduced fecal microbiota diversity in preterm infants treated with antibiotics. *J. Pediatr.* **2014**, *165*, 8–10. [CrossRef]
56. Greenwood, C.; Morrow, A.L.; Lagomarcino, A.J.; Altaye, M.; Taft, D.H.; Yu, Z.; Newburg, D.S.; Ward, D.V.; Schibler, K.R. Early empiric antibiotic use in preterm infants is associated with lower bacterial diversity and higher relative abundance of Enterobacter. *J. Pediatr.* **2014**, *165*, 23–29. [CrossRef]
57. Tanaka, S.; Kobayashi, T.; Songjinda, P.; Tateyama, A.; Tsubouchi, M.; Kiyohara, C.; Shirakawa, T.; Sonomoto, K.; Nakayama, J. Influence of antibiotic exposure in the early postnatal period on the development of intestinal microbiota. *FEMS Immunol. Med. Microbiol.* **2009**, *56*, 80–87. [CrossRef]
58. Rigo-Adrover, M.d.M.; Franch, À.; Castell, M.; Pérez-Cano, F.J. Preclinical immunomodulation by the probiotic Bifidobacterium breve M-16V in early life. *PLoS ONE* **2016**, *11*, e0166082. [CrossRef]
59. Izumi, H.; Minegishi, M.; Sato, Y.; Shimizu, T.; Sekine, K.; Takase, M. Bifidobacterium breve alters immune function and ameliorates DSS-induced inflammation in weanling rats. *Pediatr. Res.* **2015**, *78*, 407. [CrossRef] [PubMed]
60. Ohtsuka, Y.; Ikegami, T.; Izumi, H.; Namura, M.; Ikeda, T.; Ikuse, T.; Baba, Y.; Kudo, T.; Suzuki, R.; Shimizu, T. Effects of Bifidobacterium breve on inflammatory gene expression in neonatal and weaning rat intestine. *Pediatr. Res.* **2012**, *71*, 46. [CrossRef] [PubMed]
61. Patole, S.K.; Keil, A.D.; Nathan, E.; Doherty, D.; Esvaran, M.; Simmer, K.N.; Conway, P. Effect of Bifidobacterium breve M-16V supplementation on faecal bifidobacteria in growth restricted very preterm infants–analysis from a randomised trial. *J. Matern. Fetal Neonatal Med.* **2016**, *29*, 3751–3755. [CrossRef] [PubMed]
62. Akiyama, K.; Hosono, S.; Takahashi, E.; Ishizeki, S.; Takigawa, I.; Imura, S.; Yamauchi, K.; Yaeshima, T.; Hayasawa, H.; Shimamura, S. Effects of oral administration of Bifidobacterium breve on development of intestinal microflora in extremely premature infants. *Acta Neonatol. Jpn.* **1994**, *30*, 130–137.
63. Li, Y.; Shimizu, T.; Hosaka, A.; Kaneko, N.; Ohtsuka, Y.; Yamashiro, Y. Effects of Bifidobacterium breve supplementation on intestinal flora of low birth weight infants. *Pediatr. Int.* **2004**, *46*, 509–515. [CrossRef]

64. Akiyama, K.; Shimada, M.; Ishizeki, S.; Takigawa, I.; Imura, S.; Yamauchi, K.; Hatano, M.; Abe, N.; Yaeshima, T.; Hayasawa, H. Effects of administration of bifidobacterium in extremely premature infants. Development of intestinal microflora by orally administered bifidobacterium longum (in comparison with bifidobacterium breve). *Acta Neonatol. Jpn.* **1994**, *30*, 257–263.
65. Athalye-Jape, G.; Rao, S.; Simmer, K.; Patole, S. Bifidobacterium breve M-16V as a Probiotic for Preterm Infants: A Strain-Specific Systematic Review. *JPEN* **2018**, *42*, 677–688. [CrossRef]
66. Avcin, S.L.; Pokorn, M.; Kitanovski, L.; Premru, M.M.; Jazbec, J. Bifidobacterium breve sepsis in child with high-risk acute lymphoblastic leukemia. *Emerg. Infect. Dis.* **2015**, *21*, 1674. [CrossRef]
67. Ohishi, A.; Takahashi, S.; Ito, Y.; Ohishi, Y.; Tsukamoto, K.; Nanba, Y.; Ito, N.; Kakiuchi, S.; Saitoh, A.; Morotomi, M. Bifidobacterium septicemia associated with postoperative probiotic therapy in a neonate with omphalocele. *J. Pediatr.* **2010**, *156*, 679–681. [CrossRef]
68. Nakazawa, T.; Kaneko, K.-I.; Takahashi, H.; Inoue, S. Neonatal meningitis caused by Bifidobacterium breve. *Brain Dev.* **1996**, *18*, 160–162. [CrossRef]
69. van den Akker, C.H.; van Goudoever, J.B.; Szajewska, H.; Embleton, N.D.; Hojsak, I.; Reid, D.; Shamir, R. Probiotics for preterm infants: A strain-specific systematic review and network meta-analysis. *J. Pediatr. Gastroenterol. Nutr.* **2018**, *67*, 103–122. [CrossRef] [PubMed]
70. Fujii, T.; Ohtsuka, Y.; Lee, T.; Kudo, T.; Shoji, H.; Sato, H.; Nagata, S.; Shimizu, T.; Yamashiro, Y. Bifidobacterium breve enhances transforming growth factor β1 signaling by regulating smad7 expression in preterm infants. *J. Pediatr. Gastroenterol. Nutr.* **2006**, *43*, 83–88. [CrossRef] [PubMed]
71. Wang, C.; Shoji, H.; Sato, H.; Nagata, S.; Ohtsuka, Y.; Shimizu, T.; Yamashiro, Y. Effects of oral administration of Bifidobacterium breve on fecal lactic acid and short-chain fatty acids in low birth weight infants. *J. Pediatr. Gastroenterol. Nutr.* **2007**, *44*, 252–257. [CrossRef] [PubMed]
72. Lin, P.W.; Nasr, T.R.; Stoll, B.J. Necrotizing enterocolitis: Recent scientific advances in pathophysiology and prevention. In *Semin Perinatol*; Elsevier: Amsterdam, The Netherlands, 2008; Volume 32, pp. 70–82.
73. Luedtke, S.A.; Yang, J.T.; Wild, H.E. Probiotics and necrotizing enterocolitis: Finding the missing pieces of the probiotic puzzle. *J. Pediatr. Pharmacol. Ther.* **2012**, *17*, 308–328. [CrossRef] [PubMed]
74. Stewart, C.J.; Embleton, N.D.; Marrs, E.C.; Smith, D.P.; Nelson, A.; Abdulkadir, B.; Skeath, T.; Petrosino, J.F.; Perry, J.D.; Berrington, J.E. Temporal bacterial and metabolic development of the preterm gut reveals specific signatures in health and disease. *Microbiome* **2016**, *4*, 67. [CrossRef] [PubMed]
75. Satoh, T.; Izumi, H.; Iwabuchi, N.; Odamaki, T.; Namba, K.; Abe, F.; Xiao, J.Z. Bifidobacterium breve prevents necrotising enterocolitis by suppressing inflammatory responses in a preterm rat model. *Benef. Microbes* **2016**, *7*, 75–82. [CrossRef] [PubMed]
76. Hackam, D.J.; Sodhi, C.P. Toll-Like Receptor–Mediated Intestinal Inflammatory Imbalance in the Pathogenesis of Necrotizing Enterocolitis. *Cell Mol. Gastroenterol. Hepatol.* **2018**, *6*, 229–238. [CrossRef] [PubMed]
77. Hodzic, Z.; Bolock, A.M.; Good, M. The role of mucosal immunity in the pathogenesis of necrotizing enterocolitis. *Front. Pediatr.* **2017**, *5*, 40. [CrossRef]
78. Rakoff-Nahoum, S.; Paglino, J.; Eslami-Varzaneh, F.; Edberg, S.; Medzhitov, R. Recognition of commensal microflora by toll-like receptors is required for intestinal homeostasis. *Cell* **2004**, *118*, 229–241. [CrossRef]
79. Hunter, C.J.; Upperman, J.S.; Ford, H.R.; Camerini, V. Understanding the susceptibility of the premature infant to necrotizing enterocolitis (NEC). *Pediatr. Res.* **2008**, *63*, 117. [CrossRef]
80. Niño, D.F.; Sodhi, C.P.; Hackam, D.J. Necrotizing enterocolitis: New insights into pathogenesis and mechanisms. *Nat. Rev. Gastroenterol. Hepatol.* **2016**, *13*, 590. [CrossRef] [PubMed]
81. Gribar, S.C.; Sodhi, C.P.; Richardson, W.M.; Anand, R.J.; Gittes, G.K.; Branca, M.F.; Jakub, A.; Shi, X.-H.; Shah, S.; Ozolek, J.A. Reciprocal expression and signaling of TLR4 and TLR9 in the pathogenesis and treatment of necrotizing enterocolitis. *J. Immunol.* **2009**, *182*, 636–646. [CrossRef] [PubMed]
82. Shimazu, T.; Villena, J.; Tohno, M.; Fujie, H.; Hosoya, S.; Shimosato, T.; Aso, H.; Suda, Y.; Kawai, Y.; Saito, T. Immunobiotic Lactobacillus jensenii elicits anti-inflammatory activity in porcine intestinal epithelial cells by modulating negative regulators of the Toll-like receptor signaling pathway. *Infect. Immun.* **2012**, *80*, 276–288. [CrossRef] [PubMed]
83. Tomosada, Y.; Villena, J.; Murata, K.; Chiba, E.; Shimazu, T.; Aso, H.; Iwabuchi, N.; Xiao, J.-Z.; Saito, T.; Kitazawa, H. Immunoregulatory effect of bifidobacteria strains in porcine intestinal epithelial cells through modulation of ubiquitin-editing enzyme A20 expression. *PLoS ONE* **2013**, *8*, e59259. [CrossRef] [PubMed]

84. Ohtsuka, Y.; Sanderson, I.R. Transforming growth factor-β: An important cytokine in the mucosal immune response. *Curr. Opin. Gastroenterol.* **2000**, *16*, 541–545. [CrossRef] [PubMed]
85. Kulkarni, A.B.; Huh, C.-G.; Becker, D.; Geiser, A.; Lyght, M.; Flanders, K.C.; Roberts, A.B.; Sporn, M.B.; Ward, J.M.; Karlsson, S. Transforming growth factor beta 1 null mutation in mice causes excessive inflammatory response and early death. *Proc. Natl. Acad. Sci. USA* **1993**, *90*, 770–774. [CrossRef] [PubMed]
86. Hsieh, C.Y.; Osaka, T.; Moriyama, E.; Date, Y.; Kikuchi, J.; Tsuneda, S. Strengthening of the intestinal epithelial tight junction by Bifidobacterium bifidum. *Physiol. Rep.* **2015**, *3*. [CrossRef]
87. Neu, J.; Pammi, M. Necrotizing enterocolitis: The intestinal microbiome, metabolome and inflammatory mediators. *Semin. Fetal Neonatal Med.* **2018**, *23*, 400–405. [CrossRef]
88. Lin, J.; Nafday, S.M.; Chauvin, S.N.; Magid, M.S.; Pabbatireddy, S.; Holzman, I.R.; Babyatsky, M.W. Variable effects of short chain fatty acids and lactic acid in inducing intestinal mucosal injury in newborn rats. *J. Pediatr. Gastroenterol. Nutr.* **2002**, *35*, 545–550. [CrossRef]
89. Waligora-Dupriet, A.-J.; Dugay, A.; Auzeil, N.; Huerre, M.; Butel, M.-J. Evidence for clostridial implication in necrotizing enterocolitis through bacterial fermentation in a gnotobiotic quail model. *Pediatr. Res.* **2005**, *58*, 629. [CrossRef]
90. Furunyan, R.D.; Ohno, Y.; MacDermott, R.P.; Sanderson, I.R. Short-chain fatty-acids enhance interleukin-1-beta induced secretion of interleukin-8 by Caco-2 cells. In *Gastroenterology*; WB Saunders Co Independence Square West Curtis Center, Ste 300: Philadelphia, PA, USA, 1995; Volume 108, p. A726.
91. Lin, J.; Peng, L.; Itzkowitz, S.; Holzman, I.R.; Babyatsky, M.W. Short-chain fatty acid induces intestinal mucosal injury in newborn rats and down-regulates intestinal trefoil factor gene expression in vivo and in vitro. *J. Pediatr. Gastroenterol. Nutr.* **2005**, *41*, 607–611. [CrossRef] [PubMed]
92. Bach Knudsen, K.; Lærke, H.; Hedemann, M.; Nielsen, T.; Ingerslev, A.; Gundelund Nielsen, D.; Theil, P.; Purup, S.; Hald, S.; Schioldan, A. Impact of diet-modulated butyrate production on intestinal barrier function and inflammation. *Nutrients* **2018**, *10*, 1499. [CrossRef] [PubMed]
93. Hiippala, K.; Jouhten, H.; Ronkainen, A.; Hartikainen, A.; Kainulainen, V.; Jalanka, J.; Satokari, R. The potential of gut commensals in reinforcing intestinal barrier function and alleviating inflammation. *Nutrients* **2018**, *10*, 988. [CrossRef] [PubMed]
94. Kelly, C.J.; Zheng, L.; Campbell, E.L.; Saeedi, B.; Scholz, C.C.; Bayless, A.J.; Wilson, K.E.; Glover, L.E.; Kominsky, D.J.; Magnuson, A. Crosstalk between microbiota-derived short-chain fatty acids and intestinal epithelial HIF augments tissue barrier function. *Cell Host Microbe* **2015**, *17*, 662–671. [CrossRef] [PubMed]
95. Pawankar, R. Allergic diseases and asthma: A global public health concern and a call to action. *World Allergy Organ J.* **2014**, *7*. [CrossRef] [PubMed]
96. West, C.E.; Jenmalm, M.C.; Prescott, S.L. The gut microbiota and its role in the development of allergic disease: A wider perspective. *Clin. Exp. Allergy* **2015**, *45*, 43–53. [CrossRef] [PubMed]
97. Noverr, M.C.; Huffnagle, G.B. The 'microflora hypothesis' of allergic diseases. *Clin. Exp. Allergy* **2005**, *35*, 1511–1520. [CrossRef] [PubMed]
98. Abrahamsson, T.R.; Jakobsson, H.E.; Andersson, A.F.; Björkstén, B.; Engstrand, L.; Jenmalm, M.C. Low diversity of the gut microbiota in infants with atopic eczema. *J. Allergy Clin. Immunol.* **2012**, *129*, 434–440. [CrossRef] [PubMed]
99. Kalliomäki, M.; Kirjavainen, P.; Eerola, E.; Kero, P.; Salminen, S.; Isolauri, E. Distinct patterns of neonatal gut microflora in infants in whom atopy was and was not developing. *J. Allergy Clin. Immunol.* **2001**, *107*, 129–134. [CrossRef]
100. Melli, L.; do Carmo-Rodrigues, M.S.; Araújo-Filho, H.B.; Solé, D.; De Morais, M.B. Intestinal microbiota and allergic diseases: A systematic review. *Allergol. Immunopathol.* **2016**, *44*, 177–188. [CrossRef] [PubMed]
101. Penders, J.; Thijs, C.; van den Brandt, P.A.; Kummeling, I.; Snijders, B.; Stelma, F.; Adams, H.; van Ree, R.; Stobberingh, E.E. Gut microbiota composition and development of atopic manifestations in infancy: The KOALA Birth Cohort Study. *Gut* **2007**, *56*, 661–667. [CrossRef] [PubMed]
102. Dong, P.; Feng, J.-j.; Yan, D.-y.; Lyu, Y.-j.; Xu, X. Early-life gut microbiome and cow's milk allergy-a prospective case-control 6-month follow-up study. *Saudi. J. Biol. Sci.* **2018**, *25*, 875–880. [CrossRef] [PubMed]
103. Ling, Z.; Li, Z.; Liu, X.; Cheng, Y.; Luo, Y.; Tong, X.; Yuan, L.; Wang, Y.; Sun, J.; Li, L. Altered fecal microbiota composition for food allergy in infants. *Appl. Environ. Microbiol.* **2014**, *80*, 2546–2554. [CrossRef] [PubMed]
104. Qi, C.-J.; Zhang, Q.; Yu, M.; Xu, J.-P.; Zheng, J.; Wang, T.; Xiao, X.-H. Imbalance of fecal microbiota at newly diagnosed type 1 diabetes in Chinese children. *Chin. Med. J.* **2016**, *129*, 1298. [CrossRef] [PubMed]

105. Hougee, S.; Vriesema, A.J.M.; Wijering, S.C.; Knippels, L.M.J.; Folkerts, G.; Nijkamp, F.P.; Knol, J.; Garssen, J. Oral treatment with probiotics reduces allergic symptoms in ovalbumin-sensitized mice: A bacterial strain comparative study. *Int. Arch. Allergy Immunol.* **2010**, *151*, 107–117. [CrossRef] [PubMed]
106. Kostadinova, A.I.; Meulenbroek, L.A.P.M.; van Esch, B.C.A.M.; Hofman, G.A.; Garssen, J.; Willemsen, L.E.M.; Knippels, L.M.J. A Specific Mixture of Fructo-Oligosaccharides and Bifidobacterium breve M-16V Facilitates Partial Non-Responsiveness to Whey Protein in Mice Orally Exposed to β-Lactoglobulin-Derived Peptides. *Front. Immunol.* **2017**, *7*, 673. [CrossRef]
107. Mortaz, E.; Adcock, I.M.; Ricciardolo, F.L.M.; Varahram, M.; Jamaati, H.; Velayati, A.A.; Folkerts, G.; Garssen, J. Anti-inflammatory effects of lactobacillus rahmnosus and bifidobacterium breve on cigarette smoke activated human macrophages. *PLoS ONE* **2015**, *10*, e0136455. [CrossRef] [PubMed]
108. Sagar, S.; Morgan, M.E.; Chen, S.; Vos, A.P.; Garssen, J.; van Bergenhenegouwen, J.; Boon, L.; Georgiou, N.A.; Kraneveld, A.D.; Folkerts, G. Bifidobacterium breve and Lactobacillus rhamnosus treatment is as effective as budesonide at reducing inflammation in a murine model for chronic asthma. *Respir. Res.* **2014**, *15*, 46. [CrossRef]
109. Sagar, S.; Vos, A.P.; Morgan, M.E.; Garssen, J.; Georgiou, N.A.; Boon, L.; Kraneveld, A.D.; Folkerts, G. The combination of Bifidobacterium breve with non-digestible oligosaccharides suppresses airway inflammation in a murine model for chronic asthma. *Biochim. Biophys. Acta.* **2014**, *1842*, 573–583. [CrossRef]
110. Schouten, B.; van Esch, B.C.A.M.; Hofman, G.A.; van Doorn, S.A.C.M.; Knol, J.; Nauta, A.J.; Garssen, J.; Willemsen, L.E.M.; Knippels, L.M.J. Cow milk allergy symptoms are reduced in mice fed dietary synbiotics during oral sensitization with whey. *J. Nutr.* **2009**, *139*, 1398–1403. [CrossRef]
111. Del Giudice, M.M.; Indolfi, C.; Capasso, M.; Maiello, N.; Decimo, F.; Ciprandi, G. Bifidobacterium mixture (B longum BB536, B infantis M-63, B breve M-16V) treatment in children with seasonal allergic rhinitis and intermittent asthma. *Ital. J. Pediatr.* **2017**, *43*, 25. [CrossRef] [PubMed]
112. Hattori, K.; Yamamoto, A.; Sasai, M.; Taniuchi, S.; Kojima, T.; Kobayashi, Y.; Iwamoto, H.; Namba, K.; Yaeshima, T. Effects of administration of bifidobacteria on fecal microflora and clinical symptoms in infants with atopic dermatitis. *Arerugi* **2003**, *52*, 20–30. [PubMed]
113. Taniuchi, S.; Hattori, K.; Yamamoto, A.; Sasai, M.; Hatano, Y.; Kojima, T.; Kobayashi, Y.; Iwamoto, H.; Yaeshima, T. Administration of Bifidobacterium to infants with atopic dermatitis: Changes in fecal microflora and clinical symptoms. *J. Appl. Res. Clin. Exp. Therapeut.* **2005**, *5*, 387.
114. Enomoto, T.; Sowa, M.; Nishimori, K.; Shimazu, S.; Yoshida, A.; Yamada, K.; Furukawa, F.; Nakagawa, T.; Yanagisawa, N.; Iwabuchi, N. Effects of bifidobacterial supplementation to pregnant women and infants in the prevention of allergy development in infants and on fecal microbiota. *Allergol. Int.* **2014**, *63*, 575–585. [CrossRef]
115. Fiocchi, A.; Pawankar, R.; Cuello-Garcia, C.; Ahn, K.; Al-Hammadi, S.; Agarwal, A.; Beyer, K.; Burks, W.; Canonica, G.W.; Ebisawa, M. World Allergy Organization-McMaster university guidelines for allergic disease prevention (GLAD-P): Probiotics. *World Allergy Organ J.* **2015**, *8*, 1. [CrossRef] [PubMed]
116. Van der Aa, L.B.; Van Aalderen, W.M.C.; Heymans, H.S.A.; Henk Sillevis Smitt, J.; Nauta, A.J.; Knippels, L.M.J.; Ben Amor, K.; Sprikkelman, A.B.; Group, S.S. Synbiotics prevent asthma-like symptoms in infants with atopic dermatitis. *Allergy* **2011**, *66*, 170–177. [CrossRef] [PubMed]
117. Inoue, Y.; Iwabuchi, N.; Xiao, J.-Z.; Yaeshima, T.; Iwatsuki, K. Suppressive effects of Bifidobacterium breve strain M-16V on T-helper type 2 immune responses in a murine model. *Biol. Pharm. Bull.* **2009**, *32*, 760–763. [CrossRef] [PubMed]
118. Cousins, D.J. Pinning allergies on pathogenic TH2 cells. *Sci. Transl. Med.* **2017**, *9*, eaao0392. [CrossRef] [PubMed]
119. Deo, S.S.; Mistry, K.J.; Kakade, A.M.; Niphadkar, P.V. Role played by Th2 type cytokines in IgE mediated allergy and asthma. *Lung India Off. Organ Indian Chest Soc.* **2010**, *27*, 66. [CrossRef] [PubMed]
120. Kubo, M. T follicular helper and TH2 cells in allergic responses. *Allergol. Int.* **2017**, *66*, 377–381. [CrossRef]

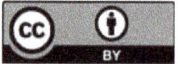

© 2019 by the authors. Licensee MDPI, Basel, Switzerland. This article is an open access article distributed under the terms and conditions of the Creative Commons Attribution (CC BY) license (http://creativecommons.org/licenses/by/4.0/).

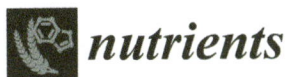 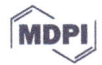

Review

Nutraceutical Potential of *Carica papaya* in Metabolic Syndrome

Lidiani F. Santana [1], Aline C. Inada [1], Bruna Larissa Spontoni do Espirito Santo [1], Wander F. O. Filiú [2], Arnildo Pott [3], Flávio M. Alves [3], Rita de Cássia A. Guimarães [1], Karine de Cássia Freitas [1,*] and Priscila A. Hiane [1]

1. Graduate Program in Health and Development in the Central-West Region of Brazil, Federal University of Mato Grosso do Sul-UFMS, MS 79079-900 Campo Grande, Brazil
2. Faculdade de Ciências Farmacêuticas, Alimentos e Nutrição, Federal University of Mato Grosso do Sul-UFMS, MS 79079-900 Campo Grande, Brazil
3. Institute of Biosciences, Federal University of Mato Grosso do Sul-UFMS, MS 79079-900 Campo Grande, Brazil
* Correspondence: kcfreitas@gmail.com; Tel.: +55-67-3345-7445

Received: 21 June 2019; Accepted: 10 July 2019; Published: 16 July 2019

Abstract: *Carica papaya* L. is a well-known fruit worldwide, and its highest production occurs in tropical and subtropical regions. The pulp contains vitamins A, C, and E, B complex vitamins, such as pantothenic acid and folate, and minerals, such as magnesium and potassium, as well as food fibers. Phenolic compounds, such as benzyl isothiocyanate, glucosinolates, tocopherols (α and δ), β-cryptoxanthin, β-carotene and carotenoids, are found in the seeds. The oil extracted from the seed principally presents oleic fatty acid followed by palmitic, linoleic and stearic acids, whereas the leaves have high contents of food fibers and polyphenolic compounds, flavonoids, saponins, pro-anthocyanins, tocopherol, and benzyl isothiocyanate. Studies demonstrated that the nutrients present in its composition have beneficial effects on the cardiovascular system, protecting it against cardiovascular illnesses and preventing harm caused by free radicals. It has also been reported that it aids in the treatment of diabetes mellitus and in the reduction of cholesterol levels. Thus, both the pulp and the other parts of the plant (leaves and seeds) present antioxidant, anti-hypertensive, hypoglycemic, and hypolipidemic actions, which, in turn, can contribute to the prevention and treatment of obesity and associated metabolic disorders.

Keywords: blood glucose; food composition; metabolic syndrome; natural products; *Carica papaya*

1. Introduction

Plants with healing properties are utilized in folk medicine and, since remote times, have been considered traditional therapeutic approaches that have effects on health. They are also advantageous from a cost–benefit point of view [1]. Synthetic drugs used to be the first option for the treatment of several diseases. However, because of the adverse effects shown by long- or even short-term consumption, studies aiming at the use of alternative therapies in the treatment and prevention of diseases have increased considerably [2].

One alternative therapy includes the use of nutraceuticals, which, in turn, according to the existing regulations, cannot be categorized or defined either as food or a drug, but can be understood in the category of food supplements, with beneficial properties for health maintenance, in particular for some pathologic conditions. Therefore, a therapeutic approach, based on nutraceuticals for maintenance of health, resulted in a worldwide "nutraceutical revolution" [3].

Among plants with beneficial properties on health is *Carica papaya*, the well-known papaya. This fruit contains considerable concentrations of vitamins, bioactive compounds and a lipidic composition that reduces inflammatory markers and anti-platelet aggregation, protects against thrombogenesis and oxidative stress, and prevents hypercholesterolemia—factors that can be triggered by obesity [4,5].

Carica papaya is a popular fruit, and its largest production occurs in tropical and subtropical regions. According to the Food and Agriculture Organization of the United Nations (FAO) [6], over 6.8 million tons of the fruit are produced in the world annually, ca. 440 thousand ha. Central and South America, especially Brazil, are responsible for 47% of the fruit yield, produced year round, being an important source of nutrients with a low cost and great availability in the market.

Carica papaya is consumed worldwide, either in natura or processed as jam, sweets and pulp, and to aggregate the nutritional value, other parts of the plant (leaves and seeds) are added to some products in the form of teas and flours [7]. The pulp composition presents three important sources of vitamins with potential antioxidant action, A, C and E [8], besides minerals, such as magnesium and potassium, and B complex vitamins, such as pantothenic acid and folate [9], as well as the presence of food fibers [10]. Besides these nutrients, papaya contains the enzyme papain, effective in increasing intestinal motility and transit time, and is also utilized in the treatment of traumas, allergies and sport lesions [5]. Some studies observed the presence of proteolytic enzymes, such as chymopapain, with anti-viral, antifungal and antibacterial properties [5,11].

The seed contains phenolic compounds, such as benzyl isothiocyanate, glucosinolates, tocopherols (α and δ), β-cryptoxanthin, β-carotene and carotenoids [12,13], while the seed oil principally presents oleic fatty acid, followed by palmitic, linoleic and stearic acids [14]. The leaves have a high content of food fibers and polyphenolic compounds, such as flavonoids, saponins, pro-anthocyanins, tocopherol and benzyl isothiocyanate [15].

Considering the nutrients present in its composition, beneficial effects have been observed, with a significant improvement in the cardiovascular system, protecting against cardiovascular illnesses, heart attack and strokes [16]. Other studies have pointed out that this fruit is an excellent source of beta-carotene (888 IU/100 g), preventing harms caused by free radicals [17], besides exerting a role in the prevention of cardiovascular illnesses, diabetes mellitus (types 1 and 2) and in the reduction of cholesterol levels through its high content of fibers, which diminish fat absorption [5,18].

Carica papaya is a plant that is easily accessed and widely available. Furthermore, scientific studies have demonstrated the biological activities and medicinal applications of different parts of the plant. However, few studies have demonstrated the therapeutic potential in metabolic dysfunctions in experimental models specific to obesity. Therefore, the present study will investigate the nutritional value and bioactive compounds of the plant, as well as the existing medicinal uses and possible application in the metabolic syndrome.

2. Nutritional Properties: *C. papaya* L.

2.1. Chemical Composition

The tree *C. papaya* is native to Central and South America and is one of the most cultivated fruit plants in the world, especially in tropical and subtropical areas [6]. It is a herbaceous perennial plant, with a milky latex that can reach 12 m in height. It has a year-round fruit production, and each fruit weighs between 1000 and 3000 g [18] (Figure 1).

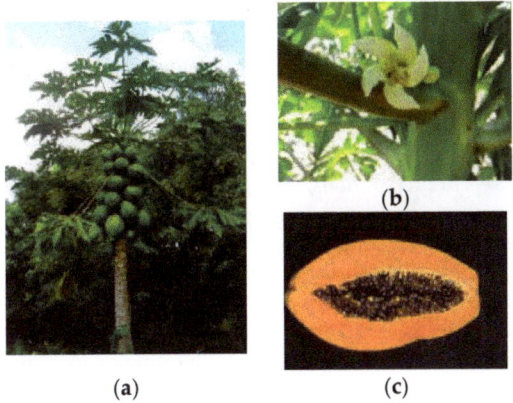

Figure 1. Images of *Carica papaya* L. (papaya CV Formosa): (**a**) Tree with leaves and green fruits, (**b**) female flower, and (**c**) ripe fruit with seeds and pulp. Photos: L. F. Santana.

The fruit of *C. papaya* is considered one of the most common fruits in relation to human consumption and provides a favorable cost benefit in consideration of its nutritional value, with a low caloric content (Table 1) and rich concentration of vitamins and minerals (Table 2) [19].

Table 1. Nutritional value of the macronutrients and fibers of *Carica papaya* L. (papaya) per 100 g of pulp of ripe fruit, seeds and leaves [5,18].

Component	Pulp	Seeds	Leaves
Proteins	0.6 g	2.6 g	5.8 g
Lipids	0.1 g	3.1 g	1.4 g
Carbohydrates	7.2 g	43.6 g	78.2 g
Fiber	0.8 g	2.1 g	13.1 g
Energy	32.1 kcal	212.7 kcal	348.6 kcal

Table 2. Value of the minerals and vitamins of *Carica papaya* L. (papaya) per 100 g of ripe fruit pulp, seeds and leaves [7,19].

Component	Pulp	Seeds	Leaves
Sodium	3 mg	ND	ND
Potassium	257 mg	344 mg	534 mg
Phosphorous	5 mg	241.5 mg	221.1 mg
Magnesium	10 mg	10.4 mg	32.4 mg
Iron	0.1 mg	0.2 mg	6.4 mg
Calcium	24 mg	54.4 mg	366.1 mg
Vitamin C	61.8 mg	11.7 mg	31.1 mg
Vitamin B9 (Folate)	38 mg	ND	ND
Vitamin B6	0.1 mg	ND	ND
Vitamin B3 (Niacin)	0.34 mg	0.26 mg	0.38 mg
Vitamin B2 (Riboflavin)	0.05 mg	0.05 mg	0.14 mg
Vitamin B1 (Thiamin)	0.04 mg	0.05 mg	0.43 mg
Vitamin A	328 mg	ND	ND
Betacarotene	888 IU	65.64 IU	659.5 IU

ND: not determined.

Among the most commercialized fruits, such as apple, banana, water melon, and orange, papaya has the highest concentrations of vitamin C (61.8 mg·100 g^{-1}), vitamin A (328 mg·100 g^{-1}), riboflavin (0.05 mg·100 g^{-1}), folate (38 mg·100 g^{-1}), thiamine (0.04 mg·100 g^{-1}), niacin (0.34 mg·100 g^{-1}), calcium (24 mg·100 g^{-1}), iron (0.1 g·100 g^{-1}), potassium (257 mg·100 g^{-1}), and fiber (0.8 g·100 g^{-1}), as well as presenting a low caloric value (32 kcal·100 g^{-1} ripe fruit) and being one of the preferred fruits for weight loss. In addition, it has a high carotene content when compared with other fruits [5,20].

The green fruit is used in preparations, such as salads, cakes, ice creams and juice, without carotene [20], but with all of the other nutrients listed in Tables 1 and 2. Besides the ripe papaya pulp, the consumption of other parts, such as the seeds and leaves, is appropriate, since they have a higher nutritional value and more fibers [7]. The leaves and seeds present a higher carbohydrate content, compared with the fruit pulp, presenting 78.2 g and 436 g·100 g^{-1}, respectively (Table 1), and the same is observed for the values of proteins (5.8 g and 2.63 g·100 g^{-1}), lipids (1.4 g and 3.1 g·100 g^{-1}) and fibers (13.1 g and 2.13 g·100 g^{-1}). Consequently, they have a higher caloric value (seeds with 212.7 kcal and leaves with 348.6 kcal) [18].

Compared with the seeds and pulp, the concentrations of vitamins and minerals are different in the leaves, because they play an important role in fruit development [21]. For example, in relation to minerals, the contents of magnesium, iron, potassium and calcium are higher in the leaves (the leaves have 366.1 mg and the seeds 54.4 mg·100 g^{-1}). Regarding vitamins, except for C, the leaves present a higher content, with the highest concentration in the pulp, as shown in Table 2 [7,22].

2.2. Phytochemical Composition

Different parts of the *C. papaya* plant, such as the fruits, seeds, roots, leaves, stem and latex were found to have important bioactive compounds, which, in turn, may exert medicinal effects. The methanolic extract of unripe fruits exerted antioxidant activity in vivo, for the presence of compounds, such as quercetin and β−sitosterol [20]. Other studies detected considerable quantities of total phenols (203 mg·100 g^{-1} extract) [22] in the methanolic extract of the papaya pulp, while terpenoids, alkaloids, flavonoids and saponins were identified in the water extract [9] (Table 3). Besides, in papaya seed extracts, the presence of benzyl isothiocyanate [13] and expressive quantities of glucosinolates were observed [12].

Table 3. Main phytochemical compounds present in *C. papaya* L. (papaya): ripe fruit pulp, seeds and leaves [14,15,19,23,24].

Phytochemical Composition		
Pulp	Seeds	Leaves
Glutathione peroxidase		
Glutathione transferase		
Glutathione reductase	Benzyl isothiocyanate glucosinolates	Polyphenols
Catalase	Fatty acids oleic, palmitic, linoleic and stearic	Flavonoids
Glucose-6-phosphate	Tocopherols (α and δ)	Saponins
Total phenols	β-cryptoxanthine	Pro-anthocyanin
Terpenols	β-carotene	Lycopene
Alkaloids	Carotenoids	Tocopherol
Flavonoids	Phenolic compounds	Benzyl isothiocyanate
Saponins		

Evaluating the oil extracted from the seeds, the main quantified fatty acid was oleic acid (71.30%), followed by palmitic (16.16%), linoleic (6.06%), and stearic acids (4.73%) (Table 3) [25]. The predominant tocopherols were α and δ-tocopherol, with 51.85 and 18.9 mg·kg^{-1}, respectively. The β-cryptoxanthin (4.29 mg·kg^{-1}) and β-carotene (2.76 mg·kg^{-1}) were the quantified carotenoids, and the content of total phenolic compounds was 957.60 mg·kg^{-1} [26].

Studies showed that *C. papaya* leaves present tocopherol [24], lycopene [14], flavonoids [25] and benzyl isothiocyanate [23]. Another important study demonstrated that the phytochemical composition of ethanolic, methanolic, acetate and water extracts of *C. papaya* leaves is independent of the type of extract, detecting polyphenols, flavonoids, saponins and pro-anthocyanins, besides the antioxidant activity, evaluated by the method 1,1-diphenyl-2-picrylhydrazyl (DPPH). However, the water extract had superior values of polyphenols (23.1 mgGAE/g) and antioxidant activity (166 µgTE/g), while the ethanolic extract had the highest concentrations of flavonoids (17.1 mgCE/g), saponins (82.8 mgAes/g) and pro-anthocyanins (7.91 mgCE/g) [15].

3. Medicinal Properties of *C. papaya*

Carica papaya contains important nutrients (Tables 1 and 2) and bioactive compounds, such as antioxidants, vitamins, and minerals (Table 3), with nutraceutical characteristics and potential beneficial effects on health [5]. Studies evaluated the actions of *C. papaya* in recovery from drug-induced hepatoxicity in rodents [27–30], e.g., by carbon tetrachloride (CCl_4), considered a potent inducer of toxic effects in the liver for being highly metabolized in bodily tissues because of the high reactivity of halogenated metabolites (CCl_3 and Cl), and such activation of metabolites liberate the active oxygen species (ROS). Another drug in question was acetaminophen (600 mg·100 g^{-1}), an analgesic and anti-pyretic, which causes acute hepatocellular damage that can be lethal if not treated [27].

Among the main effects that extracts of different parts of *C. papaya* demonstrated, in recovery from toxic effects on the liver, are the decrease in hepatic damage with the increase in antioxidant enzymes such as superoxide dismutase (SOD), glutathione (GSH), and catalase in the liver and decreases in the enzymes alanine aminotransferase (ALT), aspartate aminotransferase (AST), and alkaline phosphatase (ALP) [27–31]. Similar data were observed in nephrotoxicity induced by CCl4 in rats treated with *C. papaya* seed water extract, depending on the dose and time of treatment. The results showed a drop in biochemical parameters, such as the serum levels of uric acid, urea, and creatinine, besides the renal protecting ion, constated by histological evaluation after recovery from renal lesions [32].

Besides the effects on hepatic and renal toxicity, *C. papaya* displayed antimicrobial [33], anti-amoebic [34], anti-parasitic [12,13], and anti-malaria actions [11]. The use of *C. papaya* leaf water extract at different concentrations (25, 50, 100, 200 mg·mL^{-1}) had antimicrobial activity on the inhibition of some human pathogens, such as *Escherichia coli*, *Pseudomonas aeruginosa*, *Kleibseilla pneumoniae*, *Staphylococcus aureus*, and *Proteus mirabilis* [33]. Another study, utilizing the same type of extract at the dose of 100 mg·mL^{-1} found anti-amebic activity against *Entamoeba histolytica* [34]. Furthermore, *C. papaya* seeds had an activity on human intestinal parasites (*Caernorhabditis elegans*), without considerable side effects, owing to the presence of B-benzylisothiocyanate, a potent anti-helminthic [12]. Studies have shown the inhibitory effects on *Plasmodium falciparum* (malaria) in vitro, while the extract from the green fruit pulp of *C. papaya* demonstrated the highest anti-malaria activity, in comparison with different extracts of other tested plants [11].

Other studies showed the action of the water extract of *C. papaya* leaves (20 mg·mL^{-1}) on proliferation inhibition in strains of solid tumor cells in trials in vitro, e.g., cervical carcinoma (Hela), breast adenocarcinoma (MCF-7), hepatocellular carcinoma (HepG2), lung adenocarcinoma (PC14), pancreatic carcinoma (Panc-1) and mesothelioma (H2452) in a dose-dependent manner, suggesting the anti-tumoral action of the extract. To determine whether the proliferation inhibition was associated with decreased cell viability, the water extract of *C. papaya* leaves was shown to inhibit proliferation responses of hematopoietic cell strains, including T-cell lymphoma (Jurkat), plasma cell leukemia (ARH77), Burkitt's lymphoma (Raji), and large-cell anaplastic lymphoma (Karpas-299). In addition, the *C. papaya* leaf extract showed immunomodulatory activity on peripheral human blood mononuclear cells [17].

Antiulcerogenic actions were verified with the use of C. *papaya* seed water extract (50–100 mg/kg), the same action being observed using the methanolic extract, showing gastro-protective activity in animals, in both prevention and treatment models of gastric ulcer [35]. In addition, the *C. papaya* seed extract was able to reduce the contractility of rabbit jejunum smooth muscle—the responsible compound being benzyl isothiocyanate [36].

Effective anti-inflammatory actions were verified by applying *C. papaya* leaf ethanolic extract (25–250 mg·kg^{-1}) on carrageenan-induced paw edema in rats. However, after the ulcerogenic activity tests, the extract with the highest concentration produced a mild irritation of the gastric mucosa [37]. Besides the effects on inflammation, *C. papaya* showed wound healing properties. It is known that diabetic patients often have persistent difficulty in healing and require the delicate handling of wounds, demanding appropriate care. The topical use of the water extract of green fruits of *C. papaya* on wounds in diabetic rats, induced by streptozotocin (STPZ, 50 mg·kg^{-1}), exhibited a 77% reduction of the wound, induced by excision, with faster epithelization, compared with the control group, which received Vaseline [10]. Similar results in the healing of wounds induced by excision were observed on alloxan-induced diabetic rats (150 mg·kg^{-1}), which received a water extract of green fruits of *C. papaya*, the healing actions being attributed to the active component, papain, which led to the enzymatic debridement of wounds, and the fruit vitamin C content, since it is essential for the conversion of proline to hydroxyproline, a specific marker and component of the granulation tissue of the extracellular matrix in wounds [38,39]. In this way, besides possessing edible and tasty fruits, different parts of *C. papaya* are characterized by the quality of nutrients and bioactive compounds with medicinal properties that may be used in traditional medicine as an alternative or adjuvant in the treatment of some pathological conditions.

4. Effects of *C. papaya* L. on Metabolic Syndrome

Obesity consists of an excessive accumulation of body fat, which can represent a serious health risk and involves several ethological factors, including social, behavioral, environmental, cultural, psychological, metabolic, and genetic factors [40]. It is known that excessive fat accumulation, mostly visceral, can be an important condition in the development of metabolic dysfunctions, such as arterial hypertension, dyslipidemia and insulin resistance, and alterations conducive to the development of diabetes mellitus type 2, cardiovascular illnesses [41] and cancer [42], such as prostate [43] and colon rectal cancer [44]. Thus, the metabolic syndrome can be defined as the set of these risk factors, i.e., a cluster of metabolic disorders associated with obesity, including insulin resistance, atherogenic dyslipidemia and hypertension, which can lead to cardiovascular illnesses [45].

Since adipose tissue is a source of a great number of adipokines, such as the tumor necrosis factor (TNF-α), interleukin 6 (IL-6), monocyte chemoattractant protein, also known as chemokine ligand 2 (MCP-1/CCL-2), leptin, adiponectin, and resistin, among others [46], the larger the accumulation of adipose tissue, the higher the production of these adipokines. This leads to an imbalance in their secretion, with increased pro-inflammatory and decreased anti-inflammatory adipokines, stimulating the systemic and local inflammatory process, contributing to the development of insulin resistance [46]. Furthermore, the metabolic syndrome, besides being associated with the inflammatory process, is also related with the high production of reactive oxygen species (ROS) and, consequently, can induce insulin resistance [47,48], which is increasingly recognized as a key factor linking metabolic syndrome and liver steatosis; the last is associated with excessive fat accumulation in ectopic tissues, such as the liver, and increased circulating free fatty acids, which can further promote inflammation and endoplasmic reticulum stress [49].

For the treatment of obesity and its metabolic disorders which characterize the metabolic syndrome, there are various therapeutic approaches, either pharmacological or non-pharmacological treatments, and other methods, used as healing adjuvants. As such, the use of plants or fruits, reported since remote times as alternatives for the treatment and prevention of diseases, stand out in view of their high concentrations of vitamins, bioactive compounds and also lipidic composition, which reduces inflammatory markers, aggregates platelet, protects against thrombogenesis and oxidative stress, and prevents hypercholesterolemia, hypertriglyceridemia and hyperglycemia, which can be triggered by obesity [5].

Considering the presence of vitamins, bioactive compounds and lipids of biological and nutritional importance in C. papaya, several studies (summarized in Table 4) evinced relevant effects of this plant in the treatment of metabolic dysfunctions, associated or not associated with obesity, which can be considered an alternative therapeutic approach in the treatment of the metabolic syndrome.

A preliminary study [50] demonstrated that the water extract of C. papaya seeds showed hypoglycemic and hypolipidemic activity in adult healthy male Wistar rats, without signs of acute toxicity. The groups received the water extract of C. papaya seeds, at concentrations of 100 mg, 200 mg and 400 mg/kg, and glibenclamide at 0.1 mg·kg^{-1} by gavage for 30 days. The treatments at all doses of the extract led to decreased serum levels of fasting glycemia, triglycerides, total cholesterol, LDL-c, and VLDL-c, with increased HDL-c levels, depending on the dose, and responses similar to the effects of the positive control group (glibenclamide). Such a relation with the extract concentration was observed in the lowered atherogenic index, compared with the group receiving distilled water (10 mL/kg/day) and glibenclamide (0.1 mg/kg/day). The phytochemical analyses of the extract revealed the presence of alkaloids, flavonoids, saponins, tannins, anthraquinones and anthocyanosides, and the monitored animals showed a decrease insugars, related to the metabolic effects.

Another study [51] evaluated the effects of the water extract of C. papaya leaves (200 mg/kg to body mass), given by gavage in adult healthy male New Zealand rabbits, treated for 24 weeks, resulting in reduced body weight, concomitant with lowered levels of fasting glycemia during the trial. Moreover, over the supplementation period, the extract had a hepatotoxic effect, manifesting an increase in serum values of aspartate transaminase (AST), aspartate aminotransferase (ALT), gamma-glutamine transferase (γ-GT) and total bilirubin. Therefore, further investigations will be necessary to evaluate toxicological effects of the extract, especially on the liver, in order to, standardize doses time of administration and side effects for a safety administration.

While such metabolic effects were observed in healthy animals, other studies elucidated the hypoglycemic action in an alloxan-induced diabetes model [52–54]. Adenowo et al. (2014) [52] investigated alloxan-induced (150 mg/kg/body mass) diabetic Wistar rats, treated with an ethanolic extract of C. papaya leaves (250 and 500 mg·kg^{-1}) by gavage for 21 days, and verified reduced levels of glycemia, total cholesterol, triglycerides and LDL-c, together with increased HDL-c levels, resulting mainly from the dose of 250 mg/kg to body mass. Furthermore, they verified that the extract diminished the serum concentrations of urea, creatinine, ALT and AST, as well as the parameters of diabetic animals receiving metformin. The data corroborate the study of Maniyar (2011) [54], where the water extract of C. papaya leaf (400 mg/kg/body mass), given by gavage for 21 days, showed a reduction in the levels of glycemia, triglycerides and total cholesterol in alloxan-induced diabetic rats (120 mg/kg/body mass), confirmed by Johnson et al. (2015) [53], who tested the water extract of seeds and leaves of C. papaya (400 mg/kg/body mass), by gavage for 28 days in an experimental model of diabetes (alloxan 150 mg/kg to body mass), having observed diminished levels of glycemia total cholesterol, hepatic enzymes, ALT, AST, urea, and creatinine. Nevertheless, regarding glycemic metabolism and hypoglycemic action, the seed extract was superior to the leaf extract.

Ezekwe et al. (2014) [55] applied the experimental model of alloxan-induced diabetes (120 mg/kg to body mass) in albino rats receiving a ration added to grated green C. papaya pulp, splitting the animals into three groups: control non-diabetic, diabetic and diabetic fed with added grated green C. papaya pulp for 28 days. The third group presented relevant effects on their metabolism, such as a reduction of weight, in the levels of glycosylated hemoglobin and in the lipidic profile, including low-density lipoprotein cholesterol (LDL-c), very low-density lipoprotein (VLDL-c), triglycerides and total cholesterol, and increased serum values of High-density lipoprotein cholesterol (HDL-c).

Metabolic effects were also observed in alloxan-induced (90 mg/kg/body mass) albino rats receiving the water extract of C. papaya root (500 mg/kg/body mass) and glibenclamide (5 mg/kg/body mass) by gavage for 21 days. The treatment with the extract showed improved parameters of glycemia already after 7 days of the trial, an improvement in the dyslipidemic parameters and recovery of hepatic tissues and renal dysfunction. The compounds identified include hexadecanoicacid, methylester, 10-octadecanoic acid, methyl ester, ergosta-5,22-dien-3-olacetate (3β, 22E), dianhydromannitol, 1,1,3,3,5,5,7,7,9,9,11,11-dodecamethylhexasiloxane, methyl-11-hexadecanoate, and octadecanoic acid. The compounds 10-octadecenoic acid, methylester, hexadecanoic acid, and methyl ester, were the phytochemicals most present in the root extract. Thus, they may have contributed to the cited metabolic effects [56].

Hypoglycemic effects were observed not only with the isolated administration of the leaf extract of C. papaya in alloxan-induced diabetic rats (180 mg/kg/body mass), but also combined with co-administrated reference antidiabetic drugs, such as metformin and glimepiride. The extract, the drug, or the combination drug + extract was administered daily by gavage in periods of a short and long duration, corresponding to 3 and 7 days, respectively. The concentrations of each product given to the animals were divided based on low and high doses, established in previous studies, as follows: extract low dose: 5 mg/kg and high dose: 10 mg/kg; glimepiride low dose: 0.2 mg/kg and high dose: 0.4 mg/kg; and metformin low dose: 50 mg/kg and high dose: 100 mg/kg, for 3 and 7 days. The same period of treatment was utilized for the combinations, glimepiride + extract and metformin + extract, and the dose combinations corresponded to high-high, high-low, low-high and low-low. The lowest concentration extract (5 mg/kg) reduced the glycemic level, but the highest concentration (10 mg/kg) accelerated the starting of the glimepiride activity, while the combination of all extracts with metformin diminished the glycemic levels after 24 h. Thus, the data demonstrated that the hypoglycemic activity of the C. papaya leaf extract was as effective as the hypoglycemic agents, metformin and glimepiride. However, the latter had a faster action onset, as the effect of the duration of application was dependent on the nature, i.e., on the activity strength, and on the dose. Besides, the interaction between the combination drug-extract was different for each group, since the action mechanisms of glimepiride differ from those of metformin [57].

In studies [58] on C. papaya on streptozotocin (STPZ)-induced diabetes, the crude ethanolic extract of C. papaya leaf (100 mg/kg/day), in comparison with the ethanolic extract of the leaves of Pandanusam aryllifolius (100 mg/kg/day) and the drug glyburide (10 mg/kg) by gavage for 6 days in albino mice with induced diabetes by STPZ (60 mg/kg/body mass), did not alter body weight. However, there was a reduction of glycemia, and the histology showed spleen cell regeneration, reduced the number of liver pyknotic nuclei and vacuoles, and recovered kidney cuboidal tissue. The phytochemical analyses indicated the presence of alkaloids, tannins, flavonoids and saponins, suggesting that these bioactive compounds are responsible for such effects.

A possible hypothesis for the metabolic actions of C. papaya extracts can be seen in the study by Juárez-Rojop et al. (2012) [59], utilizing the water extract of C. papaya leaves at three doses (0.75, 1.5 and 3 g·100 mL^{-1}) in the drinking water of animals with induced diabetes by STPZ (60 mg/kg to body mass) and non-diabetic animals for a 4-week period. The results demonstrated that the extracts at 0.75 and 1.5 g·100 mL^{-1} diminished the levels of glycemia, as well as the serum levels of total cholesterol and triglycerides. The regeneration of pancreatic islets, with a preserved cell size, was demonstrated, and yet, a rupture of hepatocytes and accumulation of glycogen and lipids was prevented. Besides, it was verified that the metabolites of nitric oxide (NO) were reduced in diabetic rats. However, with the application of the extracts, the NO levels rose. It is known that hyperglycemia and hyperlipidemia are characterized by the inhibition of endothelial NO Synthase (eNOS) and, consequently, can result in the formation of reactive oxygen species (ROS) in relaxation, depending on the damaged endothelium, with a high formation of free radicals, concomitant with a low effectiveness of antioxidant enzymes, leading to an imbalance between the formation and the protection against free radicals in the organism.

Thus, the metabolic actions in that study could be related to the increased antioxidant activity of the extract, exerted in diabetic animals.

Previous studies [60] evaluated the phytochemical composition of *C. papaya* leaf extracts on the basis of chloroform, n-hexane and ethanol and verified that the chloroform extract presented steroids and quinones among its main components, which led to the choosing of this extract for the screening of biological activity in STPZ-induced diabetic rats (60 mg/kg/body mass).

Different doses of a chloroform extract (0, 31, 62, 125 mg/kg/body mass) of *C. papaya* leaf were given by gavage to diabetic and non-diabetic rats, and as the positive control group, diabetic rats were treated with insulin (5 U/kg, intraperitoneal) for 20 days. The data proved that the extract reduced the glycemic levels, the serum concentrations of triglycerides and total cholesterol and maintained the HDL-c at levels similar to those observed in non-diabetic rats. Furthermore, the concentrations of 31 and 62 mg/kg/body mass of the extract reduced the body weight and the levels of AST and ALT, without differences for the extract with the highest concentration (125/mg/kg/body mass).

Considering not just the systemic and biochemical actions, the extract was able to act on specific tissues, such as the pancreatic islets, either in diabetic rats induced by STPZ (60 mg/kg/body mass) and in vitro in cell cultures of pancreatic islets, which were found to be the actions of the chloroform extract of *C. papaya* leaves (31, 62, 125 mg/kg/body mass), applied by gavage for 20 days. The animals receiving the extract at concentrations of 31 and 62 mg/kg/body mass showed a reduction in fastening glycemia. On the other hand, the serum levels of insulin increased in non-diabetic rats receiving 62 mg/kg/body mass, compared with the non-diabetic group, without the extract. In cell cultures of pancreatic islets treated with STPZ (6 mg in 30 μL polyethylene glycol), a decrease in the liberation of the basal insulin culture with glucose (2 g/L) occurred. Besides, when added to the extract (6 mg in 30 μL polyethylene glycol) applied to cells with STPZ, more insulin liberation occurred. However, when STPZ was added simultaneously with the extracts (3, or 6, or 12 mg in 30 μL), insulin liberation was diminished in the three conditions, independently of the dose. However, when STPZ was added after 5 days of using the extracts, the insulin liberated from the pancreatic islets was superior to the cells of the control group, normal and similar to cells with the 6 mg extract, suggesting that the extracts have a protective action on pancreatic islets. The results are confirmed by an immune histochemical trial of the spleen, in which it was verified that the diameters and areas were larger in the groups treated with *C. papaya* extract, compared with the diabetic group [61].

Among the bioactive compounds of the major proportion in the chloroform extract are the steroids. In diabetes, changes occur in the structure and function of the absorption of intestinal glucose, e.g., an increase in glucose uptake that could cause postprandial hyperglycemia. Thus, the hypothesis is that the steroids hinder the hydrolysis of carbohydrates and the absorption of intestinal glucose by hydrolyzing enzymes limiting the levels of post prandial glucose [61–63].

It is known that diabetes mellitus is characterized by a deficiency in insulin secretion and by a low response of the organs in the action of insulin [64]. The compounds present in the *C. papaya* extract may be related to effects similar to those of insulin in glycemic metabolism, promoting glucose uptake in peripherical tissues or in the skeletal muscle and adipose tissues by a process of regeneration and revitalization of their main β-cells [60,65].

Another mechanism, which may be related to the effects of *C. papaya* on glycemic metabolism, may be the inhibition of important enzymes involved in the digestion of carbohydrates, such as α-amylase and α-glycosidase. Oboh et al. (2013) [66] demonstrated that the water extract of different parts of the green fruit of *C. papaya* was able to promote the inhibition of α-amylase and α-glycosidase in a dose-dependent way (0 to 2.0 mg/mL), and the combination of different parts of the green fruit, such as seeds, pulp and peel, in equal proportions had the best inhibitory effects on both enzymes. The α-amylase degrades complex carbohydrates in the diet into oligosaccharides and disaccharides, which are converted into monosaccharides by α-glycosidase. The liberated glucose is absorbed by the intestine, resulting in post prandial hyperglycemia. A higher inhibition of these enzymes thereby occurs, and the rise of post prandial glucose from a carbohydrate-rich diet will be significantly diminished, slowing the process of hydrolysis and uptake of carbohydrates [67,68].

Oxidative stress is also one of the mechanisms conducive to the development and progression of diabetes mellitus, since an exacerbated increase in the production of free radicals occurs simultaneously with the decreased mechanisms of antioxidant defenses, which can result in the cell damage of organelles and enzymes, increased lipidic peroxidation and, consequently, the development of insulin resistance [69,70]. In this way, *C. papaya* was also able to present antioxidant activity [68]. Different parts of the green fruits of *C. papaya* inhibited the lipidic peroxidation induced by sodium nitroprusside in rat pancreatic cells in vitro [66]. Sodium nitroprusside is an anti-hypertensive drug, which causes cytotoxicity by the liberation of cyanide and/or NO. Under conditions of oxidative stress, NO, together with other ROSs, such as the radical superoxide, lead to the formation of the radical peroxynitrite (ONOO-), which is a potent oxidant agent that can harm most cell components, such as proteins, DNA and membrane phospholipids [71,72]. Thus, the study showed that the extract of the pulp with the peel of green fruits can have a strong inhibitory effect on the production of malondialdehyde (MDA) and a greater ability of NO radical scavenging than seeds. Such effects are attributed to the phenolic compounds and alkaloids present in the pulp, seed and peel extracts of *C. papaya*, which are biocomponents with a high antioxidant action in removing free radicals, catalyzing chelating metals, activating antioxidant enzymes, reducing the radicals of α-tocopherol and inhibiting oxidases [64,73].

Corroborating the antioxidant actions of *C. papaya*, Salla et al. (2016) [74] reported on the antioxidant activity of the methanolic and hexanic extracts at concentrations of 50, 100 and 250 μg/mL of *C. papaya* seed on HepG2 cells, the cell strain of the human hepatoma, which incurred an induction of oxidative stress by the application of hydrogen peroxide (H_2O_2) (500μM). The activity of the antioxidant enzyme superoxide dismutase (SOD), catalase (CAT) and glutathione peroxidase (GPx) and levels of glutathione (GSH) were lower after the induction of oxidative stress by H_2O_2, and after the use of methanolic and hexanic extracts, the activity of SOD was restored, except with 50 μg/mL. The GSH levels increased with the concentration of 250 μg/mL methanolic extract and 100 and 250 μg/mL hexanic extract, and the CAT activity rose with the concentrations of 250 and 500 μg/mL, with GPx only at 250 μg/mL of methanolic extract. Besides, the highest concentrations of both extracts diminished cell viability, but this could be verified in higher proportion with the hexanic extract. The levels of flavonoids in the extracts were superior in the methanolic extract, compared with the hexanic, confirming that the antioxidant activity is related to the presence of these polyphenols.

Like glycemic metabolism, the bioactive compounds present in the *C. papaya* extracts can exert effects similar to insulin in the lipidic metabolism, as under normal conditions the insulin activates the lipoprotein lipase, hydrolyses triglycerides and inhibits the lipolysis process. Insulin deficiency, in turn, stimulates lipolysis in the adipose tissue, leading to hyperlipidemia and an accumulation of hepatic fat, decreasing the content of the enzyme lipoprotein lipase, which hydrolyses lipids, resulting in increased concentrations of serum triglycerides. Increased LDL-c levels occur because of the inhibition of the insulin action in the activity of the enzyme, β-hydroxy-β-methyl glutaryl CoA reductase (HMG-CoA reductase), which exerts an important role in cholesterol metabolism [53,66].

The action of the *C. papaya* extract on the enzyme, HMG-CoA reductase, is reported by Hasimun et al. (2018) [75], assessing specifically the actions in the lipidic metabolism of the ethanolic extract of *C. papaya* leaves (50, 100, 200 mg/kg/body mass) by gavage in Wistar rats, receiving 25% of D-fructose in drinking water for 21 days. The results showed an anti-hyperlipidemic activity of the extract at a dose of 200 mg/kg/body mass, leading to decreased total levels of cholesterol, triglycerides, and LDL-c and an increase in HDL-c. The mechanism involved is related to the inhibition of the enzyme, HMG-CoA reductase, activity in the liver, an enzyme with an important role in the synthesis of endogenous cholesterol, the inhibition of which is similar to the effects of drugs of the class of statins, such as simvastatin, used as a positive control. Besides, the phytochemical analyses revealed secondary metabolites, such as alkaloids, flavonoids, tannin, saponins, steroids/triterpenoids and quinones, suggesting that the flavonoids contained in the leaf extract, especially quercetin, could be the responsible for exerting the same mechanism as that of the statins in inhibiting HMG CoA reductase [75–77].

Similar data in the lipidic metabolism of *C. papaya* extract were observed in albino Wistar rats, fed with hyperlipidic diet. The effects on dyslipidemia were observed, testing the water extract of papaya seed (200 and 300 mg/body mass/day) by gavage for 5 weeks, which led to a significant reduction of total cholesterol, triglycerides, and LDL-c and an increase in HDL-c in hypercholesterolemic animals. However, the antilipidemic effects of different extract concentrations were not superior to the group receiving the reference drug, simvastatin (1.8 mg/bodymass/day) [78].

Besides the effects on glycemia and lipidic series, *C. papaya* showed actions on the systemic arterial hypertension (SAH) in animal models. After evaluating the inhibitory action of the extracts on the activity of the angiotensin-converting enzyme (ACE) in vitro, the methanolic extract of *C. papaya* leaves was chosen for the study by Brasil et al. (2014) [79]. The methanolic extract (100 mg/body mass/twice a day) was given by gavage in spontaneously hypertense Wistar rats (SHR) for 30 days. Like the reference drug (enalapril 10 mg/body mass/day), an ACE inhibitor, the methanolic extract inhibited plasmatic ACE activity, enhanced cardiac hypertrophy and normalized baroreflex sensibility, suggesting the efficiency of this extract as an anti-hypertensive [79]. The systemic arterial pressure is controlled by both the renin-angiotensin system (RAS) and baroreflex. The latter is an important short-term reflex, which controls the responses of the heart beats [80]. The uncontrolled activation of RAS has an important role in the development of cardiac hypertrophy, the ACE inhibitors being important treatment options, since ACE is an important component of RAS, which leads to the formation of angiotensin II, the main vasoconstrictor of RAS, and to the reduction of baroreflex sensibility for rising blood pressure and sympathetic regulation [81,82]. In that study, the extract effects on arterial pressure could result from the presence of different bioactive compounds, especially flavonoids, e.g., ferulic acid, caffeic acid, gallic acid and quercetin, with a suggested action on ACE inhibition [79]. Previous studies demonstrated the presence of quercetin, luteolin and kaempferol in apple peel extract, which acted as inhibitors of ACE activity in vitro [83,84].

In a model of arterial hypertension induced by deoxycorticosterone acetate (DOCA, 15 mg·100 g^{-1}) in Wistar rats, the crude extract of *C. papaya* fruit (20 mg/kg), besides not presenting toxic effects, was able to generate a fast drop of arterial blood pressure and heart rate, compared with normotensive rats, and had a more potent anti-hypertensive action than hydralazine (200 mg/100 g, intravenous), a vasodilator and anti-hypertensive agent [85]. Earlier studies revealed a higher activity in the synthesis of catecholamines, e.g., a higher activity of tyrosine hydroxylase in the adrenal glands of DOCA-induced hypertense rats and in rats with renal hypertension [86,87]. Therefore, the capacity of the extract to depress the arterial pressure and the heart rate may be caused by the reduction of levels of catecholamines, liberated in response to the extract [88].

While the reviewed studies hitherto were not performed in specific models of metabolic syndrome or obesity, the achieved results demonstrated that *C. papaya* has a therapeutic potential for various types of metabolic dysfunctions, such as diabetes mellitus type 1, leading to alterations in both glycemic and lipidic metabolism, oxidative stress and in models of arterial hypertension. After those studies on the actions of *C. papaya* in metabolism, further investigations on this plant in models of obesity and metabolic syndrome are needed, which would facilitate the search for new therapeutic approaches and a better understanding of the mechanisms of action in the metabolic dysfunctions associated with obesity.

Table 4. Summary of effects of the use of *Carica papaya* L. against metabolic dysfunctions.

Reference	Host	Used Part	Treatments	Main Effects
[50]	Healthy rats	Seed	Group 1: 10 mL distilled water Group 2: glibenclamide 0.1 mg/kg Group 3: water extract 100 mg Group 4: water extract 200 mg/kg Group 5: water extract 400 mg/kg Duration: 30 days	-Reduced glycemia -Reduced triglycerides, total cholesterol, LDL-c, VLDL-c and increase HDL-c -Reduced atherogenic index and coronary arteries
[51]	Healthy rabbits	Leaves	Group 1: control Group 2: water extract 200 mg/kg Duration: 24 weeks	-Reduced weight -Reduced glycemia -Increased AST, ALT, γ-GT and total bilirubin
[52]	Rats, non-diabetic and diabetic (Alloxan 150 mg/kg)	Leaves	Grupo A: non-diabetic + 1 mL distilled water Grupo B: diabetic Grupo C: diabetic + 250 mg/kg ethanolic extract Grupo D: diabetic + 500 mg/kg ethanolic extract Grupo E: diabetic + 300 mg/kg metformin Duration: 21 days	-Reduced glycemia -Reduced total cholesterol, triglycerides, LDL-c and increased HDL-c especially at 250 mg/kg -Reduced urea, creatinine, ALT and AST
[53]	Rats, non-diabetic and diabetic (Alloxan 150 mg/kg)	Seeds and leaves	Grupo 1: non-diabetic Grupo 2: diabetic + 1 mL saline Grupo 3: diabetic + 400 mg/kg seed water extract Grupo 4: diabetic + 400 mg/kg leaf water extract Duration: 28 days	-Reduced glycemic levels -Reduced total cholesterol -Reduced ALT, AST, urea and creatinine
[54]	Rats, non-diabetic and diabetic (Alloxan 120 mg/kg)	Leaves	Group 1: non-diabetic Grupo 2: diabetic Group 3: diabetic + glibenclamide (0.1 mg/kg/day) Group 4, 5 and 6: diabetic + C. papaya water extract (100, 200 and 400 mg/kg) Duration: 21 days	-Reduced glycemia -Improved lipidic profile and C-reactive protein
[55]	Rats, non-diabetic and diabetic (Alloxan 120 mg/kg)	Green pulp	Group 1: non-diabetic + standard ration Group 2: diabetic + standard ration Group 3: diabetic + grated C. papaya Duration: 28 days	-Reduced weight -Reduced glycated hemoglobin -Reduced LDL-c, VLDL-c, triglycerides, total cholesterol and increased HDL-c
[56]	Rats, non-diabetic and diabetic (Alloxan 90 mg/kg)	Root	Group 1: non-diabetic Group 2: diabetic Group 3: diabetic + 500 mg/kg C. papaya root water extract Group 4: diabetic + 5 mg/kg glibenclamide Duration: 21 days	-Reduced glycemia after 7 days with extract -Reduced dyslipidemia -Recovery of hepatic tissues and renal dysfunction

Table 4. Cont.

Reference	Host	Used Part	Treatments	Main Effects
[57]	Rats, non-diabetic and diabetic (Alloxan 180 mg/kg)	Leaves	* Combinations: comparison between low and high dose Group extract: diabetic + low dose (5 mg/kg) and diabetic high dose (10 mg/kg) Group glimepiride: diabetic + low dose (0.2 mg/kg) and diabetic high dose (0.4 mg/kg) Group metformin: diabetic + low dose (50 mg/kg) and high dose (100 mg/kg) *Combinations: glimepiride + extract = comparison between doses: high-high, high-low, low-high, low-low *Combinations: metformin + extract = comparison between doses: high-high, high-low, low-high, low-low Duration: short—3 days Long—7 days	-The low dose extract (5 mg/kg) reduced glycemic levels -The high dose extract (10 mg/kg) accelerated the starting of glimepiride activity -The combination extracts + metformin decreased glycemic levels after 24 h
[58]	Mice, diabetic and non-diabetic (streptozotocin 60 mg/kg)	Leaves	Group 1: non-diabetic + carboxy methylcellulose (5 mL/kg) Grupo 2: diabetic mice Group 3: diabetic + 10 mg/kg glyburide Group 4: diabetic + 100 mg/kg C. papaya ethanolic extract Group 5: diabetic + 100 mg/kg P. amaryllifolius ethanolic extract Duration: 6 days	-No weight change -Reduced glycemia -Regeneration of pancreatic cells -Reduced number of liver vacuoles and pyknotic nuclei -Recovery of kidney cuboid tissue
[59]	Rats, non-diabetic and diabetic	Seeds	Groups 1, 2 and 3: non-diabetic + water extract (0.75, 1.5, 3.0 g/100 mL) Groups 4, 5 and 6: diabetic + water extract (0.75, 1.5, 3.0 g/100 mL). Duration: 30 days	-Reduced glycemia -Reduced total cholesterol and triglycerides
[60]	Rats, non-diabetic and diabetic (streptozotocin 60 mg/kg)	Leaves	Groups 1, 2, 3: non-diabetic + chloroform extract (31, 62 and 125 mg/kg,) Groups 4, 5, 6: diabetic + chloroform extract (31, 62 and 125 mg/kg) Group 7: diabetic + insulin (5 U/kg) Duration: 20 days	-Reduced glycemic levels -Reduced triglycerides and total cholesterol and maintained HDL-c levels similar to those of the non-diabetic control -Reduced body mass at 31 and 62 mg extract/kg/body mass -Reduced AST and ALT levels at 31 and 62 mg extract/kg/body mass
[62]	(1) In vivo: Rats, non-diabetic and diabetic (streptozotocin 60 mg/kg) (2) In vitro: rat pancreatic islets	Leaves	Group 1: non-diabetic Group 2: non-diabetic + chloroform extract (62 mg/kg) Group 3: diabetic Group 4: diabetic + chloroform extract (31 mg/kg) Group 5: diabetic + chloroform extract (62 mg/kg) Group 6: diabetic + chloroform extract (125 mg/kg) Group 7: diabetic + insulin (5 U/kg) Duration: 20 days	-Reduced fastening glycemia at 31 and 62 mg extract/kg -Increased insulin in non-diabetic animals + 62 mg/kg compared with non-diabetic animals, without extract -Protecting action on pancreatic islets cells

Table 4. Cont.

Reference	Host	Used Part	Treatments	Main Effects
[66]	In vitro: rat spleen	Parts of green fruit -Seeds -Peel -Pulp -Pulp + peel Seeds + Peel + Pulp	Cells + (0 to 2 mg/mL) water extract	-Inhibition of the enzymatic activity of α-amylase and β-glycosidase, dose dependent (0–2 mg/mL) -Greater inhibitory action of water extracts of pulp + peel on lipidic peroxidation induced by nitroprusside -Greater ability of NO radical scavenging of pulp + peel extracts, dose dependent (0 to 0.75 mg/mL)
[74]	In vitro: HepG2 cells	Fruits	Hexanic and methanolic extracts (50, 100 and 250 μg/mL)	-Increased antioxidant activity of SOD, CAT, GPx and GSH, dose dependent and dependent on extract type -1 mg/mL methanolic extract inhibited 50% DPPH (2,2-diphenyl-1-picrylhydrazyl) -Reduced cell viability, dose dependent
[75]	Rats	Leaves	Group 1: without D-fructose Group 2: added D-fructose Group 3, 4 and 5: added D-fructose + ethanolic extract (50, 100, 200 mg/kg) Duration: 21 days	-Reduced total levels of cholesterol, triglycerides, LDL-c and increased HDL-cat 200 mg/kg/ -Inhibition of HMG-CoA reductase activity in the liver
[78]	Rats	Seed	Group 1: common + saline diet Group 2: hyperlipidic diet Group 3: hyperlipidic diet + 200 mg/kg water extract Group 4: hyperlipidic diet + 300 mg/kg water extract Group 5: hyperlipidic diet + simvastatin (1.8 mg/kg/day). Duration: 5 weeks	-Reduced total cholesterol, triglycerides, and LDL-c and increased HDL-c -No differences from positive control (simvastatin 1.8 mg/kg)
[79]	Rats	Leaves	Group 1: normotensive Group 2: hypertensive (SHR) Group 3: hypertensive (SHR) + methanolic extract 100 mg/kg Group 4: hypertensive (SHR) + enalapril 10 mg/kg Duration: 30 days	-Inhibition of activity of plasmatic ACE -Improvement of cardiac hypertrophy -Normalization of baroreflex sensibility
[85]	Rats (DOCA-induced hypertension 15 mg/100 g)	Fruits	Group 1: normotensive Group 2: hypertensive + fruit juice crude extract (20 mg/kg) Group 3: hypertensive + hydralazine (200 mg/100 g)	-Anti-hypertensive action, more potent than hydralazine

5. Conclusions

This review evaluated the nutritional and phytochemical composition of *C. papaya* as well as the effects of the use of several types of extract from different parts of the plant. *C papaya* exhibits curative properties, such as improvements in hepatotoxicity and nephrotoxicity induced by drugs, antimicrobial, antimalarial, anti-parasitic, antitumor, anti-inflammatory actions and wound healing effects. In relation to the metabolic dysfunctions, *C. papaya* displays hypoglycemic, hypolipidemic and antihypertensive potential and demonstrates increased antioxidant activity in experimental models in vivo and in vitro. Therefore, further studies including researches on diet-induced and genetic obesity models in addition to the isolation of specific substances from different parts of *C. papaya* will be important for the development of novel natural products on the treatment and prevention of obesity and metabolic disturbances.

Author Contributions: L.F.S., A.P., F.M.A. and W.F.O.F.: assistance with structuring the review, writing, and literature review; A.C.I., B.L.S.d.E.S., R.d.C.A.G., P.A.H. and K.d.C.F.: assistance with structuring the review.

Funding: This research received no external funding.

Acknowledgments: We thank the graduate program in Health and Development in the Central-West Region of Brazil, Federal University of Mato Grosso do Sul-UFMS, for support.

Conflicts of Interest: The authors declare no conflict of interest.

References

1. Kumar, G.; Loganathan, K.; Rao, B. Hemolytic activity of Indian medicinal plants towards human erythrocytes: An in vitro study. *Elixir Appl. Bot.* **2011**, *40*, 5534–5537.
2. Gooda Sahib, N.; Saari, N.; Ismail, A.; Khatib, A.; Mahomoodally, F.; Abdul Hamid, A. Plants' metabolites as potential antiobesity agents. *Sci. World J.* **2012**, *2012*, 436039. [CrossRef] [PubMed]
3. Quagliariello, V.; Vecchione, R.; Coppola, C.; Di Cicco, C.; De Capua, A.; Piscopo, G.; Paciello, R.; Narciso, V.; Formisano, C.; Taglialatela-Scafati, O.; et al. Cardioprotective effects of nanoemulsions loaded with anti-inflammatory nutraceuticals against doxorubicin-induced cardiotoxicity. *Nutrients* **2018**, *10*, 1304. [CrossRef] [PubMed]
4. Teixeira, L.G.; Lages, P.C.; Jascolka, T.L.; Aguilar, E.C.; Soares, F.L.P.; Pereira, S.S.; Beltrão, N.R.M.; de Oliveira Matoso, R.; do Nascimento, A.M.; de Castilho, R.O.; et al. White tea (*Camellia sinensis*) extract reduces oxidative stress and triacylglycerols in obese mice. *Food Sci. Technol.* **2012**, *32*, 733–741. [CrossRef]
5. Vij, T.; Prashar, Y. A review on medicinal properties of *Carica papaya* Linn. *Asian Pac. J. Trop. Dis.* **2015**, *5*, 1–6. [CrossRef]
6. FAO. FAOSTAT. Available online: http://www.fao.org/faostat/en/#data/QC (accessed on 24 April 2019).
7. Nwofia, E.; Ojimelukwe, P.; Eji, C. Chemical composition of leaves, fruit pulp and seeds in some *Carica papaya* (L) morphotypes. *Int. J. Med. Aromat. Plants* **2012**, *2*, 200–206.
8. Marfo, E.K.; Oke, O.L.; Afolabi, O.A. Chemical composition of papaya (*Carica papaya*) seeds. *Food Chem.* **1986**, *22*, 259–266. [CrossRef]
9. Aravind, G.; Bhowmik, D.S.D.; Harish, G. Traditional and Medicinal Uses of *Carica papaya*. *J. Med. Plants Stud.* **2013**, *1*, 7–15.
10. Nayak, S.B.; Pinto Pereira, L.; Maharaj, D. Wound healing activity of *Carica papaya* L. in experimentally induced diabetic rats. *Indian J. Exp. Biol.* **2007**, *45*, 739–743.
11. Bhat, G.P.; Surolia, N. In vitro antimalarial activity of extracts of three plants used in the traditional medicine of India. *Am. J. Trop. Med. Hyg.* **2001**, *65*, 304–308. [CrossRef]
12. Kermanshai, R.; McCarry, B.E.; Rosenfeld, J.; Summers, P.S.; Weretilnyk, E.A.; Sorger, G.J. Benzyl isothiocyanate is the chief or sole anthelmintic in papaya seed extracts. *Phytochemistry* **2001**, *57*, 427–435. [CrossRef]
13. Tang, C.-S. Benzyl isothiocyanate of papaya fruit. *Phytochemistry* **1971**, *10*, 117–121. [CrossRef]
14. Van Breemen, R.B.; Pajkovic, N. Multitargeted therapy of cancer by lycopene. *Cancer Lett.* **2008**, *269*, 339–351. [CrossRef] [PubMed]

15. Vuong, Q.V.; Hirun, S.; Roach, P.D.; Bowyer, M.C.; Phillips, P.A.; Scarlett, C.J. Effect of extraction conditions on total phenolic compounds and antioxidant activities of *Carica papaya* leaf aqueous extracts. *J. Herb. Med.* **2013**, *3*, 104–111. [CrossRef]
16. Wilson, R.K.; Kwan, T.K.; Kwan, C.Y.; Sorger, G.J. Effects of papaya seed extract and benzyl isothiocyanate on vascular contraction. *Life Sci.* **2002**, *71*, 497–507. [CrossRef]
17. Otsuki, N.; Dang, N.H.; Kumagai, E.; Kondo, A.; Iwata, S.; Morimoto, C. Aqueous extract of *Carica papaya* leaves exhibits anti-tumor activity and immunomodulatory effects. *J. Ethnopharmacol.* **2010**, *127*, 760–767. [CrossRef] [PubMed]
18. Krishna, K.L.; Paridhavi, M.; Patel, J.A. Review on nutritional, medicinal and pharmacological properties of papaya *(Carica papaya Linn.)*. *Nat. Prod. Radiance* **2008**, *7*, 364–373.
19. Parle, M.; Gurditta, A. Basketful benefits of papaya. *Int. Res. J. Pharm.* **2011**, *2*, 6–12.
20. Oloyede, O.I. Chemical Profile of Unripe Pulp of *Carica papaya*. *Pak. J. Nutr.* **2005**, *4*, 379–381. [CrossRef]
21. Bari, L.; Hassan, P.; Absar, N.; Haque, M.E.; Khuda, M.I.I.E.; Pervin, M.M.; Khatun, S.; Hossain, M.I. Nutritional Analysis of two Local Varieties of Papaya (*Carica papaya* L.) at Different Maturation Stages. *Pak. J. Biol. Sci.* **2006**, *9*, 137–140. [CrossRef]
22. Bouanga-Kalou, G.; Kimboguila, A.; Nzikou, J.M.; Ganongo, P.F.B.; Moutoula, F.E.; Panyoo Akdowa, E.; Siliou, T.; Desobry, S. Extraction and characteristics of seed oil from Papaya (*Carica papaya*) in Congo-Brazzaville. *Asian J. Agric. Sci.* **2011**, *3*, 132–137.
23. Basu, A.; Haldar, S. Dietary isothiocyanate mediated apoptosis of human cancer cells is associated with Bcl-xL phosphorylation. *Int. J. Oncol.* **2008**, *33*, 657–663. [PubMed]
24. Ching, L.S.; Mohamed, S. Alpha-tocopherol content in 62 edible tropical plants. *J. Agric. Food Chem.* **2001**, *49*, 3101–3105. [CrossRef] [PubMed]
25. Miean, K.H.; Mohamed, S. Flavonoid (myricetin, quercetin, kaempferol, luteolin, and apigenin) content of edible tropical plants. *J. Agric. Food Chem.* **2001**, *49*, 3106–3112. [CrossRef] [PubMed]
26. Neuza, J.; Malacrida, C. Extratos de sementes de mamão (*Carica papaya* L.) como fonte de antioxidantes naturais. *Alim. Nutr. Araraquara* **2009**, *19*, 337–340.
27. Awodele, O.; Yemitan, O.; Ise, P.U.; Ikumawoyi, V.O. Modulatory potentials of aqueous leaf and unripe fruit extracts of *Carica papaya* Linn. (Caricaceae) against carbon tetrachloride and acetaminophen-induced hepatotoxicity in rats. *J. Intercult. Ethnopharmacol.* **2016**, *5*, 27–35. [CrossRef] [PubMed]
28. Pandit, A.; Sachdeva, T.; Bafna, P. Ameliorative effect of leaves of *Carica papaya* in ethanol and antitubercular drug induced hepatotoxicity. *Br. J. Pharm. Res.* **2013**, *3*, 648–661. [CrossRef]
29. Rajkapoor, B.; Jayakar, B.; Kavimani, S.; Murugesh, N. Effect of dried fruits of *Carica papaya* Linn on hepatotoxicity. *Biol. Pharm. Bull.* **2002**, *25*, 1645–1646. [CrossRef]
30. Sule, O.; Elekwa, I.; Joffa, P. Morphological and Biochemical Effects of Dried Leaves of *Carica papaya* Linn.(Pawpaw) on the Liver in Wistar Rats. *J. Pharm. Biomed. Sci.* **2012**, *15*, 1–5.
31. Sadeque, M.Z.; Begum, Z.A. Protective effect of dried fruits of *Carica papaya* on hepatotoxicity in rat. *Bangladesh J. Pharmacol.* **2010**, *5*, 48–50. [CrossRef]
32. Olagunju, J.; Adeneye, A.; Fagbohunka, B.; Bisuga, N.; Ketiku, A.; Benebo, A.; Olufowobi, O.; Adeoye, A.; Alimi, M.; Adeleke, A. Nephroprotective activities of the aqueous seed extract of *Carica papaya* Linn. In carbon tetrachloride induced renal injured Wistar rats: A dose-and time-dependent study. *Biol. Med.* **2009**, *1*, 11–19.
33. Anibijuwon, I.; Udeze, A. Antimicrobial activity of *Carica papaya* (pawpaw leaf) on some pathogenic organisms of clinical origin from South-Western Nigeria. *Ethnobot. Leafl.* **2009**, *2009*, 4.
34. Tona, L.; Kambu, K.; Ngimbi, N.; Cimanga, K.; Vlietinck, A.J. Antiamoebic and phytochemical screening of some Congolese medicinal plants. *J. Ethnopharmacol.* **1998**, *61*, 57–65. [CrossRef]
35. Okewumi, T.A.; Oyeyemi, A.W. Gastro-protective activity of aqueous *Carica papaya* seed extract on ethanol induced gastric ulcer in male rats. *Afr. J. Biotechnol.* **2012**, *11*, 8612–8615.
36. Adebiyi, A.; Adaikan, P.G. Modulation of jejunal contractions by extract of *Carica papaya* L. seeds. *Phytother. Res.* **2005**, *19*, 628–632. [CrossRef]
37. Owoyele, B.V.; Adebukola, O.M.; Funmilayo, A.A.; Soladoye, A.O. Anti-inflammatory activities of ethanolic extract of *Carica papaya* leaves. *Inflammopharmacology* **2008**, *16*, 168–173. [CrossRef]
38. Anyakudo, M.M.C.; Erinfolami, A.B. Glycemic and Wound Healing Effects of Aqueous Mesocarp Extract of Unripe *Carica papaya* (Linn) in Diabetic and Healthy Rats. *World J. Nutr. Health* **2015**, *3*, 47–52.

39. Kamer, E.; Recai Unalp, H.; Gundogan, O.; Diniz, G.; Ortac, R.; Olukman, M.; Derici, H.; Ali Onal, M. Effect of ascorbic acid on incisional wound healing in streptozotocin-induced diabetic rats. *Wounds* **2010**, *22*, 27–31. [PubMed]
40. WHO. Obesity and Overweight. Available online: https://www.who.int/news-room/fact-sheets/detail/obesity-and-overweight (accessed on 24 April 2019).
41. Rodriguez-Lopez, C.P.; Gonzalez-Torres, M.C.; Cruz-Bautista, I.; Najera-Medina, O. Visceral obesity, skeletal muscle mass and resistin in metabolic syndrome development. *Nutr. Hosp.* **2019**, *36*, 43–50. [CrossRef]
42. Asrih, M.; Jornayvaz, F.R. Metabolic syndrome and nonalcoholic fatty liver disease: Is insulin resistance the link? *Mol. Cell. Endocrinol.* **2015**, *418*, 55–65. [CrossRef]
43. Esposito, K.; Chiodini, P.; Colao, A.; Lenzi, A.; Giugliano, D. Metabolic syndrome and risk of cancer: A systematic review and meta-analysis. *Diabetes Care* **2012**, *35*, 2402–2411. [CrossRef] [PubMed]
44. Quagliariello, V.; Rossetti, S.; Cavaliere, C.; Di Palo, R.; Lamantia, E.; Castaldo, L.; Nocertinos, F.; Ametranos, G.; Cappuccio, F.; Malzone, M.M.; et al. Metabolic syndrome, endocrine disruptors and prostate cancer associations: Biochemical and pathophysiological evidences. *Oncotarget* **2017**, *8*, 30606–30616. [CrossRef] [PubMed]
45. Samson, S.L.; Garber, A.J. Metabolic syndrome. *Endocrinol. Metab Clin. N. Am.* **2014**, *43*, 1–23. [CrossRef] [PubMed]
46. Anderson, E.J.; Lustig, M.E.; Boyle, K.E.; Woodlief, T.L.; Kane, D.A.; Lin, C.T.; Price, J.W., III; Kang, L.; Rabinovitch, P.S.; Szeto, H.H.; et al. Mitochondrial H_2O_2 emission and cellular redox state link excess fat intake to insulin resistance in both rodents and humans. *J. Clin. Investig.* **2009**, *119*, 573–581. [CrossRef] [PubMed]
47. Ando, K.; Fujita, T. Metabolic syndrome and oxidative stress. *Free Radic. Biol. Med.* **2009**, *47*, 213–218. [CrossRef] [PubMed]
48. Feillet-Coudray, C.; Fouret, G.; Vigor, C.; Bonafos, B.; Jover, B.; Blachnio-Zabielska, A.; Rieusset, J.; Casas, F.; Gaillet, S.; Landrier, J.F.; et al. Long-Term Measures of Dyslipidemia, Inflammation, and Oxidative Stress in Rats Fed a High-Fat/High-Fructose Diet. *Lipids* **2019**, *54*, 81–97. [CrossRef]
49. Ottaiano, A.; Nappi, A.; Tafuto, S.; Nasti, G.; De Divitiis, C.; Romano, C.; Cassata, A.; Casaretti, R.; Silvestro, L.; Avallone, A.; et al. Diabetes and body mass index are associated with neuropathy and prognosis in colon cancer patients treated with capecitabine and oxaliplatin adjuvant chemotherapy. *Oncology* **2016**, *90*, 36–42. [CrossRef] [PubMed]
50. Adeneye, A.; Olagunju, J. Preliminary hypoglycemic and hypolipidemic activities of the aqueous seed extract of *Carica papaya* Linn in Wistar rats. *Biol. Med.* **2009**, *1*, 1–10.
51. Omonkhua, A.A.; Onoagbe, I.O. Long-term hepatotoxicity and hypoglycaemic study of aqueous extracts of *Carica papaya* leaves on normal rabbits. *Glob. J. Pure Appl. Sci.* **2011**, *17*, 241–247.
52. Adenowo, A.F.; Ilori, M.F.; Balogun, F.O.; Kazeem, M.I. Protective effect of ethanol leaf extract of *Carica papaya* Linn (Caricaceae) in alloxan-induced diabetic rats. *Trop. J. Pharm. Res.* **2014**, *13*, 1877–1882. [CrossRef]
53. Johnson, O.R.; Samuel, S.; Elnathan, W.D.; John, M.H. Biochemical effect of Aqueous *Carica papaya* Seed and Leaf Extracts on Serum Biochemistry of Alloxan Induced Diabetic Rats. *IOSR J. Pharm. Biol. Sci.* **2015**, *10*, 18–22.
54. Maniyar, Y.; Bhixavatimath, P. Antihyperglycemic and hypolipidemic activities of aqueous extract of *Carica papaya* Linn. leaves in alloxan-induced diabetic rats. *J. Ayurveda Integr. Med.* **2012**, *3*, 70–74. [CrossRef] [PubMed]
55. Ezekwe, A.S.; Elekwa, I.; Osuocha, K. Hypoglycemic, hypolipidemic and body weight effects of unripe pulp of *Carica papaya* using diabetic Albino rat model. *J. Pharm. Phytochem.* **2014**, *2*, 109–114.
56. Ezekwe, S.A.; Chikezie, P.C. GC-MS Analysis, Hypoglycemic Activity of Aqueous Root Extract of *Carica papaya* and Its Effects on Blood Lipid Profile and Hepatorenal Tissues Biomarkers of Diabetic Rats. *J. Diabetes Metab.* **2017**, *8*, 5. [CrossRef]
57. Fakeye, T.O.; Oladipupo, T.; Showande, O.; Ogunremi, Y. Effects of Coadministration of Extract of *Carica papaya* Linn (family Cariaceae) on Activity of Two Oral Hypoglycemic Agents. *Trop. J. Pharm. Res.* **2007**, *6*, 671–678. [CrossRef]
58. Sasidharan, S.; Sumathi, V.; Jegathambigai, N.R.; Latha, L.Y. Antihyperglycaemic effects of ethanol extracts of *Carica papaya* and Pandanus amaryfollius leaf in streptozotocin-induced diabetic mice. *Nat. Prod. Res.* **2011**, *25*, 1982–1987. [CrossRef] [PubMed]

59. Juarez-Rojop, I.E.; Diaz-Zagoya, J.C.; Ble-Castillo, J.L.; Miranda-Osorio, P.H.; Castell-Rodriguez, A.E.; Tovilla-Zarate, C.A.; Rodriguez-Hernandez, A.; Aguilar-Mariscal, H.; Ramon-Frias, T.; Bermudez-Ocana, D.Y. Hypoglycemic effect of *Carica papaya* leaves in streptozotocin-induced diabetic rats. *BMC Complement Altern. Med.* **2012**, *12*, 236. [CrossRef]
60. Juárez-Rojop, I.E.; A.Tovilla-Zárate, C.; Aguilar-Domínguez, D.E.; Roa-de la Fuentec, L.F.; Lobato-García, C.E.; Blé-Castillo, J.L.; López-Meraz, L.; Díaz-Zagoya, J.C.; Bermúdez-Ocaña, D.Y. Phytochemical screening and hypoglycemic activity of *Carica papaya* leaf in streptozotocin-induced diabetic rats. *Rev. Bras. Farmacogn.* **2014**, *24*, 341–347.
61. Miranda-Osorio, P.H.; Castell-Rodriguez, A.E.; Vargas-Mancilla, J.; Tovilla-Zarate, C.A.; Ble-Castillo, J.L.; Aguilar-Dominguez, D.E.; Juarez-Rojop, I.E.; Diaz-Zagoya, J.C. Protective Action of *Carica papaya* on beta-Cells in Streptozotocin-Induced Diabetic Rats. *Int. J. Environ. Res. Public Health* **2016**, *13*, 446. [CrossRef]
62. Hamden, K.; Jaouadi, B.; Zarai, N.; Rebai, T.; Carreau, S.; Elfeki, A. Inhibitory effects of estrogens on digestive enzymes, insulin deficiency, and pancreas toxicity in diabetic rats. *J. Physiol. Biochem.* **2011**, *67*, 121–128. [CrossRef]
63. Liu, S.Z.; Deng, Y.X.; Chen, B.; Zhang, X.J.; Shi, Q.Z.; Qiu, X.M. Antihyperglycemic effect of the traditional Chinese scutellaria-coptis herb couple and its main components in streptozotocin-induced diabetic rats. *J. Ethnopharmacol.* **2013**, *145*, 490–498. [CrossRef] [PubMed]
64. Matsui, T.; Tanaka, T.; Tamura, S.; Toshima, A.; Tamaya, K.; Miyata, Y.; Tanaka, K.; Matsumoto, K. alpha-Glucosidase inhibitory profile of catechins and theaflavins. *J. Agric. Food Chem.* **2007**, *55*, 99–105. [CrossRef] [PubMed]
65. Gray, A.M.; Abdel-Wahab, Y.H.; Flatt, P.R. The traditional plant treatment, Sambucus nigra (elder), exhibits insulin-like and insulin-releasing actions in vitro. *J. Nutr.* **2000**, *130*, 15–20. [CrossRef] [PubMed]
66. Oboh, G.; Olabiyi, A.A.; Akinyemi, A.J.; Ademiluyi, A.O. Inhibition of key enzymes linked to type 2 diabetes and sodium nitroprusside-induced lipid peroxidation in rat pancreas by water-extractable phytochemicals from unripe pawpaw fruit (*Carica papaya*). *J. Basic Clin. Physiol. Pharmacol.* **2014**, *25*, 21–34. [CrossRef] [PubMed]
67. Adefegha, A.S.; Oboh, G.; Akinyemi, A.J.; Ademiluyi, A.O. Inhibitory effects of aqueous extract of two varieties of ginger on some key enzymes linked to type-2 diabetes in vitro. *J. Food Nutr. Res.* **2010**, *49*, 14–20.
68. Shim, Y.J.; Doo, H.K.; Ahn, S.Y.; Kim, Y.S.; Seong, J.K.; Park, I.S.; Min, B.H. Inhibitory effect of aqueous extract from the gall of Rhus chinensis on alpha-glucosidase activity and postprandial blood glucose. *J. Ethnopharmacol.* **2003**, *85*, 283–287. [CrossRef]
69. Baynes, J.W. Role of oxidative stress in development of complications in diabetes. *Diabetes* **1991**, *40*, 405–412. [CrossRef]
70. Ceriello, A. Oxidative stress and glycemic regulation. *Metabolism* **2000**, *49*, 27–29. [CrossRef]
71. Beckman, J.S.; Koppenol, W.H. Nitric oxide, superoxide, and peroxynitrite: The good, the bad, and ugly. *Am. J. Physiol.* **1996**, *271*, C1424–C1437. [CrossRef]
72. Pacher, P.; Szabo, C. Role of the peroxynitrite-poly(ADP-ribose) polymerase pathway in human disease. *Am. J. Pathol.* **2008**, *173*, 2–13. [CrossRef]
73. Amić, D.; Davidović-Amić, D.; Bešlo, D.; Trinajstić, N. Structure-radical scavenging activity relationships of flavonoids. *Croat. Chem. Acta* **2003**, *76*, 55–61.
74. Salla, S.; Sunkara, R.; Ogutu, S.; Walker, L.T.; Verghese, M. Antioxidant activity of papaya seed extracts against H2O2 induced oxidative stress in HepG2 cells. *LWT Food Sci. Technol.* **2016**, *66*, 293–297. [CrossRef]
75. Hasimun, P.; Sulaeman, A.; Mahakam, H.; Esde, S. Potential Role of *Carica papaya* Leaves in Regulating Cholesterol as Inhibitor HMG COA Reductase in the Liver on Wistar Rats Hyperlipidemia. *Int. J. Pharm. Phytochem. Res.* **2018**, *10*, 317–321.
76. Canini, A.; Alesiani, D.; D'Arcangelo, G.; Tagliatesta, P. Gas chromatography–mass spectrometry analysis of phenolic compounds from *Carica papaya* L. leaf. *J. Food Compos. Anal.* **2007**, *20*, 584–590. [CrossRef]
77. Leopoldini, M.; Malaj, N.; Toscano, M.; Sindona, G.; Russo, N. On the inhibitor effects of bergamot juice flavonoids binding to the 3-hydroxy-3-methylglutaryl-CoA reductase (HMGR) enzyme. *J. Agric. Food Chem.* **2010**, *58*, 10768–10773. [CrossRef] [PubMed]
78. Nwangwa, E.; Ekhoye, E. Anti-hyperlipidemic activity of aqueous extract of *Carica papaya* seed in albino rats fed with high fat diet. *Curr. Trends Technol. Sci.* **2013**, *3*, 262–266.

79. Brasil, G.A.; Ronchi, S.N.; do Nascimento, A.M.; de Lima, E.M.; Romao, W.; da Costa, H.B.; Scherer, R.; Ventura, J.A.; Lenz, D.; Bissoli, N.S.; et al. Antihypertensive effect of *Carica papaya* via a reduction in ACE activity and improved baroreflex. *Planta Med.* **2014**, *80*, 1580–1587. [CrossRef]
80. Guyton, A.C.; Hall, J.E.; Lohmeier, T.E.; Jackson, T.E.; Kastner, P.R. Blood pressure regulation: Basic concepts. *Fed. Proc.* **1981**, *40*, 2252–2256.
81. Franquni, J.V.; do Nascimento, A.M.; de Lima, E.M.; Brasil, G.A.; Heringer, O.A.; Cassaro, K.O.; da Cunha, T.V.; Musso, C.; Silva Santos, M.C.; Kalil, I.C.; et al. Nandrolone decanoate determines cardiac remodelling and injury by an imbalance in cardiac inflammatory cytokines and ACE activity, blunting of the Bezold-Jarisch reflex, resulting in the development of hypertension. *Steroids* **2013**, *78*, 379–385. [CrossRef]
82. Minami, N.; Head, G.A. Relationship between cardiovascular hypertrophy and cardiac baroreflex function in spontaneously hypertensive and stroke-prone rats. *J. Hypertens.* **1993**, *11*, 523–533. [CrossRef]
83. Balasuriya, N.; Rupasinghe, H.P. Antihypertensive properties of flavonoid-rich apple peel extract. *Food Chem.* **2012**, *135*, 2320–2325. [CrossRef] [PubMed]
84. Guerrero, L.; Castillo, J.; Quinones, M.; Garcia-Vallve, S.; Arola, L.; Pujadas, G.; Muguerza, B. Inhibition of angiotensin-converting enzyme activity by flavonoids: Structure-activity relationship studies. *PLoS ONE* **2012**, *7*, e49493. [CrossRef] [PubMed]
85. Eno, A.E.; Owo, O.I.; Itam, E.H.; Konya, R.S. Blood pressure depression by the fruit juice of *Carica papaya* (L.) in renal and DOCA-induced hypertension in the rat. *Phytother. Res.* **2000**, *14*, 235–239. [CrossRef]
86. Grobecker, H.; Saavedra, J.; Roizen, M.; Weise, V.; Kopin, I.; Axelrod, J. *Peripheral and Central Catecholaminergic Neurons in Genetic and Experimental Hypertension in Rats*; Portland Press Limited: London, UK, 1976.
87. Osunkwo, U.; Eferakeya, A. Plasma-Catecholamine levels during development of doca, renal and spontaneous hypertension in rats. *Med. Sci. Res. Biochem.* **1987**, *15*, 971–972.
88. Osunkwo, U.; Eferakeya, A. Attenuated hypothalamic secondary pressor responsiveness and the effect of gallopamil or hydrallazine in DOCA-salt and renal hypertensive rats. *Niger. J. Physiol. Sci.* **1994**, *1*, 1–5.

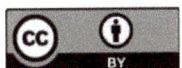 © 2019 by the authors. Licensee MDPI, Basel, Switzerland. This article is an open access article distributed under the terms and conditions of the Creative Commons Attribution (CC BY) license (http://creativecommons.org/licenses/by/4.0/).

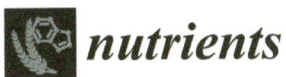

Article

Use of an Extract of *Annona muricata* Linn to Prevent High-Fat Diet Induced Metabolic Disorders in C57BL/6 Mice [†]

Sandramara Sasso [1], Priscilla Cristovam Sampaio e Souza [2], Lidiani Figueiredo Santana [1], Claudia Andréa Lima Cardoso [3], Flávio Macedo Alves [4], Luciane Candeloro Portugal [4], Bernardo Bacelar de Faria [5], Anderson Fernandes da Silva [1], Ana Rita Coimbra Motta-Castro [6,7], Luana Silva Soares [6], Larissa Melo Bandeira [6], Rita de Cássia Avellaneda Guimarães [1] and Karine de Cássia Freitas [1,*]

1. Posgraduate Program in Health and Development in the Midwest Region, Medical School, Federal University of Mato Grosso do Sul, Campo Grande, 79070-900 Mato Grosso do Sul, Brazil
2. Faculty of Pharmaceutical Sciences, Food and Nutrition, Federal University of Mato Grosso do Sul, Campo Grande, 79070-900 Mato Grosso do Sul, Brazil
3. Course of Chemistry, State University of Mato Grosso do Sul, Dourados, 79070-900 Mato Grosso do Sul, Brazil
4. Institute of Biosciences, Federal University of Mato Grosso do Sul, Campo Grande, 79070-900 Mato Grosso do Sul, Brazil
5. Medicina Diagnóstica Laboratory-Scapulatempo, Campo Grande, 79002-170 Mato Grosso do Sul, Brazil
6. Laboratory of Clinical Immunology, Faculty of Pharmaceutical Sciences, Food and Nutrition, Federal University of Mato Grosso do Sul, Campo Grande, 79070-900 Mato Grosso do Sul, Brazil
7. Oswaldo Cruz Foundation, Campo Grande, 79074-460 Mato Grosso do Sul, Brazil
* Correspondence: kcfreitas@gmail.com; Tel.: +55-67-3345-7882
† This paper is an extended version of master's thesis of the former student Sandramara Sasso.

Received: 4 May 2019; Accepted: 30 June 2019; Published: 2 July 2019

Abstract: *Annona muricata* Linn, commonly known as graviola, is one of the most popular plants used in Brazil for weight loss. The aim of this study is to evaluate the therapeutic effects of three different doses (50 mg/kg, 100 mg/kg, and 150 mg/kg) of aqueous graviola leaf extract (AGE) supplemented by oral gavage, on obese C57BL/6 mice. Food intake, body weight, an oral glucose tolerance test (OGTT), an insulin sensitivity test, quantification of adipose tissue cytokines, weight of fat pads, and serum biochemical and histological analyses of the liver, pancreas, and epididymal adipose tissue were measured. AGE had an anti-inflammatory effect by increasing IL-10 at doses of 50 and 100 mg/kg. Regarding the cholesterol profile, there was a significant decrease in LDL-cholesterol levels in the AGE 150 group, and VLDL-cholesterol and triglycerides in the AGE 100 and 150 groups. There was an increase in HDL cholesterol in the AGE 150 group. The extract was able to reduce the adipocyte area of the epididymal adipose tissue in the AGE 100 and 150 groups. According to the histological analysis of the liver and pancreas, no significant difference was found among the groups. There were no significant effects of AGE on OGTT and serum fasting glucose concentration. However, the extract was effective in improving glucose tolerance in the AGE 150 group.

Keywords: graviola; weight loss; obesity

1. Introduction

Obesity is a worldwide public health problem. It increases the risk of metabolic diseases such as hypercholesterolemia, hypertriglyceridemia, insulin resistance, heart disease, type 2 diabetes, atherosclerosis, and cancer [1,2].

The etiology of obesity is complex and multifactorial. Obesity results from the interaction of genetic/epigenetic, environmental, emotional, lifestyle factors and that technically obesity results from a positive energy balance: More energy intake than energy expenditure [3]. Although genetic factors are determinant in the development of obesity, metabolic factors, an unhealthy diet, and a sedentary lifestyle provide conditions for the development of this disorder [4].

Obesity is an increased deposition of white adipose tissue and phenotypic changes in this tissue. It is associated with metabolic changes such as increased production of pro-inflammatory mediators. This leads to organs dysfunction and chronic low-grade inflammation with high levels of proinflammatory cytokines, such as interleukin-6 (IL-6) and tumor necrosis factor-α (TNF-α), and chemokines, such as monocyte chemotactic protein 1 (MCP1), which in turn promotes migration of macrophages into the adipose tissue and increases the release of cytokines. In parallel, low levels of interleukin 10 (IL-10) are observed in obese individuals, and worsens their metabolic profile, since IL-10 inhibits the synthesis of pro-inflammatory cytokines [2,5–8].

To control such abnormalities, several methods have been suggested to regulate obesity and weight gain, including agents that could inhibit fat absorption, control biochemical parameters, such as, serum glucose, serum triglyceride, total cholesterol, high-density lipoprotein (HDL), low-density lipoprotein (LDL), and very low-density lipoprotein (VLDL) levels, reduce systemic inflammation, and induce weight loss [9]. Medicinal plants, popularly indicated for the treatment of obesity, have been used in many countries to control weight gain and obesity [10].

For these reasons, anti-obesity agents, including infusions and extracts, are widely used for weight control in obese individuals, in addition to reducing biochemical parameters [11].

Tropical countries have a wide variety of flora and a high number of food and medicinal plants. There is information available on the potential functional properties of several of these plants [12]. The investigation of such properties may be of interest for both the pharmaceutical and the food industry [13].

Among the species of pharmaceutical interest, the leaf of *Annona muricata* Linn (Annonaceae), commonly known as soursop or graviola, is used routinely for weight control. It is used in traditional medicine as an antihypertensive, vasodilator, antidiabetic, and hypolipidemic agent due to the presence of several bioactive compounds, such as acetogenins, flavonoids, tannins, alkaloids, coumarins, and terpenoids [14,15]. Therefore, considering the popular use of tea from graviola leaves to prevent obesity and its complications, it is important to verify whether treatment using an aqueous extract of *Annona muricata* Linn could also be beneficial for the treatment of obesity. Thus, the objective of this study is to verify the effects of three different doses of aqueous extract of *Annona muricata* on obese C57BL/6 mice induced by a high-fat diet.

2. Materials and Methods

2.1. Extraction of Plant Material

Leaves of *Annona muricata* Linn were collected in June 2015 from an adult specimen that produces flowers and fruits, in the municipality of Campo Grande, Mato Grosso do Sul state, Brazil. The tree was properly identified. The geographical coordinates defined by manual GPS were 22°29′42.6″ S and 054°37′1.6″ W. A voucher specimen (number 53,928) was deposited at the Herbarium CGMS of the Federal University of Mato Grosso do Sul, Brazil. The extract of leaves of *Annona muricata* Linn was prepared by immersing 1 kg of leaf powder into 3 L of distilled water for 48 h, then lyophilizing this until a dry powder was obtained. Then, the extract was stored at room temperature and protected from light until use [14].

2.2. Quantification of Total Phenols and Flavonoids

The total phenols of aqueous graviola leaf extract (AGE) were determined by the Folin-Ciocalteu reagent method [16]. Samples and a standard curve of gallic acid were read at 760 nm. The result was expressed as mg of gallic acid per g of extract. For the quantification of the flavonoids, the colorimetric method of aluminum chloride was used [17]. The absorbances were read at 415 nm with a UV-Vis spectrophotometer. To calculate the concentration of flavonoids, an analytical curve was prepared using quercetin as standard. The results are expressed as mg quercetin per g of extract.

2.3. Quantification of Condensed Tannins

The extract was dissolved in water at a concentration of 50 µg·mL^{-1} using the valinine reaction [18]. The absorbance reading was performed using a spectrophotometer at 510 nm. The quantification was performed using an external calibration curve with catechin as standard. The results are expressed as mg equivalent of catechin per g of extract.

2.4. Assay of Antioxidant Activity Using the 2,2-Diphenyl-1-Picrylhydrazyl Free Radical (DPPH)

The sequestering capacity was measured using DPPH solution. The absorbances were read at 517 nm with a spectrophotometer. The percentage of DPPH radical sequestration inhibition was calculated according to the equation:

$$\text{Percent inhibition activity (\%)} = [(A0 - A1)/A0]\, 100 \qquad (1)$$

where A_0 is the absorbance of the control, and A_1 is the absorbance in the presence of the compound. Subsequently, the mean inhibitory concentration (IC 50) was calculated. It represents the concentration of the sample required to capture 50% of the DPPH [19].

2.5. Isolation and Identification of Compounds

The extract was fractionated by XAD-2 (Supelco, Bellefonte, PA, USA) on column chromatography (30 cm × 3 cm). The extract (3.16 g) was eluted with 0.5 L of water, followed by 0.5 L of methanol, and again eluted with 0.2 L of ethyl acetate. An aliquot of 0.89 g of the methanolic fraction was dissolved into 50 mL of methanol and fractionated by chromatography using a Sephadex LH-20 (Amersham Pharmacia Biotech, Uppsala, Sweden) on column chromatography (70 cm × 3 cm) at a rate of 0.2 mL·min^{-1}. Twenty-five fractions of 2 mL were collected. The fractions were combined according to their chemical behavior on thin layer chromatography (silica gel plates) using ethyl acetate:n-propanol:water (123:7:70 v/v/v) as the eluent. The fractions 2–4, 6–8 and 11–14 were purified using polyvinylpolypyrrolidone (Sigma, St. Louis, MO, USA) on column chromatography (10 cm × 2 cm) by eluting them with methanol. The result is the identification of compounds. An aliquot of 0.54 g of the ethyl acetate fraction was dissolved into 10 mL of methanol and fractionated by chromatography using a Sephadex LH-20 (Amersham Pharmacia Biotech, Uppsala, Sweden) on column chromatography (80 cm × 2 cm) by eluting it with methanol at a rate of 0.3 mL·min^{-1}. Twenty-eight fractions of 5 mL were collected. The fractions were combined according to their chemical behavior on thin layer chromatography (silica gel plates) using ethyl acetate:methanol (60:40 v/v) as the eluent. The fractions 10–13, 18–19 and 22–25 resulted in the isolation of the other compounds. The identification of the compounds was carried out using ^{1}H and ^{13}C nuclear resonance (Advance 300 MHz, Brucher, Ettlingen, Germany) and mass spectrometry (Shimadzu Corp. Shimadzu, Kyoto). Their chemical structures were confirmed by comparison with literature data [20–22].

2.6. Ethics Statement

All animal experiments were submitted and approved by the Ethics Committee on Animal Use, Federal University of Mato Grosso do Sul (Protocol n°. 682/2015).

2.7. Acute Oral Toxicity

The acute toxicity test of the AGE was performed in female Wistar rats (*Rattus norvegicus*) based on the OECD Guidelines 425 (Organization for Economic Co-operation and Development) [23]. For the test, the animals were divided into two groups (n = 5): A control group that received saline solution, and the treatment group that received the aqueous extract of *Annona muricata* Linn orally (gavage) at a dose of 2000 mg/kg. After treatment, the animals were observed at 30 min, 1 h, 2 h, 3 h, 4 h, 6 h, 12 h, 24 h, and then daily for 14 days.

At the same time, the hippocratic screening test was carried out to quantify the effects of abnormal morphological and behavioral signs of toxicity. Furthermore, changes in body weight, water and food intake, as well as excreta production, were also evaluated [24].

At the end of 14 days, the animals were euthanized (ketamine and xylazine). The organs (heart, lung, liver, spleen, pancreas, and kidneys) were removed, weighed, and analyzed macroscopically to investigate possible changes [25].

2.8. Animals and Experimental Design

C57BL/6 adult male mice (n = 55, 12 weeks of age) were divided into two groups based on body weight, as follows: SHAM group (n = 11), treated with standard diet AIN-93M [26], and HFD group (n = 44), treated with a hyperlipidic diet. After 12 weeks, the animals of the HFD group were divided into four homogenous groups according to weight and value of fasting blood glucose and concomitantly supplemented (oral gavage) with aqueous graviola leaf extract in different doses: HFD SALINE group (HFD + saline), AGE 50 mg/kg group (HFD + aqueous graviola leaf extract of 50 mg/kg) (n = 11), AGE 100 mg/kg group (HFD + aqueous graviola leaf extract of 100 mg/kg) (n = 11), and AGE 150 mg/kg group (HFD + aqueous graviola leaf extract of 150 mg/kg) (n = 11). The SHAM group also received saline solution at this stage of the study. Each group had ad libitum access to water and food during the experimental period. The composition of the experimental diets is show in the Table 1 below.

Table 1. Composition of experimental diets (g/kg diet).

Experimental Groups	AIN-93M Diet	High-Fat Diet (HFD)
Composition (g/kg)		
Cornstarch	620.69	320.69
Casein	140.00	140.00
Fat	-	320.00
Sucrose	100.00	100.00
Soybean oil	40.00	20.00
Fiber	50.00	50.00
Mineral mix	35.00	35.00
Vitamin mix	10.00	10.00
L-cystine	1.80	1.80
Choline bitartrate	2.50	2.50
Tert-butylhydroquinone	0.008	0.008
Energy (kcal/kg)	3802.8	5302.8
Carbohydrates (%)	75.81	31.73
Protein (%)	14.73	10.56
Lipids (%)	9.47	57.71
Calories/g of diet	3.80	5.30

The mice were anesthetized (Ketamine and xylazine, 75 and 10 mg/kg, respectively), and euthanized by cardiac puncture when they reached 35 weeks of age. The blood and the organs were collected for subsequent analyses.

2.9. Body Weight and Diet Intake

The mice were weighed weekly to observe weight changes until the end of the study. Food intake was measured three times per week.

The energy intake was calculated by multiplying the amount of diet ingested (g/day/animal) by the energy density of each diet, expressed in kcal/day per animal. In addition, the calculation of the feed efficiency index (FEI) was performed using the following equation:

$$\text{Free efficiency index} = \frac{(FW - IW)}{TF} \qquad (2)$$

where FW is the final body weight in grams, IW is the initial body weight in grams, and TF is the total amount of food ingested in grams [27].

2.10. Biochemical Analysis

Serum glucose, serum triglyceride, total cholesterol, high-density lipoprotein (HDL), low-density lipoprotein (LDL), and very low-density lipoprotein (VLDL) levels were analyzed by the enzymatic colorimetric test, according to the manufacturer's instructions (Labtest®, Lagoa Santa, Minas Gerais, Brazil). The atherogenic index was determined by the ratio between total cholesterol and HDL cholesterol [14].

2.11. Oral Glucose Tolerance Test

The oral glucose tolerance test (OGTT) was performed one day prior to initiating treatment with the AGE or saline solution, and three days prior to the euthanasia of animals after six hours of fasting. Fasting glucose was verified via flow rate (time 0) using a G-Tech® glucometer (G-TECH Free, Infopia Co., Ltd. South Korea). Then, the animals received a D-glucose solution (Sigma Aldrich, Duque de Caxias, Rio de Janeiro, Brazil), at 2 g/kg of body weight, by gavage. A blood glucose reading was performed 15, 30, 60 and 120 min after glucose application. The area under the curve (AUC) was calculated for each mouse, and the mean was calculated for each experimental group [28].

2.12. Insulin Sensitivity Test

The insulin sensitivity test was performed five days before euthanasia. Glycemia was verified with the animals in a fed state (time 0). Then, 0.75 units of insulin (NovoRapid®, 100 U/mL, Novo Nordisk, Bagsvaerd, Denmark) per kg of animal weight was injected intraperitoneally. The blood glucose reading was performed at 15, 30 and 60 min using a G-Tech® glucometer (G-TECH Free, Korea). The area under the curve (AUC) was calculated for each animal, and the mean was calculated for each experimental group [28].

2.13. Quantification of Cytokines in the Adipose Tissue

Epididymal adipose tissue was collected, weighed (100 mg) and stored at −80 °C. For protein extraction, the epididymal adipose tissue was thawed on ice and homogenized in 1 mL of RIPA (RIPA Lysis Buffer, 10×, Cat. n°. 20–188, MERCK, Darmstadt, Germany). A cocktail of protease inhibitors was added (Protease Inhibitor Cocktail Set Calbiochem, Cat. n°. 539131, MERCK, Darmstadt, Germany).

The supernatant was collected after centrifugation at 4 °C and stored again at −80 °C until cytokine analysis, according to the recommendations of the manufacturer (MILLIPLEX MAP/Mouse Cytokine/Chemokine and Adipocyte Magnetic Bead panel) (Millipore, Billerica, MA, USA). The concentrations of the following cytokines were analyzed: IL-10, IL-6, MCP-1, and TNF-α using the MCYTOMAG-70K kit, and adiponectin using the MADCYMAG-72K kit. The concentration of the cytokines IL-10, IL-6, MCP-1, and TNF-α in the adipose tissue was expressed as cytokine picograms in relation to protein content (mg of protein). For adiponectin, the values were expressed as nanograms of cytokines in relation to protein content (mg of protein). Protein quantification was based on the bicinchoninic acid assay (BCA) following the manufacturer's recommendations (BCA Protein Assay kit) (MERCK, Darmstadt, Germany) [29,30].

2.14. Assessment of Body Fat and Liver Weight

After euthanasia, the liver and fat pads of white adipose tissue (omental, epididymal, perirenal, retroperitoneal, and mesenteric) were dissected and weighed. The adiposity index was calculated as the total sum of visceral white adipose tissue (g) divided by the final body weight of the animal × 100 and expressed as percentage of adiposity [31].

2.15. Histopathological Analysis

Samples of the liver, pancreas, and epididymal adipose tissue were fixed with 10% formalin solution. After fixation, the specimens were dehydrated, embedded in paraffin, cut in a microtome to a thickness of 5 mm each, and stained with hematoxylin-eosin. An expert pathologist performed the histological analysis of the liver and pancreas. For the analysis of treatment effects on the hepatocytes, a scoring system was used [32]. In the evaluation of the architecture of the pancreas, there were changes in the Islets of Langerhans and pancreatic acini, and inflammation was observed [33,34]. For the analysis of the adipocyte area of the epididymal adipose tissue, the images were initially taken using a LEICA DFC 495 digital camera system (Leica Microsystems, Wetzlar, Germany) integrated into a LEICA DM 5500B microscope (Leica Microsystems, Wetzlar, Germany), with a magnification of 20X. The images were analyzed using the LEICA Application Suite software, version 4.0 (Leica Microsystems, Wetzlar, Germany), and the mean area of 100 adipocytes per sample was determined [35].

2.16. Statistical Analyses

The results were expressed as mean ± MSE (mean standard error). For multiple comparisons of parametric results, an ANOVA followed by a Tukey post-test were performed. The Student t-test was performed for comparison between two groups. The chi-square test was used to evaluate associations in histological analyses. A significance level of $p < 0.05$ was adopted. Statistical analysis was performed using the software Jandel Sigma Stat, version 3.5 (Systat software, Incs., San Jose, CA, USA), and Sigma Plot, version 12.5 (Systat Software Inc., San Jose, CA, USA).

3. Results

3.1. Chemical Composition

The content of phenols, flavonoids, and tannins in AGE was 156.37 ± 1.2 mg/g, 92.07 ± 1.8 mg/g and 42.99 ± 0.6 mg/g, respectively. The antioxidant activity of IC_{50} was 12 ± 0.1 µg·mL^{-1}. In addition, six compounds were isolated and identified in the extract: kaempferol-3-O-a-l-rhamnopyranoside, quercetin 3-O-rutinoside, kaempferol 3-O-rutinoside, luteolin, quercetin, and sitosterol-3-O-β-D-glucopyranoside.

3.2. Acute Oral Toxicity

The results showed no signs of systemic toxicity. There are no changes in body weight, water consumption, food intake, and excretion of urine and feces. In addition, no changes in the Hippocratic screening test were observed, such as motor and/or sensory and neurological changes, as no animals died. The weight of the liver, spleen, pancreas, lungs, heart, and kidneys did not show significant differences among groups. Macroscopic changes in the organs of the animals were not visualized (Supplementary Material Figure S1).

3.3. Effects of AGE on Body Weight and Food Intake

At the beginning of the experiment, the animals in the HFD group did not present significant differences in body weight when compared to animals in the SHAM group ($p = 0.971$) (Table 2).

Table 2. Initial and final weight, weight gain and food intake assessment during obesity induction between the first and the 12th week.

Parameter	Experimental Group	
	SHAM (n = 11)	HFD (n = 44)
Initial weight (g)	26.55 ± 0.55	26.52 ± 0.28
Final weight (g)	32.91 ± 0.99	37.87 ± 0.60 ***
Weight gain (g)	6.36 ± 0.95	11.34 ± 0.68 **
Food intake (g/day)	3.47 ± 0.05	2.73 ± 0.03 ***
Food intake (kcal/day)	13.18 ± 0.19	14.54 ± 0.16 ***
Feed efficiency index	0.0216 ± 0.0031	0.0501 ± 0.0033 ***

SHAM: Standard diet. HFD: Hyperlipidic diet. Values represent the mean ± mean standard error;, ** $p \leq 0.01$, *** $p \leq 0.001$ vs. SHAM SALINE. Student t test.

However, with the HFD, the weight evolution evidenced a greater gain of body weight in the HFD group, with maintenance of a significant difference from the fourth week up to the 12th week ($p = 0.005$) compared to the control group ($p \leq 0.001$) (Figure 1A).

Then, the animals of groups receiving a hyperlipidic diet began treatments with different doses of the extract or saline solution. At the 12th week, there was a significant difference in body weight in relation to the SHAM SALINE group (Table 3). However, this difference was not stable throughout the treatment. At the end of the 24th week, this group had a statistically similar body weight compared to the other groups (Figure 1B).

Table 3. Initial and final weight, weight gain, and food intake of control animals and animals treated with AGE between the 13th and the 24th week.

Parameter	Experimental Group				
	SHAM SALINE	HFD SALINE	AGE 50	AGE 100	AGE 150
Initial weight (g)	32.89 ± 0.94	38.09 ± 1.42 *	37.91 ± 1.09 *	37.82 ± 0.91 *	37.64 ± 1.43 *
Final weight (g)	35.91 ± 1.26	40.27 ± 1.42	37.82 ± 1.05	36.82 ± 1.33	38.27 ± 1.94
Weight gain (g)	3.09 ± 0.60	2.18 ± 0.26	−0.09 ± 0.53 *	−1.00 ± 1.14 **,§	0.64 ± 0.92
Food intake (g/day)	3.40 ± 0.43	2.62 ± 0.62 ***	2.76 ± 0.05 ***	2.70 ± 0.98 ***	2.83 ± 0.07 ***
Food intake (kcal/day)	12.89 ± 0.16	13.89 ± 0.33	14.65 ± 0.25 **	14.30 ± 0.52 *	14.99 ± 0.37 ***
Feed efficiency index	0.0109 ± 0.0021	0.010 ± 0.00128	−0.0006 ± 0.0023	−0.0036 ± 0.0050 *,§	0.0031 ± 0.0040

SHAM SALINE: standard diet + saline solution. HFD SALINE: hyperlipidic diet + saline solution. AGE 50: hyperlipidic diet + 50 mg/kg of aqueous graviola leaf extract. AGE 100: hyperlipidic diet + 100 mg/kg of aqueous graviola leaf extract. AGE 150: hyperlipidic diet + 150 mg/kg of aqueous graviola leaf extract. Values represent the mean ± mean standard error. In the same line, * $p \leq 0.05$, ** $p \leq 0.01$, *** $p \leq 0.001$ vs. SHAM SALINE; § $p \leq 0.05$ vs. HFD SALINE; ANOVA followed by post Tukey test.

At the end of the treatment with the extract, the groups AGE 50 mg/kg and AGE 100 mg/kg presented a lower weight gain in comparison to the other groups (Table 3). The group AGE 50 mg/kg presented a statistical difference in relation to the SHAM SALINE group ($p = 0.034$). The group AGE 100 mg/kg had a significant body weight loss compared to the SHAM SALINE ($p = 0.003$) and HFD SALINE ($p = 0.034$) groups.

Food intake during the induction period was significantly higher in the SHAM group than in the HFD group ($p \leq 0.001$). However, the caloric intake and the FEI were significantly higher in the HFD group than in the SHAM group ($p \leq 0.001$) (Table 2). During the treatment period with the extract, similar results were observed for food intake, but daily caloric intake was significantly higher in the groups AGE 50 mg/kg ($p = 0.007$), AGE 100 mg/kg ($p = 0.048$) and AGE 150 mg/kg ($p \leq 0.001$), compared to the SHAM SALINE group. However, the FEI was significantly lower in the group AGE 100 mg/kg when compared to the SHAM SALINE group ($p = 0.021$) and the HFD SALINE ($p = 0.035$) group (Table 3). That is, there was a lower feed conversion capacity into body mass in the group AGE 100 mg/kg.

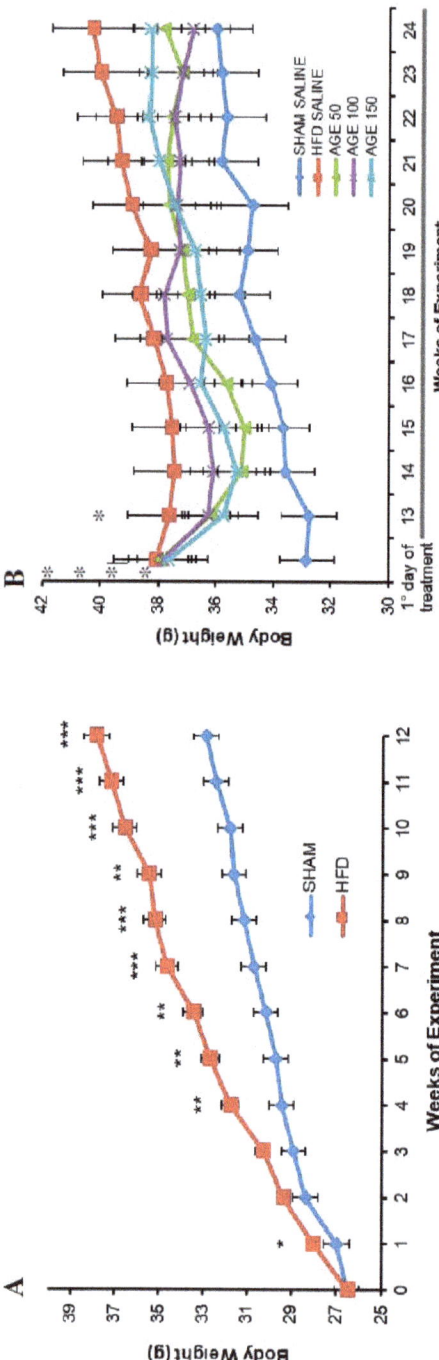

Figure 1. Effects of a hyperlipidic diet and AGE on weight gain. (**A**) Body weight of animals fed on the standard diet (SHAM) and on the hyperlipidic diet (HFD) during obesity induction for 12 consecutive weeks (0: initial weight). (**B**) Weight of control animals (SHAM SALINE: standard diet + saline solution. HDF SALINE: hyperlipidic diet + saline solution) and of animals treated with aqueous graviola leaf extract (AGE) (AGE 50: hyperlipidic diet + 50 mg/kg AGE. AGE 100: hyperlipidic diet + 100 mg/kg AGE. AGE 150: hyperlipidic diet + 150 mg/kg AGE) (depicted on the graph from the first day of treatment up to the 24th week). Values represent mean ± mean standard error. * $p \leq 0.05$, ** $p \leq 0.01$ and *** $p \leq 0.001$ vs. SHAM SALINE. Student t-test (Figure 1A) and ANOVA followed by post Tukey test (Figure 1B).

3.4. Effects of AGE on Serum Biochemical Parameters

In this experimental model, the AGE was not able to decrease serum fasting glucose concentrations at the end of the study ($p = 0.242$) (Figure 2A).

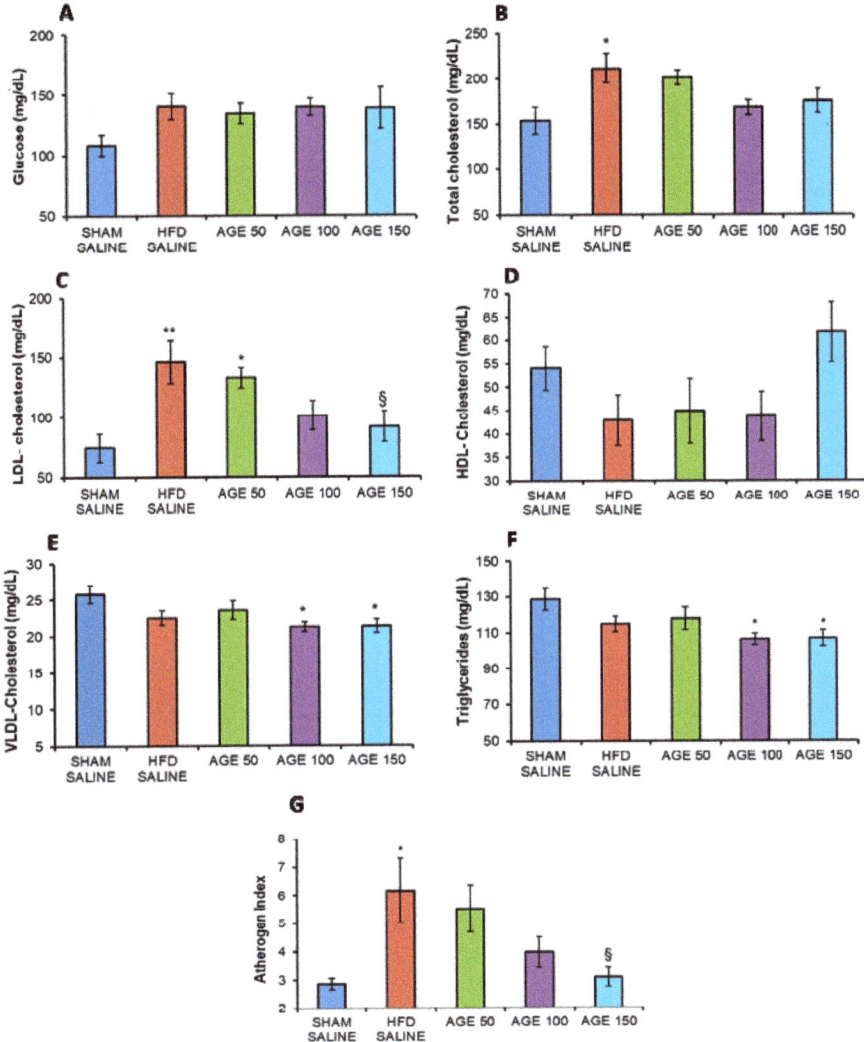

Figure 2. Evaluation of serum parameters. (**A**) Blood glucose (mg/dL), (**B**) total cholesterol (mg/dL), (**C**) LDL-cholesterol (mg/dL), (**D**) HDL-cholesterol (mg/dL), (**E**) VLDL-cholesterol (mg/dL), (**F**) triglycerides (mg/dL), and (**G**) atherogenic index of control animals (SHAM SALINE: standard diet + saline solution, HFD SALINE: hyperlipidic diet + saline solution), and of animals treated with aqueous graviola leaf extract (AGE) at 50, 100, and 150 mg/kg + hyperlipidic diet between the 13th and the 24th week of study. Values represent mean ± mean standard error. * $p < 0.05$, ** $p < 0.01$ vs. SHAM SALINE; § $p < 0.05$ vs. HFD SALINE. ANOVA followed by post Tukey test.

The AGE was also not able to significantly change the total serum cholesterol and HDL concentration (Figure 2B,D). However, serum HDL-cholesterol levels showed a 30.35% increase in concentration in the group treated with AGE 150 mg/kg (61.57 ± 6.47 mg/dL), compared to the HFD SALINE group (42.88 ± 5.40 mg/dL) (Figure 2D). For total serum cholesterol, the percentage decrease in AGE-treated groups was 4.92% for AGE 50 mg/kg (200.84 ± 8.30 mg/dL), 20.54% for AGE 100 mg/kg (167.85 ± 8.22 mg/dL), and 17.49% for AGE 150 mg/kg (174.30 ± 13.10 mg/dL) compared to the HFD SALINE group (211.24 ± 16.33 mg/dL) (Figure 2B).

In this study, the decrease in LDL-cholesterol concentration in the AGE-treated groups seems to be directly associated with the dose given. That is, the higher the AGE dose, the greater the decrease. There was a significant difference ($p = 0.038$) between AGE 150 mg/kg in relation to the HFD SALINE group (Figure 2C). In addition, AGE was able to significantly decrease triglyceride concentrations in the treated groups at doses of 100 mg/kg ($p = 0.026$) and 150 mg/kg ($p = 0.025$) compared to the SHAM SALINE group (Figure 2F). There was also a decrease in VLDL cholesterol using AGE 100 mg/kg and 150 mg/kg ($p = 0.030$) compared to the SHAM SALINE group (Figure 2E). Regarding the atherogenic index, which evaluates the risk of developing cardiovascular diseases, the group AGE 150 mg/kg presented a significantly lower mean value ($p = 0.025$) than the HFD SALINE group. In addition, the HFD SALINE group presented a significantly higher value in relation to the SHAM SALINE group (Figure 2G).

3.5. Effects of AGE on Insulin Sensitivity and Glucose Tolerance

The OGTT was performed prior to the beginning of the AGE treatment. No significant increases in fasting glycemia were observed between the hyperlipidic and the normolipidic diet groups. However, there was a significant increase ($p \leq 0.05$) in the glycemia of animals at 15 min in the groups HFD SALINE and AGE 150 mg/kg, in relation to the group fed on a normolipidic diet (SHAM SALINE). At 30 min, all groups fed on a hyperlipidic diet had a significant increase in glycemia in relation to the SHAM SALINE group (Figure 3A).

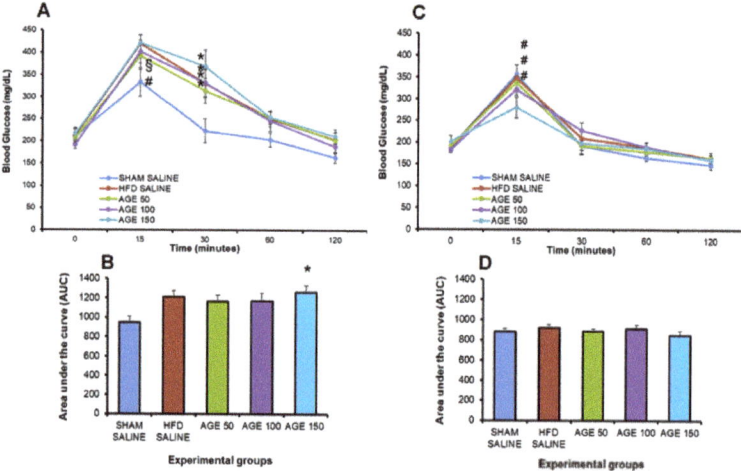

Figure 3. Evaluation of the glycemic profile before and at the end of the treatment with AGE. (**A**) Oral glucose tolerance test prior to the beginning of treatment (12th week). (**B**) Area under the curve (AUC) of blood glucose of animals evaluated prior to the beginning of treatment (12th week). (**C**) Oral glucose tolerance test at the end of treatment (24th week). (**D**) Area under the curve (AUC) of glycemia of animals evaluated at the end of treatment (24th week). SHAM SALINE: standard diet + saline solution. HFD SALINE: hyperlipidic diet + saline solution. AGE 50: hyperlipidic diet + 50 mg/kg of aqueous graviola leaf extract. AGE 100: hyperlipidic diet + 100 mg/kg of aqueous graviola leaf extract. AGE 150: hyperlipidic diet + 150 mg/kg of aqueous graviola leaf extract. Values represent mean ± mean standard error. * $p < 0.05$ vs. SHAM SALINE, § $p < 0.05$ vs. HFD SALINE, # $p < 0.05$ vs. AGE 150. ANOVA followed by post Tukey test.

The OGTT performed at the end of the experiment indicated that the AGE 150 mg/kg dose was able to significantly reduce blood glucose ($p \leq 0.05$) at 15 min, in relation to the groups SHAM SALINE, HFD SALINE and AGE 50 mg/kg. However, there was no significant difference between AGE 100 mg/kg and AGE 150 mg/kg. The area under the curve did not indicate a significant difference for the comparison among groups (Figure 3B).

The insulin sensitivity test performed at the end of the treatment with AGE or saline solution did not present a statistical difference in glycemia at the times analyzed after administration of insulin. This result is confirmed by observing the total area under the curve among the groups that received AGE or SALINE during the experimental period (Figure 4A,B).

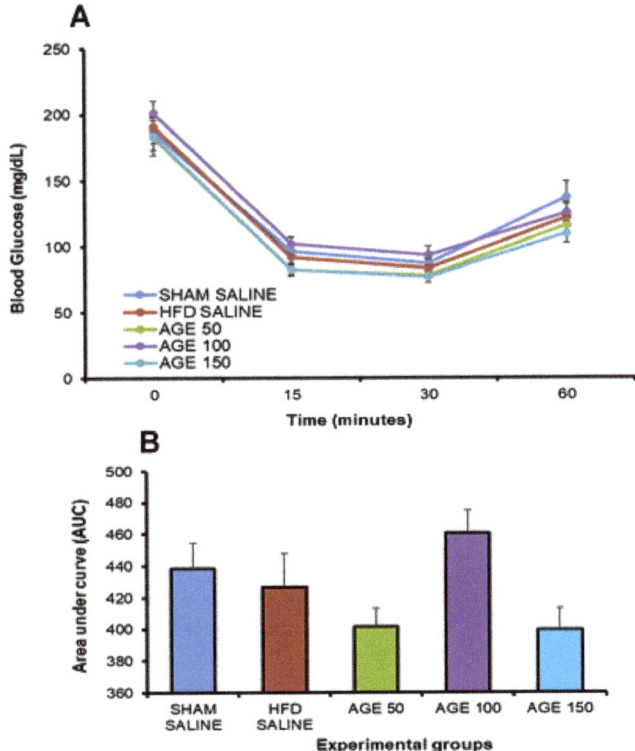

Figure 4. Evaluation of the glycemic profile at the end of the treatment with AGE. (**A**) Insulin sensitivity test performed at the end of treatment. (**B**) Area under the curve (AUC) of the insulin sensitivity test at the end of treatment. SHAM SALINE: standard diet + saline solution. HFD SALINE: hyperlipidic diet + saline solution. AGE 50: hyperlipidic diet + 50 mg/kg of aqueous graviola leaf extract. AGE 100: hyperlipidic diet + 100 mg/kg of aqueous graviola leaf extract. AGE 150: hyperlipidic diet + 150 mg/kg of aqueous graviola leaf extract. Each column represents the mean, and the bar represents the mean standard error. ANOVA.

3.6. Effects of AGE on Anti- and Pro-inflammatory Cytokines, Chemokines and Adiponectin

The animals treated with AGE showed an increase in IL-10 concentration, with a significant difference for the groups AGE 100 mg/kg ($p = 0.021$) and AGE 50 mg/kg ($p = 0.042$) when compared to the HFD SALINE group (Figure 5A). In analyzing MCP-1, no significant changes were observed between the groups studied ($p = 0.840$) (Figure 5B). As shown in Figure 5C,D, the levels of proinflammatory cytokines TNF-α ($p = 0.640$) and IL-6 ($p = 0.768$) also did not differ between study groups. Furthermore, there was no significant difference ($p = 0.244$) in the levels of adiponectin in the adipose tissue of mice (Figure 5D).

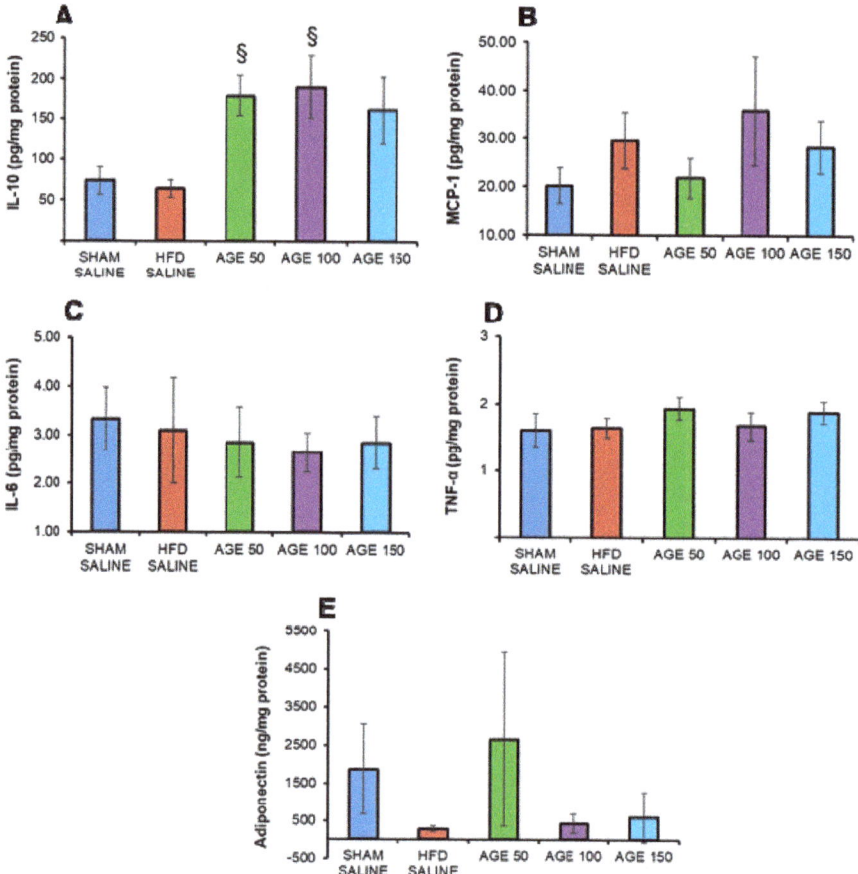

Figure 5. Effects of AGE on anti- and pro-inflammatory cytokines, chemokines and adiponectin. (**A**) Interleukin-10 (pg/mg protein). (**B**) Interleukin-6 (pg/mg protein). (**C**) Monocyte-1 chemotactic protein (pg/mg protein). (**D**) Tumor necrosis factor alpha (pg/mg protein). (**E**) Adiponectin (ng/mg protein) of control animals (SHAM SALINE: standard diet + saline solution. HFD SALINE: hyperlipidic diet + saline solution) and of animals treated with aqueous graviola leaf extract (AGE) at 50, 100 and 150 mg/kg + hyperlipidic diet between the 13th and the 24th week of study. The cytokines are measured in adipose tissue. Values represent mean ± mean standard error. § $p < 0.05$ vs. HFD SALINE. ANOVA/Tukey. Kruskal-Wallis test.

3.7. Effects of AGE on Fat Pads, Adiposity Index and Liver Weight

The AGE at the doses studied was not able to reduce the rate of adiposity of the animals. However, there was a decrease, although not significant, in the weight of fat pads of groups treated with aqueous graviola leaf extract: AGE 50 mg/kg: omental (22.22%), mesenteric (6.79%), retroperitoneal (8.79%), perirenal (9.41%); AGE 100 mg/kg: omental (11.11%), epididymal (14.34%), mesenteric (21.36%), retroperitoneal (31.04%); and AGE 150 mg/kg: omental (33.33%), epididymal (6.17%), mesenteric (6.08%), retroperitoneal (3.16%), and perirenal (2.35%), all compared to the HFD SALINE group (Table 4).

Table 4. Effects of AGE on fat pads, adiposity index, and liver weight.

Parameter	Experimental Group				
	SHAM SALINE	HFD SALINE	AGE 50	AGE 100	AGE 150
Omental weight (g)	0.028 ± 0.009	0.018 ± 0.005	0.014 ± 0.004	0.016 ± 0.004	0.012 ± 0.004
Epididymal weight (g)	1.068 ± 0.127	1.506 ± 0.112	1.543 ± 0.783	1.290 ± 0.149	1.413 ± 0.169
Mesenteric weight (g)	0.496 ± 0.634	0.707 ± 0.092	0.659 ± 0.049	0.556 ± 0.122	0.664 ± 0.136
Retroperitoneal weight (g)	0.360 ± 0.053	0.728 ± 0.087 *	0.664 ± 0.053	0.502 ± 0.090	0.705 ± 0.125
Perirenal weight (g)	0.198 ± 0.039	0.255 ± 0.039	0.231 ± 0.026	0.275 ± 0.061	0.198 ± 0.036
Adiposity index (%)	6.080 ± 0.514	10.893 ± 0.481 ***	11.620 ± 0.387 ***	10.212 ± 0.797 ***	10.713 ± 0.779 ***
Liver (g)	1.225 ± 0.066	1.236 ± 0.056	1.213 ± 0.030	1.200 ± 0.058	1.185 ± 0.047

Values represent mean ± mean standard error. * $p \leq 0.05$, *** $p \leq 0.001$ vs. SHAM SALINE; ANOVA followed by post Tukey test.

3.8. Effects of AGE on Liver, Pancreas, and Epididymal Adipose Tissue

The histological analysis of the pancreas showed no statistical differences among groups regarding pancreatic acini ($p = 0.400$), Islet of Langerhans ($p = 0.291$), and inflammation ($p = 0.458$) (Table 5, Figure 6). However, the atrophy/necrosis was less frequent in the pancreas of animals treated with AGE, especially in the AGE 100 mg/kg group (Table 5).

Table 5. Results for changes observed in the pancreas of the animals in each experimental group.

Variable	Experimental Group				
	SHAM SALINE	HFD SALINE	AGE 50	AGE 100	AGE 150
Changes in the pancreas					
Islet of Langerhans ($p = 0.291$)					
No change	36.4 (4)	45.5 (5)	72.7 (8)	80.0 (8)	54.5 (6)
Discrete atrophy	9.1 (1)	0.0 (0)	0.0 (0)	0.0 (0)	9.1 (1)
Atrophy	18.2 (2)	36.4 (4)	9.1 (1)	0.0 (0)	0.0 (0)
Discrete hypertrophy	18.2 (2)	9.1 (1)	0.0 (0)	20.0 (2)	27.3 (3)
Hypertrophy	18.2 (2)	9.1 (1)	18.2 (2)	0.0 (0)	9.1 (1)
Pancreatic acini ($p = 0.400$)					
No change	81.8 (9)	72.7 (8)	90.9 (10)	100.0 (10)	90.9 (10)
Necrosis/Atrophy	18.2 (2)	27.3 (3)	9.1 (1)	0.0 (0)	9.1 (1)
Inflammatory cells ($p = 0.458$)					
No change	90.9 (10)	81.8 (9)	90.9 (10)	100.0 (10)	100.0 (11)
Insulitis	0.0 (0)	0.0 (0)	0.0 (0)	0.0 (0)	0.0 (0)
Perinsulitis	9.1 (1)	18.2 (2)	9.1 (1)	0.0 (0)	0.0 (0)

Data presented as relative frequency (absolute frequency). Value of p in the chi-square test.

Similarly, the liver histological analysis also showed that the treatment with AGE did not change the quantification of steatosis ($p = 0.881$), microvesicular steatosis ($p = 0.501$), lobular inflammation ($p = 0.501$), balloonization ($p = 0.192$), Mallory's Hyaline ($p = 0.408$), apoptosis ($p = 1.00$), and glycogenate nucleus ($p = 0.408$) (Table 5, Figure 6). However, ballooning was more frequent in the HFD SALINE group compared to the groups that received AGE at different concentrations when fed on a hyperlipidic diet. Furthermore, hepatic steatosis was also frequent in the experimental groups that received a hyperlipidic diet or a normolipidic diet. However, the carbohydrate content in normolipidic diet was high, which may have contributed to this result (Table 6).

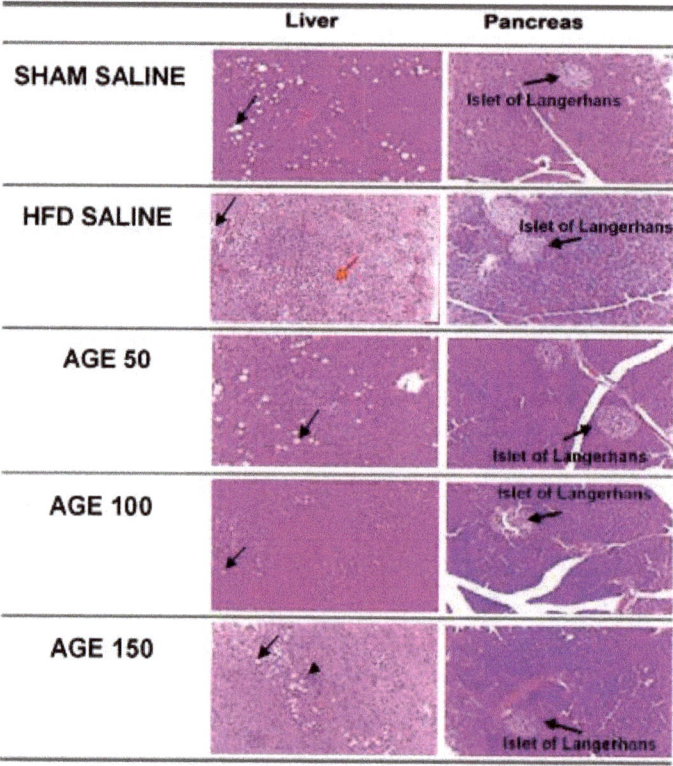

Figure 6. Histological analysis of the liver (Black arrows indicate hepatic steatosis, arrow head lobular inflammation and red arrows indicate ballooning) and pancreas of each experimental group. 20× magnification. Bar scale: 100 μm.

Table 6. Results for changes observed in the liver of animals in each experimental group.

Variable	Experimental Group				
	SHAM SALINE	HFD SALINE	AGE 50	AGE 100	AGE 150
	Liver Changes				
Steatosis ($p = 0.881$)					
< 5%	54.5 (5)	36.4 (4)	54.5 (6)	60.0 (6)	54.5 (6)
5 to 33%	36.4 (4)	36.4 (4)	36.4 (4)	10.0 (1)	36.4 (4)
34 to 66%	9.1 (1)	18.2 (2)	9.1 (1)	20.0 (2)	9.1 (1)
>66%	0.0 (0)	9.1 (1)	0.0 (0)	10.0 (1)	0.0 (0)
Microvesicular steatosis ($p = 0.501$)					
Absent	45.5 (5)	18.2 (2)	54.5 (6)	40.0 (4)	36.4 (4)
Present	54.5 (6)	81.8 (9)	45.5 (5)	60.0 (6)	63.6 (7)

Table 6. Cont.

Variable	Experimental Group				
	SHAM SALINE	HFD SALINE	AGE 50	AGE 100	AGE 150
Liver Changes					
Lobular inflammation ($p = 0.919$)					
Absent	63.6 (7)	72.7 (8)	81.8 (9)	70.7 (7)	72.7 (8)
<1 focus/field	36.4 (4)	27.3 (3)	18.2 (2)	30.0 (3)	27.3 (3)
2–4 focuses/field	0.0 (0)	0.0 (0)	0.0 (0)	0.0 (0)	0.0 (0)
> 4 focuses/field	0.0 (0)	0.0 (0)	0.0 (0)	0.0 (0)	0.0 (0)
Ballooning ($p = 0.91$)					
Absent	72.7 (8)	36.4 (4)	81.8 (9)	70.7 (7)	72.7 (8)
Few cells	27.3 (3)	63.6 (7)	18.2 (2)	30.0 (3)	27.3 (3)
Many cells	0.0 (0)	0.0 (0)	0.0 (0)	0.0 (0)	0.0 (0)
Mallory's hyaline ($p = 0.91$)					
Absent	100.0 (11)	100.0 (11)	100.0 (11)	100.0 (10)	90.9 (10)
Present	0.0 (0)	0.0 (0)	0.0 (0)	0.0 (0)	9.1 (1)
Apoptosis					
Absent	100.0 (11)	100.0 (11)	100.0 (11)	100.0 (10)	100.0 (11)
Present	0.0 (0)	0.0 (0)	0.0 (0)	0.0 (0)	0.0 (0)
Glycogenate nucleus ($p = 0.408$)					
None/rare	100.0 (11)	100.0 (11)	100.0 (11)	100.0 (10)	90.9 (10)
Some	0.0 (0)	0.0 (0)	0.0 (0)	0.0 (0)	9.1 (1)

Data presented as relative frequency (absolute frequency). Value of p in the chi-square test.

Regarding adipocytes, AGE at the dose of 100 mg/kg (4682.52 ± 476.91 µm^2) and at the dose of 150 mg/kg (4410.54 ± 426.73 µm^2) was able to significantly reduce the adipocyte area of the epididymal adipose tissue compared to the HFD SALINE group (6675.10 ± 736.87 µm^2) (Figure 7).

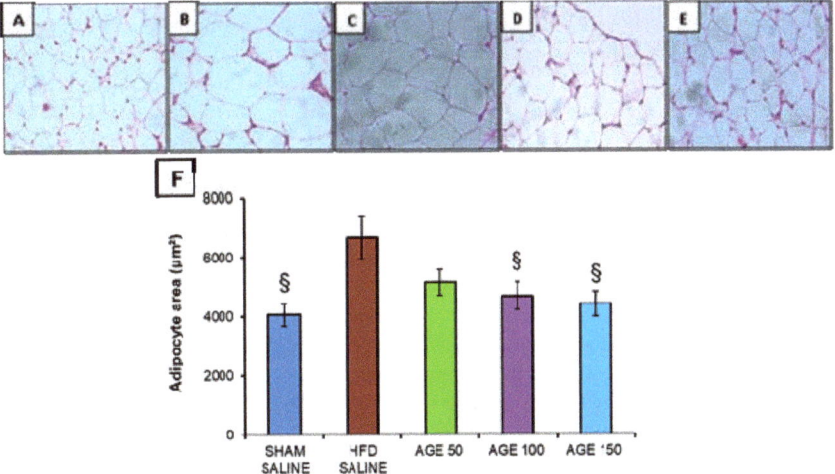

Figure 7. Histological analysis of the epididymal adipose tissue of each experimental group. (A) SHAM SALINE group. (B) HFD SALINE group. (C) AGE 50 mg/kg group. (D) AGE 100 mg/kg group. (E) AGE 150 mg/kg group. 20× magnification. Bar scale: 100 µm. (F) Adipocyte area (µm^2) of the groups studied. Values represent mean ± mean standard error. § $p < 0.05$ vs. HFD SALINE. ANOVA followed by post Tukey test.

4. Discussion

The choice of *Annona muricata* Linn for this study is because this plant is used for the treatment of obesity and its comorbidities. However, more scientific evidence is needed to support the notion that this plant extract can be used for treating obese patients [36].

Plants interact with the environment to survive and are influenced by many factors, such as pathogen attacks, temperature, circadian rhythm, water availability, nutrients, pollutants, and pesticides, all of which can cause stress. In response, plants produce secondary metabolites such as flavonoids, coumarins, saponins, alkaloids, tannins, and glucosinolates, among others. Thus, plants of the same species grown in different environments may present different concentrations of a certain secondary metabolic compound [37]. In a previous study, a high concentration of tannins and a medium concentration of flavonoids and saponins were identified in the methanolic and aqueous leaf extracts of *A. muricata* [38]. These substances were absent from the aqueous graviola leaf extract produced in this study. However, another study identified a low concentration of flavonoids and a high concentration of tannins, alkaloids, phenols, saponins, and phytosterols in AGE [39]. Thus, the different concentrations of the chemical composition of *Annona muricata* Linn leaves found in the literature and in our study may be related to the mentioned factors.

Studies have indicated that two hundred and twelve bioactive compounds have already been identified in *Annona muricata* Linn. Phenolic compounds are the major phytochemicals responsible for the antioxidant activity of *Annona muricata* Linn [36,40–42].

Acute toxicity tests using AGE found in the literature corroborate the results presented here. In the literature, the administration of a single dose of 2000 mg/kg and 5000 mg/kg of AGE to mice was not able to induce changes in animal behavior or mortality, or visible macroscopic changes in organs after euthanasia on the 14th day of the experiment [14].

Experimental models with modified diets can simulate pathophysiological changes in rodents that are similar to what occurs in humans. Such experiments allow understanding of the specific mechanisms of obesity and its metabolic changes. However, the feed composition and duration of experimental period have not been consistently established in the literature. In general, high-fat diets and physical inactivity are used in these models and are also the main risk factors for humans [40,43].

In experimental models with a high-fat diet, the increase in body weight is significant after two weeks of treatment, and after four weeks of induction this model shows different obesity phenotypes. However, long-term induction leads to obesity-related comorbidities such as moderate hyperglycemia and glucose intolerance [43]. Furthermore, in another model using C57BL/6J mice fed on a high-fat diet and 10% fructose after 16 weeks of treatment, the animals developed central obesity, dyslipidemia, arterial hypertension, insulin resistance, systemic oxidative stress, inflammation, and steatohepatitis. These are the main characteristics of metabolic syndrome [44].

In our study, we exposed mice to a 58% lipid diet for 12 weeks to induce obesity. After this period, our results indicated a significant increase in the weight of the HFD group compared to the SHAM group. The weight gain in the HFD group is consistent with the higher caloric intake evidenced by the FEI. Furthermore, at the end of the experimental period, we verified a significant increase in total and LDL cholesterol, and in the atherogenic index, of the HFD group in relation to the control group, which indicates that the model allowed the desired changes.

Among the various medicinal plants used for weight reduction, *Annona muricata* Linn is the second most used by the Brazilian population [16]. In our study, AGE at the doses 50 mg/kg and 100 mg/kg represented the popularly understood relationship between graviola and weight loss. Despite an observed decrease in body weight, no reduction in caloric intake was observed in the groups treated with AGE during the experimental period. Thus, weight reduction in this study is probably not related to a lower caloric intake.

Effective medicinal plants for weight loss have phenolic compounds among their chemical constituents, such as flavonoids, which modulate lipid metabolism and increase the rate of basal metabolism [45]. Quercetin and kaempferol stand out among flavonoids with an antiobesity effect. These were identified in AGE in the literature. We also found them in our study [42,46].

In the current study, regarding the cholesterol profile, no significant effects of the aqueous extract were observed on total cholesterol and HDL in two of the groups that received AGE. However, a significant increase in HDL cholesterol was observed in the group treated with AGE 150 mg/kg compared to the HFD SALINE group. We also observed a significant ($p = 0.038$) decrease in LDL-cholesterol, VLDL-cholesterol ($p = 0.030$), and triglyceride ($p = 0.026$) concentrations. In a study with streptozotocin-induced diabetic rats, AGE was able to significantly reduce plasma lipid concentrations. However, no difference was observed in relation to the diabetic group treated with 10 IU/kg of insulin [14].

The mechanisms of action of the aqueous extract of graviola on metabolism are not fully understood. However, several studies have reported isolated chemical compounds such as tannins, flavonoids, saponins, and coumarins, among other constituents, as being responsible for hypoglycemic, hypolipidemic, hypotensive, anti-inflammatory, and hepatic tissue changes, among other properties [47].

In our study, we observed a decrease in the atherogenic index after treatment with AGE, mainly in the group treated with 150 mg/kg. This decrease is directly related to the decrease in the development of cardiovascular diseases. This was associated with a decrease in triglycerides and LDL-cholesterol, and an increase in HDL-cholesterol, mainly in the 150 mg/kg group. Previous studies have shown that the antioxidant capacity of some substances can modify lipid metabolism and reduce inflammation, suggesting positive effects on cardiovascular diseases mainly by modulating oxidative stress. Furthermore, the high plasma level of the atherogenic index is related to small LDL-cholesterol particles. This is a predictor of conditions such as obesity, insulin resistance and inflammation, and consequently coronary artery disease, diabetes mellitus, and metabolic syndrome [48,49].

In our study, there were no significant effects of aqueous graviola leaf extract on capillary fasting glycemia evaluated in the oral glucose tolerance test performed at the end of treatment, and in the serum concentration of fasting glucose. When we calculated the area under the curve at the end of the experiment, we did not observe a significant difference in the comparison between the groups. However, there was a reduction in blood glucose levels at 15 min according to the oral glucose tolerance test in group 150 mg/kg. Some studies have demonstrated a significant decrease in plasma glucose concentrations after treatment with graviola extract in diabetic animals induced by streptozotocin or monohydrate aloxane [14,47,50,51].

Thus, the results found in our study do not indicate the effectiveness of aqueous graviola leaf extract on insulin resistance and diabetes mellitus type 2, in relation to the intake of a high calorie diet, high in saturated fat and simple carbohydrates and low in dietary fiber associated with sedentary lifestyle. However, further studies with AGE concentrations above 150 mg/kg may prove effective in reducing blood glucose, and therefore should be conducted.

Evidence shows that a greater fluctuation of glycemia induces endothelial dysfunction in diabetic or non-diabetic individuals, through oxidative stress resulting from an increase in free radicals [52,53].

Pro-inflammatory cytokines and chemokines, such as TNF-α, IL-6 and MCP-1, are required to initiate an inflammatory response. TNF-α is a cytokine that initiates the inflammatory response since it triggers the production of other cytokines, such as IL-6. On the other hand, anti-inflammatory cytokines, such as IL-10, are required to inhibit the synthesis of proinflammatory cytokines [54].

Previous studies have demonstrated that secondary metabolites present in plants, such as triterpenes, flavonoids and steroids, can modulate the inflammation and metabolic dysfunctions associated with obesity [55]. In our study, AGE did not change the levels of the inflammatory markers TNF-α, IL-6 and MCP-1 in adipose tissue. On the other hand, the AGE showed an anti-inflammatory effect due to a significant increase in IL-10 levels at the AGE doses of 50 and 100 mg/kg. In this study, the increased doses of AGE did not significantly interfere with TNF-α, IL-6 and MCP-1 levels. However, recent studies have demonstrated that IL-10 can exert anti-inflammatory effects via Janus kinase (JAK) signal transducer of activation 3 (JAK-STAT3), by binding IL-10 to the receptor on the target of the cell membrane—tyrosine kinase 2—leading to activation of the signal transducer and activator of transcription 3 (STAT3). However, further studies are needed to evaluate the possible effects of AGE on this pathway [56].

Adiponectin is a protein secreted by adipocytes. It exerts anti-diabetic, anti-atherogenic and anti-inflammatory effects directly. An increased expression may prevent and/or assist in the treatment of metabolic diseases related to obesity [57]. In our study, no significant effects of AGE were observed on adiponectin in adipose tissue. However, an increase of this protein was noticed in the group treated with AGE 50 mg/kg in relation to the other groups treated with AGE. Furthermore, the HFD SALINE group presented the lowest levels of adiponectin among the groups in our study.

Although the aqueous graviola leaf extract is able to induce a significant reduction in body weight according to the experimental model studied, and although there was a decrease in the weight percentage of all fat pads evaluated without significant differences in the comparison among groups, no decrease of visceral adiposity was observed at the end of the experiment when analyzing the weight of fat pads and the adiposity index. It is also possible to observe a significant decrease in the epididymal adipocyte area in the animals treated with AGE. Therefore, AGE attenuates the accumulation of lipids in mice, as was reported by another study after administration of blueberry and mulberry juice to C57BL/6 mice fed on a hyperlipidic diet for 12 weeks [58]. It should be noted that epididymal adipose tissue in mice is one of the major deposit areas of visceral fat [44].

In our experimental model, aqueous graviola leaf extract at the doses studied is not sufficient to prevent accumulation of liver fat and lesions to hepatocytes, as well as lesions to the pancreas. However, the ballooning of hepatocytes is less frequent in animals receiving treatment with the extract, as well as necrosis/atrophy of pancreatic acini. Thus, treatment with AGE is not able to avoid hepatic changes. However, it seems to protect the hepatocytes from morphological changes.

This may be related to a decrease in oxidative stress. In yet another study, the aqueous graviola leaf extract of *Annona muricata* Linn was able to protect pancreatic β-cells, and hence improve glucose metabolism, which was not visualized in our results [14].

5. Conclusions

In conclusion, no neurotoxic, behavioral, or mortality effects are produced by AGE in the acute toxicity test immediately after or during the post-treatment period. In addition, this study confirms the popular knowledge that graviola leaf tea reduces body weight and may also reduce cardiovascular risks, due to its beneficial effects in reducing plasma concentrations of LDL-cholesterol, VLDL-cholesterol, triglycerides, and the atherogenic index, while also attenuating the accumulation of body fat. In addition, in our experimental model, the results found do not indicate the effectiveness of aqueous graviola leaf extract on insulin resistance and diabetes mellitus type 2. However, the extract was effective in improving glucose tolerance in the higher concentration of the AGE. Furthermore, AGE has anti-inflammatory activity due to the increase in IL-10. However, it does not inhibit the expression of TNF-α, IL-6 and MCP-1. These data support the utility of conducting further studies aimed at identifying the active compounds of the aqueous extract of the aqueous graviola leaf extract, and at clarifying its mechanism of action.

Supplementary Materials: The following are available online at http://www.mdpi.com/2072-6643/11/7/1509/s1, Figure S1: Body weight, weight of organs, food intake and water intake of animals in the control group and animals treated with AGE during the acute toxicity test.

Author Contributions: Conceptualization: S.S., K.d.C.F.; methodology: S.S., P.C.S.e.S., L.F.S., C.A.L.C., L.C.P., B.B.d.F., L.S.S., L.M.B., A.R.C.M.-C., A.F.d.S.; F.M.A.; R.d.C.A.G., K.d.C.F.; validation: S.S., RCAG KCF; formal analysis: S.S., P.C.S.e.S., L.F.S., C.A.L.C., L.C.P., R.d.C.A.G., K.d.C.F.; writing—review and editing: S.S., L.F.S., C.A.L.C., F.M.A.; L.C.P., B.B.d.F., A.F.d.S.; A.R.C.M.-C., R.d.C.A.G., K.d.C.F.; data curation: S.S., R.d.C.A.G., KCF; project administration S.S., R.d.C.A.G., K.d.C.F.; software: KCF R.d.C.A.G.; visualization: S.S., R.d.C.A.G., KCF; supervision: S.S., L.F.S., C.A.L.C., R.d.C.A.G., K.d.C.F.

Funding: This research received no external funding.

Acknowledgments: The authors would like to thank CAPES for the scholarship awarded.

Conflicts of Interest: The authors declare no conflict of interest.

References

1. Maki, C.; Funakoshi-Tago, M.; Aoyagi, R.; Ueda, F.; Kimura, M.; Kobata, K.; Tago, K.; Tamura, H. Coffee extract inhibits adipogenesis in 3T3-L1 preadipocyes by interrupting insulin signaling through the downregulation of IRS1. *PLoS ONE* **2017**, *12*, e0173264. [CrossRef] [PubMed]
2. Sung, Y.Y.; Kim, D.S.; Kim, S.H.; Kim, H.K. Anti-obesity activity, acute toxicity, and chemical constituents of aqueous and ethanol Viola mandshurica extracts. *BMC Complement. Altern. Med.* **2017**, *17*, 297. [CrossRef] [PubMed]
3. Han, T.S.; Lean, M.E. A clinical perspective of obesity, metabolic syndrome and cardiovascular disease. *JRSM Cardiovasc. Dis.* **2016**, *5*, 2048004016633371. [CrossRef] [PubMed]
4. Vucenik, I.; Stains, J.P. Obesity and cancer risk: Evidence, mechanisms, and recommendations. *Ann. N. Y. Acad. Sci.* **2012**, *1271*, 37–43. [CrossRef]
5. Hoving, L.R.; van der Zande, H.J.P.; Pronk, A.; Guigas, B.; Willems van Dijk, K.; van Harmelen, V. Dietary yeast-derived mannan oligosaccharides have immune-modulatory properties but do not improve high fat diet-induced obesity and glucose intolerance. *PLoS ONE* **2018**, *13*, e0196165. [CrossRef]
6. Li, S.; Tan, H.Y.; Wang, N.; Zhang, Z.J.; Lao, L.; Wong, C.W.; Feng, Y. The Role of Oxidative Stress and Antioxidants in Liver Diseases. *Int. J. Mol. Sci.* **2015**, *16*, 26087–26124. [CrossRef]
7. Showalter, M.R.; Nonnecke, E.B.; Linderholm, A.L.; Cajka, T.; Sa, M.R.; Lonnerdal, B.; Kenyon, N.J.; Fiehn, O. Obesogenic diets alter metabolism in mice. *PLoS ONE* **2018**, *13*, e0190632. [CrossRef]
8. Zhang, C.; Ward, J.; Dauch, J.R.; Tanzi, R.E.; Cheng, H.T. Cytokine-mediated inflammation mediates painful neuropathy from metabolic syndrome. *PLoS ONE* **2018**, *13*, e0192333. [CrossRef]
9. Gu, M.; Zhang, Y.; Fan, S.; Ding, X.; Ji, G.; Huang, C. Extracts of Rhizoma polygonati odorati prevent high-fat diet-induced metabolic disorders in C57BL/6 mice. *PLoS ONE* **2013**, *8*, e81724. [CrossRef]
10. Tan, S.; Li, M.; Ding, X.; Fan, S.; Guo, L.; Gu, M.; Zhang, Y.; Feng, L.; Jiang, D.; Li, Y.; et al. Effects of Fortunella margarita fruit extract on metabolic disorders in high-fat diet-induced obese C57BL/6 mice. *PLoS ONE* **2014**, *9*, e93510. [CrossRef]
11. Donado-Pestana, C.M.; Dos Santos-Donado, P.R.; Daza, L.D.; Belchior, T.; Festuccia, W.T.; Genovese, M.I. Cagaita fruit (Eugenia dysenterica DC.) and obesity: Role of polyphenols on already established obesity. *Food Res. Int.* **2018**, *103*, 40–47. [CrossRef] [PubMed]
12. Costa, A.G.V.; Garcia-Diaz, D.F.; Jimenez, P.; Silva, P.I. Bioactive compounds and health benefits of exotic tropical red–black berries. *J. Funct. Foods* **2013**, *5*, 539–549. [CrossRef]
13. Khan, W.; Parveen, R.; Chester, K.; Parveen, S.; Ahmad, S. Hypoglycemic Potential of Aqueous Extract of Moringa oleifera Leaf and In Vivo GC-MS Metabolomics. *Front. Pharmacol.* **2017**, *8*, 577. [CrossRef] [PubMed]
14. Florence, N.T.; Benoit, M.Z.; Jonas, K.; Alexandra, T.; Desire, D.D.; Pierre, K.; Theophile, D. Antidiabetic and antioxidant effects of Annona muricata (Annonaceae), aqueous extract on streptozotocin-induced diabetic rats. *J. Ethnopharmacol.* **2014**, *151*, 784–790. [CrossRef] [PubMed]
15. Justino, A.B.; Miranda, N.C.; Franco, R.R.; Martins, M.M.; Silva, N.M.D.; Espindola, F.S. Annona muricata Linn. leaf as a source of antioxidant compounds with in vitro antidiabetic and inhibitory potential against alpha-amylase, alpha-glucosidase, lipase, non-enzymatic glycation and lipid peroxidation. *Biomed. Pharmacother.* **2018**, *100*, 83–92. [CrossRef] [PubMed]
16. Djeridane, A.; Yousfi, M.; Nadjemi, B.; Boutassouna, D.; Stocker, P.; Vidal, N. Antioxidant activity of some algerian medicinal plants extracts containing phenolic compounds. *Food Chem.* **2006**, *97*, 654–660. [CrossRef]
17. Lin, J.-Y.; Tang, C.-Y. Determination of total phenolic and flavonoid contents in selected fruits and vegetables, as well as their stimulatory effects on mouse splenocyte proliferation. *Food Chem.* **2007**, *101*, 140–147. [CrossRef]
18. Broadhurst, R.B.; Jones, W.T. Analysis of condensed tannins using acidified vanillin. *J. Sci. Food Agric.* **1978**, *29*, 788–794. [CrossRef]

19. Kumaran, A.; Karunakaran, R.J. Nitric oxide radical scavenging active components from *Phyllanthus emblica* L. *Plant Foods Hum. Nutr.* **2006**, *61*, 1–5. [CrossRef]
20. Berrondo, L.F.; Gabriel, F.T.; Fernandes, S.B.d.O.; Menezes, F.d.S.; Moreira, D.d.L. Dirhamnosyl flavonoid and other constituents from Brillantaisia palisatii. *Química Nova* **2003**, *26*, 922–923. [CrossRef]
21. Harborne, J.B. The Flavonoids: Advances in Research Since 1986 (Harborne, J.B.). *J. Chem. Educ.* **1995**, *72*, 73.
22. Agrawal, P.K. *Carbon-13 NMR of Flavonoids*, 1st ed.; Agrawal, P.K., Ed.; Elsevier Science: Amsterdam, The Netherlands, 1989; Volume 39, pp. 283–364.
23. OECD. *Test No. 425: Acute Oral Toxicity: Up-and-Down Procedure*; OECD Publishing: Paris, France, 2008. [CrossRef]
24. Malone, M.H.; Robichaud, R.C. A Hippocratic screen for pure or crude drug materials. *Lloydia* **1962**, *25*, 320–322.
25. Da Silva, E.R.; Salmazzo, G.R.; da Silva Arrigo, J.; Oliveira, R.J.; Kassuya, C.A.; Cardoso, C.A. Anti-inflammatory Evaluation and Toxicological Analysis of Campomanesia xanthocarpa Berg. *Inflammation* **2016**, *39*, 1462–1468. [CrossRef] [PubMed]
26. Reeves, P.G.; Nielsen, F.H.; Fahey, G.C., Jr. AIN-93 purified diets for laboratory rodents: Final report of the American Institute of Nutrition ad hoc writing committee on the reformulation of the AIN-76A rodent diet. *J. Nutr.* **1993**, *123*, 1939–1951. [CrossRef] [PubMed]
27. Hargrove, R.E.; Alford, J.A. Growth Rate and Feed Efficiency of Rats Fed Yogurt and Other Fermented Milks. *J. Dairy Sci.* **1978**, *61*, 11–19. [CrossRef]
28. Santos, S.H.; Fernandes, L.R.; Mario, E.G.; Ferreira, A.V.; Porto, L.C.; Alvarez-Leite, J.I.; Botion, L.M.; Bader, M.; Alenina, N.; Santos, R.A. Mas deficiency in FVB/N mice produces marked changes in lipid and glycemic metabolism. *Diabetes* **2008**, *57*, 340–347. [CrossRef] [PubMed]
29. Donatto, F.F.; Neves, R.X.; Rosa, F.O.; Camargo, R.G.; Ribeiro, H.; Matos-Neto, E.M.; Seelaender, M. Resistance exercise modulates lipid plasma profile and cytokine content in the adipose tissue of tumour-bearing rats. *Cytokine* **2013**, *61*, 426–432. [CrossRef] [PubMed]
30. Lira, F.S.; Rosa, J.C.; Pimentel, G.D.; Tarini, V.A.; Arida, R.M.; Faloppa, F.; Alves, E.S.; do Nascimento, C.O.; Oyama, L.M.; Seelaender, M.; et al. Inflammation and adipose tissue: Effects of progressive load training in rats. *Lipids Health Dis.* **2010**, *9*, 109. [CrossRef] [PubMed]
31. White, P.A.; Cercato, L.M.; Batista, V.S.; Camargo, E.A.; De Lucca, W.; Oliveira, A.S.; Silva, F.T.; Goes, T.C.; Oliveira, E.R.; Moraes, V.R.; et al. Aqueous extract of Chrysobalanus icaco leaves, in lower doses, prevent fat gain in obese high-fat fed mice. *J. Ethnopharmacol.* **2016**, *179*, 92–100. [CrossRef] [PubMed]
32. Kleiner, D.E.; Brunt, E.M.; Van Natta, M.; Behling, C.; Contos, M.J.; Cummings, O.W.; Ferrell, L.D.; Liu, Y.C.; Torbenson, M.S.; Unalp-Arida, A.; et al. Design and validation of a histological scoring system for nonalcoholic fatty liver disease. *Hepatology* **2005**, *41*, 1313–1321. [CrossRef] [PubMed]
33. Chandran, R.; Parimelazhagan, T.; Shanmugam, S.; Thankarajan, S. Antidiabetic activity of Syzygium calophyllifolium in Streptozotocin-Nicotinamide induced Type-2 diabetic rats. *Biomed. Pharmacother.* **2016**, *82*, 547–554. [CrossRef] [PubMed]
34. Wang, H.; Xue, Y.; Wang, B.; Zhao, J.; Yan, X.; Huang, Y.; Du, M.; Zhu, M.J. Maternal obesity exacerbates insulitis and type 1 diabetes in non-obese diabetic mice. *Reproduction* **2014**, *148*, 73–79. [PubMed]
35. Pereira, S.S.; Teixeira, L.G.; Aguilar, E.C.; Matoso, R.O.; Soares, F.L.; Ferreira, A.V.; Alvarez-Leite, J.I. Differences in adipose tissue inflammation and oxidative status in C57BL/6 and ApoE-/- mice fed high fat diet. *Anim. Sci. J.* **2012**, *83*, 549–555. [CrossRef] [PubMed]
36. Cercato, L.M.; White, P.A.; Nampo, F.K.; Santos, M.R.; Camargo, E.A. A systematic review of medicinal plants used for weight loss in Brazil: Is there potential for obesity treatment? *J. Ethnopharmacol.* **2015**, *176*, 286–296. [CrossRef] [PubMed]
37. Verma, N.; Shukla, S. Impact of various factors responsible for fluctuation in plant secondary metabolites. *J. Appl. Res. Med. Aromat. Plants* **2015**, *2*, 105–113. [CrossRef]
38. George, V.C.; Kumar, D.R.; Suresh, P.K.; Kumar, R.A. Antioxidant, DNA protective efficacy and HPLC analysis of Annona muricata (soursop) extracts. *J. Food Sci. Technol.* **2015**, *52*, 2328–2335.
39. Gavamukulya, Y.; Abou-Elella, F.; Wamunyokoli, F.; AEl-Shemy, H. Phytochemical screening, anti-oxidant activity and in vitro anticancer potential of ethanolic and water leaves extracts of Annona muricata (Graviola). *Asian Pac. J. Trop. Med.* **2014**, *7*, S355–S363. [CrossRef]

40. Coria-Téllez, A.V.; Montalvo-Gónzalez, E.; Yahia, E.M.; Obledo-Vázquez, E.N. Annona muricata: A comprehensive review on its traditional medicinal uses, phytochemicals, pharmacological activities, mechanisms of action and toxicity. *Arab. J. Chem.* **2018**, *11*, 662–691. [CrossRef]
41. Moghadamtousi, S.Z.; Fadaeinasab, M.; Nikzad, S.; Mohan, G.; Ali, H.M.; Kadir, H.A. Annona muricata (Annonaceae): A Review of Its Traditional Uses, Isolated Acetogenins and Biological Activities. *Int. J. Mol. Sci.* **2015**, *16*, 15625–15658. [CrossRef]
42. Nawwar, M.; Ayoub, N.; Hussein, S.; Hashim, A.; El-Sharawy, R.; Wende, K.; Harms, M.; Lindequist, U. A flavonol triglycoside and investigation of the antioxidant and cell stimulating activities of Annona muricata Linn. *Arch. Pharm. Res.* **2012**, *35*, 761–767. [CrossRef]
43. Panchal, S.K.; Brown, L. Rodent models for metabolic syndrome research. *J. Biomed. Biotechnol.* **2011**, *2011*, 351982. [PubMed]
44. Della Vedova, M.C.; Muñoz, M.D.; Santillan, L.D.; Plateo-Pignatari, M.G.; Germanó, M.J.; Tosi, M.E.R.; Garcia, S.; Gomez, N.N.; Fornes, M.W.; Mejiba, S.E.G.; et al. A Mouse Model of Diet-Induced Obesity Resembling Most Features of Human Metabolic Syndrome. *Nutr. Metab. Insights* **2016**, *9*, NMI.S32907.
45. Rupasinghe, H.P.; Sekhon-Loodu, S.; Mantso, T.; Panayiotidis, M.I. Phytochemicals in regulating fatty acid beta-oxidation: Potential underlying mechanisms and their involvement in obesity and weight loss. *Pharmacol. Ther.* **2016**, *165*, 153–163. [PubMed]
46. Boadi, W.Y.; Lo, A. Effects of Quercetin, Kaempferol, and Exogenous Glutathione on Phospho- and Total-AKT in 3T3-L1 Preadipocytes. *J. Diet Suppl.* **2018**, *15*, 814–826. [PubMed]
47. Adewole, S.O.; Ojewole, J.A. Protective effects of Annona muricata Linn. (Annonaceae) leaf aqueous extract on serum lipid profiles and oxidative stress in hepatocytes of streptozotocin-treated diabetic rats. *Afr. J. Tradit. Complement. Altern. Med.* **2008**, *6*, 30–41.
48. Chernukha, I.M.; Fedulova, L.V.; Kotenkova, E.A.; Takeda, S.; Sakata, R. Hypolipidemic and anti-inflammatory effects of aorta and heart tissues of cattle and pigs in the atherosclerosis rat model. *Anim. Sci. J.* **2018**, *89*, 784–793. [PubMed]
49. Mazaherioun, M.; Djalali, M.; Koohdani, F.; Javanbakht, M.H.; Zarei, M.; Beigy, M.; Ansari, S.; Rezvan, N.; Saedisomeolia, A. Beneficial Effects of n-3 Fatty Acids on Cardiometabolic and Inflammatory Markers in Type 2 Diabetes Mellitus: A Clinical Trial. *Med. Princ. Pract.* **2017**, *26*, 535–541.
50. Adeyemi, D.O.; Komolafe, O.A.; Adewole, O.S.; Obuotor, E.M.; Adenowo, T.K. Anti hyperglycemic activities of Annona muricata (Linn). *Afr. J. Tradit. Complement. Altern. Med.* **2008**, *6*, 62–69.
51. Ahalya, B.; Shankar, K.R.; Kiranmayi, G.V.N. Exploration of anti-hyperglycemic and hypolipidemic activities of ethanolic extract of Annona muricata bark in alloxan induced diabetic rats. *Int. J. Pharm. Sci. Rev. Res.* **2014**, *25*, 21–27.
52. Cavalot, F. Do data in the literature indicate that glycaemic variability is a clinical problem? Glycaemic variability and vascular complications of diabetes. *Diabetes Obes. Metab.* **2013**, *15* (Suppl. 2), 3–8. [CrossRef]
53. Ceriello, A.; Esposito, K.; Piconi, L.; Ihnat, M.; Thorpe, J.; Testa, R.; Bonfigli, A.R.; Giugliano, D. Glucose "peak" and glucose "spike": Impact on endothelial function and oxidative stress. *Diabetes Re. Clin. Pract.* **2008**, *82*, 262–267.
54. Galan, A.; Mayer, I.; Rafaj, R.B.; Bendelja, K.; Susic, V.; Ceron, J.J.; Mrljak, V. MCP-1, KC-like and IL-8 as critical mediators of pathogenesis caused by Babesia canis. *PLoS ONE* **2018**, *13*, e0190474. [CrossRef] [PubMed]
55. Veloso, C.C.; Oliveira, M.C.; Rodrigues, V.G.; Oliveira, C.C.; Duarte, L.P.; Teixeira, M.M.; Ferreira, A.V.M.; Perez, A.C. Evaluation of the effects of extracts of Maytenus imbricata (Celastraceae) on the treatment of inflammatory and metabolic dysfunction induced by high-refined carbohydrate diet. *Inflammopharmacology* **2018**, *27*, 539–548. [CrossRef] [PubMed]
56. Liu, Y.; Xu, D.; Yin, C.; Wang, S.; Wang, M.; Xiao, Y. IL-10/STAT3 is reduced in childhood obesity with hypertriglyceridemia and is related to triglyceride level in diet-induced obese rats. *BMC Endocr. Disord.* **2018**, *18*, 39. [CrossRef] [PubMed]

57. Scoditti, E.; Massaro, M.; Carluccio, M.A.; Pellegrino, M.; Wabitsch, M.; Calabriso, N.; Storelli, C.; De Caterina, R. Additive regulation of adiponectin expression by the mediterranean diet olive oil components oleic Acid and hydroxytyrosol in human adipocytes. *PLoS ONE* **2015**, *10*, e0128218.
58. Wu, T.; Tang, Q.; Gao, Z.; Yu, Z.; Song, H.; Zheng, X.; Chen, W. Blueberry and mulberry juice prevent obesity development in C57BL/6 mice. *PLoS ONE* **2013**, *8*, e77585.

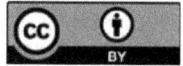

© 2019 by the authors. Licensee MDPI, Basel, Switzerland. This article is an open access article distributed under the terms and conditions of the Creative Commons Attribution (CC BY) license (http://creativecommons.org/licenses/by/4.0/).

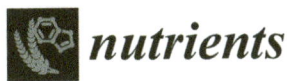

Article

Polyphenol-Enriched Plum Extract Enhances Myotubule Formation and Anabolism while Attenuating Colon Cancer-induced Cellular Damage in C2C12 Cells

Faten A. Alsolmei [1,2], Haiwen Li [1], Suzette L. Pereira [3], Padmavathy Krishnan [4], Paul W. Johns [3] and Rafat A. Siddiqui [1,*]

[1] Food Chemistry and Nutrition Science Research Laboratory, Agricultural Research Station, College of Agriculture, Petersburg, VA 23806, USA; fatenalsolmei@gmail.com (F.A.A.); hali@vsu.edu (H.L.)
[2] Department of Biology, College of Natural and Health Sciences, Virginia State University, Petersburg, VA 23806, USA
[3] Abbott-Nutrition Division, Research and Development, 3300 Stelzer Road, Columbus, OH 43219, USA; suzette.pereira@abbott.com (S.L.P.); paul.johns@abbott.com (P.W.J.)
[4] Valley Children's Hospital, Madera, CA 93636, USA; padmakrishnan@hotmail.com
* Correspondence: rsiddiqui@vsu.edu; Tel.: +(804)-524-5957

Received: 5 April 2019; Accepted: 11 May 2019; Published: 15 May 2019

Abstract: Preventing muscle wasting in certain chronic diseases including cancer is an ongoing challenge. Studies have shown that polyphenols derived from fruits and vegetables shows promise in reducing muscle loss in cellular and animal models of muscle wasting. We hypothesized that polyphenols derived from plums (*Prunus domestica*) could have anabolic and anti-catabolic benefits on skeletal muscle. The effects of a polyphenol-enriched plum extract (PE60) were evaluated in vitro on C2C12 and Colon-26 cancer cells. Data were analyzed using a one-way ANOVA and we found that treatment of myocytes with plum extract increased the cell size by ~3-fold ($p < 0.05$) and stimulated myoblast differentiation by ~2-fold ($p < 0.05$). Plum extract induced total protein synthesis by ~50% ($p < 0.05$), reduced serum deprivation-induced total protein degradation by ~30% ($p < 0.05$), and increased expression of Insulin-Like Growth Factor-1 (IGF-1) by ~2-fold ($p < 0.05$). Plum extract also reduced tumor necrosis factor α (TNFα)-induced nuclear factor κB (NFκB) activation by 80% ($p < 0.05$) in A549/NF-κB-luc cells. In addition, plum extract inhibited the growth of Colon-26 cancer cells, and attenuated cytotoxicity in C2C12 myoblasts induced by soluble factors released from Colon-26 cells. In conclusion, our data suggests that plum extract may have pluripotent health benefits on muscle, due to its demonstrated ability to promote myogenesis, stimulate muscle protein synthesis, and inhibit protein degradation. It also appears to protect muscle cell from tumor-induced cytotoxicity.

Keywords: cachexia; plum; cancer; muscle wasting; myoblasts; protein synthesis

1. Introduction

Skeletal muscle weakness and wasting, which is also referred as cachexia, is a major clinical problem for advanced cancer patients [1]. In 1932, Warren described cachexia as the most common cause of death across a variety of cancers in a post mortem study of 500 patients [2]. The term "Cachexia" is derived from the Greek words "kakos" and "hexis," meaning "bad condition." It is a multi-organ syndrome associated with and characterized by at least 5% body weight loss due to muscle and adipose tissue wasting [3]. Cancer cachexia is a multifactorial syndrome that is common in advanced malignancy occurring in 80% of patients, which cannot be reversed by nutritional support and leads to significant function deficits [4], and which is responsible for an estimated 20% of cancer-related deaths [5].

Colorectal cancer (CRC) patients are often presented with cachexia syndrome, which is a major contributor to colorectal cancer-related morbidity and mortality [4–8]. About 35 to 60% of CRC patients show some degree of muscle wasting and 28% lose >5% of their body weight in the six months preceding diagnosis [9]. Blocking muscle wasting can prolong life even in the absence of effects on tumor growth [10].

Oxidative stress through activating initial steps in protein degradation via the ubiquitin-proteasome pathway and the activation of caspases contributes to muscular atrophy [11–13]. In addition, inflammation also leads to muscle atrophy and this is mediated through cytokine (e.g., tumor necrosis factor α (TNFα), interleukin-6 (IL-6), and interferon γ (IFNγ)) induced activation of the nuclear factor κB (NF-κB) pathway [14].

Recent studies have shown that polyphenol-rich plant extracts prevent oxidative stress, reduce inflammation, and help reduce muscle atrophy. We have previously shown that curcumin treatment attenuated muscle wasting in cancer cachectic mice [15]. Supplementation with red grape polyphenols mitigated muscular atrophy in transforming growth factor (TGF) mice, a model of chronic inflammation, by reducing mitochondrial oxidative stress and by inhibiting caspase activation [16]. Grape seed extract supplementation effectively prevented muscle wasting in IL10-knock out mice [17]. Green tea polyphenol, catechins, protected normal and dystrophic muscle cells from oxidative damage [18]. Epigallocatechin-3-gallate (EGCG) supplementation preserved muscle in sarcopenic rats [19] and attenuated skeletal muscle atrophy caused by experimentally induced cancer cachexia in in mice [20]. More recently, ursolic acid—a polyphenol present in apple peels, basil leaves, prunes, and cranberries [21]—has been shown to increase muscle mass in mice exhibiting fasting-induced muscle atrophy [22]; it has also increased muscle mass, fast and slow fiber size, grip strength, and exercise capacity in mice with diet-induced obesity [23]. These observations clearly suggest that intake of polyphenols can be beneficial in preserving muscle mass.

The common plum (*Prunus domestica*) is well known to be rich in polyphenols and contains unique phytonutrients called neochlorogenic and chlorogenic acid which have high antioxidant activities. Among functional foods, plums are also considered "super foods" since their consumption has been associated with the decrease in chronic degenerative diseases and circulatory and digestive issues [24]. Dried plums have been shown to reduce symptoms of arthritis in an inflammation model [25]. These effects are attributed to their high polyphenolic composition and related high antioxidant activity [26]. Plums have several health benefits and studies have found that plums also initiate anti-cancer mechanisms that may help prevent the growth of cancerous cells and tumors [27–29].

In addition, plums have been extensively studied for their effects on bone health [30,31]. Plums contain caffeic acid (the polyphenol component of neochlorogenic and chlorogenic acids) and rutin, which have been shown to inhibit the deterioration of bone tissues and prevent diseases such as osteoporosis in postmenopausal women [32]. Research has also shown that regular consumption of dried plums helps in the restoration of bone density lost to aging [33].

Formation of bone and much of the skeletal tissues is derived from the proliferation and differentiation of skeletal stem cells. As dried plum was found to be a potent regulator of bone health, it is possible that plum and its associated polyphenols may have benefits on other cells of musculoskeletal system. Thus, in the present study, we sought to investigate the effect of a polyphenol-enriched plum extract on muscle cell growth and differentiation, and on muscle protein synthesis and degradation *in vitro*. In addition, we explored the effect of plum extract on inflammation as well as studied its effect on colon cancer cells.

2. Materials and Methods

2.1. Materials

Dulbecco's modified Eagle's medium (DMEM), fetal bovine serum (FBS), horse serum, and Penicillin-Streptomycin solution were purchased from Gibco-Thermo-Fisher Scientific (Grand Island, NY, USA). L-[2,3,4,5,6-3H] Phenylalanine and L-[Ring-3, 5-3H]-Tyrosine was purchased from Perkin-Elmer (Waltham, MA, USA), Prune extract-60% enriched polyphenol extract (PE60) was purchased from PL Thomas (Morristown, NJ, USA). All other chemicals were of reagent grade, and were purchased from Sigma Chemical Co. (St. Louis, MO, USA).

2.2. Composition of the PE60-Plum Extract

Free gallic acid, 3-cholorogenic acid, rutin, free quercetin, and proanthocyanidins were determined with an Agilent Technologies (Wilmington, DE, USA) Model 1200 HPLC System equipped with a Model G1311A quaternary pump, Model G1322A vacuum degasser, Model G1329A autosampler, Model G1316A thermostatted column compartment, a Model G1315B diode array detector, and a Chem Station data processor. The separations were performed with a YMC-Pack ODS-AQ analytical column (4.6 × 250 mm, 5 µm, P/N AQ12S05-2546WT, Waters Corporation, Milford, MA, USA), using mobile phase A = 1000/100 (v/v) 0.05 M KH2PO4, pH 2.9/acetonitrile, and mobile phase B = 200/800 (v/v) Milli-Q Plus water/acetonitrile, a column temperature of 40 °C, an injection volume of 5 µL, and the analytes were quantified at signals of 280 nm/590 nm (for gallic acid and the proanthocyanidins), 330 nm/590 nm (for 3-chlorogenic acid), and 375 nm/590 nm (for rutin and quercetin). The elution program was 0% mobile phase B from 0 to 5 min, 0 to 60% (linear gradient) mobile phase B from 5 to 35 min, 100% mobile phase B from 35 to 40 min, and 0% mobile phase B from 40 to 55 min (end). The PE60 extract was prepared for analysis by stirring (at room temperature for 15 min) 0.250 g in 100 mL of 50/50 (v/v) 0.05 M citric acid/methanol. The determinations were calibrated with standard solutions of gallic acid, 3-chlorogenic acid, rutin hydrate, and quercetin dihydrate (all obtained from Sigma-Aldrich, St. Louis, MO, USA), also prepared in the citric acid/methanol medium. The proanthocyanidin content was estimated by peak area proportionation vs. the corresponding peak areas (at 280 nm/590 nm) of grapeseed extracts (from Kikkoman, Polyphenolics, and Seppic) of known (i.e., label claim) proanthocyanidin content, included in the analysis. The anthocyanin concentration was estimated by a published colorimetric method [34]. During present investigation, minor isomers of chlorogenic acid (4-chlorogenic acid, 5-chlorogenic acid) were not determined.

2.3. Characterization of Anti-Oxidation Capacity of the Plum Extract

The PE60 (Lot PE6009-1601) extract was dissolved in water (10 mg/mL) and then centrifuged at 1500 × g for 10 min to remove any insoluble material. The dissolved material was sterile filtered and the filtrate was assayed for total polyphenols by the Folin Ciocalteu method [35], for total flavonoids by the AlCl3 complexation method [36], for anti-oxidant activity by the DPPH assay [37], and for oxygen scavenging activity by the ABTS assay [38], as described.

2.4. Cell Culture

C2C12 cell line (mouse myoblasts) were obtained from American Type Culture Collection (Manassas, VA, USA). The undifferentiated cells were grown in complete media consisting of Dulbecco's modified Eagle's medium (DMEM, 4.5 mg/mL glucose) supplemented with heat-inactivated fetal calf serum (10%), penicillin (100 units/mL), and streptomycin (100 µg/mL) at 37 °C in the presence of 5% CO_2. The myoblasts were differentiated into myotubes by culturing them into differentiation medium, consisting of DMEM supplemented with heat-inactivated horse serum (5%), penicillin (100 units/mL), and streptomycin (100 µg/mL) for five days.

2.5. Determination of C2C12 Myoblast Cell Size

Muscles cells were grown in a 96-well plate for 24 h in 100 µL complete media. Cells were then treated with 0, 50, 100, 150, and 200 µg/mL of extract for 48 h to evaluate a dose-response effect of plum extract. After incubations, the cells were observed under a microscope and pictures (100 × magnification) were taken using a Nikon microscope with calibrated objectives. The size of cells was determined using Element-BR software (Nikon Instruments Inc, Melville, NY, USA).

2.6. Assaying C2C12 Myoblast Differentiation

Muscle cells were initially cultured in a 96-well plate for 24 h in 100 µL complete media. Cells were then incubated with 0, 50, 100, and 200 µg/mL plum extract for five days and the medium containing corresponding concentration of plum extract was changed every 24 h. After treatment, the cells were washed once with PBS, and then fixed with cold 4% paraformaldehyde for 10 min on ice. The cells were washed three times with PBS and the monolayer was treated with blocking solution containing 2% albumin. The cells were then incubated with anti-myosin antibody at room temperature for 2 h. Cell were washed again and then incubated with anti-mouse Alexa-488 antibody (Abcam, Cambridge, MA) for two hours. Cells were washed again three times with PBS and the nuclei were stained briefly with Hoechst 33342 dye (1:2000 dilution). Pictures were taken at 200 × magnification using a Nikon Fluorescent Microscope (Nikon Instruments Inc, Melville, NY 11747, USA). Myotubes were defined as myosin positive cells with 2 or more fused nuclei.

2.7. Protein Synthesis in Cultured C2C12 Myotubules

C2C12 cells (375,000) were initially plated on a 12-well tissue culture plate that was initially coated with 2% gelatin. Cells were differentiated for five days in 5% horse serum (media was changed every two days) and then starved for 30 min by replacing the media with 1 ml PBS. The cells were then treated with 0, 50, 100, and 200 µg/mL of plum extract in PBS, spiked with [^{3}H] phenylalanine (1µCi/well), and incubated for 2 h at 37 °C. The reaction was stopped by placing the plates on ice. Wells were washed two times with DPBS-media containing 2 mM cold phenylalanine. Further, 1 mL of 20% cold trichloroacetic acid (TCA) solution was added to each well and plates were incubated on ice for 1 h for protein precipitation. Wells were washed two times with cold TCA and then the precipitated proteins were dissolved in 0.5 mL of 0.5N NaOH containing 0.2% Triton X-100 overnight in a refrigerator. An aliquot (5 µL) of the NaOH solubilized material was used for protein determination and the rest of the dissolved proteins were mixed with scintillation fluid and counted. Data is computed as cpm/mg of proteins and then % change over control is calculated.

2.8. Protein Degradation in C1C12 Myotubules

C2C12 myoblasts were cultured and differentiated as described above. Cells were then labelled with [^{3}H] Tyrosine 1 µCi/1 mL in serum free-DMEM (SF-DMEM) for 24 h. The unincorporated [^{3}H] Tyrosine was removed by washing the cell monolayer three times with SF-DMEM containing 50 µM cycloheximide (protein synthesis inhibitor) and 2 mM non-labelled Tyrosine. Proteolysis was induced by serum deprivation for 48 h in the presence or absence of 50, 100, 200 µg/mL of plum extract in serum-free DMEM containing 50 µM cycloheximide. The extent of protein degradation was assayed by monitoring release of radioactive tyrosine in the media after 48 h of incubation and was expressed as protein degradation in comparison to control (normalized to 100%).

2.9. Determination of Insulin-Like Growth Factor-1 (IGF-1) Expression

Total RNA was extracted from C2C12 myotubules with RNeasy Plus Universal Mini Kit (Qiagen, Hilden, Germany), according to the manufacturer's instructions. The concentration and purity of RNA was determined by measuring the absorbance in a Nano drop spectrophotometer. RT2 First Strand Kit from Qiagen (Qiagen, Hilden, Germany) was used to synthesize first strand complementary DNA (cDNA). The gene expression levels were analyzed by Quantitative real-time RT-PCR conducted on the Bio-Rad CFX-96 Real-Time PCR System using RT2 SYBR Green Master mix (Bio-Rad Laboratories, Hercules, CA). The primers (*IGF*: forward primer GGACCAGAGACCCTTTGCGGGG and reverse primer, AGCTCAGTAACAGTCCGCCTAGA; *GAPDH*: forward primer ATCCCATCACCATCTTCCAG and reverse primer CCATCACGCCACAGTTTCC) were designed. Hot-Start DNA Taq Polymerase was activated by heating at 95 °C for 10 min and real time PCR was conducted for 40 cycles (15 s for 95 °C, 1 min for 60 °C). All results were obtained from at least three independent biological repeats. Data were analyzed using the $\Delta\Delta CT$ method. Glyceraldehyde-3-phosphate dehydrogenase (*GAPDH*) genes were used as house-keeping genes for expression calculation.

2.10. Determination of NFκB Activation

A549/NFkB-luc cells (Panomics Catalog No. RC0002) at 3×10^5/well were seeded in 1 mL of Initial Growth Media (Dulbecco's Modified Eagle's medium containing 10% FBS and 1% Pen-Strep) in a 12-well plate. The cells were incubated in a humidified incubator at 37 °C and 5% CO_2 for 24 h to allow cells to recover and attach. After washing the cells once with serum-free media containing penicillin (100 units/mL), and streptomycin (100 mg/mL), 1 mL of this media was added to each well. Cells were pretreated with varying concentrations of plum extracts for 1 h at 37 °C and 5% CO_2, and then TNFα was added to achieve a final concentration of 2 ng/mL to all wells except control untreated cells. The cells were incubated in a humidified incubator at 37 °C and 5% CO_2 for 6 h. After treatment, the media was carefully removed. Cells were washed with PBS once and then lysed by 100 µL of 1× lysis buffer. Assay for luciferase activity was performed according to assay manufacturer's (Promega P/N E1500) recommendations. The average relative luminescence units (RLU) were calculated and corrected for baseline quenching for each set of triplicate wells, using WinGlow software (PerkinElmer, Waltham, MA 02451, USA and Microsoft Excel (Microsoft Corporation, Redmond, WA 98073, USA). The data is reported as the relative percent inhibition of TNFα mediated NFκB activation on A549 cells.

2.11. Effect of Plum Extract on Colon-26 Proliferation and its' Soluble Factor Induced Cytotoxicity on C2C12 Myotubules

Colon 26 cells, a mouse colon carcinoma cell line, was obtained from American Type Culture Collection (Manassas, VA, USA). Effect of plum extract on Colon-26 cell proliferation was assayed using a Water-Soluble Tetrazolium-1 (WST-1) (Talkara, Shiga, Japan) assay as described previously [39]. To determine the effects of soluble factors released from Colon-26 on C2C12 myotubules, conditioned media from Colon-26 culture was collected after 24 h. of cultivation. The media was centrifuged at $2500 \times g$ for 20 min to remove cellular material. The clear supernatant (conditioned media) was diluted 1:10 with normal complete media. The C2C12 differentiated myoblasts were then treated with normal complete medium or with Colon-26 conditioned medium with or without 50 µg/mL plum extract. A lower dose of plum extract (50 µg/mL) was used to avoid a direct effect of higher dose of plum extract (100 µg/mL or 200 µg/mL) on protein synthesis and degradation. The cell viability was assayed using a WST-1 assay. Control cells were subjected to equal amounts of non-conditioned media.

2.12. Data Analysis

The data is expressed as mean ± SD for at least three replicates. All comparisons were made by one-way ANOVA with Tukey's -HSD-post-hoc test using SPSS Statistics 20 software. All significant differences are reported at $p < 0.05$ and indicated by "*".

3. Results

3.1. Characterization of PE60 Plum Extract Composition and Anti-Oxidation Properties

As shown in Table 1, the major components identified in the polyphenol-enriched PE60 plum extract are proanthocyanidins, along with minor components such as anthocyanidins, 3-chlorogenic acid, rutin, quercetin (free), and gallic acid (free).

The PE60 was also characterized by determining total phenolic content (TPC), total flavonoid content (TFC), anti-oxidant activity (DPPH assay), and oxygen scavenging activity (ABTS). The data in Table 2 shows that the content of TPC was in the same range as reported by the commercial vendor (60%). The data indicate that the PE60 contained TPC in range 525–575 mg/g of dry extract. The TFC was in 480–560 mg/g dry weight range. The anti-oxidation effects as determined by inhibition of DPPH oxidation and ABTS assay ranged from 3280–3460 and 4000–4500 µM Trolox equivalents/g, respectively.

Table 1. Characterization of composition of polyphenol-enriched plum extract (PE60).

Component	Concentration (g per 100 g) $n = 3$	Flavonoid Type (USDA)	Analytical Method
Anthocyanins	0.391 ± 0.020 (rsd = 5.1%)	Anthocyanidin	Colorimetric
3-chlorogenic acid	1.76 ± 0.01 (rsd = 0.6%)	Hydroxycinnamic acid	LC/UV *
Rutin	1.12 ± 0.01 (rsd = 0.6%)	Flavanol	LC/UV *
Quercetin (free)	0.718 ± 0.005 (rsd = 0.7%)	Flavanol	LC/UV *
Gallic acid (free)	0.381 ± 0.004 (rsd = 1.1%)	Hydroxybenzoic	LC/UV *
Proanthocyanidins	60 ± 10 (rsd < 2%)	Flavan-3-ol	LC/UV *

Contents in PE60 plum extract were determined either using an Agilent Technologies Model 1200 HPLC System (Wilmington, DE, USA) or a colorimetric method as described in Section 2.2 in the text. Values are mean ± SD of three experiments. * LC/UV = liquid chromatography/ultraviolet light detection

Table 2. Characterization of anti-oxidation properties of PE60.

Assays	Units	Mean ± SD
Total Phenolic Content (TPC)	mg/g	542.44 ± 24.75
Total Flavonoid Content (TFC)	mg/g	520.00 ± 40.10
Anti-oxidant activity (DPPH)	µM Trolox Equivalent/g	3375 ± 90
Oxygen Scavenging Activity (ABTS)	µM Trolox Equivalent/g	4250 ± 250

The anti-oxidation properties of PE60 plum extract were determined using specific assays (TPC: total phenolic content, TFC: total flavonoid content, DPPH: 2,2-diphenyl-1-picrylhydrazyl, ABTS: 2,2′-azino-bis(3-ethylbenzothiazoline-6-sulfonic acid)) as described in Section 2.3 in the text. Values are mean ± SD of three experiments.

3.2. Effect of PE60 Plum Extract on C2C12 Myoblast Size and Differentiation

Plum extract had no cytotoxic effect on myoblast when used even at a high dose of 250 µg/mL (data not shown). It is evident from images that plum extract has some effect on cell proliferation; however, it was interesting to note that the plum extract increased the size of undifferentiated myoblasts cells in a dose-dependent manner (Figure 1a). The size of myoblast increased ~two-fold ($p < 0.05$) after treating cells with 50 µg/mL of plum extract when compared to that of untreated-control cells. Increase in myoblast size plateaued to a maximum increase of three-fold at 200 µg/mL concentration (Figure 1b). The effect of plum extract was also assessed on myoblast differentiation. Figure 2a indicates that the plum extract stimulated differentiation of myoblast in a dose-dependent manner using expression of myosin heavy chain as a marker for differentiation. The number of myotubes formed resulting from fusion of differentiated cells was increased by two-fold in cells treated with

100 µg/mL plum extract ($p < 0.05$) and by three-fold at 200 µg/mL ($p < 0.05$) compared to that of control cells (Figure 2b).

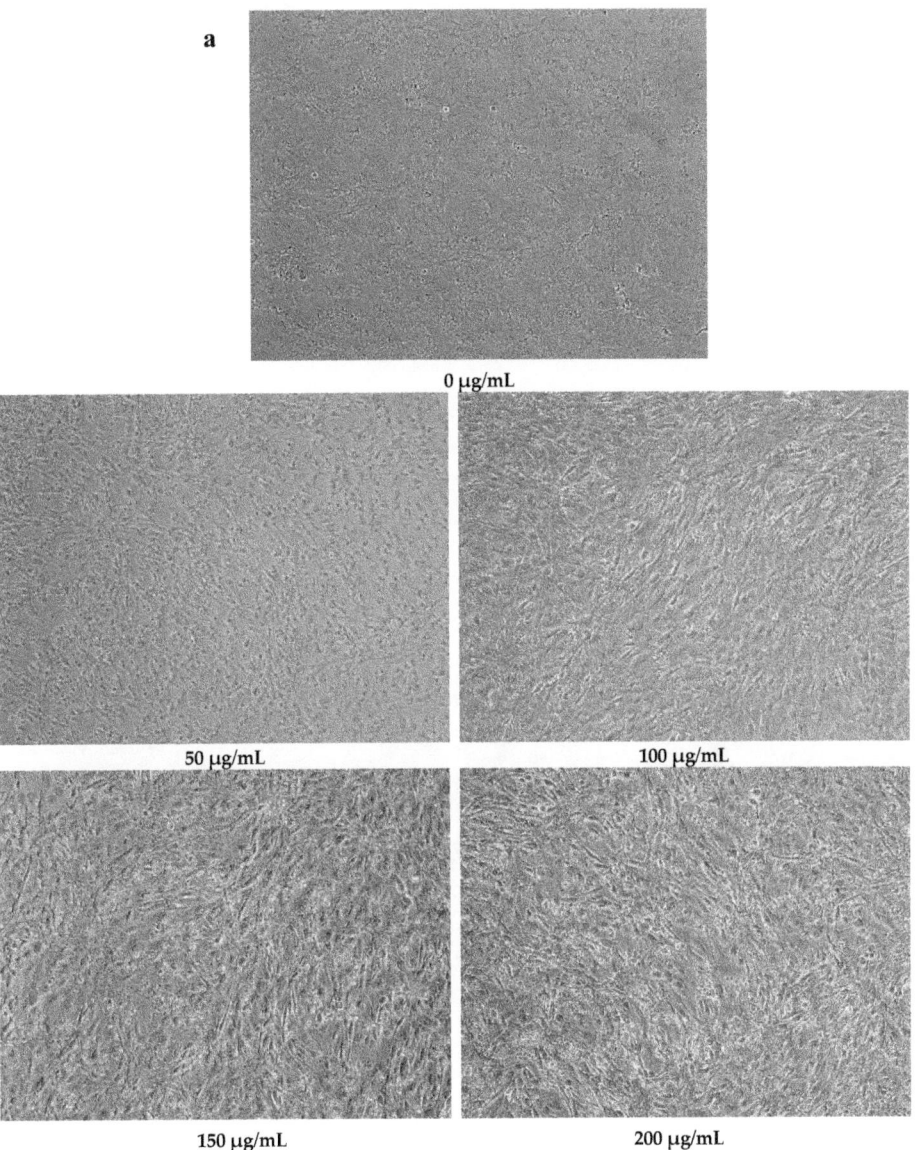

Plum Extract

Figure 1. *Cont.*

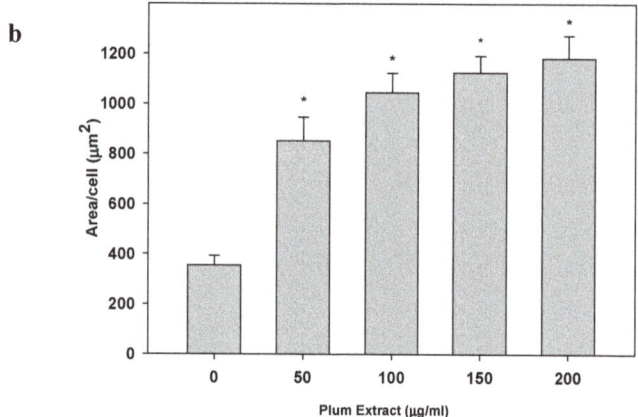

Figure 1. The effect of plum extract on C2C12 myoblast cell size. (**a**) The representative pictures of myoblast after treatment with varying concentration of plum extract (100 × magnified images) taken by a Nikon Microscope. The bar represents a length of 500 μm. (**b**) The size of myoblast was determined using Element-BR software as described in "Materials and Methods". The data are expressed as mean ± SD for at least three experiments. All comparisons were made to control (untreated cells) using one-way ANOVA; significant differences are reported at * $p < 0.05$.

(**a**)

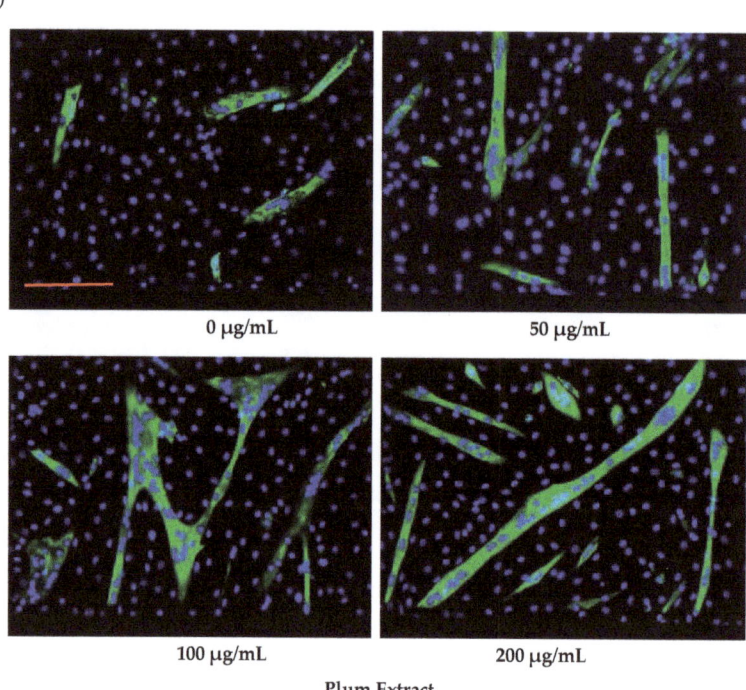

Plum Extract

Figure 2. *Cont.*

(b)

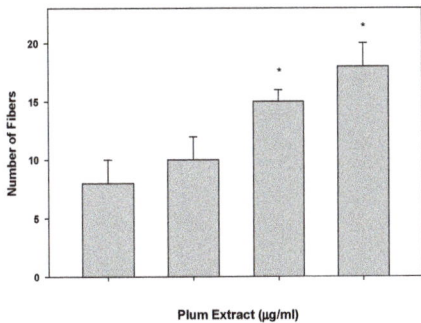

Figure 2. The effect of plum extract on C2C12 myoblast differentiation. (**a**) Images of differentiated cells after treatment with varying concentration of plum extract showing nuclei stained in blue (Hoechst 33342) and myofibers stained in green (Alexa 488). Pictures were taken at 200× magnification using a Nikon Fluorescent Microscope. The bar represents a length of 300 µm. (**b**) Fused cells from five random fields were counted manually under 200× as described in "Materials and Methods". The data are expressed as mean ± SD for at least three experiments. All comparisons were made to control (untreated cells) using one-way ANOVA; significant differences are reported at * $p < 0.05$.

3.3. Effect of PE60 Plum Extract on Myotubule Protein Synthesis

Plum extract showed almost a linear increase in [^{3}H] phenylalanine incorporation into proteins in a dose dependent manner in C2C12 myotubules (Figure 3). Doses of 100 µg/mL and 200 µg/mL of plum extract caused a significant increase in protein synthesis by 30% and 50%, respectively ($p < 0.05$).

3.4. Effect of PE60 Plum Extract on Myotubules Protein Degradation

We also examined if plum extract could reduce myotubule protein degradation induced by serum starvation. Figure 4 revealed that plum extract did inhibit protein degradation in a dose-dependent manner. Doses of 100 µg/mL and 200 µg/mL significantly inhibited protein degradation by 20% and 30%, respectively ($p < 0.05$).

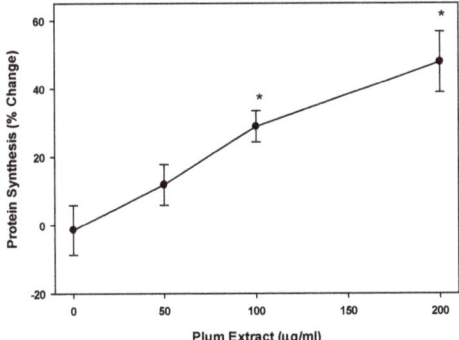

Figure 3. The effect of plum extract on myotubule protein synthesis. Protein synthesis was measure by the incorporation of labeled phenylalanine into total myotubule proteins in response to various levels of plum extract. Data were computed as cpm/mg of proteins followed by calculation of % change over control. The data were expressed as mean ± SD for at least three experiments. All comparisons were made to control (untreated cells) using one-way ANOVA; significant differences are reported at * $p < 0.05$.

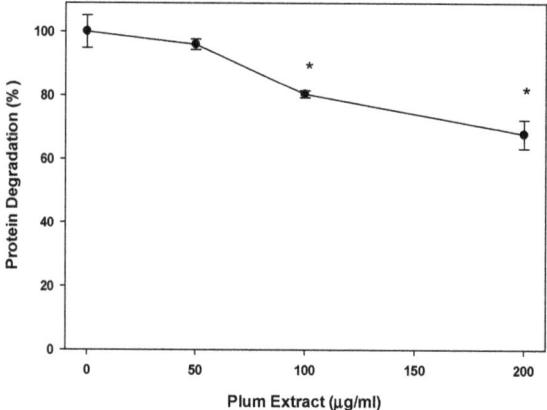

Figure 4. The effect of plum extract on myotubule protein degradation. Proteolysis was induced by 48 h-serum starvation in the presence or absence of plum extract, and monitored by release of radioactive tyrosine from pre-labelled cells. Data were computed as cpm/mg of proteins and then % change over control was calculated. The data were expressed as mean ± SD for at least three experiments. All comparisons were made to control (untreated cells) using one-way ANOVA; significant differences are reported at * $p < 0.05$.

3.5. Effect of PE60 Plum Extract on IGF-1 Expression in Myotubules

Expression of IGF-1 mRNA in C2C12 myotubules upon treatment with plum extract is shown in Figure 5. Compared to that of untreated cells, low concentration of plum extract (50 µg/mL) has no significant effect on IGF-1 mRNA expression; however, it significantly stimulated IGF-1 expression when cells were treated at a higher dose (100 or 200 µg/mL) plum extract.

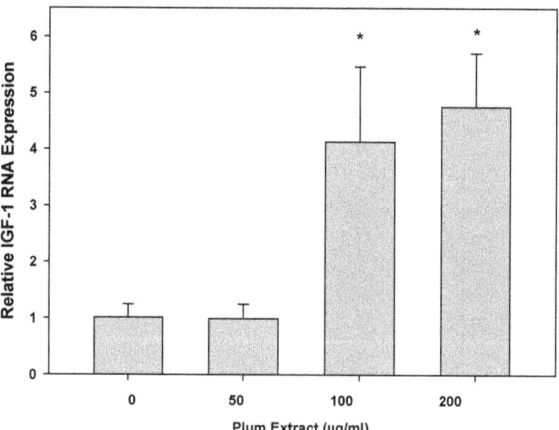

Figure 5. The effect of plum extract of IGF-1 gene expression. Total RNA was extracted from C2C12 myotubules treated with various concentrations of plum extract and compared to untreated control. All results were obtained from at least three independent biological repeats. Data were analyzed using the ΔΔCT method. Glyceraldehyde-3-phosphate dehydrogenase (*GAPDH*) genes were used as house-keeping genes for expression calculation. All comparisons were made to control (untreated cells) using one-way ANOVA; significant differences are reported at * $p < 0.05$.

3.6. Anti-Inflammatory Effect of PE60 plum Extract in Vitro

We evaluated the anti-inflammatory activity of plum extract by assessing its effect on TNF-α-induced NFkB activation where the activity was measured in terms of luciferase activity of NFkB reporter system assay. Plum extract inhibited NFkB activation in a dose dependent manner (Figure 6). A dose response assay indicated that ~40% inhibition ($p < 0.05$) of TNF-α-mediated NFkB activation was achieved at 25 µg/mL plum extract, and >80% inhibition ($p < 0.05$) of TNF-α-mediated NFkB activation was achieved at 50 µg/mL plum extract.

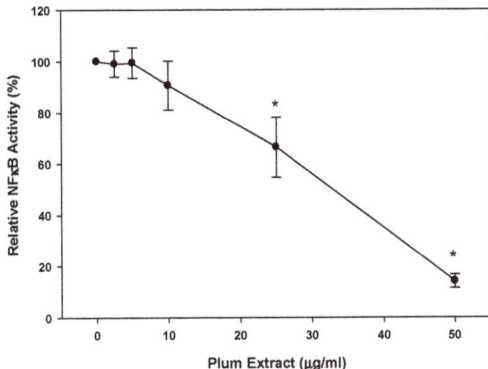

Figure 6. Effects of plum extract on NFkB activation. The effect of plum extract on TNFα-mediated NFkB activation was measured in the A549/NFκB-luc reporter stable cell line. Activity was measured in terms of luciferase activity. The data are reported as the relative percent inhibition of TNFα-mediated NFkB activation. The data are expressed as mean ± SD for at least three experiments. All comparisons were made to control (untreated cells) using one-way ANOVA; significant differences are reported at * $p < 0.05$.

3.7. Effect of PE60 Plum Extract on Colon-26 Mouse Adenocarcinoma Cell Line

When Colon-26 cells were treated with plum extract, the cells viability was reduced in a dose-dependent manner reaching ~80% reduction ($p < 0.05$) at 150 µg/mL. Upon further increasing the concentration of plum extract, the cell viability was further reduced 90% ($p < 0.05$) at 200 µg/mL (Figure 7).

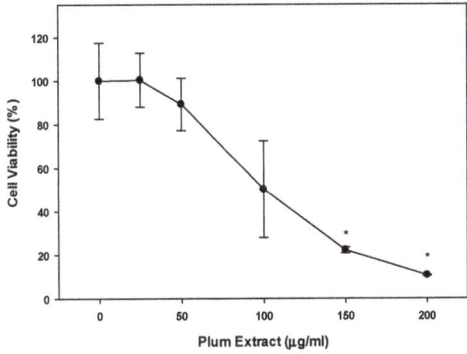

Figure 7. Effect of plum extract on Colon-26 adenocarcinoma cells. Data were calculated as % inhibition of cell growth in response to various concentrations of plum extract. The data are expressed as mean ± SD for at least three replicates. All comparisons were made to control (untreated cells) using one-way ANOVA; the significant differences are reported at * $p < 0.05$.

3.8. Effect of PE60 Plum Extract on C2C12 Cell Viability in Response to Colon-26 Cells Cytotoxicity-Inducing Factors

Mouse derived Colon-26 adenomacarcinoma cells are known to induce muscle wasting in rodents [40]. The effect of these circulating soluble factors released by Colon-26 was examined on growth of C2C12 myotubules in vitro in presence or absence of plum extract. Figure 8a,b shows that in the absence of plum extract, soluble factors released in media derived from Colon-26 cells caused a significant reduction of C2C12 cell viability by ~25% ($p < 0.05$). However, in the presence of plum extract, the negative effects of Colon-26-derived media on C2C12 viability was prevented and the cell viability was maintained to a similar level that was seen in the untreated cells.

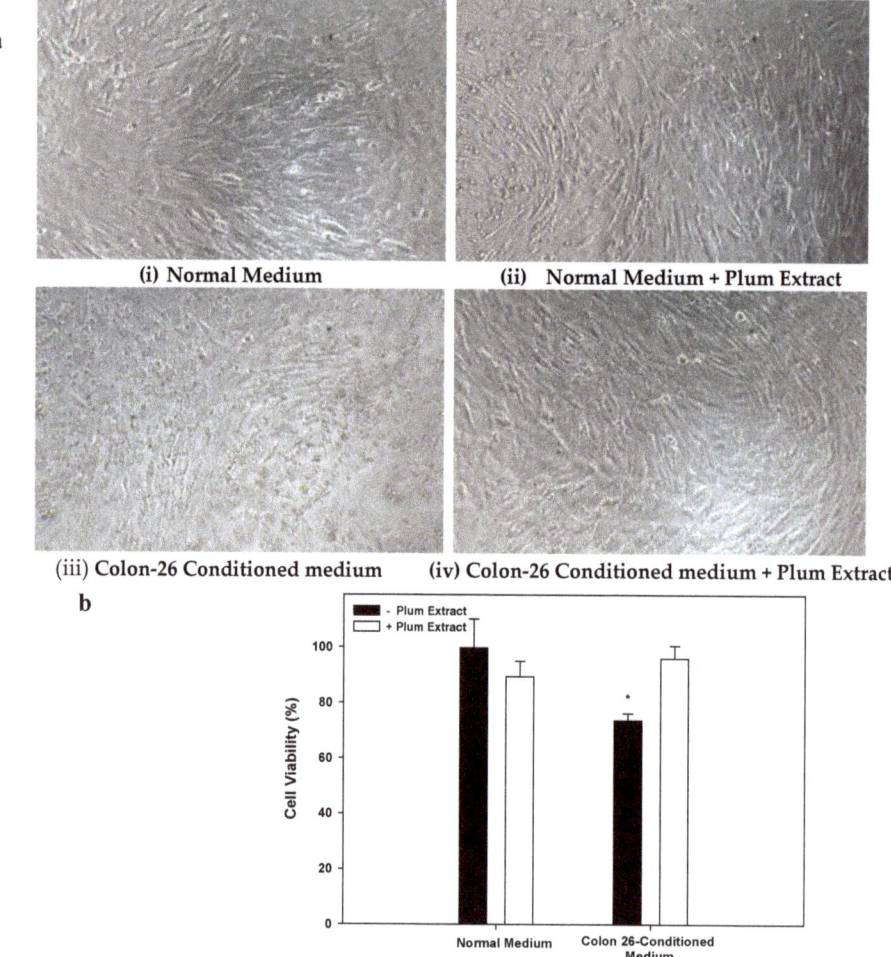

Figure 8. The effect of plum extract on C2C12 viability in response to Colon-26-induced cytotoxicity. (**a**) Differentiated C2C12 myotubes were treated with normal medium (i & ii) or Colon-26-conditioned medium (iii & iv) in the absence (i & iii) or presence (ii & iv) of plum extract (50 µg/mL). (**b**) The viability of C2C12 myotubules were determined using WST-1 assay. The data is expressed as mean ± SD for at least three experiments. All comparisons were made to control (untreated cells) using one-way ANOVA; significant differences are reported at * $p < 0.05$.

4. Discussion

In our study, we sought to investigate if plums had benefits on skeletal muscle. Specifically, we selected to use a plum extract that was enriched in polyphenols (~60% polyphenols) because the health benefits of plum have been partly attributed to its high polyphenol content [41–43]. Our data indicates that about 95% of total phenolic content in the plum extract used was present in the form of flavonoids. This data is not surprising as fruits are often reported to have phenolic compounds which are high in flavonoids with a range of 90–100% [44]. The anti-oxidant activity in the plum extract was found to be in range of 3–4 mM of Trolox equivalent/g, which is higher than that of turmeric (0.27–0.35 mM Trolox eq/g) and mulberry (1–2 mM Tolox eq/g), but lower than green tea (13–17 mM Trolox eq/g) and pomegranate (20–25 mM Trolox eq/g) [45–49].

Dried plum has previously been reported to have health benefits on bone. In rat models of osteoporosis, dried plum intake resulted in prevention and reversal of bone loss [50,51]. A three-month clinical intervention study showed that dried plum intake improved biomarkers of bone formation in postmenopausal women, whereas longer-term intake of dried plum resulted in mitigating loss of bone mineral density [31]. The present study was designed to analyze the effects of plum extract on muscle metabolism in C2C12 myotubules. In our initial experiments, the effect of plum extract was tested on myoblast viability. The data show that this plum extract has no toxicity on the muscle cells, even at very high doses. These results are consistent with prior literature on plum effects on non-diseased cells [52]. The maintenance of muscle mass is dependent on synthesis of new proteins and breakdown of old or damaged proteins. If these processes are balanced, the muscle mass is maintained; however, with aging and under certain catabolic condition including cancer, renal failure or trauma, muscle protein degradation exceeds the synthesis of new proteins, and results in muscle atrophy [53]. One interesting observation was that that plum extract increased the size of growing myoblast under un-differentiated conditions, suggestive of inducing increase in cytoplasmic volumes by stimulating protein synthesis. We also measured effect of plum extract on protein synthesis and degradation in differentiated myotubules. Our data clearly demonstrated that plum extract not only increased protein synthesis but also inhibited myotubules protein degradation in response to serum starvation, demonstrating both an anabolic and anti-catabolic effect.

The activity of the plum extract appears to be at least partly mediated through IGF-1 stimulation. Several studies have shown that IGFs stimulated both proliferation and differentiation of myoblasts, and also play a role in regenerating damaged skeletal muscle [54–58]. In line with our results, prior studies have also demonstrated that plums can increase IGF-1 levels in both humans [58] and animal models [51,59]. One of the manifestations of muscle loss is associated with decreased production of IGF-1 [60]. The signaling pathway IGF-1/PI3K/Akt (Insulin like growth factor -1/phosphatidyl inositol 3-kinase/protein kinase) is considered the main mediator of normal muscle development and one of the most studied signaling molecular systems involved in muscle metabolism [61]. Akt activation leads to activation of mTOR (mammalian target of rapamycin), which is responsible for promoting protein synthesis. The Akt-mTOR signaling pathway and its downstream components (p70s6k and 4E-BPI) are attenuated with muscle wasting [62]. Further studies need to be performed to confirm the if plum extract is indeed regulating Akt activity. The identification of compound or compounds in plum responsible for stimulating IGF-1 levels in myoblast was beyond the scope of the present study. As discussed earlier, ursolic acid has been shown to increase muscle mass in mice exhibiting fasting-induced muscle atrophy [22] or diet-induced obesity [23]. Interestingly, ursolic acid has also been shown to induce IGF-1 levels in the skeletal muscle of these mice with an increased Akt phosphorylation [22,23]. During present investigation, we were not able to detetect ursolic acid in PE60 extracts due to technical limitation for detecting all polyphenols; however, other studies have reported presence of ursolic acid in plums [21]. Therefore, it is possible that ursolic to some extent may have contributed in IGF-1 mediated muscle growth in our studies.

Studies have demonstrated the anti-inflammatory effect of dried-plum or plum juice in several cellular system including lipopolysaccharide-induced macrophages [63,64], splenocytes from ovariectomized mice [65], colorectal cells in azoxymethane-treated rats [66], heart tissues in obese rats [67] and joints of TNF-over expressing mice [25]. The antioxidation activities of plum appeared to be mediated through the inhibition of NFκB activation [25,66,67]. Based on these reported studies, we decided to test the effect of plum extract on NFκB activation, since oxidative stress and inflammatory responses through activation of NFκB play an important part in muscle atrophy. Activation of NFκB plays a central role in muscle atrophy in several catabolic situations including cancer cachexia [68,69]. We found that even a small dose of plum extract was able to almost completely inhibit (>80% inhibition) TNF-α-induced NFκB activity *in vitro*. It is likely that the proanthocyanidins, which comprise over 70% of the polyphenols, may be involved in suppressing the inflammatory cytokine (TNF)-induced activation of NFκB, although this has not been systematically tested with the individual components of the extract.

Cancer cachexia-related morbidity and mortality are often accompanied by whole body and muscle loss [4,7,8] and it is suggested that blocking muscle wasting can prolong life despite tumor growth [10]. The effect of plum extract on colon cancer cell viability, as well as its ability to protect muscle cells from colon-cancer cell induced cytotoxicity, were, therefore, also investigated. We used Colon-26 adenocarcinoma cells, which is a widely used preclinical model because it induces clinical cachexia, including its development as well as the resultant physiological and metabolic impairment [40,69,70]. Treating the Colon-26 colon cancer cells with plum extract caused a significant decrease in the Colon-26 cell's viability, indicating potential anti-tumor activity.

It is known that muscle wasting in cancer patients is mediated through factors released from tumor in circulation [71–74]. Studies have shown that elevated circulating levels of IL-6 mediated skeletal muscle cell death in severely cachectic mice with colon cancer [75]. Our studies found that plum extract can protect C2C12 myotubules from cytotoxicity induced by soluble factors released by the Colon-26 cells. The exact pathways leading to reduced cell viability in response to tumor induced soluble factors are not known, but it is possible that both atrophy and apoptosis may be attenuated by the plum extract. It is also possible that compound(s) in plum extract may directly affect colon cells to inhibit secretion of inflammatory cytokines. Future studies need to be conducted to elucidate the molecular mechanism involved in the anti-cytotoxic activity of the plum extract.

Our current studies have several limitations. The study was performed using an *in vitro* system that may not represent the complexities of an *in vivo* system. Furthermore, polyphenols in the plum extract can undergo biotransformation in vivo, which could either enhance or diminish the anabolic of plum extract on muscle as well as its anti-inflammatory benefit. However, previous human studies with dried plum still demonstrated its ability to activate IGF-1 as well as its anti-inflammatory benefits, indicating that biotransformation may not result in loss of these effects observed in our study.

5. Conclusions

In conclusion, the polyphenol-enriched plum extract has both anti-catabolic and anabolic effects on muscle cells, as well as myogenic potential. In addition, this plum extract exhibited anti-cytotoxic properties in response to soluble factors released from cancer cells. Thus, plum extract may be a useful intervention to be considered for cancer cachexia or other chronic disease-induced cachexia involving inflammation. These results need to be confirmed in an animal model of cachexia, followed by clinical translation.

Author Contributions: Conceptualization: R.A.S., and S.L.P.; Experimentation and Data collection: F.A.A., H.L., P.K., P.W.J.; Manuscript writing: R.A.S., P.W.J., and S.L.P.

Funding: The study was partly funded by a grant from Abbott-Nutrition, Columbus, OH, and by Evans-Allen grant from USDA.

Acknowledgments: The financial support to Faten A. Alsolmei was provided by Saudi Arabian Culture Mission, Kingdom of Saudi Arabia.

Conflicts of Interest: Suzette Pereira and Paul Johns are currently employed by Abbott. Padmavathy Krishnan is an ex-Abbott employee. Rafat Siddiqui, Haiwen Li, and Faten Alsolmei have no conflict of interest.

References

1. Nixon, D.W.; Heymsfield, S.B.; Cohen, A.E.; Lutne, M.H.; Ansley, J.; Lawson, D.H.; Rudman, D. Protein calorie under-nutrition in hospitalized cancer patients. *Am. J. Med.* **1980**, *68*, 683–690. [CrossRef]
2. Warren, S. The immediate causes of death in cancer. *Am. J. Med. Sci.* **1932**, *184*, 610–616. [CrossRef]
3. Evans, W.J.; Morley, J.E.; Argiles, J.; Bales, C.; Baracos, V.; Guttridge, D.; Jatoi, A.; Kalantar-Zadeh, K.; Lochs, H.; Mantovani, G.; et al. Cachexia: A new definition. *Clin. Nutr.* **2008**, *27*, 793–799. [CrossRef]
4. Fearon, K.C.; Glass, D.J.; Guttridge, D.C. Cancer cachexia: Mediators, signaling, and metabolic pathways. *Cell Metab.* **2012**, *16*, 153–166. [CrossRef] [PubMed]
5. Fearon, K.; Strasser, F.; Anker, S.D.; Bosaeus, I.; Bruera, E.; Fainsinger, R.L.; Jatoi, A.; Loprinzi, C.; MacDonald, N.; Mantovani, G.; et al. Definition and classification of cancer cachexia: An international consensus. *Lancet Oncol.* **2011**, *12*, 489–495. [CrossRef]
6. Lieffers, J.R.; Mourtzakis, M.; Hall, K.D.; McCargar, L.J.; Prado, C.M.; Baracos, V.E. A viscerally driven cachexia syndrome in patients with advanced colorectal cancer: Contributions of organ and tumor mass to whole-body energy demands. *Am. J. Clin. Nutr.* **2009**, *89*, 1173–1179. [CrossRef]
7. Ravasco, P.; Monteiro-Grillo, I.; Vidal, P.M.; Camilo, M.E. Dietary counseling improves patient outcomes: A prospective, randomized, controlled trial in colorectal cancer patients undergoing radiotherapy. *J. Clin. Oncol.* **2005**, *23*, 1431–1438. [CrossRef] [PubMed]
8. Bapuji, S.B.; Sawatzky, J.A. Understanding weight loss in patients with colorectal cancer: A human response to illness. *Oncol. Nurs. Forum* **2010**, *37*, 303–310. [CrossRef]
9. Houten, L.; Reilley, A.A. An investigation of the cause of death from cancer. *J. Surg. Oncol.* **1980**, *13*, 111–116. [CrossRef] [PubMed]
10. Benny Klimek, M.E.; Aydogdu, T.; Link, M.J.; Pons, M.; Koniaris, L.G.; Zimmers, T.A. Acute inhibition of myostatin-family proteins preserves skeletal muscle in mouse models of cancer cachexia. *Biochem. Biophys. Res. Commun.* **2010**, *391*, 1548–1554. [CrossRef]
11. Gomes-Marcondes, M.C.; Tisdale, M.J. Induction of protein catabolism and the ubiquitin-proteasome pathway by mild oxidative stress. *Cancer Lett.* **2002**, *180*, 69–74. [CrossRef]
12. Powers, S.K.; Kavazis, A.N.; McClung, J.M. Oxidative stress and disuse muscle atrophy. *J. Appl. Phys.* **2007**, *102*, 2389–2397.
13. Powers, S.K.; Kavazis, A.N.; DeRuisseau, K.C. Mechanisms of disuse muscle atrophy: Role of oxidative stress. *Am. J. Physiol. Regul. Integr. Comp. Physiol.* **2005**, *288*, 337–344. [CrossRef] [PubMed]
14. Reid, M.B.; Moylan, J.S. Beyond atrophy: Redox mechanisms of muscle dysfunction in chronic inflammatory disease. *J. Physiol.* **2011**, *589*, 2171–2179. [CrossRef]
15. Siddiqui, R.A.; Hassan, S.; Harvey, K.A.; Rasool, T.; Das, T.; Mukerji, P.; DeMichele, S. Attenuation of proteolysis and muscle wasting by curcumin C3 complex in MAC16 colon tumour-bearing mice. *Br. J. Nutr.* **2009**, *102*, 967–975. [CrossRef]
16. Lambert, K.; Coisy-Quivy, M.; Bisbal, C.; Sirvent, P.; Hugon, G.; Mercier, J.; Avignon, A.; Sultan, A. Grape polyphenols supplementation reduces muscle atrophy in a mouse model of chronic inflammation. *Nutrition* **2015**, *31*, 275–283. [CrossRef] [PubMed]
17. Wang, B.; Yang, G.; Liang, X.; Zhu, M.; Du, M. Grape seed extract prevents skeletal muscle wasting in interleukin 10 knockout mice. *BMC Complement. Altern. Med.* **2014**, *14*, 162. [CrossRef]
18. Dorchies, O.M.; Wagner, S.; Buetler, T.M.; Ruegg, U.T. Protection of dystrophic muscle cells with polyphenols from green tea correlates with improved glutathione balance and increased expression of 67LR, a receptor for (-)-epigallocatechin gallate. *BioFactors* **2009**, *35*, 279–294. [CrossRef]
19. Meador, B.M.; Mirza, K.A.; Tian, M.; Skelding, M.B.; Reaves, L.A.; Edens, N.K.; Pereira, S.L. The green tea polyphenol Epigallocatechin-3-Gallate (EGCg) attenuates skeletal muscle atrophy in a rat model of sarcopenia. *J. Frailty Aging* **2015**, *4*, 209–215.
20. Wang, H.; Lai, Y.J.; Chan, Y.L.; Li, T.L.; Wu, C.J. Epigallocatechin-3-gallate effectively attenuates skeletal muscle atrophy caused by cancer cachexia. *Cancer Lett.* **2011**, *305*, 40–49. [CrossRef]
21. Liu, J. Pharmacology of oleanolic acid and ursolic acid. *J. Ethnopharmacol.* **1995**, *49*, 57–68. [CrossRef]
22. Kunkel, S.D.; Suneja, M.; Ebert, S.M.; Bongers, K.S.; Fox, D.K.; Malmberg, S.E.; Alipour, F.; Shields, R.K.; Adams, C.M. mRNA expression signatures of human skeletal muscle atrophy identify a natural compound that increases muscle mass. *Cell Metab.* **2011**, *8*, 627–638. [CrossRef]

23. Kunkel, S.D.; Elmore, C.J.; Bongers, K.S.; Ebert, S.M.; Fox, D.K.; Dyle, M.C.; Bullard, S.A.; Adams, C.M. Ursolic acid increases skeletal muscle and brown fat and decreases diet-induced obesity, glucose intolerance and fatty liver disease. *PLoS One* **2012**, *7*, e39332. [CrossRef]
24. Stacewicz-Sapuntzakis, M. Dried plums and their products: Composition and health effects–an updated review. *Crit. Rev. Food Sci. Nutr.* **2013**, *53*, 277–302. [CrossRef]
25. Mirza, F.; Lorenzo, J.; Drissi, H.; Lee, F.Y.; Soung, D.Y. Dried plum alleviates symptoms of inflammatory arthritis in TNF transgenic mice. *J. Nutr. Biochem.* **2018**, *52*, 54–61. [CrossRef] [PubMed]
26. Kim, D.-O.; Jeong, S.W.; Lee, C.Y. Antioxidant capacity of phenolic phytochemicals from various cultivars of plums. *Food Chem.* **2003**, *81*, 321–326. [CrossRef]
27. Ramos, S.; Alia, M.; Bravo, L.; Goya, L. Comparative effects of food-derived polyphenols on the viability and apoptosis of a human hepatoma cell line (HepG2). *J. Agric. Food Chem.* **2005**, *53*, 1271–1280. [CrossRef] [PubMed]
28. Yu, M.H.; Im, H.G.; Kim, H.I.; Lee, I.S. Induction of apoptosis by immature plum in human hepatocellular carcinoma. *J. Med. Food* **2009**, *12*, 518–527. [CrossRef]
29. Yu, M.H.; Gwon, I.H.; Gyu, L.S.; Kim, D.I.; Jeong, S.H.; Lee, I.S. Inhibitory effect of immature plum on PMA-induced MMP-9 expression in human hepatocellular carcinoma. *Nat. Prod. Res.* **2009**, *23*, 704–718. [CrossRef] [PubMed]
30. Rendina, E.; Hembree, K.D.; Davis, M.R.; Marlow, D.; Clarke, S.L.; Halloran, B.P.; Lucas, E.A.; Smith, B.J. Dried plum's unique capacity to reverse bone loss and alter bone metabolism in postmenopausal osteoporosis model. *PLoS One* **2013**, *8*, e60569. [CrossRef]
31. Arjmandi, B.H.; Johnson, S.A.; Pourafshar, S.; Navaei, N.; George, K.S.; Hooshmand, S.; Sheau, C.; Chai, S.C.; Akhavan, N.S. Bone-protective effects of dried plum in postmenopausal women: Efficacy and possible mechanisms. *Nutrients* **2017**, *9*, 496. [CrossRef] [PubMed]
32. Hooshmand, S.; Brisco, J.R.; Arjmandi, B.H. The effect of dried plum on serum levels of receptor activator of NF-κB ligand, osteoprotegerin and sclerostin in osteopenic postmenopausal women: A randomised controlled trial. *Br. J. Nutr.* **2014**, *112*, 55–60. [CrossRef]
33. Halloran, B.P.; Wronski, T.J.; VonHerzen, D.C.; Chu, V.; Xia, X.; Pingel, J.E.; Williams, A.A.; Smith, B.J. Dietary dried plum increases bone mass in adult and aged male mice. *J. Nutr.* **2010**, *140*, 1781–1787. [CrossRef] [PubMed]
34. Niketic-Aleksic, G.K.; Hrazdina, G. Quantitative analysis of the anthocyanin content in grape juices and wines. *LWT-FOOD. SCI. TECHNOL.* **1972**, *5*, 163–165.
35. Yu, L.; Haley, S.; Perret, J.; Harris, M. Antioxidant properties of extracts from hard winter wheat. *Food Chem.* **2002**, *78*, 457–461. [CrossRef]
36. Parry, J.W.; Su, L.; Moore, J.; Cheng, Z.; Luther, M.; Jaladanki, R.; Wang, J.; Yu, L. Chemical Compositions, Antioxidative Capacities, and Anti-Proliferative Activities of Selected Fruit Seed Flours. *J. Agric. Food Chem.* **2006**, *54*, 3773–3778. [CrossRef]
37. Cheng, Z.; Moore, J.; Yu, L. High-throughput relative DPPH radical scavenging capacity assay. *J. Agric. Food Chem.* **2006**, *54*, 7429–7436. [CrossRef] [PubMed]
38. Re, R.; Pellegrini, N.; Proteggente, A.; Pannala, A.; Yang, M.; Rice-Evens, C. Antioxidant activity applying an improved ABTS radical cation decolorization assay. *Free Radic. Bio. Med.* **1999**, *26*, 1231–1237. [CrossRef]
39. Siddiqui, R.A.; Harvey, K.A.; Xu, Z.; Natarajan, S.K.; Davisson, V.J. Characterization of lovastatin-docosahexaenoate anticancer properties against breast cancer cells. *Bioorg. Med. Chem.* **2014**, *22*, 1899–1908. [CrossRef]
40. Yuan, L.; Hani, J.; Mmeng, Q.; Xi, Q.; Zhuang, Q.; Jiang, Y.; Han, Y.; Zhang, B.; Fang, Z.; Wu, G. Muscle-specific E3 ubiquitin ligases are involved in muscle atrophy of cancer cachexia: An *in vitro* and *in vivo* study. *Oncol. Rept.* **2015**, *33*, 2261–2268. [CrossRef]
41. Nakatani, N.; Kayano, S.; Kikuzaki, H.; Sumino, K.; Katagiri, K.; Mitani, T. Identification, quantitative determination, and antioxidative activities of chlorogenic acid isomers in prune (*Prunus domestica* L.). *J Agric. Food Chem* **2000**, *48*, 5512–5516. [CrossRef]
42. Graef, J.L.; Rendina-Ruedya, E.; Crocketta, E.K.; Ouyanga, P.; King, J.B.; Cichewiczb, R.H.; Lucasa, E.A.; Smitha, B.J. Select polyphenolic fractions from dried plum enhance osteoblast activity through BMP-2 signaling. *J. Nutr. Biochem.* **2018**, *55*, 59–67. [CrossRef]

43. Graef, J.L.; Ouyanga, P.; Wanga, Y.; Rendina-Ruedya, E.; Lernerc, M.R.; Marlowb, D.; Lucasa, E.A.; Smith, B.J. Dried plum polyphenolic extract combined with vitamin K and potassium restores trabecular and cortical bone in osteopenic model of postmenopausal bone loss. *J. Funct. Foods* **2018**, *42*, 262–270. [CrossRef] [PubMed]
44. Ferreyra, M.L.F.; Rius, S.P.; Casati, P. Flavonoids: Biosynthesis, biological functions, and biotechnological applications. *Front Plant Sci.* **2012**, *3*, 222.
45. Bener, M.; Ozyurek, M.; Guçlu, K.; Apak, P. Optimization of microwave-assisted extraction of curcumin from *Curcuma longa* L. (turmeric) and evaluation of antioxidant activity in multi-test systems. *Rec. Nat. Prod.* **2016**, *10*, 542–554.
46. Pekal, A.; Drozdz, P.; Pyrzynska, K. Comparison of the antioxidant properties of commonly consumed commercial teas. *Int. J. Food Prop.* **2012**, *15*, 1101–1109. [CrossRef]
47. Forester, S.C.; Lambert, J.D. Antioxidant effects of green tea. *Mol. Nutr. Food Res.* **2011**, *55*, 844–854. [CrossRef] [PubMed]
48. Arfan, M.; Khan, R.; Rybarczyk, A.; Amarowicz, R. Antioxidant activity of mulberry fruit extracts. *Int. J. Mol. Sci.* **2012**, *13*, 2472–2480. [CrossRef] [PubMed]
49. Gil, M.I.; Tomas-Barberan, F.A.; Hess-Pierce, B.; Holcroft, D.M.; Kader, A.A. Antioxidant activity of pomegranate juice and its relationship with phenolic composition and processing. *J. Agric. Food Chem.* **2000**, *48*, 4581–4589. [CrossRef]
50. Deyhim, F.; Stoecker, B.J.; Brusewitz, G.H.; Devareddy, L.; Arjmandi, B.H. Dried plum reverses bone loss in an osteopenic rat model of osteoporosis. *Menopause* **2005**, *2*, 755–762. [CrossRef]
51. Franklin, M.; Bu, S.Y.; Lerner, M.R.; Lancaster, E.A.; Bellmer, D.; Marlow, D.; Lightfoot, S.A.; Arjmandi, B.H.; Brackett, D.J.; Lucas, E.A.; et al. Dried plum prevents bone loss in a male osteoporosis model via IGF-I and the RANK pathway. *Bone* **2006**, *39*, 1331–1342. [CrossRef]
52. Vizzotto, M.; Porter, W.; Byrne, D.; Cisneros-Zevallos, L. Polyphenols of selected peach and plum genotypes reduce cell viability and inhibit proliferation of breast cancer cells while not affecting normal cells. *Food Chem.* **2014**, *164*, 363–370. [CrossRef]
53. Cohen, S.; Nathan, J.A.; Goldberg, A.L. Muscle wasting in disease: Molecular mechanisms and promising therapies. *Nat. Rev. Drug Discov.* **2015**, *14*, 58–74. [CrossRef]
54. Florini, J.R.; Ewton, D.Z.; Coolican, S.A. Growth hormone and the insulin-like growth factor system in myogenesis. *Endocr. Rev.* **1996**, *17*, 481–517.
55. Coleman, M.E.; DeMayo, F.; Yin, K.C.; Lee, H.M.; Geske, R.; Montgomery, C.; Schwartz, R.J. Myogenic vector expression of insulin-like growth factor 1 stimulates muscle cell differentiation and myofiber hypertrophy in transgenic mice. *J. Biol. Chem.* **1995**, *270*, 12109–12116. [CrossRef] [PubMed]
56. Jennische, E.; Skottner, A.; Hansson, H.A. Satellite cells express the trophic factor IGF-1 in regenerating skeletal muscle cell. *Acta Physiol. Scand.* **1987**, *129*, 9–15. [CrossRef]
57. Jannische, E.; Hansson, H.A. Regenerating skeletal muscle cells express insulin-like growth factor I. *Acta Physiol. Scand.* **1987**, *130*, 327–332. [CrossRef]
58. Arjmandi, B.H.; Khalil, D.A.; Lucas, E.A.; Georgis, A.; Stoecker, B.J.; Hardin, C.; Payton, M.E.; Wild, R.A. Dried plums improve indices of bone formation in postmenopausal women. *J. Womens Health Gend. Based Med.* **2002**, *11*, 61–68. [CrossRef] [PubMed]
59. Smith, B.J.; Bu, S.Y.; Wang, Y.; Rendina, E.; Lim, Y.F.; Marlow, D.; Clarke, S.L.; Cullen, D.M.; Lucas, E.A. A comparative study of the bone metabolic response to dried plum supplementation and PTH treatment in adult, osteopenic ovariectomized rat. *Bone* **2014**, *58*, 151–159. [CrossRef]
60. Costelli, P.; Muscaritoli, M.; Bossola, M.; Penna, F.; Reffo, P.; Bonetto, A.; Busquets, S.; Bonelli, G.; Lopez-Soriano, F.J.; Doglietto, G.B.; et al. IGF-1 is downregulated in experimental cancer cachexia. *Am. J. Physiol. Regul. Integr. Comp Physiol.* **2006**, *291*, R674–R683. [CrossRef]
61. Schiaffino, S.; Mammucari, C. Regulation of skeletal muscle growth by the IGF1-Akt/PKB pathway: Insights from genetic models. *Skeletal Muscle* **2011**. [CrossRef] [PubMed]
62. Eley, H.L.; Russell, S.T.; Tisdale, M.J. Effect of branched-chain amino acids on muscle atrophy in cancer cachexia. *Biochem. J.* **2007**, *407*, 113–120. [CrossRef] [PubMed]
63. Bu, S.Y.; Lerner, M.; Stoecker, B.J.; Boldrin, E.; Brackett, D.J.; Lucas, E.A.; Smith, B.J. Dried plum polyphenols inhibit osteoclastogenesis by downregulating NFATc1 and inflammatory mediators. *Calcif. Tissue Int.* **2008**, *82*, 475–488. [CrossRef] [PubMed]

64. Hooshmand, S.; Kumar, A.; Zhang, J.Y.; Johnson, S.A.; Chai, S.C.; Bahram, H.; Arjmandi, B.H. Evidence for anti-inflammatory and antioxidative properties of dried plum polyphenols in macrophage RAW 264.7 cells. *Food Funct.* **2015**, *6*, 1719–1725. [CrossRef]
65. Rendina, E.; Lima, Y.F.; Marlowb, D.; Wanga, Y.; Clarkea, S.L.; Kuvibidilaa, S.; Lucasa, E.A.; Brenda, J.; Smith, B.J. Dietary supplementation with dried plum prevents ovariectomy-induced bone loss while modulating the immune response in C57BL/6J mice. *J. Nutr. Biochem.* **2012**, *23*, 60–68. [CrossRef]
66. Banerjee, N.; Kim, H.; Talcott, S.T.; Turner, N.D.; Byrne, D.H.; Mertens-Talcott, S.U. Plum polyphenols inhibit colorectal aberrant crypt foci formation in rats: Potential role of the miR-143/protein kinase B/mammalian target of rapamycin axis. *Nutr. Res.* **2016**, *36*, 1105–1113. [CrossRef] [PubMed]
67. Noratto, G.; Martino, H.S.D.; Simbo, S.; Byrne, D.; Mertens-Talcott, S.U. Consumption of polyphenol-rich peach and plum juice prevents risk factors for obesity-related metabolic disorders and cardiovascular disease in Zucker rats. *J. Nutr. Biochem.* **2015**, *26*, 633–641. [CrossRef]
68. Guttridge, D.C.; Mayo, M.W.; Madrid, L.V.; Wang, C.-Y.; Baldwin, A.S., Jr. NF-κB-induced loss of MyoD messenger RNA: Possible role in muscle decay and cachexia. *Science* **2000**, *289*, 2363–2366. [CrossRef] [PubMed]
69. Aulino, P.; Berardi, E.; Cardillo, V.M.; Rizzuto, E.; Perniconi, B.; Ramina, C.; Padula, F.; Spugnini, E.P.; Baldi, A.; Faiola, F.; et al. Molecular, cellular and physiological characterization of the cancer cachexia-inducing C26 colon carcinoma in mouse. *BMC Cancer* **2010**, *10*, 363. [CrossRef]
70. Tian, M.; Kliewer, K.L.; Asp, M.L.; Stout, M.B.; Belury, M.A. c9t11-Conjugated linoleic acid-rich oil fails to attenuate wasting in colon-26 tumor-induced late-stage cancer cachexia in male CD2F1 mice. *Mol. Nutr. Food Res.* **2010**, *55*, 268–277. [CrossRef]
71. Siddiqui, R.; Pandya, D.; Harvey, K.; Zaloga, G.P. Nutrition modulation of cachexia/proteolysis. *Nutr. Clin. Pract.* **2006**, *21*, 55–67. [CrossRef]
72. Siddiqui, R.A.; Williams, J.F. Tentative identification of the toxohormones of cancer cachexia: Roles of vasopressin, prostaglandin E2 and cachectic-TNF. *Biochem. Int.* **1990**, *20*, 787–797.
73. Tisdale, M.J. Mechanisms of Cancer Cachexia. *Physiol Rev.* **2009**, *89*, 381–410. [CrossRef]
74. Lorite, M.J.; Smith, H.J.; Arnold, J.A.; Morris, A.; Thompson, M.G.; Tisdale, M.J. Activation of ATP-ubiquitin-dependent proteolysis in skeletal muscle in vivo and murine myoblasts in vitro by a proteolysis-inducing factor (PIF). *Brit. J. Cancer* **2001**, *85*, 297–302. [CrossRef] [PubMed]
75. Baltgalvis, K.A.; Berger, F.G.; Peña, M.M.O.; Davis, J.M.; White, J.P.; Carson, J.A. Activity level, apoptosis, and development of cachexia in Apc mice. *J. Appl. Physiol.* **2010**, *109*, 1155–1161. [CrossRef] [PubMed]

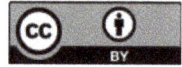

© 2019 by the authors. Licensee MDPI, Basel, Switzerland. This article is an open access article distributed under the terms and conditions of the Creative Commons Attribution (CC BY) license (http://creativecommons.org/licenses/by/4.0/).

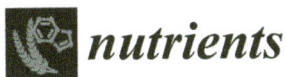

Article

Rectal and Vaginal Eradication of *Streptococcus agalactiae* (GBS) in Pregnant Women by Using *Lactobacillus salivarius* CECT 9145, A Target-specific Probiotic Strain

Virginia Martín [1,†], Nivia Cárdenas [2,‡], Sara Ocaña [2,3], María Marín [1], Rebeca Arroyo [1], David Beltrán [4], Carlos Badiola [5], Leónides Fernández [2] and Juan M. Rodríguez [1,*]

1. Department of Nutrition and Food Science, Complutense University of Madrid, 28040 Madrid, Spain; vmartinmerino@gmail.com (V.M.); mlmarin@vet.ucm.es (M.M.); rebecaa@vet.ucm.es (R.A.)
2. Department of Galenic Pharmacy and Food Technology, Complutense University of Madrid, 28040 Madrid, Spain; niviacu@yahoo.com (N.C.); saripsima@yahoo.es (S.O.); leonides@vet.ucm.es (L.F.)
3. Unidad de Reproducción, Fundación Hospital Alcorcón, 28922 Alcorcón, Spain
4. Centro de Diagnóstico Médico, Ayuntamiento de Madrid, 28006 Madrid, Spain; beltrangine@gmail.com
5. Laboratorios Casen Recordati S.L., Vía de las Dos Castillas, 33, 28224 Pozuelo de Alarcón, Madrid, Spain; cjbadiola@casenrecordati.com
* Correspondence: jmrodrig@ucm.es; Tel.: +34-913943749
† Current address: Centro Nacional de Microbiología, Instituto de Salud Carlos III, Ctra. de Pozuelo, 28; 28222 Majadahonda, Madrid, Spain.
‡ Current address: Probisearch S.L.U., C/ Santiago Grisolía, 2, 28760 Tres Cantos, Spain.

Received: 13 March 2019; Accepted: 5 April 2019; Published: 10 April 2019

Abstract: *Streptococcus agalactiae* (Group B Streptococci, GBS) can cause severe neonatal sepsis. The recto-vaginal GBS screening of pregnant women and intrapartum antibiotic prophylaxis (IAP) to positive ones is one of the main preventive options. However, such a strategy has some limitations and there is a need for alternative approaches. Initially, the vaginal microbiota of 30 non-pregnant and 24 pregnant women, including the assessment of GBS colonization, was studied. Among the *Lactobacillus* isolates, 10 *Lactobacillus salivarius* strains were selected for further characterization. In vitro characterization revealed that *L. salivarius* CECT 9145 was the best candidate for GBS eradication. Its efficacy to eradicate GBS from the intestinal and vaginal tracts of pregnant women was evaluated in a pilot trial involving 57 healthy pregnant women. All the volunteers in the probiotic group (n = 25) were GBS-positive and consumed ~9 $\log_{10}$ cfu of *L. salivarius* CECT 9145 daily from week 26 to week 38. At the end of the trial (week 38), 72% and 68% of the women in this group were GBS-negative in the rectal and vaginal samples, respectively. *L. salivarius* CECT 9145 seems to be an efficient method to reduce the number of GBS-positive women during pregnancy, decreasing the number of women receiving IAP during delivery.

Keywords: Lactobacillus salivarius; Streptococcus agalactiae; GBS; probiotic; pregnancy

1. Introduction

Neonatal sepsis contributes substantially to neonatal morbidity and mortality and is a major global public health challenge worldwide. According to the age of onset, neonatal sepsis is divided into early-onset sepsis (EOS) and late-onset sepsis (LOS). EOS has been variably defined based on the age at onset, with bacteremia or bacterial meningitis occurring at ≤72 h in infants hospitalized in the neonatal intensive care unit versus <7 days in term infants, and usually reflects transplacental or ascending infections from the maternal genitourinary tract [1].

Streptococcus agalactiae (Group B Streptococci, GBS) is one of the microorganisms most frequently involved in severe neonatal EOS cases [2–4]. Women, men and children of all ages can be asymptomatically colonized with GBS, acting the gastrointestinal tract, vagina and urethra as reservoirs. A recent systematic review and meta-analyses found that adjusted estimate for maternal GBS colonization worldwide was 18% (95% confidence interval [CI], 17%–19%), with regional variations (11%–35%) [5]. GBS vaginal and/or intestinal colonization is considered as a risk factor for ascending infection during pregnancy [6].

The relevance of GBS as an agent of neonatal infections soon prompted the finding of strategies for its eradication from the intestinal and genitourinary mucosal surfaces of pregnant women [7], including the use of chlorhexidine, which showed no effect [8] and, particularly, the development of vaccines. Unfortunately, no GBS vaccine is available at present despite the strong research efforts made in the last decades [9]. At present, two main approaches have been recommended for the prevention of neonatal GBS infections in Western countries: (a) a risk-based strategy; and (b) a screening-based strategy [10]. The second approach, involving recto-vaginal GBS screening at week 35–38 of pregnancy and subsequent intrapartum antibiotic prophylaxis (IAP) to positive mothers, is the preventive option followed in the USA and some European countries.

However, such a strategy also faces some limitations: (a) it does not guarantee GBS eradication [11]; (b) it does not prevent GBS-related abortions, stillbirths and preterm births [4]; (c) it may lead to increasing rates of antibiotic resistance among GBS and other clinically relevant microorganisms [12–14]; and (d), it has a very negative impact on the acquisition, composition and development of the infant microbiota. Perinatal antibiotic use affects the gut microbiota development during the critical first weeks of life [15,16]. The composition of the gut microbiota of neonates whose mothers received IAP has been described as aberrant in comparison with that of non-treated neonates [17,18]. The detrimental impact of perinatal antibiotics, mainly IAP, on early life microbiota may have a lasting effect on the host's health [19]. Therefore, there is a need for alternative strategies to avoid GBS colonization during pregnancy.

In this context, the objective of this work was, first, the assessment of the presence of GBS in the vaginal exudate of healthy pregnant and non-pregnant women; and, second, the selection of a safe probiotic strain with the ability to eradicate GBS from the intestinal and genitourinary tracts of pregnant women.

2. Material and Methods

2.1. Microbiological Analysis of Vaginal Swabs Obtained from Pregnant and Non-pregnant Women

A total of 54 women (30 non-pregnant women and 24 pregnant women), aged 25–35, participated in this part of the study. In accordance with the Declaration of Helsinki, all volunteers gave written informed consent to the protocol, which had been approved (protocol 10/017-E) by the Ethical Committee of Clinical Research of the Hospital Clínico San Carlos Madrid (Spain). In relation to non-pregnant women, 4 vaginal exudates samples were collected within a menstrual cycle (days 0, 7, 14 and 21). Pregnant women provided a single sample in week 35–37 of pregnancy. All women claimed to be completely healthy.

Samples were diluted in peptone water and spread onto Columbia Nalidixic Acid (CNA), Mac Conkey (MCK), Sabouraud Dextrose Chloramphenicol (SDC), Gardnerella (GAR) and Mycoplasma agar plates (BioMerieux, Marcy l'Etoile, France) for selective isolation and quantification of the main agents involved in vaginal infections. They were also spread onto agar plates of MRS (Oxoid, Basingstoke, UK) supplemented with either L-cysteine (2.5 g/L) (MRS-C) or horse blood (5%) (MRS-B) for isolation of lactobacilli. All the plates were incubated for 48 h at 37 °C in aerobic conditions, with the exception of the MRS-C and MRS-B ones, which were incubated anaerobically (85% nitrogen, 10% hydrogen, 5% carbon dioxide) in an anaerobic workstation (DW Scientific, Shipley, UK). Parallel, all the samples were submitted to an enrichment step in Todd Hewitt broth (Oxoid) to facilitate the isolation of *S. agalactiae* in CNA plates.

Initially, identification of the bacterial strains (at least one isolate of each colony morphology per medium and per sample) was performed by 16S rDNA sequencing using the primers and PCR conditions described by Kullen et al. [20]. Sequencing reactions were prepared using the ABI PRISM® BigDye™ Terminator Cycle Sequencing kit with AmpliTaq DNA polymerase according to the manufacturer's instructions (Applied Biosystems, Foster City, CA, USA) and were run on an ABI 377A automated sequencer (Applied Biosystems). The resulting sequences were used to search sequences deposited in the EMBL database using the BLAST algorithm. The identity of the strain was determined on the basis of the highest (>98%) scores.

Identification of yeasts and confirmation of the initial 16S rDNA-based bacterial identifications was performed by MALDI-TOF (VITEK MS, BioMerieux, Marcy-L'Étoile, France) [21]. Identification of *S. agalactiae* isolates was also confirmed by using a latex agglutination test (Streptococcal grouping kit, Oxoid, Basingstoke, UK), following the instructions of the manufacturer.

Those isolates identified as belonging to the genus *Lactobacillus* were preserved for further studies. For such a purpose, an MRS-C broth culture of each isolate was mixed with glycerol (30%, v/v) and kept at $-80\ °C$ until required. A total of 89 different *Lactobacillus* strains were isolated from the vaginal swabs and submitted to the Random Amplification of Polymorphic DNA (RAPD) genotyping as described [22] in order to avoid duplication of isolates. Among them, 10 *Lactobacillus salivarius* strains were selected for further characterization on the basis of the following criteria: (1) absence of *S. agalactiae*, *Gardnella vaginalis*, *Candida* spp., *Ureaplasma* spp. and *Mycoplasma* spp in the vaginal samples from which the lactobacilli were originally isolated; (2) Qualified Presumption of Safety (QPS) status conceded by EFSA; and (3) the ability of the strain to grow rapidly in MRS broth under aerobic conditions ($\geq 1 \times 10^6$ cfu/mL after 16 h at 37 °C).

2.2. Antimicrobial Activity of the Lactobacilli Strains against GBS

Initially, an overlay method [23] was used to determine the ability of the lactobacilli strains to inhibit the growth of 12 different *S. agalactiae* strains. Among them, 6 strains had been isolated from blood or cerebrospinal fluid in clinical cases of neonatal sepsis (Hospital Universitario Ramón y Cajal, Madrid, Spain) while the remaining 6 had been isolated from vaginal samples of pregnant women (our own collection). It was performed using MRS agar plates, on which the lactobacilli strains were inoculated as approximately 2 cm-long lines and incubated at 37 °C for 48 h. The plates were then overlaid with the indicator *S. agalactiae* strains vehiculated in 10 mL of Brain Heart Infusion (BHI, Oxoid) broth supplemented with soft agar (0.7%), at a concentration of $\sim 10^4$ colony-forming units (cfu)/mL. The overlaid plates were incubated at 37 °C for 48 h and, then, examined for clear zones of inhibition (>2 mm) around the lactobacilli streaks. All experiments assaying inhibitory activity were performed in triplicate.

2.3. Production of Specific Antimicrobials (Bacteriocins, Lactic Acid, Hydrogen Peroxide) by the Lactobacilli Strains

Bacteriocin production was assayed using an agar diffusion method as described by Dodd et al. [24] and modified by Martín et al. [25], using the *S. agalactiae* strains as the indicator bacteria employed for the overlay method. The lactobacilli strains were screened for hydrogen peroxide production following the procedure described by Song et al. [26]. In the case of positive strains, hydrogen peroxide production was also measured by the quantitative method of Yap and Gilliland [27]. The concentration of L- and D-lactic acid in the supernatants of MRS cultures of the lactobacilli strains was quantified using an enzymatic kit (Roche Diagnostics, Mannheim, Germany), following the manufacturer's instructions. The pH values of the supernatants were also measured. All these assays were performed in triplicate and the values were expressed as the mean $\pm$ SD.

2.4. Coaggregation and Co-culture Assays

The ability of the lactobacilli strains to aggregate with cells of the *S. agalactiae* strains was investigated following the procedure of Younes et al. [28]. The suspensions were observed under a phase-contrast microscope after Gram staining.

To test the anti-*S. agalactiae* activity of the lactobacilli in a broth assay format, tubes containing 20 mL of MRS broth were co-inoculated with 1 mL of a *Lactobacillus* strain culture (7 $\log_{10}$cfu/mL) and 1 mL of an *S. agalactiae* strain (7 $\log_{10}$ cfu/mL). Subsequently, the cultures were incubated for 6 h at 37 °C in aerobic conditions. Immediately after the co-inoculation and after the incubation period, aliquots were collected, serially diluted and plated on MRS-C plates and CHROMagar StrepB agar plates (CHROMagar, París, France) for the selective enumeration of lactobacilli and streptococci, respectively. Correct taxonomic assignment was confirmed by the MALDI-TOF analysis as described previously.

2.5. Survival After In Vitro Exposure to Saliva and Gastrointestinal-Like Conditions

The survival of the strain to conditions resembling those found in the human digestive tract (saliva, human stomach and small intestine) was assessed in the in vitro system described by Marteau et al. [29], with the modifications reported by Martín et al. [25]. For this purpose, the strain was vehiculated in UHT-treated milk (25 mL) at a concentration of 10^9 CFU/mL. The values of the pH curve in the stomach-like compartment were those recommended by Conway et al. [30]. Different fractions were taken at 20, 40, 60, and 80 min from this compartment, and exposed for 120 minutes to a solution with a composition similar to that of human duodenal juice [30]. The survival rate of the strain was determined by culturing the samples on MRS agar plates, which were incubated at 37 °C for 48 h.

2.6. Adhesion to Caco-2, HT-29 and Vaginal Cells and to Mucin

The ability of the strains to adhere to HT-29 and Caco-2 cells was evaluated as described by Coconnier et al. [31] with the modifications reported by Martín et al. [25]. HT-29 and Caco-2 were cultured to confluence in 2 mL of DMEM medium (PAA, Linz, Austria) containing 25 mM of glucose, 1 mM of sodium pyruvate and supplemented with 10% heat-inactivated fetal calf serum, 2 mM of L-glutamine and 1% non-essential amino acid preparation. At day 10 after confluence, 1 mL of the medium was replaced with 1 mL of DMEM containing 10^8 CFU/mL of the strains. Adherence was measured as the number of lactobacilli adhered to the cells in 20 random microscopic fields. The assay was performed by triplicate.

Adherence to vaginal epithelial cells collected from healthy premenopausal women was performed as described previously [32].

The adhesion of the lactobacilli strains to mucin was determined according to the method described by Cohen and Laux [33].

2.7. Sensitivity to Antibiotics

The sensitivity of the strains to antibiotics was tested using the lactic acid bacteria susceptibility test medium (LSM) [34] and the microtiter VetMIC plates for lactic acid bacteria (National Veterinary Institute of Sweden, Uppsala, Sweden), as described previously [35]. Parallel, minimum inhibitory concentrations (MICs) were also determined by the E-test [AB BIODISK, Solna, Sweden) following the instructions of the manufacturer. Results were compared to the cut-off levels proposed by the European Food Safety Authority [36].

2.8. Hemolysis, Formation of Biogenic Amines and Degradation of Mucin

For investigation of hemolysis, strains were streaked onto layered fresh horse blood agar plates and grown for 24 h at 37 °C. Zones of clearing around colonies indicated hemolysin production. The capacity of the strains to synthesize biogenic amines (tyramine, histamine, putrescine and cadaverine) from their respective precursor amino acids (tyrosine, histidine, ornithine and lysine; Sigma-Aldrich) was evaluated using the method described by Bover-Cid and Holzapfel [37]. The potential of the strains to degrade gastric mucine (HGM; Sigma) was evaluated in vitro as indicated by Zhou et al. [38].

2.9. Acute and Repeated Dose (4-Weeks) Oral Toxicity Studies in a Rat Model

Wistar male and female rats (Charles River Inc., Marget, Kent, UK) were used to study the acute and repeated dose (4-weeks) oral toxicity of *L. salivarius* CECT 9145 in a rat model. Acclimation, housing and management (including feeding) of the rats was performed as previously described [39]. The rats were 56-days old at the initiation of treatment. Acute (limit test) and repeated dose (4 weeks) studies were conducted in accordance with the European Union guidelines (EC Council Regulation No. 440), and authorized by the Ethical Committee on Animal Research of the Complutense University of Madrid (protocol 240111).

In the acute (limit test) study, 24 rats (12 males, 12 females) were distributed into two groups of 6 males and 6 females each. After an overnight of fasting, each rat received skim milk (500 µL) orally (control group or Group 1), or a single oral dose of 1×10^{10} CFU of *L. salivarius* CECT 9145 dissolved in 500 µL of skim milk (treated group or Group 2). Doses of the test and control products were administered by gavage. At the end of a 14 days observation period, the rats were weighed, euthanized by CO_2 inhalation, exsanguinated, and necropsied.

The repeated dose (4 weeks) (limit test) study was conducted in 48 rats (24 males, 24 females) divided in four groups of 6 males and 6 females each (control group or Group 3; treated group or Group 4; satellite control group or Group 5; and satellite treated group or Group 6). Rats received a daily oral dose of either skim milk (Groups 3 and 5) or 1×10^9 CFU of *L. salivarius* CECT 9145 dissolved in 500 µL of skim milk (Groups 4 and 6) for 4 weeks. All rats of Groups 3 and 4 were deprived of food for 18 h, weighed, euthanized by CO_2 inhalation, exsanguinated, and necropsied on Day 29. All animals of the satellite groups (Groups 5 and 6) were kept a further 14 days without treatment to detect the delayed occurrence, persistence or recovery from potential toxic effects. All rats of the Groups 5 and 6 were deprived of food for 18 h, weighed, euthanized by CO_2 inhalation, exsanguinated, and necropsied on day 42.

Behavior and clinical observations, blood biochemistry and hematology analysis, organ weight ratios and histopathological analysis were carried as described previously [39]. Bacterial translocation to blood, liver or spleen, and total liver glutathione (GSH) concentration was evaluated following the methods described by Lara-Villoslada et al. [40].

2.10. Efficacy of L. salivarius CECT 9145 to Eradicate GBS from the Intestinal and Vaginal Tracts of Pregnant Women: A Pilot Clinical Trial

In this prospective pilot clinical assay, 57 pregnant women (39 rectal and vaginal GBS-positive women; 18 rectal and vaginal GBS-negative women at the start of the intervention), aged 25–36, participated in this study. All met the following criteria: a normal pregnancy and a healthy status. Women ingesting probiotic supplements or receiving antibiotic treatment in the previous 30 days were excluded. Women with lactose intolerance or a cow's milk protein allergy were also excluded because of the excipient used to administer the strain. All volunteers gave written informed consent to the protocol (10/017-E), which had been approved by the Ethical Committee of Clinical Research of the Hospital Clínico San Carlos Madrid (Spain).

Volunteers were distributed into 3 groups (1 probiotic group and 2 placebo groups). All the volunteers in the probiotic group ($n = 25$) were GBS-positive and consumed a daily sachet with ~50 mg of freeze-dried probiotic (~9 $\log_{10}$ cfu of *L. salivarius* CECT 9145) from week 26 to week 38 of the pregnancy. Placebo subgroup 1 ($n = 14$) included GBS-positive women (pregnancy week ranging from 19 to 30) that were going to receive IAP because they had a previous baby that suffered a GBS sepsis. Placebo subgroup 2 ($n = 18$) included GBS-negative women (pregnancy week ranging from 14 to 26). Women in both placebo subgroups received a daily sachet containing 50 mg of the excipient used to carry the probiotic strain. In all cases, the intervention lasted from the start of the intervention to week

38. Probiotic- and excipient-containing sachets were kept at 4 °C throughout the study. All volunteers were provided with diaries to record compliance with the study product intake. Minimum compliance rate (% of the total treatment doses) was set at 86%.

Recto-vaginal GBS screening was performed at 28, 32 and 38 weeks. Rectal and vaginal exudates samples collected during the trial were serially diluted and plated on Granada (Biomerieux; isolation of hemolytic GBS, which appear as orange colonies), and CHROMagar StrepB (CHROMagar; for isolation of hemolytic and non- hemolytic GBS, which appear as purple colonies) agar plates. To avoid sensitivity-related problems, samples were submitted to a GBS enrichment step in Todd-Hewitt broth (Oxoid). After 24 h at 37 °C, the broth cultures were spread on CHROMagar agar plates. Correct taxonomic assignment was confirmed by MALDI-TOF and latex agglutination analyses, as described previously. At the last sampling time (week 38), recto-vaginal GBS screening was performed not only in our laboratory but also in those of the hospitals in which the respective women were going to deliver their babies.

Microbiological data were recorded as CFU/mL and transformed to logarithmic values before statistical analysis. Two-way ANOVA was used to investigate the effect of the individual (woman) and sampling time on the semiquantitative *S. agalactiae* counts in vaginal swabs. Statistical significance was set at $P < 0.05$. Statgraphics Centurion XVI version 17.0.16 (Statpoint Technologies Inc, Warrenton, Virginia) was used to carry out statistical analyses.

3. Results

3.1. Microbiological Analysis of Vaginal Swabs Obtained from Pregnant and Non-Pregnant Women

Bacterial growth was detected in all the samples when they were inoculated on MRS (2.70–8.08 $\log_{10}$ colony-forming units (cfu); mean 5.36 $\log_{10}$ cfu); CNA (3.00–7.92 $\log_{10}$ cfu; mean 5.13 $\log_{10}$ cfu) and GAR (2.70–8.10 $\log_{10}$ cfu; mean 5.24 $\log_{10}$ cfu) agar plates. Similar bacterial groups grew in these three media. Growth on MCK, SDC or Mycoplasma plates was only detected in a few percentages of samples (from 0% in Mycoplasma plates to ~40% in SDC plates).

S. agalactiae could be isolated from both non-pregnant (~25%) and pregnant (~19%) women. *Candida albicans* and other yeasts were isolated from approximately 7 and 36% of the non-pregnant and pregnant women, respectively. *Gardnerella vaginalis* was isolated in ~7% of the pregnant women. In both groups, *Lactobacillus* was the dominant genus since it was detected in ~93% of the participating women.

In relation to the samples provided by non-pregnant women, a total of 433 isolates (including at least one representative of each colony and cell morphology) were submitted to taxonomical analyses. The highest number of isolates corresponded to the genus *Lactobacillus* (28% of the total isolates), followed by *Staphylococcus* (17%), *Enterococcus* (11%), *Corynebacterium* (7%), and *Streptococcus* (4%). Among the *Lactobacillus* isolates, the main species were *L. gasseri* (24%), *L. crispatus* (23%), *L. salivarius* (21%), *L. vaginalis* (12%), *L. plantarum* (13%), *L. coleohominis* (5%), and *L. jensenii* (2%). Isolates belonging to the species *L. crispatus*, *L. gasseri*, *L. salivarius*, *L. vaginalis*, and *L. plantarum* could be isolated from the 4 phases of the menstrual cycle sampled in this study.

From the samples provided by pregnant women, 120 isolates were submitted to taxonomical analyses. Again, the genus *Lactobacillus* was associated to the highest number of isolates (17%), followed by *Staphylococcus* (15%), *Streptococcus* (8%), yeasts (8%), *Enterococcus* (5%), *Bifidobacterium* (3%) and *Corynebacterium* (1%). Among the *Lactobacillus* isolates, the main species were *L. gasseri* (41%), *L. casei* (19%), *L. salivarius* (16%), *L. fermentum* (8%), *L. vaginalis* (6%), *L. reuteri* (5%) and *L. jensenii* (5%).

Among the *Lactobacillus* isolates obtained in this study, a few were selected to evaluate their potential as probiotics to control GBS populations on the basis of the following criteria: (1) absence of *S. agalactiae*, *Gardnella vaginalis*, *Candida* spp., *Ureaplasma* spp., and *Mycoplasma* spp. in the vaginal samples from which the lactobacilli were originally isolated; (2) Qualified Presumption of Safety (QPS) status (European Authority of Food Safety, EFSA); and (3) ability of the strain to grow rapidly in MRS broth under aerobic conditions ($\geq 1 \times 10^6$ cfu/mL after 16 h at 37 °C). In fact, only 10 strains (V3III-1,

V4II-90, V7II-1, V7II-62, V7IV-1, V7IV 60, V8III-62, V11I-60, V11III-60 y, V11IV-60) met all the criteria and all of them belonged to the same species (*Lactobacillus salivarius*). These strains were then selected for further characterization. Later, *L. salivarius* V4II-90 was deposited in the Spanish Collection of Type Cultures (CECT) as *L. salivarius* CECT 9145 and, therefore, this is the name used for this strain in this article.

3.2. Antimicrobial Activity of the Lactobacilli Strains Against GBS and the Production of Potential Antimicrobial Compounds

Initially, the antimicrobial activity of the 10 selected lactobacilli against the *S. agalactiae* strains was determined by an overlay method. Clear inhibition zones (ranging from 2 to 20 mm) were observed around the lactobacilli streaks.

In relation to the antimicrobial compounds that may be responsible for such activity, the concentration of L- and D-lactic acid and the pH of the supernatants obtained from MRS cultures of the lactobacilli are shown in Table 1. The global concentration of L-lactic acid was similar (~10 mg/mL) in all the supernatants. In contrast, D-lactic acid was not detected in the supernatants of the tested strains. In addition, all the strains acidified the MRS-broth medium to a final pH of ~4 after 16 h of incubation; among them, *L. salivarius* V7IV-1 showed the highest acidifying capacity (final pH of 3.8). No bacteriocin-like activity could be detected against the tested *S. agalactiae* strains. Two strains (*L. salivarius* CECT 9145 and V7IV-1) were able to produce hydrogen peroxide (7.29 µg/mL ± 0.69 and 7.46 µg/mL ± 0.58, respectively) (Table 1).

Table 1. The pH and concentrations of L- and D-lactic acid (mg/mL; mean ± SD), and hydrogen peroxide (µg/mL; mean ± SD) in the supernatants obtained from the MRS cultures of the lactobacilli ($n = 4$).

Strain	pH	L-lactic Acid	D-lactic Acid	Hydrogen Peroxide
L. salivarius V3III-1	4.00	9.66 ± 0.57	Nd	Nd
L. salivarius CECT 9145	4.01	10.03 ± 0.60	Nd	7.29 ± 0.69
L. salivarius V7II-1	4.02	9.82 ± 0.69	Nd	Nd
L. salivarius V7II-62	4.01	9.76 ± 0.54	Nd	Nd
L. salivarius V7IV-1	3.85	10.47 ± 0.58	Nd	7.46 ± 0.58
L. salivarius V7IV-60	4.02	9.72 ± 0.63	Nd	Nd
L. salivarius V8III-62	4.04	9.91 ± 0.55	Nd	Nd
L. salivarius V11I-60	4.03	9.84 ± 0.43	Nd	Nd
L. salivarius V11III-60	4.07	9.61 ± 0.47	Nd	Nd
L. salivarius V11IV-60	4.03	10.02 ± 0.62	Nd	Nd
L. salivarius CECT 5713	3.93	10.26 ± 0.62	Nd	-

The initial pH value of MRS broth was 6.2. Nd: not detectable.

The capacity of the lactobacilli strains to form large well-defined co-aggregates with *S. agalactiae* was strain-dependent. Strains V3III-1, V7IV-60 and V11IV-60 coaggregated with 5 *S. agalactiae* strains; strains V8III-62, V11I-60 and V11III-60 with 7; strain V7II-62 with 9 *S. agalactiae* strains; and strains CECT 9145, V7II-1 and V7IV-1 with 10 *S. agalactiae* strains (Figure 1). The ability of the lactobacilli strains to interfere or inhibit the growth of four *S. agalactiae* strains was evaluated using MRS broth co-cultures. Co-cultures with *S. agalactiae* seemed not to affect the growth of any of the *L. salivarius* strains (Table 2). In contrast, most of the *L. salivarius* strains were able to interfere at a higher or lower degree with the growth of the different *S. agalactiae* strains included in this assay. Among them, *L. salivarius* CECT 9145 showed the highest ability to inhibit the growth of *S. agalactiae* since the presence of two of the four *S. agalactiae* strains was not detectable in the co-cultures and the concentration of the other two showed a ~2.5 log10 decrease after an incubation period of only 6 h at 37 °C (Table 2). Interestingly, no viable streptococci could be detected when the co-cultures were incubated for 24 h (Table 2).

Table 2. The bacterial counts ($\log_{10}$ cfu/mL) of the *S. agalactiae* strains when co-cultured with the *L. salivarius* strains in MRS broth for 0, 6 and 24 h at 37 °C.

L. salivarius (Strain)	S. agalactiae (Strain)	0 h	6 h	24 h
V3III-1	RC5	7.10	6.44	Nd
	RC6	7.24	7.04	Nd
	V2I-80	7.10	7.04	Nd
	V14I-63	7.27	7.10	Nd
CECT 9145	RC5	7.04	4.48	Nd
	RC6	7.23	Nd	Nd
	V2I-80	7.10	4.70	Nd
	V14I-63	7.34	Nd	Nd
V7II-1	RC5	7.15	7.27	Nd
	RC6	7.15	6.70	Nd
	V2I-80	7.04	7.10	Nd
	V14I-63	7.35	5.65	Nd
V7II-62	RC5	7.24	7.04	Nd
	RC6	6.98	7.49	Nd
	V2I-80	7.35	7.92	Nd
	V14I-63	7.10	6.93	Nd
V7IV-1	RC5	7.32	7.58	Nd
	RC6	7.34	6.90	Nd
	V2I-80	7.15	7.38	Nd
	V14I-63	7.23	6.04	Nd
V7IV-60	RC5	7.24	7.32	Nd
	RC6	7.32	8.06	Nd
	V2I-80	7.04	7.15	Nd
	V14I-63	7.35	8.34	Nd
V8III-62	RC5	7.15	7.90	Nd
	RC6	7.34	7.23	Nd
	V2I-80	7.24	6.90	Nd
	V14I-63	7.20	8.77	Nd
V11I-60	RC5	7.31	7.44	Nd
	RC6	7.01	6.94	Nd
	V2I-80	7.23	7.07	Nd
	V14I-63	6.93	6.60	Nd
V11 III-60	RC5	7.27	6.44	Nd
	RC6	6.95	6.88	Nd
	V2I-80	7.28	6.52	Nd
	V14I-63	7.37	6.85	Nd
V11IV-60	RC5	7.26	6.74	Nd
	RC6	7.42	6.60	Nd
	V2I-80	7.10	6.60	Nd
	V14I-63	7.06	5.32	Nd
Control cultures (no *L. salivarius* strain)	RC5	7.20	9.32	9.34
	RC6	7.31	9.20	9.27
	V2I-80	7.04	9.15	9.23
	V14I-63	7.10	9.02	9.15

Nd: *S. agalactiae* was not detected.

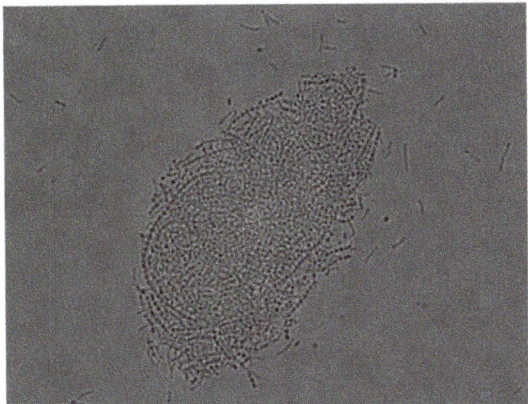

Figure 1. The strong co-aggregation between *L. salivarius* CECT 9145 (rods) and an *S. agalactiae* strain (cocci chains).

3.3. Survival After In Vitro Exposure to Saliva and Gastrointestinal-Like Conditions

The viability of the strains after exposition to conditions simulating those found in the gastrointestinal tract varied from ~64% (*L. reuteri* CR20, *L. salivarius* CECT 9145) to 30% (*L. salivarius* V3III-1) (Table 3).

Table 3. The percentage (%) of initial lactobacilli (9 $\log_{10}$ cfu/mL) that survived to conditions simulating those of the gastrointestinal tract.

Strain	% Total *
L. salivarius V3III-1	30.2 [a]
L. salivarius CECT 9145	64.3 [b]
L. salivarius V7II-1	59.8 [b]
L. salivarius V7II-62	50.5 [b]
L. salivarius V7IV-1	48.1 [b]
L. salivarius V7IV-60	53.3 [b]
L. salivarius V8III-62	41.3 [c]
L. salivarius V11I-60	40.8 [c]
L. salivarius V11III-60	41.1 [c]
L. salivarius V11IV-60	42.3 [c]
L. salivarius CELA2	64.4 [b]

*, different letters mean statistically different values.

3.4. Adhesion to Caco-2, HT-29 and Vaginal Cells and to Mucin

In this study, the lactobacilli strains tested were strongly adhesive to both Caco-2 and HT-29 cells, with the exception of the negative control strain (*L. casei imunitas*) which showed a low adhesive potential (Table 4). In addition, all showed adhesion to vaginal epithelial cells. Among the *L. salivarius* strains, *L. salivarius* CECT 9145 globally displayed the highest ability to adhere to both intestinal and vaginal epithelial cells (Table 4). The lactobacilli strains tested showed a variable ability to adhere to porcine mucin (Table 4). *L. salivarius* CECT 9145 and *L. salivarius* V7IV-1 were the strains that showed the highest adherence ability.

3.5. Sensitivity to Antibiotics

The MIC values of the lactobacilli strains for 16 antibiotics assayed are shown in Table 5. All the strains were sensitive to most of the antibiotics tested, including those considered clinically relevant antibiotics such as gentamycin, tetracycline, clindamycin, chloramphenicol, and ampicillin, showing MICs equal to or lower than the breakpoints defined by EFSA (EFSA, 2018). All the strains were resistant to vancomycin and kanamycin, which is an intrinsic property of the *L. salivarius* at the species level.

Table 4. The ability of the lactobacilli to adhere to HT-29, Caco-2 and vaginal epithelial cells, and to porcine mucin.

Strain	HT-29 [a]	Caco-2 [a]	Vaginal Cells [b]	Adhesion [c]
L. salivarius V3III-1	877.3 ± 303.2	259.1 ± 67.1	+	9.3 ± 2.0
L. salivarius CECT 9145	905.2 ± 297.0	345.1 ± 72.8	+++	10.9 ± 1.8
L. salivarius V7II-1	900.5 ± 336.2	297.8 ± 84.5	++	8.9 ± 1.9
L. salivarius V7II-62	911.7 ± 250.9	321.5 ± 80.2	++	9.0 ± 1.6
L. salivarius V7IV-1	884.0 ± 226.3	252.3 ± 67.1	++	8.5 ± 1.2
L. salivarius V7IV-60	799.7 ± 210.1	255.9 ± 60.3	++	9.6 ± 1.7
L. salivarius V8III-62	623.4 ± 200.2	108.7 ± 24.3	+	3.3 ± 0.7
L. salivarius V11I-60	593.2 ± 191.5	121.6 ± 22.0	+	2.9 ± 0.8
L. salivarius V11III-60	612.4 ± 188.2	153.2 ± 26.7	+	2.4 ± 1.0
L. salivarius V11IV-60	601.6 ± 172.0	159.5 ± 23.4	+	3.4 ± 0.8

[a] The adherent lactobacilli in 20 random microscopic fields were counted for each test ($n = 4$). [b] Semiquantitative scale: 0, no adhesion; +, low adhesion; ++, middle adhesion; +++, high adhesion. [c] Values are expressed as the percentage of the fluorescence retained in the wells after the washing steps of the assay.

3.6. Hemolysis, the Formation of Biogenic Amines and the Degradation of Mucin

The strains did not show the ability to produce biogenic amines, and they were neither hemolytic nor able to degrade gastric mucin *in vitro*.

3.7. Acute and Repeated Dose (4 Weeks) Oral Toxicity Studies in a Rat Model

All animals survived both oral toxicity trials. The development of the treated animals during the experimental periods corresponded to their species and age. There were no significant differences in body weight or body weight gain among groups treated with *L. salivarius* CECT 9145 (including the satellite ones) in comparison to the control groups at any time point of the experimental period. No abnormal clinical signs, behavioral changes, body weight changes, hematological and clinical chemistry parameters, macroscopic or histological findings, or organ weight changes were observed. There were no statistical differences in body weights among groups. Similarly, no statistically significant differences in body weight gain, food and water consumption were observed between the groups. No significant differences in liver GSH concentration were observed between the control and treated groups (9.54 ± 1.21 vs. 9.37 ± 1.39 mmol/g, $P > 0.1$). *L. salivarius* CECT 9145 could be isolated from colonic material and vaginal swabs samples of all the treated animals (probiotic groups) at the end of the treatment. The concentration oscillated between 5.39 and 8.85 $\log_{10}$ cfu/g of the colonic material, and between 3.34 and 6.14 $\log_{10}$ cfu/swab in the vaginal samples. The strain could not be detected in any sample from the placebo group.

3.8. The Efficacy of L. salivarius CECT 9145 to Eradicate GBS from the Intestinal and Vaginal Tracts of Pregnant Women: A Pilot Clinical Trial

At the inclusion in the study, GBS was detected in both rectal and vaginal swabs obtained from 39 women, out of a total of 57 participating women, while the rest of the women ($n = 18$) were GBS-negative (Table 6). This last group of GBS-negative women, who did not ingest the *L. salivarius* strain also had negative GBS cultures from rectal and vaginal swabs taken regularly at 28, 32 and 36–38 weeks (Table 6). A group of GBS-positive women at the start of the study ($n = 14$) did not receive the probiotic and the routine screening results for vaginal and rectal GBS at 28, 32 and 36–38 weeks were found to be all positive (Table 6).

Table 5. The minimal inhibitory concentration (MIC, mg/mL) values of 16 antibiotics [a] to the *L. salivarius* strains.

Strain	Antibiotic [a]															
	GEN	KAN	STP	NEO	TET	ERY	CLI	CHL	AMP	PEN	VAN	VIR	LIN	TRM	CIP	RIF
V3III-1	4	64	32	8	2	0.12	0.5	2	0.5	0.12	>128	0.5	0.5	0.5	2	0.5
CECT 9145	4	256	32	8	2	0.12	0.5	2	0.5	0.12	>128	0.5	1	0.25	4	1
V7II-1	4	128	32	4	2	0.12	0.5	4	0.5	0.12	>128	0.5	0.5	0.5	2	0.25
V7II-62	2	128	32	8	2	0.25	0.5	2	0.5	0.25	>128	0.25	1	0.25	2	0.5
V7IV-1	8	256	32	4	2	0.12	0.5	2	0.5	0.25	>128	0.5	1	0.5	2	0.5
V7IV-60	8	128	32	8	2	0.12	0.4	4	0.5	0.25	>128	0.5	1	0.5	2	0.5
V8III-62	8	128	32	2	2	0.25	0.5	4	0.5	0.25	>128	1	1	0.5	2	0.5
V1II-60	8	128	32	8	2	0.12	0.5	2	0.5	0.25	>128	1	1	0.5	2	0.5
V1III-60	8	256	32	4	2	0.12	0.5	2	0.5	0.25	>128	0.5	1	0.5	2	0.5
V1IV-60	4	128	32	8	2	0.12	0.5	2	0.5	0.25	>128	1	1	0.5	2	0.5
Breakpoint [b]	16	64 (R)	nr	nr	8	1	4	4	4	nr	nr (R)	nr	nr	nr	nr	nr

[a] Abbreviations: GEN, gentamycin; KAN, kanamycin; STP, streptomycin; NEO, neomycin; TET, tetracycline; ERY, erythromycin; CLI, clindamycin; CHL, chloramphenicol; AMP, ampicillin; PEN, penicillin; VAN, vancomycin; VIR, virginiamycin; LIN, linezolid; TRM, trimethoprim; CIP, ciprofloxacin; RIF, rifampicin; nr, not required by EFSA. R, the species *L. salivarius* is intrinsically resistant. [b] Breakpoint: microbiological breakpoints (mg/mL) that categorise *Lactobacillus salivarius* as resistant (microbiological breakpoints are defined as the MIC values that clearly deviate from those displayed by the normal susceptible populations; EFSA, 2018).

Table 6. The qualitative assessment (Group B Streptococci (GBS)-positive/GBS-negative) of *Streptococcus agalactiae* in rectal and vaginal swabs of participants ($N = 57$).

Initial GBS Status	Probiotic Intake	GBS Status	Rectal Swabs (Week)				Vaginal Swabs (Week)			
			12-26	28 [a]	32 [b]	36-38	12-26	28 [a]	32 [b]	36-38
Negative ($n = 18$)	NO	GBS-positive	0	0	0	0	0	0	0	0
		GBS-negative	18	17	16	18	18	17	16	18
		GBS-negative (%)	100	100	100	100	100	100	100	100
Positive ($n = 14$)	NO	GBS-positive	14-17	28 [b]	32 [a]	36-38	14-17	28 [b]	32 [a]	36-38
		GBS-negative	14	12	13	14	14	12	13	14
		GBS-negative (%)	0	0	0	0	0	0	0	0
			0	0	0	0	0	0	0	0
Positive ($n = 25$)	YES	GBS-positive	26	28	32	38	28	30	32	38
		GBS-negative	25	25	12	7	25	25	15	8
			0	0	9	18	0	0	10	17
		GBS-negative (%)	0	0	16	18	0	0	15	15
			0	0	52	72	0	0	40	60	68

[a]: sample from one participant was missing at this sampling time. [b]: samples from two participants were missing at this sampling time.

Significantly, the group of GBS-positive women that started using the probiotic (9 $\log_{10}$ cfu/daily) since they were enrolled in this study (from 26 weeks) also tested positive for GBS at 28 weeks, but an increasing number of GBS-negative results appeared in the successive swabs collected until delivery (Table 6). At 30 weeks, the culture of rectal swabs taken from four women of this group rendered a negative result and the number of these samples increased to 18 (72% of the participants) at 38 weeks. Similar results were obtained by culturing vaginal swabs obtained from this group, although the proportion of women testing negative for GBS were always slightly higher when analyzing the rectal swabs than in vaginal swabs (Table 6).

The estimation of the concentration of GBS in vaginal swabs taken regularly up to the delivery from all participants is shown in Figure 2. There were no significant changes in both GBS-negative women (n = 18) and GBS-positive women (n = 14) without oral administration of *L. salivarius* CECT 9145 regarding the semiquantitative estimation of GBS. However, the number of vaginal swabs where GBS could not be detected increased in successive sampling times in the group that initially tested positive for GBS taking 9 $\log_{10}$cfu of *L. salivarius* CECT 9145 (n = 25). The mean value for *S. agalactiae* counts decreased significantly with the administration time of *L. salivarius* CECT 9145 (Figure 2) from a mean value of 5.14 cfu/mL at 26 weeks (n = 25) to 3.80 cfu/mL at 38 weeks (n = 9) (Figure 2).

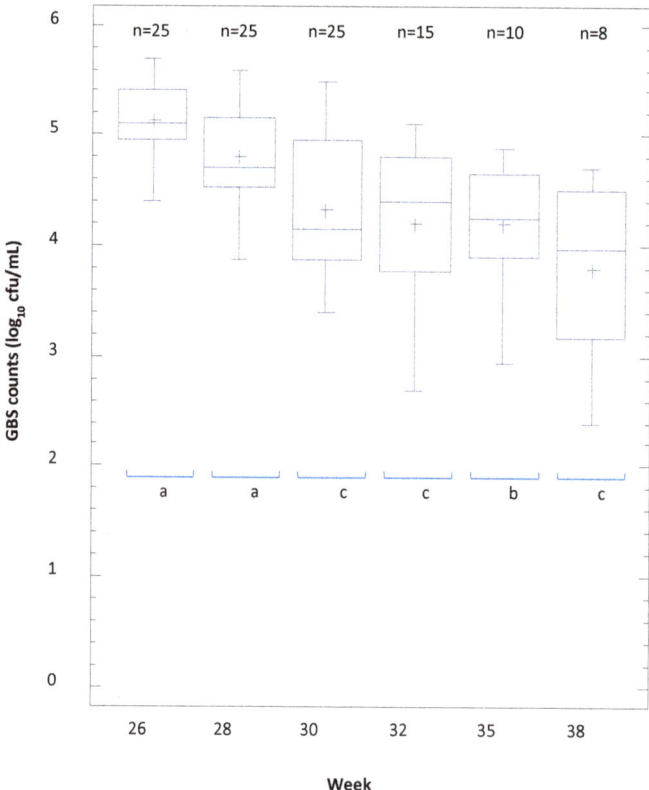

Figure 2. The mean concentrations (CFU/mL) of *S. agalactiae* (GBS) in vaginal swabs sampled regularly up to the delivery from Group B Streptococci (GBS)-positive women taking 9 $\log_{10}$ cfu of *L. salivarius* CECT 9145 daily. Statistically significant differences between samples taking at different sampling times are indicated by letters (Bonferroni post-hoc test).

No adverse effects arising from the intake of *L. salivarius* CECT 9145 were reported by any of the women who participated in this study. The results of the GBS status obtained in our laboratory at week 38 were identical to those obtained in the hospitals were the recruited women were screened for GBS and, as a result, none of the women who became GBS-negative in this study received IAP.

4. Discussion

In this work, the GBS colonization rates were 25% and 20% among non-pregnant and pregnant women, respectively. In pregnant women, GBS colonization is found in up to 30% of rectovaginal samples [2,41] and stable colonization with the same clone for several years has been demonstrated [41]. Previous studies have shown that the presence of GBS is not linked to an abnormal microbiome or a reduction of the predominant *Lactobacillus* genus in the vaginal tract of the mother [42–44].

In contrast, a study involving a low number of participants found significant taxonomic differences in stools of 6-month infants, when mothers were GBS carriers, as compared to non-carriers [45]. Anyway, there is no epidemiological evidence for a correlation between neonatal colonization with GBS and specific shifts in the maternal intestinal or vaginal microbiome.

In the USA and many other countries (including Spain), women are routinely screened in the late third trimester (between 35 and 37 weeks' gestation) for GBS colonization by rectovaginal swabs and subsequent cultures. If the rectovaginal swab is culture-positive, or if the patient has GBS in the urine, or has a prior history of GBS perinatal infection, intrapartum prophylactic antibiotics are administered to prevent vertical transmission of GBS to the neonate during labor and delivery. Some European countries (e.g., UK) have not adopted the GBS screening program but, instead, administer antibiotics upon the development of a risk factor for GBS neonatal disease (e.g., prolonged rupture of membranes). However, none of these approaches has eliminated neonatal GBS infections. This is because these prevention strategies do not address the risk of ascending infection, which can potentially occur anytime during pregnancy, leading to preterm birth or stillbirth.

Overall, the prevention of GBS infection in pregnancy is still a complex question, with risk likely associated to several factors, including the pathogenicity of the GBS strain, host factors, influence of the vaginal/rectal microbiome, false-negative screening results, and/or changes in GBS antibiotic resistance [6,46]. Currently, strategies are mainly focused on the prevention of GBS transmission during labor and delivery through the use of antibiotics. This strategy does not fully capture the biology of the GBS infection, nor does it completely address the full burden of the GBS disease. Moreover, antibiotic resistance is increasing and the use of antibiotics during pregnancy has consequential effects for neonatal health that are only now being appreciated [47]. To successfully eradicate the burden of disease, interventions need to be specifically targeted while having minimal detrimental effects on the microbiome. Therefore, there is a need for alternatives that are respectful with the neonatal and infant microbiota, and that do not compromise the health of future generations. In this context, the final objective of this work was the selection of safe probiotic strains with the in vitro and in vivo ability to eradicate GBS from the intestinal and genitourinary tracts of pregnant women and/or their infants.

The genus *Lactobacillus* constitutes the dominant bacterial group of the vaginal tract in most healthy women, playing a key role in the genitourinary homeostasis [48–52]. In this study, all the vaginal isolates (from either pregnant or non-pregnant healthy women) that fulfilled the initial selection criteria belonged to the species *L. salivarius*. This species is part of the indigenous microbiota of the human gastrointestinal tract, oral cavity, genitourinary tract and milk, and some strains have been studied as probiotics because of their in vitro and in vivo antimicrobial, anti-inflammatory and immunomodulatory properties [53–64]. Previous studies have shown the ability of *L. salivarius* strains to inhibit the growth of vaginal pathogens, including *Gardnerella vaginalis* and *Candida albicans* and, therefore, we have suggested their potential to be used as probiotics for the treatment or prevention of vaginal infections [65,66].

Administration of probiotic bacteria benefits the host through a wide array of mechanisms that are increasingly recognized as being either species- and/or strain-specific [67]. A comparative genomics study that included 33 *L. salivarius* strains isolated from humans, animals or food revealed that this species displays a high level of genomic diversity [68]. Therefore, the selection of *L. salivarius* strains for probiotic use requires the experimental validation of target-tailored phenotypic traits. Some *L. salivarius* strains have shown to be efficient in preventing infectious diseases such as mastitis caused by staphylococci and streptococci, when administered during late pregnancy [69]. Moreover, the oral administration of *L. salivarius* strains is also a valid strategy for the treatment of such a condition during lactation and, in fact, one of the strains was more efficient than antibiotics for this target [70]. In this work, the target was the antagonism towards GBS and, as a consequence, properties such as antimicrobial activity against *S. agalactiae* strains or coaggregation with this species were considered particularly relevant.

The production of antagonistic substances such as bacteriocins, hydrogen peroxide or organic acids represents an important contribution to the defense mechanisms exerted by intestinal and vaginal lactobacilli [59,71]. Some *L. salivarius* strains produce bacteriocins or display bacteriocin-like activity against a variable spectrum of Gram-positive bacteria, including *S. agalactiae* strains [72]. However, none of the *L. salivarius* strains selected in our study displayed bacteriocin-like activity against *S. agalactiae* strains. Therefore, the antimicrobial activity that the selected *L. salivarius* strains exhibited against *S. agalactiae* must be related to the production of other antimicrobial compounds, such as organic acids. The ability of lactobacilli to acidify the vaginal milieu contributes to the displacement and inhibition of pathogens proliferation [73] and, more specifically, the acid production by lactobacilli has been directly correlated with the inhibition of GBS growth [74]. Another antimicrobial defense mechanism attributed to some intestinal or vaginal lactobacilli is the production of peroxide hydrogen, a compound that is toxic for catalase-negative bacteria, such as streptococci [75]. The production of this compound by *L. salivarius* has already been reported [59,76,77]. In our study, *L. salivarius* CECT 9145 (the strain that showed the highest anti-GBS activity) produced high amounts of lactic acid and, in addition, was able to produce peroxide hydrogen.

The ability to adhere to intestinal or vaginal epithelial cells or to mucin, and to co-aggregate with potential pathogens constitutes one of the main mechanisms for preventing their adhesion and colonization of mucosal surfaces. Therefore, it is not strange that such properties are considered relevant to the selection of probiotic strains [28]. The high adherence of *L. salivarius* strains to Caco-2 and HT-29 cells or to mucin has been previously observed [53,59,78]. Globally, *L. salivarius* CECT 9145 showed the best combination of adherence to epithelial cells, co-aggregation with *S. agalactiae* and the inhibition of *S. agalactiae* strains in broth co-cultures. This strain showed a high survival rate during transit through an in vitro gastrointestinal model and survival of lactobacilli when exposed to conditions found in the gastrointestinal tract seems to be a critical pre-requisite for a probiotic strain when its use as a food supplement is pursued, as it was the case.

Some vaginal strains of *L. gasseri* and *L reuteri* have also been reported to co-aggregate with GBS [78]. In contrast, no co-aggregation activity between *S. agalactiae* and other vaginal lactobacilli belonging to the species *L. acidophilus*, *L. gasseri* and *L. jensenii* was observed in another study [32], a fact suggesting that such property is a highly strain-specific trait. In relation to broth co-cultures, the capacity to antagonize the growth of *S. agalactiae* by lactobacilli strains belonging to different species, including *L. salivarius*, has been previously reported [79,80]. Similar to our results, this activity was strain-dependent [79].

One of the most important criteria for the selection of probiotic strains is the assessment of their safety, particularly to the target population. In this work, no adverse effect was reported by any of the women who participated in the clinical trial and ascribed to the probiotic group [thus, receiving *L. salivarius* CECT 9145 at 9 $\log_{10}$ cfu daily for several weeks). Previously, other *L. salivarius* strains have been shown to be well-tolerated and safe in animal models [40] and in human clinical assays [70,81–83], including one involving pregnant women [69].

The *L. salivarius* strains included in this study were very susceptible to most of the antimicrobials tested. In fact, their MICs were lower than the cut-offs established for lactobacilli to seven out of the eight antibiotics required for this species by the European Food Safety Authority [36]. The only exception was kanamycin. The intrinsic resistance of lactobacilli to kanamycin and other aminoglycosides (such as neomycin or streptomycin) has been repeatedly reported [84,85], and this is thought to be an *L. salivarius* species-specific trait due to the lack of cytochrome-mediated transport of this class of antibiotics [86]. The *L. salivarius* strains were also resistant to vancomycin but the assessment of vancomycin sensitivity is not required by EFSA in the case of homofermentative lactobacilli (including *L. salivarius*) since they are intrinsically resistant to this antibiotic probably due to the presence of D-Ala-D-lactate in their peptidoglycan structure [87]. Therefore, *L. salivarius* CECT 9145 and the other strains evaluated in this study can be considered as safe from this point of view.

Lactobacilli are among the Gram-positive bacteria with the potential to produce biogenic amines and these substances can cause several toxicological problems and/or may act as potential precursors of carcinogenic nitrosamines [37]. The screened *L. salivarius* strains neither produced histamine, tyramine, putrescine or cadaverine nor harbored the gene determinants required for their biosynthesis. Additionally, they were unable to degrade gastric mucin in vitro.

Some studies have been focused on the potential of different lactic acid bacteria strains or their metabolites to inhibit the growth of *S. agalactiae* in vitro or in murine models [74,80,88–95]. However, few studies have evaluated the efficacy of probiotic strains for the rectal and vaginal eradication of GBS in pregnant women. Ho et al. [96] examined the effect of *Lactobacillus rhamnosus* GR-1 and *Lactobacillus reuteri* RC-14 taken orally on GBS-positive pregnant women at 35–37 weeks of gestation, and found that GBS colonization changed from positive to negative in 42.9% of the women in the probiotic group. The rate of women that became GBS-negative was lower than in our study and this might be due to the fact that, in the cited study, the recruited women started the probiotic intake many weeks later. A second study using the same two strains (*L. rhamnosus* GR-1 and *L. reuteri* RC-14) provided non-conclusive results due to the low adherence to the probiotic treatment since only seven of 21 women in the intervention group completed the entire 21 days of probiotics [97].

It is important to highlight that nutrition may also play a key role in creating mucosal conditions favoring the action of bacterial strains that are able to improve the rectal and vaginal environments, as it is the case of *L. salivarius* CECT 9145. Such conditions may include the selective fermentation of dietary fiber, the production of relevant bioactive compounds, such as short-chain fatty acids [98], or the use of hyaluronic acid, which has been shown to be useful in the treatment of female recurrent genitourinary infections [99]. The impact of diet on the outcomes of clinical assays involving probiotic-interventions is often underrated and should be taken into account in future studies.

Our study includes the whole process from strain isolation to a pilot clinical study specifically targeting GBS eradication in pregnant women. The criteria followed for the selection of the best candidate for such a target (*L. salivarius* CECT 9145) allowed a notable reduction in the rate of GBS-colonized women and led to a reduction in the use of antibiotics during the peripartum period. As a conclusion, the administration of *L. salivarius* CECT 9145 to GBS-positive pregnant women is a safe and successful strategy to significantly decrease the rates of GBS colonization during pregnancy and, therefore, to reduce the exposure of pregnant women and their infants to intrapartum prophylaxis. Work is in progress to study the mechanisms involving GBS antagonism, including the study of the strain genome and to initiate a multicenter well-designed clinical trial involving a higher number of women.

Author Contributions: J.M.R., L.F., D.B. and C.B. designed the study; N.C., V.M., M.M. and R.A. characterized the strain and performed the microbial analyses. S.O. collected the biological samples and coordinated the pilot clinical study. L.F. did the statistical analysis. J.M.R. wrote, edited and revised the manuscript. All the authors approved the final version of the manuscript.

Funding: This work was supported by Laboratorios Casen Recordati SL. The funding agency had no role in study design, data collection and analysis.

Acknowledgments: We acknowledge all the women, gynaecologists and midwives that participated in this study.

Conflicts of Interest: NC is an employee of Probisearch SLU. CB is employee of Casen Recordati SL. The remaining authors declare that the research was conducted in the absence of any commercial or financial relationships that could be construed as a potential conflict of interest.

References

1. Romero, R.; Dey, S.K.; Fisher, S.J. Preterm labor: One syndrome, many causes. *Science* **2014**, *345*, 760–765. [CrossRef]
2. Stoll, B.J.; Hansen, N.I.; Sanchez, P.J.; Faix, R.G.; Poindexter, B.B.; Van Meurs, K.P.; Bizzarro, M.J.; Goldberg, R.N.; Frantz, I.D., III; Hale, E.C.; et al. Early onset neonatal sepsis: The burden of group B streptococcal and *E. coli* disease continues. *Pediatrics* **2011**, *127*, 817–826. [CrossRef] [PubMed]
3. Le Doare, K.; Heath, P.T. An overview of global GBS epidemiology. *Vaccine* **2013**, *31* (Suppl. 4), D7–D12. [CrossRef] [PubMed]
4. Lawn, J.E.; Bianchi-Jassir, F.; Russell, N.J.; Kohli-Lynch, M.; Tann, C.J.; Hall, J.; Madrid, L.; Baker, C.J.; Bartlett, L.; Cutland, C.; et al. Group B streptococcal disease worldwide for pregnant women, stillbirths, and children: Why, what, and how to undertake estimates? *Clin. Infect. Dis.* **2017**, *65* (Suppl. 2), S89–S99. [CrossRef] [PubMed]
5. Russell, N.J.; Seale, A.C.; O'Driscoll, M.; O'Sullivan, C.; Bianchi-Jassir, F.; Gonzalez-Guarin, J.; Lawn, J.E.; Baker, C.J.; Bartlett, L.; Cutland, C.; et al. Maternal colonization with group B *Streptococcus* and serotype distribution worldwide: Systematic review and meta-analyses. *Clin. Infect. Dis.* **2017**, *65* (Suppl. 2), S100–S111. [CrossRef]
6. Vornhagen, J.; Adams Waldorf, K.M.; Rajagopal, L. Perinatal group B streptococcal infections: Virulence factors, immunity, and prevention strategies. *Trends Microbiol.* **2017**, *25*, 919–931. [CrossRef]
7. Puopolo, K.M.; Madoff, L.C.; Eichenwald, E.C. Early-onset group B streptococcal disease in the era of maternal screening. *Pediatrics* **2005**, *115*, 1240–1246. [CrossRef] [PubMed]
8. Stade, B.; Shah, V.; Ohlsson, A. Vaginal chlorhexidine during labour to prevent early-onset neonatal group B streptococcal infection. *Cochrane Database Syst. Rev.* **2004**. [CrossRef]
9. Kobayashi, M.; Schrag, S.J.; Alderson, M.R.; Madhi, S.A.; Baker, C.J.; Sobanjo-Ter Meulen, A. WHO consultation on group B *Streptococcus* vaccine development: Report from a meeting held on 27–28 April 2016. *Vaccine* **2016**. [CrossRef]
10. Akker-van Marle, M.E.; Rijnders, M.E.B.; Dommelen, P.; Fekkes, M.; Wouwe, J.P.; Amelink-Verburg, M.P.; Verkerk, P.H. Cost-effectiveness of different treatment strategies with intrapartum antibiotic prophylaxis to prevent early-onset group B streptococcal disease. *BJOG* **2005**, *112*, 820–826. [CrossRef] [PubMed]
11. Baecher, L.; Grobman, W. Prenatal antibiotic treatment does not decrease group B *Streptococcus* colonization at delivery. *Int. J. Gynaecol. Obstet.* **2008**, *101*, 125–128. [CrossRef]
12. Chu, Y.W.; Tse, C.; Tsang, G.K.; So, D.K.; Fung, J.T.; Lo, J.Y. Invasive group B *Streptococcus* isolates showing reduced susceptibility to penicillin in Hong Kong. *J. Antimicrob. Chemother.* **2007**, *60*, 1407–1409. [CrossRef] [PubMed]
13. Dahesh, S.; Hensler, M.E.; Van Sorge, N.M.; Gertz, R.E.; Schrag, S.; Nizet, V.; Beall, B.W. Point mutation in the group B streptococcal *pbp2x* gene conferring decreased susceptibility to beta-lactam antibiotics. *Antimicrob. Agents Chemother.* **2008**, *52*, 2915–2918. [CrossRef] [PubMed]
14. Gao, K.; Guan, X.; Zeng, L.; Qian, J.; Zhu, S.; Deng, Q.; Zhong, H.; Pang, S.; Gao, F.; Wang, J.; et al. An increasing trend of neonatal invasive multidrug-resistant group B *streptococcus* infections in southern China, 2011–2017. *Infect. Drug Resist.* **2018**, *11*, 2561–2569. [CrossRef]
15. Arboleya, S.; Sánchez, B.; Solís, G.; Fernández, N.; Suárez, M.; Hernández-Barranco, A.; Milani, C.; Margolles, A.; de los Reyes-Gavilán, C.; Ventura, M.; et al. Impact of prematurity and perinatal antibiotics on the developing intestinal microbiota: A functional inference study. *Int. J. Mol. Sci.* **2016**, *17*, 649. [CrossRef]
16. Cotten, C.M. Adverse consequences of neonatal antibiotic exposure. *Curr. Opin. Pediatr.* **2016**, *28*, 141–149. [CrossRef] [PubMed]
17. Tanaka, S.; Kobayashi, T.; Songjinda, P.; Tateyama, A.; Tsubouchi, M.; Kiyohara, C.; Shirakawa, T.; Sonomoto, K.; Nakayama, J. Influence of antibiotic exposure in the early postnatal period on the development of intestinal microbiota. *FEMS Immunol. Med. Microbiol.* **2009**, *56*, 80–87. [CrossRef]

18. Aloisio, I.; Quagliariello, A.; de Fanti, S.; Luiselli, D.; de Filippo, C.; Albanese, D.; Corvaglia, L.T.; Faldella, G.; Di Gioia, D. Evaluation of the effects of intrapartum antibiotic prophylaxix on newborn intestinal microbiota using a sequencing approach targeted to multi hypervariate 16S rDNA regions. *Appl. Microbiol. Biotechnol.* **2016**, *100*, 5537–5546. [CrossRef]
19. Cox, L.M.; Yamanishi, S.; Sohn, J.; Alekseyenko, A.V.; Leung, J.M.; Cho, I.; Kim, S.G.; Li, H.; Gao, Z.; Mahana, D.; et al. Altering the intestinal microbiota during a critical developmental window has lasting metabolic consequences. *Cell* **2014**, *158*, 705–721. [CrossRef]
20. Kullen, M.J.; Sanozky-Dawes, R.B.; Crowell, D.C.; Klaenhammer, T.R. Use of DNA sequence of variable regions of the 16SrRNA gene for rapid and accurate identification of bacteria in the *Lactobacillus acidophilus* complex. *J. Appl. Microbiol.* **2000**, *89*, 511–518. [CrossRef]
21. Marín, M.; Arroyo, R.; Espinosa-Martos, I.; Fernández, L.; Rodríguez, J.M. Identification of emerging human mastitis pathogens by MALDI-TOF and assessment of their antibiotic resistance patterns. *Front. Microbiol.* **2017**, *8*, 1258. [CrossRef]
22. Ruiz-Barba, J.L.; Maldonado, A.; Jiménez-Díaz, R. Small-scale total DNA extraction from bacteria and yeast for PCR applications. *Anal. Biochem.* **2005**, *347*, 333–335. [CrossRef]
23. Magnusson, J.; Schnürer, J. *Lactobacillus coryniformis* subsp. *coryniformis* strain Si3 produces a broad-spectrum proteinaceous antifungal compound. *Appl. Environ. Microbiol.* **2001**, *67*, 1–5. [CrossRef]
24. Dodd, H.M.; Horn, N.; Zhang, H.; Gasson, M.J. A lactococcal expression system for engineered nisins. *Appl. Environ. Microbiol.* **1992**, *58*, 3683–3693.
25. Martín, R.; Olivares, M.; Marín, M.L.; Fernández, L.; Xaus, J.; Rodríguez, J.M. Probiotic potential of 3 Lactobacilli strains isolated from breast milk. *J. Hum. Lact.* **2005**, *21*, 8–17. [CrossRef]
26. Song, Y.L.; Kato, N.; Matsumiy, Y.; Lu, C.X.; Kato, H.; Watanabe, K. Identification of an hydrogen peroxide production by fecal and vaginal lactobacilli isolated from Japanese women and newborn infants. *J. Clin. Microbiol.* **1999**, *37*, 3062–3064.
27. Yap, P.S.; Gilliland, S.E. Comparison of newly isolated strains of *Lactobacillus delbrueckii* susp. *lactis* for hydrogen peroxide production at 5 °C. *J. Dairy Sci.* **2000**, *83*, 628–632. [CrossRef]
28. Younes, J.A.; van der Mei, H.C.; van den Heuvel, E.; Busscher, H.J.; Reid, G. Adhesion forces and coaggregation between vaginal staphylococci and lactobacilli. *PLoS ONE* **2012**, *7*, e36917. [CrossRef]
29. Marteau, P.; Minekus, M.; Havenaar, R.; Huis In't Veld, J.H.J. Survival of lactic acid bacteria in a dynamic model of the stomach and small intestine: Validation and the effects of bile. *J. Dairy Sci.* **1997**, *80*, 1031–1037. [CrossRef]
30. Conway, P.L.; Gorbach, S.L.; Goldin, B.R. Survival of lactic acid bacteria in the human stomach and adhesion to intestinal cells. *J. Dairy Sci.* **1987**, *70*, 1–12. [CrossRef]
31. Coconnier, M.H.; Klaenhammer, T.R.; Kernéis, S.; Bernet, M.F.; Servin, A.L. Protein-mediated adhesion of *Lactobacillus acidophilus* BG2FO4 on human enterocyte and mucus-secreting cell lines in culture. *Appl. Environ. Microbiol.* **1992**, *58*, 2034–2039.
32. Boris, S.; Suárez, J.E.; Vázquez, F.; Barbés, C. Adherence of human vaginal lactobacilli to vaginal epithelial cells and interaction with uropathogens. *Infect. Immun.* **1998**, *66*, 1985–1989.
33. Cohen, P.S.; Laux, D.C. Bacterial adhesion to and penetration of intestinal mucus in vitro. *Methods Enzymol.* **1995**, *253*, 309–314.
34. Klare, I.; Konstabel, C.; Müller-Bertling, S.; Reissbrodt, R.; Huys, G.; Vancanneyt, M.; Swings, J.; Goossens, H.; Witte, W. Evaluation of new broth media for microdilution antibiotic susceptibility testing of lactobacilli, lactococci, pediococci, and bifidobacteria. *Appl. Environ. Microbiol.* **2005**, *71*, 8982–8986. [CrossRef]
35. Langa, S.; Maldonado-Barragán, A.; Delgado, S.; Martín, R.; Martín, V.; Jiménez, E.; Ruíz-Barba, J.L.; Mayo, B.; Connor, R.I.; Suárez, J.E.; et al. Characterization of *Lactobacillus salivarius* CECT 5713, a strain isolated from human milk: From genotype to phenotype. *Appl. Microbiol. Biotechnol.* **2012**, *94*, 1279–1287. [CrossRef]
36. EFSA. Guidance on the characterisation of microorganisms used as feed additives or as production organisms. *EFSA J.* **2018**, *16*, e05206.
37. Bover-Cid, S.; Holzapfel, W.H. Improved screening procedure for biogenic amine production by lactic acid bacteria. *Int. J. Food Microbiol.* **1999**, *53*, 33–41. [CrossRef]
38. Zhou, J.S.; Gopal, P.K.; Hill, H.S. Potential probiotic lactic acid bacteria *Lactobacillus rhamnosus* (HN001), *Lactobacillus acidophilus* (HN017) and *Bifidobacterium lactis* (HN019) do not degrade gastric mucin in vitro. *Int. J. Food Microbiol.* **2001**, *63*, 81–90. [CrossRef]

39. Anadón, A.; Martínez, M.A.; Ares, I.; Ramos, E.; Martínez-Larrañaga, M.R.; Contreras, M.M.; Ramos, M.; Recio, I. Acute and repeated dose (4 weeks) oral toxicity studies of two antihypertensive peptides, RYLGY and AYFYPEL, that correspond to fragments (90–94) and (143–149) from alpha(s1)-casein. *Food Chem. Toxicol.* **2010**, *48*, 1836–1845.
40. Lara-Villoslada, F.; Sierra, S.; Martín, R.; Delgado, S.; Rodríguez, J.M.; Olivares, M.; Xaus, J. Safety assessment of two probiotic strains, *Lactobacillus coryniformis* CECT5711 and *Lactobacillus gasseri* CECT5714. *J. Appl. Microbiol.* **2007**, *103*, 175–184. [CrossRef]
41. Hansen, S.M.; Uldbjerg, N.; Kilian, M.; Sorensen, U.B.S. Dynamics of *Streptococcus agalactiae* colonization in women during and after pregnancy and in their infants. *J. Clin. Microbiol.* **2004**, *42*, 83–89. [CrossRef]
42. Brzychczy-Wloch, M.; Pabian, W.; Majewska, E.; Zuk, M.G.; Kielbik, J.; Gosiewski, T.; Bulanda, M.G. Dynamics of colonization with group B streptococci in relation to normal flora in women during subsequent trimesters of pregnancy. *New Microbiol.* **2014**, *37*, 307–319.
43. Rick, A.M.; Aguilar, A.; Cortes, R.; Gordillo, R.; Melgar, M.; Samayoa-Reyes, G.; Frank, D.N.; Asturias, E.J. Group B streptococci colonization in pregnant guatemalan women: Prevalence, risk factors, and vaginal microbiome. *Open Forum Infect. Dis.* **2017**, *4*, ofx020. [CrossRef]
44. Rosen, G.H.; Randis, T.M.; Desai, P.V.; Sapra, K.J.; Ma, B.; Gajer, P.; Humphrys, M.S.; Ravel, J.; Gelber, S.E.; Ratner, A.J. Group B *Streptococcus* and the vaginal microbiota. *J. Infect. Dis.* **2017**, *216*, 744–751. [CrossRef]
45. Cassidy-Bushrow, A.E.; Sitarik, A.; Levin, A.M.; Lynch, S.V.; Havstad, S.; Ownby, D.R.; Johnson, C.C.; Wegienka, G. Maternal group B *Streptococcus* and the infant gut microbiota. *J. Dev. Orig. Health Dis.* **2016**, *7*, 45–53. [CrossRef]
46. Patras, K.A.; Nizet, V. Group B streptococcal maternal colonization and neonatal disease: Molecular mechanisms and preventative approaches. *Front. Pediatr.* **2018**, *6*, 27. [CrossRef]
47. Bokulich, N.A.; Chung, J.; Battaglia, T.; Henderson, N.; Jay, M.; Li, H.; Lieber, A.; Wu, F.; Perez-Perez, G.I.; Chen, Y.; et al. Antibiotics, birth mode, and diet shape microbiome maturation during early life. *Sci. Transl. Med.* **2016**, *8*, 343ra382. [CrossRef]
48. Boris, S.; Barbés, C. Role played by lactobacilli in controlling the population of vaginal pathogens. *Microbes Infect.* **2000**, *2*, 543–546. [CrossRef]
49. Reid, G.; Burton, J. Use of *Lactobacillus* to prevent infection by pathogenic bacteria. *Microbes Infect.* **2002**, *4*, 319–324. [CrossRef]
50. Ravel, J.; Gajer, P.; Abdo, Z.; Schneider, G.M.; Koenig, S.S.; McCulle, S.L.; Karlebach, S.; Gorle, R.; Russell, J.; Tacket, C.O.; et al. Vaginal microbiome of reproductive-age women. *Proc. Natl. Acad. Sci. USA* **2011**, *108* (Suppl. 1), 4680–4687. [CrossRef]
51. Ma, B.; Forney, L.J.; Ravel, J. Vaginal microbiome: Rethinking health and diseases. *Ann. Rev. Microbiol.* **2012**, *66*, 371–389. [CrossRef]
52. Reid, G.; Kumar, H.; Khan, A.I.; Rautava, S.; Tobin, J.; Salminen, S. The case in favour of probiotics before, during and after pregnancy: Insights from the first 1500 days. *Benef. Microbes* **2016**, *3*, 1–10.
53. Dunne, C.; Murphy, L.; Flynn, S.; O'Mahony, L.; O'Halloran, S.; Feeney, M.; Morrissey, D.; Thornton, G.; Fitzgerald, G.; Daly, C.; et al. Probiotics: From myth to reality. Demonstration of functionality in animal models of disease and in human clinical trials. *Antonie van Leeuwenhoek* **1999**, *76*, 279–292. [CrossRef]
54. Mattila-Sandholm, T.; Blum, S.; Collins, J.K.; Crittenden, R.; de Vos, W.M.; Dunne, C.; Fondén, R.; Grenov, G.; Isolauri, E.; Kiely, B.; et al. Probiotics: Towards demonstrating efficacy. *Trends Food Sci. Technol.* **1999**, *10*, 393–399. [CrossRef]
55. Dunne, C.; O'Mahony, L.; Murphy, L.; Thornton, G.; Morrissey, D.; Halloran, S.; Feeney, M.; Flynn, S.; Fitzgerald, G.; Daly, C.; et al. In vitro selection criteria for probiotic bacteria of human origin: Correlation with in vivo findings. *Am. J. Clin. Nutr.* **2001**, *73*, 386S–392S. [CrossRef]
56. McCarthy, J.; O'Mahony, L.; O'Callaghan, L.; Sheil, B.; Vaughan, E.E.; Fitzsimons, N.; Fitzgibbon, J.; O'Sullivan, G.C.; Kiely, B.; Collins, J.K.; et al. Double blind; placebo controlled trial of two probiotic strains in interleukin 10 knockout mice and mechanistic link with cytokine balance. *Gut* **2003**, *52*, 975–980. [CrossRef]
57. Dunne, C.; Kelly, P.; O'Halloran, S.; Soden, D.; Bennett, M.; von Wright, A.; Vilpponen-Salmela, T.; Kiely, B.; O'Mahony, L.; Collins, J.K.; et al. Mechanisms of adherence of a probiotic *Lactobacillus* strain during and after in vivo assessment in ulcerative colitis patients. *Microb. Ecol. Health Dis.* **2004**, *16*, 96–104. [CrossRef]

58. Sheil, B.; McCarthy, J.; O'Mahony, L.; Bennett, M.W.; Ryan, P.; Fitzgibbon, J.; Kiely, B.; Collins, J.K.; Shanahan, F. Is the mucosal route of administration essential for probiotic function? Subcutaneous administration is associated with attenuation of murine colitis and arthritis. *Gut* **2004**, *53*, 694–700. [CrossRef]
59. Martín, R.; Jiménez, E.; Olivares, M.; Marín, M.; Fernández, L.; Xaus, J.; Rodríguez, J.M. *Lactobacillus salivarius* CECT 5713, a potential probiotic strain isolated from infant feces and breast milk of a mother-child pair. *Int. J. Food Microbiol.* **2006**, *112*, 35–43. [CrossRef]
60. Olivares, M.; Díaz-Ropero, M.P.; Martín, R.; Rodríguez, J.M.; Xaus, J. Antimicrobial potential of four *Lactobacillus* strains isolated from breast milk. *J. Appl. Microbiol.* **2006**, *101*, 72–79. [CrossRef]
61. Pérez-Cano, F.J.; Dong, H.; Yaqoob, P. In vitro immunomodulatory activity of *Lactobacillus fermentum* CECT5716 and *Lactobacillus salivarius* CECT5713: Two probiotic strains isolated from human breast milk. *Inmunobiology* **2010**, *12*, 996–1004. [CrossRef] [PubMed]
62. Neville, B.A.; O'Toole, P.W. Probiotic properties of *Lactobacillus salivarius* and closely related *Lactobacillus* species. *Future Microbiol.* **2010**, *5*, 759–774. [CrossRef] [PubMed]
63. Messaoudi, S.; Manai, M.; Kergourlay, G.; Prévost, H.; Connil, N.; Chobert, J.M.; Dousset, X. *Lactobacillus salivarius*: Bacteriocin and probiotic activity. *Food Microbiol.* **2013**, *36*, 296–304. [CrossRef] [PubMed]
64. Sun, E.; Ren, F.; Liu, S.; Ge, S.; Zhang, M.; Guo, H.; Jiang, L.; Zhang, H.; Zhao, L. Complete genome sequence of *Lactobacillus salivarius* Ren, a probiotic strain with anti-tumor activity. *J. Biotechnol.* **2015**, *210*, 57–58. [CrossRef]
65. Kang, C.H.; Han, S.H.; Kim, Y.; Paek, N.S.; So, J.S. In vitro probiotic properties of *Lactobacillus salivarius* mg242 isolated from human vagina. *Probiotics Antimicrob. Proteins* **2018**, *10*, 343–349. [CrossRef] [PubMed]
66. Pino, A.; Bartolo, E.; Caggia, C.; Cianci, A.; Randazzo, C.L. Detection of vaginal lactobacilli as probiotic candidates. *Sci. Rep.* **2019**, *9*, 3355. [CrossRef] [PubMed]
67. Hill, C.; Guarner, F.; Reid, G.; Gibson, G.R.; Merenstein, D.J.; Pot, B.; Morelli, L.; Canani, R.B.; Flint, H.J.; Salminen, S.; et al. Expert consensus document. The International Scientific Association for Probiotics and Prebiotics consensus statement on the scope and appropriate use of the term probiotic. *Nat. Rev. Gastroenterol. Hepatol.* **2014**, *11*, 506–514. [CrossRef]
68. Raftis, E.J.; Salvetti, E.; Torriani, S.; Felis, G.E.; O'Toole, P.W. Genomic diversity of *Lactobacillus salivarius*. *Appl. Environ. Microbiol.* **2011**, *77*, 954–965. [CrossRef]
69. Fernández, L.; Cárdenas, N.; Arroyo, R.; Manzano, S.; Jiménez, E.; Martín, V.; Rodríguez, J.M. Prevention of infectious mastitis by oral administration of Lactobacillus salivarius PS2 during late pregnancy. *Clin. Infect. Dis.* **2016**, *62*, 568–573. [CrossRef]
70. Arroyo, R.; Martin, V.; Maldonado, A.; Jimenez, E.; Fernández, L.; Rodríguez, J.M. Treatment of infectious mastitis during lactation: Antibiotics versus oral administration of lactobacilli isolated from breast milk. *Clin. Infect. Dis.* **2010**, *50*, 1551–1558. [CrossRef]
71. Martín, R.; Soberón, N.; Vázquez, F.; Suárez, J.E. Vaginal microbiota: Composition, protective role, associated pathologies, and therapeutic perspectives. *Enferm. Infecc. Microbiol. Clin.* **2008**, *26*, 160–167. [CrossRef] [PubMed]
72. Ruiz, F.O.; Gerbaldo, G.; Garcia, M.J.; Giordano, W.; Pascual, L.; Barberis, I.L. Synergistic effect between two bacteriocin-like inhibitory substances produced by lactobacilli strains with inhibitory activity for *Streptococcus agalactiae*. *Curr. Microbiol.* **2012**, *64*, 349–356. [CrossRef] [PubMed]
73. Charlier, C.; Cretenet, M.; Even, S.; Le Loir, Y. Interactions between *Staphylococcus aureus* and lactic acid bacteria: An old story with new perspectives. *Int. J. Food Microbiol.* **2009**, *131*, 30–39. [CrossRef]
74. Açikgöz, Z.C.; Gamberzade, S.; Göçer, S.; Ceylan, P. Inhibitor effect of vaginal lactobacilli on group B streptococci. *Mikrobiyoloji Bulteni* **2005**, *39*, 17–23.
75. Borges, S.; Silva, J.; Teixeira, P. The role of lactobacilli and probiotics in maintaining vaginal health. *Arch. Gynecol. Obstet.* **2014**, *289*, 479–489. [CrossRef] [PubMed]
76. Ocaña, V.S.; Pesce De Ruiz Holgado, A.A.; Nader-Macías, M.E. Characterization of a bacteriocin-like substance produced by a vaginal *Lactobacillus salivarius* strain. *Appl. Environ. Microbiol.* **1999**, *65*, 5631–5635.
77. Cárdenas, N.; Martín, V.; Arroyo, R.; López, M.; Carrera, M.; Badiola, C.; Jiménez, E.; Rodríguez, J.M. Prevention of recurrent acute otitis media in children through the use of *Lactobacillus salivarius* PS7, a target-specific probiotic strain. *Nutrients* **2019**, *11*, 376. [CrossRef]

78. Martín, R.; Delgado, S.; Maldonado, A.; Jiménez, E.; Olivares, M.; Fernández, L.; Sobrino, O.J.; Rodríguez, J.M. Isolation of lactobacilli from sow milk and evaluation of their probiotic potential. *J. Dairy Res.* **2009**, *76*, 418–425. [CrossRef]
79. De Gregorio, P.R.; Juárez Tomás, M.S.; Leccese Terraf, M.C.; Nader-Macías, M.E. In vitro and in vivo effects of beneficial vaginal lactobacilli on pathogens responsible for urogenital tract infections. *J. Med. Microbiol.* **2014**, *63*, 685–696. [CrossRef]
80. Bodaszewska, M.; Brzychczy-Włoch, M.; Gosiewski, T.; Adamski, P.; Strus, M.; Heczko, P.B. Evaluation of group B streptococcus susceptibility to lactic acid bacteria strains. *Medycyna Doswiadczalna i Mikrobiologia* **2010**, *62*, 153–161.
81. Maldonado, J.; Lara-Villoslada, F.; Sierra, S.; Sempere, L.; Gómez, M.; Rodríguez, J.M.; Boza, J.; Xaus, J.; Olivares, M. Safety and tolerance of the human milk probiotic strain *Lactobacillus salivarius* CECT5713 in 6-month-old children. *Nutrition* **2010**, *26*, 1082–1087. [CrossRef]
82. Vázquez-Fresno, R.; Llorach, R.; Marinic, J.; Tulipani, S.; Garcia-Aloy, M.; Espinosa-Martos, I.; Jiménez, E.; Rodríguez, J.M.; Andres-Lacueva, C. Urinary metabolomic fingerprinting after consumption of a probiotic strain in women with mastitis. *Pharmacol. Res.* **2014**, *87*, 160–165. [CrossRef]
83. Espinosa-Martos, I.; Jiménez, E.; de Andrés, J.; Rodríguez-Alcalá, L.M.; Tavárez, S.; Manzano, S.; Fernández, L.; Alonso, E.; Fontecha, J.; Rodríguez, J.M. Milk and blood biomarkers associated to the clinical efficacy of a probiotic for the treatment of infectious mastitis. *Benef. Microbes* **2016**, *7*, 305–318. [CrossRef]
84. Danielsen, M.; Wind, A. Susceptibility of *Lactobacillus* spp. to antimicrobial agents. *Int. J. Food Microbiol.* **2003**, *26*, 1–11. [CrossRef]
85. Gueimonde, M.; Sánchez, B.; de los Reyes-Gavilán, C.G.; Margolles, A. Antibiotic resistance in probiotic bacteria. *Front. Microbiol.* **2013**, *4*, 1–6. [CrossRef]
86. Bryan, L.E.; Kwan, S. Mechanisms of aminoglycoside resistance of anaerobic bacteria and facultative bacteria grown anaerobically. *J. Antimicrob. Chemother.* **1981**, *8*, S1–S8. [CrossRef]
87. Handwerger, S.; Pucci, M.J.; Volk, K.J.; Liu, J.; Lee, M.S. Vancomycin-resistant *Leuconostoc mesenteroides* and *Lactobacillus casei* synthesize cytoplasmic peptidoglycan precursors that terminate in lactate. *J. Bacteriol.* **1994**, *176*, 260–264. [CrossRef]
88. Marsalková, S.; Cízek, M.; Vasil, M.; Bomba, A.; Nad', P.; Datelinka, I.; Jonecová, Z.; Rimková, S.; Kalinácová, V.; Styriak, I. Testing two *Lactobacillus plantarum* and *Lactobacillus acidophilus* strains for their suitability as a lipoid probiotic. *Berliner und Munchener Tierarztliche Wochenschrift* **2004**, *117*, 145–147.
89. Lee, Y. Characterization of *Weissella kimchii* PL9023 as a potential probiotic for women. *FEMS Microbiol. Lett.* **2005**, *250*, 157–162. [CrossRef]
90. Zárate, G.; Nader-Macias, M.E. Influence of probiotic vaginal lactobacilli on in vitro adhesion of urogenital pathogens to vaginal epithelial cells. *Lett. Appl. Microbiol.* **2006**, *43*, 174–180. [CrossRef]
91. Ermolenko, E.I.; Chernysh, A.I.; Martsinkovskaia, I.V.; Suvorov, A.N. Influence of probiotic enterococci on the growth of *Streptococcus agalactiae*. *Zhurnal Mikrobiol. Epidemiol. Immunobiol.* **2007**, *5*, 73–77.
92. Tsapieva, A.; Duplik, N.; Suvorov, A. Structure of plantaricin locus of *Lactobacillus plantarum* 8P-A3. *Benef. Microbes* **2011**, *2*, 255–261. [CrossRef]
93. Aloisio, I.; Mazzola, G.; Corvaglia, L.T.; Tonti, G.; Faldella, G.; Biavati, B.; Di Gioia, D. Influence of intrapartum antibiotic prophylaxis against group B *Streptococcus* on the early newborn gut composition and evaluation of the anti-*Streptococcus* activity of *Bifidobacterium* strains. *Appl. Microbiol. Biotechnol.* **2014**, *98*, 6051–6060. [CrossRef]
94. De Gregorio, P.R.; Juárez Tomas, M.S.; Leccese Terraf, M.C.; Nader-Macias, M.E. Preventive effect of *Lactobacillus reuteri* CRL1324 on Group B streptococcus vaginal colonization in an experimental mouse model. *J. Appl. Microbiol.* **2015**, *118*, 1034–1047. [CrossRef]
95. Patras, K.A.; Wescombe, P.A.; Rosler, B.; Hale, J.D.; Tagg, J.R.; Doran, K.S. *Streptococcus salivarius* K12 limits group B *Streptococcus* vaginal colonization. *Infect. Immun.* **2015**, *83*, 3438–3444. [CrossRef]
96. Ho, M.; Chang, Y.Y.; Chang, W.C.; Lin, H.C.; Wang, M.H.; Lin, W.C.; Chiu, T.H. Oral *Lactobacillus rhamnosus* GR-1 and *Lactobacillus reuteri* RC-14 to reduce Group B *Streptococcus* colonization in pregnant women: A randomized controlled trial. *Taiwan J. Obstet. Gynecol.* **2016**, *55*, 515–518. [CrossRef]

97. Olsen, P.; Williamson, M.; Traynor, V.; Georgiou, C. The impact of oral probiotics on vaginal Group B Streptococcal colonisation rates in pregnant women: A pilot randomised control study. *Women Birth* **2018**, *31*, 31–37. [CrossRef]
98. Quagliariello, V.; Masarone, M.; Armenia, E.; Giudice, A.; Barbarisi, M.; Caraglia, M.; Barbarisi, A.; Persico, M. Chitosan-coated liposomes loaded with butyric acid demonstrate anticancer and anti-inflammatory activity in human hepatoma HepG2 cells. *Oncol. Rep.* **2019**, *41*, 1476–1486. [CrossRef]
99. Ciani, O.; Arendsen, E.; Romancik, M.; Lunik, R.; Costantini, E.; Di Biase, M.; Morgia, G.; Fragalà, E.; Roman, T.; Bernat, M.; et al. Intravesical administration of combined hyaluronic acid (HA) and chondroitin sulfate (CS) for the treatment of female recurrent urinary tract infections: A European multicentre nested case-control study. *BMJ Open.* **2016**, *6*, e009669. [CrossRef]

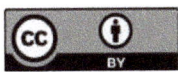 © 2019 by the authors. Licensee MDPI, Basel, Switzerland. This article is an open access article distributed under the terms and conditions of the Creative Commons Attribution (CC BY) license (http://creativecommons.org/licenses/by/4.0/).

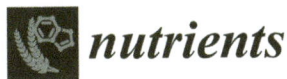

Article

Decaffeinated Green Tea Extract Does Not Elicit Hepatotoxic Effects and Modulates the Gut Microbiome in Lean B6C3F$_1$ Mice

Bill J. Gurley [1,2], Isabelle R. Miousse [3,4], Intawat Nookaew [5], Laura E. Ewing [3,6], Charles M. Skinner [2,3], Piroon Jenjaroenpun [5], Thidathip Wongsurawat [5], Stefanie Kennon-McGill [3], Bharathi Avula [7], Ji-Yeong Bae [7], Mitchell R. McGill [2,3,6], David Ussery [5], Ikhlas A. Khan [7] and Igor Koturbash [2,3,*]

[1] Department of Pharmaceutical Sciences, University of Arkansas for Medical Sciences, Little Rock, AR 72205-7199, USA; GurleyBillyJ@uams.edu
[2] Center for Dietary Supplements Research, University of Arkansas for Medical Sciences, Little Rock, AR 72205-7199, USA; CMSkinner@uams.edu (C.M.S.); MMcgill@uams.edu (M.R.M.)
[3] Department of Environmental and Occupational Health, University of Arkansas for Medical Sciences, Little Rock, AR 72205-7199, USA; IRacinemiousse@uams.edu (I.R.M.); LEEwing@uams.edu (L.E.E.); SKennonmcgill@uams.edu (S.K.-M.)
[4] Department of Biochemistry and Molecular Biology, University of Arkansas for Medical Sciences, Little Rock, AR 72205-7199, USA
[5] Department of Biomedical Informatics, University of Arkansas for Medical Sciences, Little Rock, AR 72205-7199, USA; INookaew@uams.edu (I.N.); PJenjaroenpun@uams.edu (P.J.); TWongsurawat@uams.edu (T.W.); DWUssery@uams.edu (D.U.)
[6] Department of Pharmacology and Toxicology, University of Arkansas for Medical Sciences, Little Rock, AR 72205-7199, USA
[7] National Center for Natural Product Research, School of Pharmacy, The University of Mississippi, University, MS 38677, USA; bavula@olemiss.edu (B.A.); jbae7@olemiss.edu (J.-Y.B.); ikhan@olemiss.edu (I.A.K.)
* Correspondence: IKoturbash@uams.edu; Tel.: +1-501-526-6638

Received: 5 March 2019; Accepted: 29 March 2019; Published: 3 April 2019

Abstract: The main purpose of this study was to investigate the hepatotoxic potential and effects on the gut microbiome of decaffeinated green tea extract (dGTE) in lean B6C3F$_1$ mice. Gavaging dGTE over a range of 1X–10X mouse equivalent doses (MED) for up to two weeks did not elicit significant histomorphological, physiological, biochemical or molecular alterations in mouse livers. At the same time, administration of dGTE at MED comparable to those consumed by humans resulted in significant modulation of gut microflora, with increases in *Akkermansia* sp. being most pronounced. Results of this study demonstrate that administration of relevant-to-human-consumption MED of dGTE to non-fasting mice does not lead to hepatotoxicity. Furthermore, dGTE administered to lean mice, caused changes in gut microflora comparable to those observed in obese mice. This study provides further insight into the previously reported weight management properties of dGTE; however, future studies are needed to fully evaluate and understand this effect.

Keywords: catechins; green tea extract; herbal dietary supplements; hepatotoxicity; microbiome

1. Introduction

The importance of dietary polyphenols for systemic health benefits is becoming increasingly recognized. Green tea, a major source of catechin polyphenols, is the second most popular beverage in the world and extracts of green tea are common ingredients in many dietary supplements. Major green tea extract (GTE) catechins include epicatechin (EC), epicatechin gallate (ECG), epigallocatechin

(EGC) and epigallocatechine gallate (EGCG), where the latter constitutes 50-80% of total catechins [1,2]. Catechins are reported to exert a number of positive effects on human health, including antioxidant, antibacterial and anti-inflammatory activities as well as reduced risks for cancer and cardiovascular disease [3–6]. Furthermore, the association of green tea or GTE consumption with weight loss and weight management, has further attracted interest to studies on catechins [7,8]. While these claims are based mostly upon the results of animal studies or equivocal clinical trial findings, the popularity of GTE and GTE-containing herbal dietary supplements (HDS) continues to grow. At the same time, GTE and its various catechin components (mainly–EGCG) are linked to a number of hepatotoxicity cases [9–15]. This hepatotoxicity has been confirmed experimentally and was shown to be further exacerbated by fasting conditions [16–19]. Therefore, the first aim of this study was to investigate potential hepatotoxicity and associated mechanisms of decaffeinated GTE (dGTE) in non-fasting mice.

The potentially beneficial effects associated with GTE and their mechanisms remain poorly understood. It has been demonstrated that short-term ingestion of GTE increases energy expenditure and promotes weight loss among lean and overweight volunteers but the long-term effects of GTE on energy expenditure were less conclusive [20–25]. Other hypotheses include GTE-mediated effects on sympathetic nervous system activity and promotion of fat oxidation [8]. Furthermore, a number of in vitro studies have indicated that EGCG inhibits adipocyte differentiation and proliferation while inducing adipocyte apoptosis [26–28]. However, it must be recognized that most in vitro studies have utilized EGCG concentrations (50–400 µM) much greater than that typically observed in humans (up to 1 µM) following GTE ingestion [29]. Furthermore, it is become increasingly recognized that intestinal absorption of catechins is at best nominal with less than 30% of ingested green tea polyphenols reaching the systemic circulation [30–34]. Poor absorption coupled with extensive first-pass metabolism likely explains the poor tissue accumulation of catechins following oral ingestion [35,36]. Therefore, the purported health benefits of GTE are not readily attributable to circulating levels of catechins.

Substantial levels of unabsorbed catechins, mainly EGCG, have been shown to reach the proximal and distal colon [37,38]. To what extent gut microbial metabolism plays a role in mediating GTE's health benefits remains to be determined. However, accumulating evidence indicates that GTE can modulate the gut microbiome in both experimental models and in humans [39–42]. Therefore, it has been proposed that GTE's health benefits may be linked to the effects catechins exert on particular bacterial species in the gut. Recent studies report similar patterns in the effects GTE causes on the gut microbiome in both experimental models and in human subjects. Those patterns are characterized by higher Shannon and Simpson microbiome diversities, increases in abundance of *Bacteroidetes* concomitant with deceases in *Firmicutes* at the phyla level and increases in *Prevotellaceae* and *Bacteroidaceae* paralleled by decreases in *Eubacteriaceae, Lachnospiraceae, Ruminococcaceae* and *Clostridiaceae* at the family level [39–41]. These studies, however, were performed on obese individuals or obese/fed high-fat diet mice; however, the effects of GTE on the gut microbiome associated with the lean phenotype remain unknown. Therefore, the second aim of this study was to investigate the effects of dGTE on the gut microbiome as a result of short-term ingestion in lean $B6C3F_1$ mice.

2. Materials and Methods

2.1. Decaffeinated Green Tea Extract (dGTE)

The studied product was a standardized dGTE manufactured by Nature's Way (Green Bay, WI, USA; lot # 20055697, expiration 11/30/18). The gavage solution was prepared by extracting the contents of 10 capsules with 10 mL of distilled water (pH = 5.3) in 20 mL round bottom, glass screw cap tubes via rotation (12 revolutions per minute) for 24 h. Tubes were then centrifuged at 10,000 rpm for 1 h, the supernatant was collected and two 1 mL aliquots were analyzed by the University of Mississippi's National Center for Natural Products Research for analysis (NCNPR).

dGTE was characterized for phytochemical content using validated analytical methods incorporating ultra-high performance liquid chromatography (UPLC) coupled with photodiode array (PDA) and mass spectrometry (MS) detection previously developed for the quantitative analysis of caffeine, theobromine and individual catechins (i.e., catechin, epicatechin, epicatechin gallate, epigallocatechin gallate) in *Camellia sinensis* leaves and GTE-containing products. Quantitative analysis was performed using a Waters Acquity UPLC™ H-class system (Waters Corp., Milford, MA, USA) including a quaternary solvent manager, sample manager, column compartment and PDA (Waters Acquity model code UPD) connected to a Waters Empower 2 data station. Separations were achieved within 15 min using a Waters C_{18} column. The injection volume was 2 μL and the PDA wavelength was 230 nm. The effluent from the LC column was directed into an electrospray ionization (ESI) probe. Compounds were confirmed under both positive and negative ionization modes.

2.2. Animals

Male $B6C3F_1/J$ mice, 8 weeks of age, were purchased from Jackson Laboratories (Bar Harbor, ME) and were housed at the UAMS Division of Laboratory Animal Medicine facility. $B6C3F_1/J$ mice are characterized by an average sensitivity to hepatotoxicants and are widely used by both the U.S. Food and Drug Administration (FDA) and industry to investigate the potential for xenobiotics to produce hepatotoxicity. Male mice were used on account of previous reports indicating a higher sensitivity to GTE-induced toxicity in male animals [17]. Animals were given one week to acclimate before the initiation of studies. Animal experiments were conducted in two stages. In the first stage, mice were gavaged with a single dose of either 1X, 3X or 10X mouse equivalent doses (MED) of dGTE with the subsequent tissue harvest at 24 h. This stage was performed in order to address the potential for acute toxicity of dGTE. During the second stage, mice were gavaged with dGTE for two weeks (Mon-Fri). The duration of this stage was chosen to investigate dGTE's sub-acute toxicity. To avoid potential fasting-exacerbated toxicity, food and water were provided *ad libitum*. Animal body weights were measured and recorded twice a week. All procedures were approved by the UAMS Institutional Animal Care and Use Committee at UAMS (protocol number: AUP #3701).

2.3. Dosage Information/Dosage Regimen

Allometric scaling for mouse equivalent doses for dGTE was determined per the recommendation of Wojcikowski and Gobe [43] which, in turn, is based upon the FDA Industry Guidance for Estimating the Maximum Safe Starting Dose in Initial Clinical Trials for Therapeutics in Adult Volunteers [44].

According to the label, each capsule 250 mg of dGTE was standardized to 95% polyphenols (75% catechins). Label recommended dose was "2 capsules daily, preferably with food." The human dose of catechins was calculated to be 375 mg catechins/70 kg = 5.36 mg/kg. MED of dGTE was calculated as 5.36 mg/kg × 12.3 = 65.9 mg/kg, where 12.3 is the scaling factor commonly used for mice weighing between 11–34 g. Concentration of total catechins per mL for the Nature's Way extraction solution as determined by NCNPR was 723.5 mg/mL. Therefore, for the 1X MED, the quantity of catechins administered was 65.9 mg/kg × 0.0235 kg (average mouse weight in our study) = 1.5 mg total catechins delivered in 300 μL of gavage solution. Consequently, 3X MED = 4.5 mg total catechins and 10X MED = 15 mg total catechins.

All extract supernatants were kept in the refrigerator and gavage doses were prepared fresh each day. After 40 days, a reanalysis of the catechin content of the supernatants was performed and the total catechin concentration was 92% of the original quantity.

2.4. Blood Sampling and Clinical Biochemistry

To measure the effects of dGTE on the panel of enzymes characteristic for liver injury, blood was collected at the end of each experimental stage. Blood was collected under isoflurane anesthesia from the retroorbital plexus. Tubes were kept on ice and centrifuged at 10,000 rpm for 20 min; serum samples were then immediately aliquoted and delivered to Arkansas Livestock and Poultry Commission Veterinary Diagnostic Laboratory (Little Rock, AR, USA) where the samples were processed same day.

2.5. Histopathological Assessment

Livers were excised, and a 1 mm section was obtained from the left lateral lobe and another from the right medial lobe. The sections were fixed in 4% formalin for 24 h, then briefly rinsed in PBS and stored in 70% ethanol for 24 h. Livers were then processed at the UAMS Pathology Core Facility, stained with hematoxylin eosin and shipped to the Heartland Veterinary Pathology Services, PLLC (Edmond, OK) where they were assessed by a board-certified veterinary pathologist in a blind fashion.

For histologic evaluation purposes, each liver was represented by two sections obtained from different lobes. Each section was initially evaluated at magnifications of 4×0 and 100X. The sections were then evaluated at 200X and 400X to better determine if significant changes were present and to check for the presence of mitotic figures and apoptotic bodies.

2.6. Glutathione Analysis

Glutathione was measured using a modified Tietze assay [45]. Briefly, liver tissue was homogenized in 3% sulfosalicylic acid. One aliquot was diluted in N-ethylmaleimide (NEM) to mask reduced glutathione (GSH) to facilitate measurement of oxidized glutathione (GSSG), while another was diluted in 0.1 M HCl for measurement of total (GSH+GSSG) glutathione. After removal of NEM by solid phase extraction with a C18 column, glutathione was measured in both aliquots using a colorimetric glutathione reductase cycling detection method [45].

2.7. Gene Expression Array

Total RNA was extracted from flash frozen liver tissue using the RNeasy Mini Kit (Qiagen, Germantown, MD, USA). Following purification, 1000 ng were reverse transcribed with the High Capacity cDNA Reverse Transcription Kit (ThermoFisher, Waltham, MA, USA). The cDNA was diluted to 5 ng/µL and 105 µL was mixed with an equal volume of 2X TaqMan® Fast Advanced Master Mix. For real-time PCR, 100 µL of the mix was applied to each of two channels on a TaqMan Low Density Hepatotoxicity Array (TLDA) (Supporting Information Table S1) (ThermoFisher, Waltham, MA, USA). Four biological samples were loaded on each array with five samples per each group analyzed. Analysis was performed using the ExpressionSuite Software v1.1 (ThermoFisher, Waltham, MA, USA).

2.8. Analysis of the Gut Microbiome

Fecal samples from individual mice were placed into collection tubes containing a nucleic acid stabilizer (Zymo Research, Irvine, CA, USA). Bacterial DNA extraction was performed using ZymoBIOMICS DNA Kits (Zymo Research). In total, 400 ng of each sample was used for tagmentation and library preparation, as directed by manufacturer's protocol of KAPA HyperPlus Kit (Roche, Madison, WI, USA). Then, each library was purified using AMPure XP bead (Beckman Coulter, Indianapolis, IN, USA). Normalized libraries were pooled and pair-end sequencing using the Illumina NextSeq 500 platform to obtain 150 bp paired-end reads was performed.

Raw Illumina fastq files were preprocessed to ensure that only the high-quality reads would be used for further bioinformatics analysis; adapter trimming and quality filtering were performed using Trimmomatic software version 0.36 with default parameters [46]. High quality fastqs were further used as the inputs for reference taxonomic classification and quantification using Centrigue version 1.0.4 with default parameters to generate species profile [47]. Profiles were then visualized on a taxonomic hierarchy using *Pavian* package for comparison purposes. The high quality reads were used for *de novo* assembly binning to construct high quality metagenomic gene profiling using the metaWRAP pipeline—a flexible pipeline for genome-resolved metagenomic data analysis with default parameters except using the mouse genome (mm10) to account for host contamination. Non-redundance gene sets were constructed as per Foong et al. from the obtained ORFs of the samples using Usearch fast clustering with identity cutoff of 95% and overlap length of 90% [48]. The constructed non-redundance gene sets were then translated into amino acid sequences for KEGG pathway annotation using ghostKOALA pipeline [48,49]. Differential abundance analysis of taxonomic and gene profiles were performed from the count data using DESeq2 package [50]. The adjusted p-values were then used for KEGG pathway enrichment analysis using piano package [51]. Pathways that had enrichment p-value of < 0.001 were selected to plot heatmaps. Raw sequence reads have been uploaded to NCBI, accession ID: PRJNA523806.

2.9. Statistical Analysis

All statistical analyses were performed with the GraphPad Prism 6 software (GraphPad Software. San Diego, CA, USA). Treatment groups were compared with their respective untreated group using ANOVA followed by Tukey's multiple comparison test. In cases where the data was not normally distributed, a Kruskal-Wallis test followed by a Dunn's multiple comparisons test was used instead.

3. Results

3.1. Phytochemical Characterization of Dgte Utilized in the Study

Phytochemical characterization of utilized dGTE is presented in Table 1. The catechin composition of the characterized product was comparable to the catechin composition in the product used in other animal studies with no more than 10% difference for each particular catechin ingredient.

Table 1. Phytochemical characterization of decaffeinated green tea extract (dGTE) product used in the study.

Ingredient	mg/Capsule
Caffeine	9.9
Gallocatechin	4.5
Epigallocatechin	17.2
Catechin	2.6
Epicatechin	14.4
Epigallocatechin gallate	180.3
Gallocatechin gallate	4.5
Epicatechin gallate	31.1
Catechin gallate	0.6
Sum of catechins	255.3
Sum of E-catechins	243.0

3.2. Studies on Acute dGTE Toxicity

Acute toxicity was investigated 24 h after a single gavage of mice with either 1X, 3X or 10X MED of dGTE to determine if dGTE can cause hepatotoxicity in a fed state. Significant decreases in body weight were observed in mice gavaged with 10X MED (12%, $p < 0.001$) (Figure 1A). The liver-to-body weight ratio was slightly but significantly decreased in all experimental groups (Figure 1B). Moderate changes in the organ-to-body weight ratios were also observed in the heart but not in the kidney (Supporting Information Figure S1A,B). No appreciable differences in cytoplasmic vacuolation, apoptotic or mitotic events, nor steatosis were observed in the livers of control versus experimental animals (Figure 1C).

Analysis of clinical biochemistry did not reveal any substantial changes in any of the evaluated parameters, besides the insignificant nearly two-fold increase in ALT and ~20% increase in AST after gavage with 1X MED (Table 2). To determine if dGTE had any effect on glutathione concentration or generation of reactive oxygen species (ROS) in the liver, we measured both total (GSH+GSSG) and oxidized (GSSG) glutathione. dGTE dose-dependently decreased hepatic GSH+GSSG content at 24 h, with ~40% ($p < 0.05$) depletion at 10X MED (Figure 1D). On the molecular level, only two genes out of 84 investigated were significantly deregulated—*Lss* and *Chrebp*. The expression of both genes was decreased; however, the extent of the changes was low (below 2-fold) (Figure 1E).

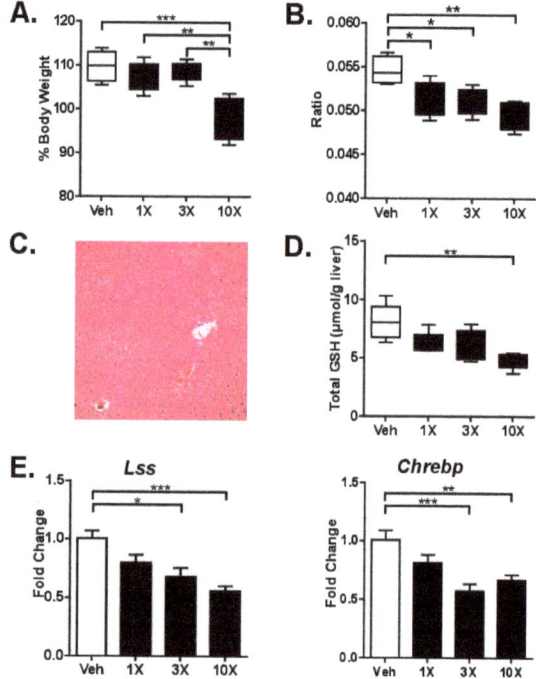

Figure 1. Analysis of dGTE acute toxicity. Body weights (**A**) and liver-to-body weight ratio (**B**). Photomicrograph of intact mouse liver after a single gavage with 10X mouse equivalent dose (MED) of dGTE (**C**). Total glutathione (**D**). mRNA levels of *Lss* and *Chrebp* genes (E). * $p < 0.05$, ** $p < 0.01$, *** $p < 0.001$; mean +/- SEM (n = 5 per group).

Table 2. Clinical chemistry parameters after dosing with dGTE for 24 h and 2 weeks.

24 h	Units	Vehicle	1X	3X	10X
Total Bilirubin	mg/dL	<0.2	<0.2	<0.2	<0.2
ALT	U/L	28.8 (±8.8)	52.6 (±20.2)	34.4 (±14.8)	32.2 (±11.9)
AST	U/L	66.2 (±5.7)	84.2 (±8.2)	65.2 (±9.8)	68.2 (±10.3)
GGT	U/L	<3.0	<3.0	<3.0	<3.0
Alkaline Phosphatase	IU/L	197 (±3.8)	196.2 (±7.3)	163.8 (±13.5) *	189.8 (±6.4)
2 weeks	Units	Vehicle	1X	3X	10X
Total Bilirubin	mg/dL	<0.2	<0.2	0.2	<0.2
ALT	U/L	28.8 (±8.8)	24.8 (±2.3)	34.2 (±14.4)	33.5 (±11.6)
AST	U/L	66.2 (±5.7)	49.2 (±12.9)	70.8 (±13.9)	67.6 (±10.4)
GGT	U/L	<3.0	4.8 (±1.3)	<3.0	<3.0
Alkaline Phosphatase	IU/L	148 (±4.5)	91.6 (±12.9) **	131.2 (±18.1)	140.2 (±6.7)

Data presented as mean +/- SEM (n = 5 per group) * $p < 0.05$, ** $p < 0.01$ compared to vehicle.

3.3. Studies on Sub-Acute dGTE Toxicity

Sub-acute toxicity was investigated after 2 weeks (Mon-Fri) of daily gavage with either 1X, 3X or 10X MED dGTE. A statistically significant decrease in body weight (8%, $p = 0.012$) was observed after gavaging mice with 1X MED dGTE compared to control mice at the end of the study (Figure 2A). No differences in body weight were observed after 3X and 10X MED dGTE. Gavaging with dGTE did not cause any changes in liver-to-body weight ratio (Figure 2B) as well as heart-to-body weight ratios (Supporting Information Figure S2A). A small increase in kidney-to-body weight ratio was observed in mice gavaged with 1X MED dGTE (Supporting Information Figure S2B).

Similar to the acute toxicity study, there were no histomorphological changes in the livers of experimental animals (Figure 2C). Furthermore, no changes were observed in the evaluated serum parameters except for the ~30% decrease in ALP in mice gavaged with 1X MED dGTE (Table 2). GSH+GSSG did not differ between groups after 2 weeks (Figure 2D), indicating compensatory GSH synthesis with prolonged exposure. Although the ratio of GSSG to GSH was significantly increased after GTE treatment at 24 h (data not shown), the absolute amount of GSSG was unchanged at both 24 h and 2 weeks (Figure 2E).

Gene expression analysis revealed only one (1) out of 84 genes significantly deregulated, *Mcm10*, increased expression of which was observed after administration of 10X MED dGTE (1.9-fold, $p < 0.01$) (Figure 2F).

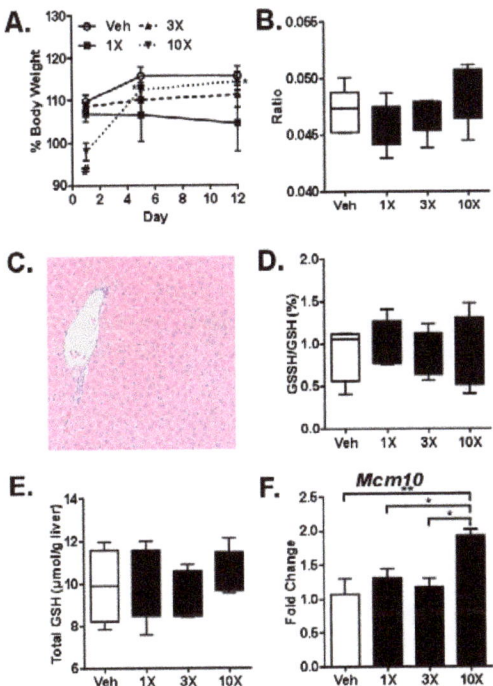

Figure 2. Analysis of dGTE sub-acute toxicity. Body weights ((**A**) # significant compared to vehicle, *significantly different from Day 1 within a dose group) and liver-to-body weight ratio (**B**). Photomicrograph of intact liver after gavaging mouse with 10X MED dGTE for 2 weeks (**C**). GSSH/GSH ratio (**D**), total glutathione (**E**) and mRNA levels of *Mcm10* gene (**F**). * $p < 0.05$, ** $p < 0.01$; # $p < 0.05$ compared to vehicle (**F**); mean +/− SEM ($n = 5$ per group).

3.4. Studies on the Gut Microbiome

Next, we sought to investigate whether or not orally administered dGTE affected the gut microbiome of lean mice. We selected 3X MED (equivalent of ~200 mg/kg/bw) since this is a dGTE dose analogous to that commonly consumed by humans [52].

We report that gavaging lean B6C3F$_1$ mice with 3X MED dGTE for the period of two weeks, caused substantial perturbations in the mouse gut ecology. Taxonomic profiling using Centrifuge software identified a clear discrimination between the control and dGTE mice (Figure 3A). At the cut-off of 0.5% relative abundance, *B. thetaiotaomicron*, a common resident bacteria in a mouse gut, was the most abundant species, followed by *L. johnsonii*, *Akkermansia muciniphila*, *Lachnoclostridium sp. YL32*, *Parabacteroides sp. YL27* and *Ruminoclostridium sp KB18* (Figure 3B). Administration of dGTE caused an increase in the *Bacteroidetes* to *Firmicutes* ratio (Figure 3C,D). Interestingly, only *A. muciniphila* abundance was dramatically increased in the dGTE group compared to control in the high abundance taxa (Figure 3C,D) with the most statistically significant adjusted *p*-value of 1.75e-7 (Supporting Information Figure S3, Table S2). Based on KEGG pathway analysis, increased abundance of genes associated with glycan degradation-related pathway in dGTE group compared to control was found (Figure 3E). As mucin is composed of different types of glycans, this correlates with the increased abundance of *A. muciniphila*, which is the main consumer of mucin in both human and animal gut [53]. On the other hand, decreased abundance of genes related with *Salmonella* infection, bacterial chemotaxis and bacterial mobility proteins in dGTE group was noted.

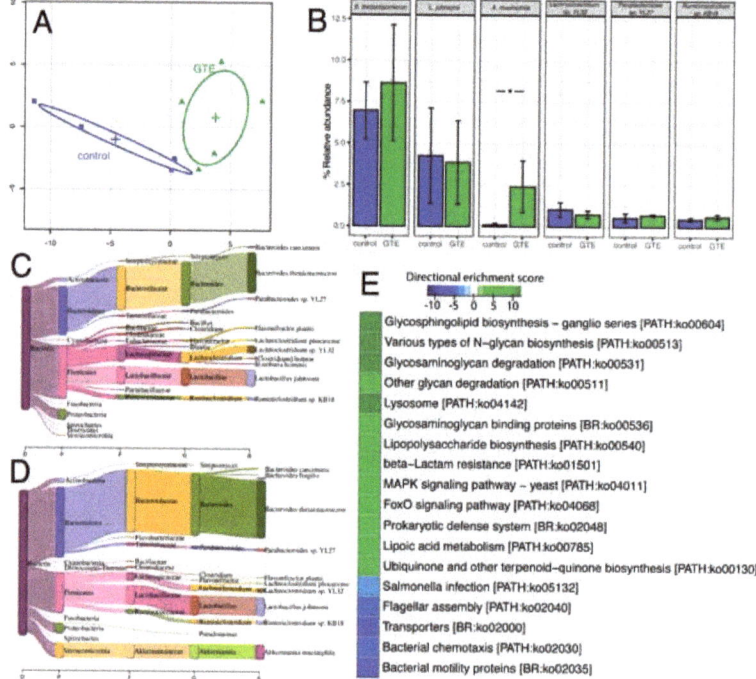

Figure 3. Shot gun metagenome analysis of dGTE (green) compare with control (blue). PCA plot of gut microbiome species abundance (**A**). Bag plots of high abundance gut bacteria (>5% relative abundance) in the study (**B**) * *p* < 0.05 compared to vehicle; mean +/- SEM (*n* = 5 per group). Sankey diagram for visualization of species abundance in a taxonomic tree of a sample control group (**C**) and dGTE (**D**). Heat map of directional enrichment score (−log10 enrichment *p*-value) for selected KEGG pathway (**E**).

4. Discussion

To assess the hepatotoxic potential of dGTE, we utilized an integrative approach similar to our other recent studies for the safety assessment of multi-ingredient botanical dietary supplement formulations [54,55]. This approach considers analyses based upon: (1) the number of end-points characteristic for liver injury; (2) a dose range of 1X to 10X MED (65.9 to 659 mg/kg bw/day of dGTE for this study); and (3) single and repeated dosing studies. This allows for a fast and comprehensive investigation of phytochemical hepatotoxicity as well as provide insight into potential toxicological mechanisms.

Our findings are in agreement with previous pre-clinical and clinical studies on dGTE hepatotoxicity that reported a lack of liver injury at doses below ~750 mg/kg bw/day [13,16,52]. Despite administering dGTE at doses as high as 10X MED, no appreciable toxicological responses were observed in experimental mice. Specifically, gavaging mice with dGTE produced no histopathological abnormalities in the livers and no significant alterations were observed in clinical biochemistry parameters indicative of liver injury. Small decreases in total glutathione were observed in mice livers 24 h after a single administration of dGTE; however, these effects were short-lived and had disappeared by day 14. The fact that dGTE had no effect on GSSG at 1X and 3X MED argues against the idea that orally administered dGTE is an antioxidant and the observed depletion of GSH+GSSG after a bolus dose of dGTE may even increase the risk of oxidative stress. This finding underscores the necessity of validating in vitro data using in vivo models and warrants further in vivo studies to investigate the potential anti- and pro-oxidant effects of GTE [56,57].

Only very modest, dose-independent changes in gene expression were detected in the livers of dGTE-gavaged mice. Analysis of expression panels for genes involved in xenobiotic metabolism or hepatocellular responses to toxicants revealed only a small subset (<5%) that was significantly dysregulated. Importantly, the magnitude of responses in those genes was minimal, with only one gene, *Mcm10*, exceeding a 1.5-fold increase from control. Furthermore, reduced expression of *Lss* and *Chrebp* genes that are associated with cholesterol and glycogen metabolism in mice may suggest potentially beneficial health effects and warrant future studies. No dGTE-induced weight-loss was observed; however, this can be explained by the lean nature of the mice and the study's short duration.

It must be noted that our study was performed under conditions that purposefully omitted other potential contributors to liver injury, such as genetics, fasting and caffeine [16,19,58]. GTE- or EGCG-induced liver injury is considered idiosyncratic by nature. While the mechanisms of this idiosyncrasy remain unknown, genetic components seem to play a significant, if not key, role [10,59]. Furthermore, in their elegant study using diversity outbred (DO) mice, Church and colleagues demonstrated that variations in select genomic loci may predispose to higher sensitivity to EGCG [19]. Therefore, our observed lack of dGTE-induced hepatotoxicity among inbred B6C3F$_1$ mice, a strain characterized by average sensitivity to hepatotoxicants, is not surprising.

Previous research hints at a contribution of fasting in GTE/catechins-induced liver injury. For instance, in two classical studies with beagle dogs, fasted animals exhibited high sensitivity to orally administered EGCG, including mortality at doses of 400 mg/kg bw with No-Observed-Adverse-Effect-Level (NOAEL) observed at 40 mg EGCG/kg bw/day [16]. At the same time, the NOAEL in dogs that received food *ad libitum* was 460 mg/kg bw/day and could potentially have been higher, as this dose of EGCG was the highest used in the study [16]. In our study, the mice received food *ad libitum*, with a NOAEL of 659 mg/kg bw/day.

Furthermore, our study utilized dGTE, thereby precluding any contributory effects from caffeine [58]. Importantly, in many GTE-associated cases of hepatotoxicity, GTE was one but not the only, constituent of the formulation. For example, GTE was present in both Hydroxycut™ and X-elles™, two dietary supplement formulations linked to multiple cases of hepatotoxicity that were voluntarily withdrawn from the market [14]. Besides GTE, both of those formulations contained caffeine and a host of other botanical ingredients. Caffeine's propensity to exacerbate the toxicity of other phytochemicals was recently recognized by the FDA, which banned the sale of pure caffeine powder and dietary supplements containing high caffeine content [60].

Finally, product adulteration with prescription medications (e.g., acetaminophen, amphetamines, etc.) or contamination with heavy metals, pesticides/herbicides or bacteria cannot be ruled as contributors to the hepatotoxicity of multi-ingredient, GTE-containing supplements [10,11]. Phytochemical characterization of the dGTE used in the present study revealed no evidence of adulteration, heavy metal or bacterial contamination.

Accumulating evidence indicates that catechin oral bioavailability is relatively low [13,15–18,34,35]. Our findings, together with a wealth of previously published data, suggest that any dGTE-derived health effects from catechins, likely stem from dGTE-mediated alterations in the distal gut microbiome and potential active metabolites generated therein, rather than from catechin absorption in the proximal intestine. Indeed, even minimal dietary interventions can substantially affect the gut microbiome and metabolome [61].

It has been proposed that GTE's health benefits may be linked to the effects catechins exert on particular bacterial species in the gut. For instance, catechins have been shown to affect the growth of *Bacteroidetes* and *Firmicutes* [62]. It is especially important to note that the relative proportion of *Bacteroidetes* to *Firmicutes* and bacterial alpha diversity are markedly decreased in both obese humans and obese mice [25,63–65]. Further studies have confirmed EGCG-induced changes to gut ecology [66]. Additionally, administration of green tea polyphenols appears to modulate gut microbiota diversity, including restoration of the *Bacteroidetes* to *Firmicutes* ratio resulting in body weight loss in mice fed a high fat diet [65]. Interestingly, another recent study that used liquid green tea reported opposite results with a decrease observed in the *Bacteroidetes* to *Firmicutes* ratio [42]. In our study, coincident with an increased *Bacteroides* to *Firmicutes* ratio, we also found an increase in *A. muciniphila*, a mucin degrading bacteria, which has been reported as a beneficial gut microbe associated with body fat reduction, correction of dyslipidemia and reduced insulin resistance [67].

In conclusion, we demonstrate that dGTE, when administered to non-fasting and genetically uncompromised mice, does not elicit hepatotoxic effects even when administered at doses as high as 659 mg/kg bw/day. Additional studies, however, will be needed to delineate the role of other confounding factors like caffeine, which may decrease tolerance to GTE. We further demonstrate that dGTE doses ~200 mg/kg bw can substantially modulate the gut microbiome, leading to increases in the health-beneficial bacteria *Akkermansia sp*. These findings may give insight into the potential weight management properties of GTE; however, future studies are needed to fully delineate this effect.

Supplementary Materials: The following are available online at http://www.mdpi.com/2072-6643/11/4/776/s1, Figure S1: Analysis of dGTE acute toxicity. Heart-to-body weight ratio (A) and kidney-to-body weight ratio (B). * $p < 0.05$, Figure S2: Analysis of dGTE sub-acute toxicity. Heart-to-body weight ratio (A) and kidney-to-body weight ratio (B). * $p < 0.05$, Figure S3: High abundance taxa in individual gut microbiome samples, Table S1: Taqman Custom Array targets, Table S2: Listing of taxa abundance.

Author Contributions: B.J.G. and I.K. designed the study; I.R.M., I.N., L.E.E., S.K.-M., C.M.S. and B.A. performed the experiments; B.J.G., I.R.M., I.N., P.J., T.W., S.K.-M., B.A., J.-Y.B., M.R.M., D.U., I.A.K. and I.K. analyzed the data; B.J.G., I.N. and I.K. wrote the manuscript.

Funding: This work was supported by the National Institute of General Medical Sciences (P20 GM109005 and P20GM125503) and Arkansas Biosciences Institute. DWU, IN, PJ and TW are supported by the Helen Adams & Arkansas Research Alliance Endowment.

Acknowledgments: The authors are thankful to Robin Mulkey for excellent animal care at the UAMS Animal Facility.

Conflicts of Interest: The authors declare no conflict of interests and did not receive any financial or other compensation from Nature's Way for this study.

References

1. Graham, H.N. Green tea composition, consumption and polyphenol chemistry. *Prev. Med.* **1992**, *21*, 334–350. [CrossRef]

2. Khan, N.; Mukhtar, H. Tea polyphenols for health promotion. *Life Sci.* **2007**, *81*, 519–533. [CrossRef]
3. Higdon, J.V.; Frei, B. Tea catechins and polyphenols: Health effects, metabolism and antioxidant functions. *Crit. Rev. Food Sci. Nutr.* **2003**, *43*, 89–143. [CrossRef]
4. Cooper, R.; Morre, D.J.; Morre, D.M. Medicinal benefits of green tea: Part i. Review of noncancer health benefits. *J. Altern. Complement. Med.* **2005**, *11*, 521–528. [CrossRef]
5. Lambert, J.D.; Hong, J.; Yang, G.Y.; Liao, J.; Yang, C.S. Inhibition of carcinogenesis by polyphenols: Evidence from laboratory investigations. *Am. J. Clin. Nutr* **2005**, *81*, 284S–291S. [CrossRef]
6. Hodgson, J.M.; Croft, K.D. Tea flavonoids and cardiovascular health. *Mol. Aspects Med.* **2010**, *31*, 495–502. [CrossRef]
7. Thielecke, F.; Boschmann, M. The potential role of green tea catechins in the prevention of the metabolic syndrome—A review. *Phytochemistry* **2009**, *70*, 11–24. [CrossRef]
8. Rains, T.M.; Agarwal, S.; Maki, K.C. Antiobesity effects of green tea catechins: A mechanistic review. *J. Nutr. Biochem.* **2011**, *22*, 1–7. [CrossRef]
9. Roytman, M.M.; Poerzgen, P.; Navarro, V. Botanicals and hepatotoxicity. *Clin. Pharmacol. Ther.* **2018**, *104*, 458–469. [CrossRef]
10. Navarro, V.J.; Khan, I.; Bjornsson, E.; Seeff, L.B.; Serrano, J.; Hoofnagle, J.H. Liver injury from herbal and dietary supplements. *Hepatology* **2017**, *65*, 363–373. [CrossRef]
11. Surapaneni, B.K.; Le, M.; Jakobovits, J.; Vinayek, R.; Dutta, S. A case of acute severe hepatotoxicity and mild constriction of common bile duct associated with ingestion of green tea extract: A clinical challenge. *Clin. Med. Insights Gastroenterol.* **2018**, *11*, 1179552218779970. [CrossRef]
12. Brown, A.C. Liver toxicity related to herbs and dietary supplements: Online table of case reports. Part 2 of 5 series. *Food Chem. Toxicol.* **2017**, *107*, 472–501. [CrossRef]
13. Isomura, T.; Suzuki, S.; Origasa, H.; Hosono, A.; Suzuki, M.; Sawada, T.; Terao, S.; Muto, Y.; Koga, T. Liver-related safety assessment of green tea extracts in humans: A systematic review of randomized controlled trials. *Eur. J. Clin. Nutr.* **2016**, *70*, 1340. [CrossRef]
14. Garcia-Cortes, M.; Robles-Diaz, M.; Ortega-Alonso, A.; Medina-Caliz, I.; Andrade, R.J. Hepatotoxicity by dietary supplements: A tabular listing and clinical characteristics. *Int. J. Mol. Sci.* **2016**, *17*, 537. [CrossRef]
15. Mazzanti, G.; Di Sotto, A.; Vitalone, A. Hepatotoxicity of green tea: An update. *Arch. Toxicol.* **2015**, *89*, 1175–1191. [CrossRef]
16. Isbrucker, R.A.; Edwards, J.A.; Wolz, E.; Davidovich, A.; Bausch, J. Safety studies on epigallocatechin gallate (egcg) preparations. Part 2: Dermal, acute and short-term toxicity studies. *Food Chem. Toxicol.* **2006**, *44*, 636–650. [CrossRef]
17. Kapetanovic, I.M.; Crowell, J.A.; Krishnaraj, R.; Zakharov, A.; Lindeblad, M.; Lyubimov, A. Exposure and toxicity of green tea polyphenols in fasted and non-fasted dogs. *Toxicology* **2009**, *260*, 28–36. [CrossRef]
18. Wu, K.M.; Yao, J.; Boring, D. Green tea extract-induced lethal toxicity in fasted but not in nonfasted dogs. *Int. J. Toxicol.* **2011**, *30*, 19–20. [CrossRef]
19. Church, R.J.; Gatti, D.M.; Urban, T.J.; Long, N.; Yang, X.; Shi, Q.; Eaddy, J.S.; Mosedale, M.; Ballard, S.; Churchill, G.A.; et al. Sensitivity to hepatotoxicity due to epigallocatechin gallate is affected by genetic background in diversity outbred mice. *Food Chem. Toxicol.* **2015**, *76*, 19–26. [CrossRef]
20. Berube-Parent, S.; Pelletier, C.; Dore, J.; Tremblay, A. Effects of encapsulated green tea and guarana extracts containing a mixture of epigallocatechin-3-gallate and caffeine on 24 h energy expenditure and fat oxidation in men. *Br. J. Nutr.* **2005**, *94*, 432–436. [CrossRef]
21. Dulloo, A.G.; Duret, C.; Rohrer, D.; Girardier, L.; Mensi, N.; Fathi, M.; Chantre, P.; Vandermander, J. Efficacy of a green tea extract rich in catechin polyphenols and caffeine in increasing 24-h energy expenditure and fat oxidation in humans. *Am. J. Clin. Nutr.* **1999**, *70*, 1040–1045. [CrossRef]
22. Rudelle, S.; Ferruzzi, M.G.; Cristiani, I.; Moulin, J.; Mace, K.; Acheson, K.J.; Tappy, L. Effect of a thermogenic beverage on 24-hour energy metabolism in humans. *Obesity* **2007**, *15*, 349–355. [CrossRef]
23. Most, J.; Goossens, G.H.; Jocken, J.W.; Blaak, E.E. Short-term supplementation with a specific combination of dietary polyphenols increases energy expenditure and alters substrate metabolism in overweight subjects. *Int. J. Obes.* **2014**, *38*, 698–706. [CrossRef]
24. Janssens, P.L.; Hursel, R.; Westerterp-Plantenga, M.S. Long-term green tea extract supplementation does not affect fat absorption, resting energy expenditure and body composition in adults. *J. Nutr.* **2015**, *145*, 864–870. [CrossRef]

25. Janssens, P.L.; Penders, J.; Hursel, R.; Budding, A.E.; Savelkoul, P.H.; Westerterp-Plantenga, M.S. Long-term green tea supplementation does not change the human gut microbiota. *PLoS ONE* **2016**, *11*, e0153134. [CrossRef]
26. Furuyashiki, T.; Nagayasu, H.; Aoki, Y.; Bessho, H.; Hashimoto, T.; Kanazawa, K.; Ashida, H. Tea catechin suppresses adipocyte differentiation accompanied by down-regulation of ppargamma2 and c/ebpalpha in 3t3-l1 cells. *Biosci. Biotechnol. Biochem.* **2004**, *68*, 2353–2359. [CrossRef]
27. Hung, P.F.; Wu, B.T.; Chen, H.C.; Chen, Y.H.; Chen, C.L.; Wu, M.H.; Liu, H.C.; Lee, M.J.; Kao, Y.H. Antimitogenic effect of green tea (-)-epigallocatechin gallate on 3t3-l1 preadipocytes depends on the erk and cdk2 pathways. *Am. J. Physiol. Cell Physiol* **2005**, *288*, C1094–C1108. [CrossRef]
28. Huang, J.; Wang, Y.; Xie, Z.; Zhou, Y.; Zhang, Y.; Wan, X. The anti-obesity effects of green tea in human intervention and basic molecular studies. *Eur. J. Clin. Nutr.* **2014**, *68*, 1075–1087. [CrossRef]
29. Yang, C.S.; Chen, L.; Lee, M.J.; Balentine, D.; Kuo, M.C.; Schantz, S.P. Blood and urine levels of tea catechins after ingestion of different amounts of green tea by human volunteers. *Cancer Epidemiol. Biomark. Prev.* **1998**, *7*, 351–354.
30. Chen, L.; Lee, M.J.; Li, H.; Yang, C.S. Absorption, distribution, elimination of tea polyphenols in rats. *Drug Metab. Dispos.* **1997**, *25*, 1045–1050.
31. Kohri, T.; Matsumoto, N.; Yamakawa, M.; Suzuki, M.; Nanjo, F.; Hara, Y.; Oku, N. Metabolic fate of (-)-[4-(3)h]epigallocatechin gallate in rats after oral administration. *J. Agric. Food Chem.* **2001**, *49*, 4102–4112. [CrossRef]
32. Kohri, T.; Suzuki, M.; Nanjo, F. Identification of metabolites of (-)-epicatechin gallate and their metabolic fate in the rat. *J. Agric. Food Chem.* **2003**, *51*, 5561–5566. [CrossRef] [PubMed]
33. Manach, C.; Williamson, G.; Morand, C.; Scalbert, A.; Remesy, C. Bioavailability and bioefficacy of polyphenols in humans. I. Review of 97 bioavailability studies. *Am. J. Clin. Nutr.* **2005**, *81*, 230S–242S. [CrossRef]
34. Stalmach, A.; Troufflard, S.; Serafini, M.; Crozier, A. Absorption, metabolism and excretion of choladi green tea flavan-3-ols by humans. *Mol. Nutr. Food Res.* **2009**, *53* (Suppl. 1), S44–S53. [CrossRef]
35. Okushio, K.; Suzuki, M.; Matsumoto, N.; Nanjo, F.; Hara, Y. Identification of (-)-epicatechin metabolites and their metabolic fate in the rat. *Drug Metab. Dispos.* **1999**, *27*, 309–316. [PubMed]
36. Donovan, J.L.; Manach, C.; Rios, L.; Morand, C.; Scalbert, A.; Remesy, C. Procyanidins are not bioavailable in rats fed a single meal containing a grapeseed extract or the procyanidin dimer b3. *Br. J. Nutr.* **2002**, *87*, 299–306. [CrossRef]
37. Jenner, A.M.; Rafter, J.; Halliwell, B. Human fecal water content of phenolics: The extent of colonic exposure to aromatic compounds. *Free Radic. Biol. Med.* **2005**, *38*, 763–772. [CrossRef] [PubMed]
38. Auger, C.; Mullen, W.; Hara, Y.; Crozier, A. Bioavailability of polyphenon e flavan-3-ols in humans with an ileostomy. *J. Nutr.* **2008**, *138*, 1535S–1542S. [CrossRef] [PubMed]
39. Zhang, X.; Chen, Y.; Zhu, J.; Zhang, M.; Ho, C.T.; Huang, Q.; Cao, J. Metagenomics analysis of gut microbiota in a high fat diet-induced obesity mouse model fed with (-)-epigallocatechin 3-o-(3-o-methyl) gallate (egcg3"me). *Mol. Nutr. Food Res.* **2018**, *62*, e1800274. [CrossRef] [PubMed]
40. Cheng, M.; Zhang, X.; Miao, Y.; Cao, J.; Wu, Z.; Weng, P. The modulatory effect of (-)-epigallocatechin 3-o-(3-o-methyl) gallate (egcg3"me) on intestinal microbiota of high fat diet-induced obesity mice model. *Food Res. Int* **2017**, *92*, 9–16. [CrossRef]
41. Henning, S.M.; Yang, J.; Hsu, M.; Lee, R.P.; Grojean, E.M.; Ly, A.; Tseng, C.H.; Heber, D.; Li, Z. Decaffeinated green and black tea polyphenols decrease weight gain and alter microbiome populations and function in diet-induced obese mice. *Eur. J. Nutr.* **2018**, *57*, 2759–2769. [CrossRef]
42. Yuan, X.; Long, Y.; Ji, Z.; Gao, J.; Fu, T.; Yan, M.; Zhang, L.; Su, H.; Zhang, W.; Wen, X.; et al. Green tea liquid consumption alters the human intestinal and oral microbiome. *Mol. Nutr. Food Res.* **2018**, *62*, e1800178. [CrossRef]
43. Wojcikowski, K.; Gobe, G. Animal studies on medicinal herbs: Predictability, dose conversion and potential value. *Phytother. Res.* **2014**, *28*, 22–27. [CrossRef]
44. Nair, A.B.; Jacob, S. A simple practice guide for dose conversion between animals and human. *J. Basic Clin. Pharm.* **2016**, *7*, 27–31. [CrossRef]
45. McGill, M.R.; Jaeschke, H. A direct comparison of methods used to measure oxidized glutathione in biological samples: 2-vinylpyridine and n-ethylmaleimide. *Toxicol. Mech. Methods* **2015**, *25*, 589–595. [CrossRef]

46. Bolger, A.M.; Lohse, M.; Usadel, B. Trimmomatic: A flexible trimmer for illumina sequence data. *Bioinformatics* **2014**, *30*, 2114–2120. [CrossRef]
47. Kim, D.; Song, L.; Breitwieser, F.P.; Salzberg, S.L. Centrifuge: Rapid and sensitive classification of metagenomic sequences. *Genome Res.* **2016**, *26*, 1721–1729. [CrossRef]
48. Foong, J.; Girdea, M.; Stavropoulos, J.; Brudno, M. Prioritizing clinically relevant copy number variation from genetic interactions and gene function data. *PLoS ONE* **2015**, *10*, e0139656. [CrossRef]
49. Kanehisa, M.; Sato, Y.; Morishima, K. Blastkoala and ghostkoala: Kegg tools for functional characterization of genome and metagenome sequences. *J. Mol. Biol.* **2016**, *428*, 726–731. [CrossRef]
50. Love, M.I.; Huber, W.; Anders, S. Moderated estimation of fold change and dispersion for rna-seq data with deseq2. *Genome Biol.* **2014**, *15*, 550. [CrossRef]
51. Varemo, L.; Nielsen, J.; Nookaew, I. Enriching the gene set analysis of genome-wide data by incorporating directionality of gene expression and combining statistical hypotheses and methods. *Nucleic Acids Res.* **2013**, *41*, 4378–4391. [CrossRef] [PubMed]
52. Dekant, W.; Fujii, K.; Shibata, E.; Morita, O.; Shimotoyodome, A. Safety assessment of green tea based beverages and dried green tea extracts as nutritional supplements. *Toxicol. Lett.* **2017**, *277*, 104–108. [CrossRef] [PubMed]
53. Derrien, M.; Vaughan, E.E.; Plugge, C.M.; de Vos, W.M. Akkermansia muciniphila gen. Nov., sp. Nov., a human intestinal mucin-degrading bacterium. *Int. J. Syst. Evol. Microbiol.* **2004**, *54*, 1469–1476. [CrossRef]
54. Skinner, C.M.; Miousse, I.R.; Ewing, L.E.; Sridharan, V.; Cao, M.; Lin, H.; Williams, D.K.; Avula, B.; Haider, S.; Chittiboyina, A.G.; et al. Impact of obesity on the toxicity of a multi-ingredient dietary supplement, oxyelite pro (new formula), using the novel nzo/hiltj obese mouse model: Physiological and mechanistic assessments. *Food Chem. Toxicol.* **2018**, *122*, 21–32. [CrossRef]
55. Miousse, I.R.; Skinner, C.M.; Lin, H.; Ewing, L.E.; Kosanke, S.D.; Williams, D.K.; Avula, B.; Khan, I.A.; ElSohly, M.A.; Gurley, B.J.; et al. Safety assessment of the dietary supplement oxyelite pro (new formula) in inbred and outbred mouse strains. *Food Chem. Toxicol.* **2017**, *109*, 194–209. [CrossRef]
56. Tan, X.L.; Shi, M.; Tang, H.; Han, W.; Spivack, S.D. Candidate dietary phytochemicals modulate expression of phase ii enzymes gstp1 and nqo1 in human lung cells. *J. Nutr.* **2010**, *140*, 1404–1410. [CrossRef]
57. Coyle, C.H.; Philips, B.J.; Morrisroe, S.N.; Chancellor, M.B.; Yoshimura, N. Antioxidant effects of green tea and its polyphenols on bladder cells. *Life Sci.* **2008**, *83*, 12–18. [CrossRef] [PubMed]
58. Gurley, B.J.; Steelman, S.C.; Thomas, S.L. Multi-ingredient, caffeine-containing dietary supplements: History, safety and efficacy. *Clin. Ther.* **2015**, *37*, 275–301. [CrossRef] [PubMed]
59. de Boer, Y.S.; Sherker, A.H. Herbal and dietary supplement-induced liver injury. *Clin. Liver Dis.* **2017**, *21*, 135–149. [CrossRef] [PubMed]
60. Gurley, B.J.; Yates, C.R.; Markowitz, J.S. " . . . Not intended to diagnose, treat, cure or prevent any disease." 25 years of botanical dietary supplement research and the lessons learned. *Clin. Pharmacol. Ther.* **2018**, *104*, 470–483. [CrossRef] [PubMed]
61. Miousse, I.R.; Pathak, R.; Garg, S.; Skinner, C.M.; Melnyk, S.; Pavliv, O.; Hendrickson, H.; Landes, R.D.; Lumen, A.; Tackett, A.J.; et al. Short-term dietary methionine supplementation affects one-carbon metabolism and DNA methylation in the mouse gut and leads to altered microbiome profiles, barrier function, gene expression and histomorphology. *Genes Nutr.* **2017**, *12*, 22. [CrossRef] [PubMed]
62. Xue, B.; Xie, J.; Huang, J.; Chen, L.; Gao, L.; Ou, S.; Wang, Y.; Peng, X. Plant polyphenols alter a pathway of energy metabolism by inhibiting fecal bacteroidetes and firmicutes in vitro. *Food Funct.* **2016**, *7*, 1501–1507. [CrossRef] [PubMed]
63. Ley, R.E.; Turnbaugh, P.J.; Klein, S.; Gordon, J.I. Microbial ecology: Human gut microbes associated with obesity. *Nature* **2006**, *444*, 1022–1023. [CrossRef] [PubMed]
64. Bajzer, M.; Seeley, R.J. Physiology: Obesity and gut flora. *Nature* **2006**, *444*, 1009–1010. [CrossRef] [PubMed]
65. Wang, L.; Zeng, B.; Zhang, X.; Liao, Z.; Gu, L.; Liu, Z.; Zhong, Q.; Wei, H.; Fang, X. The effect of green tea polyphenols on gut microbial diversity and fat deposition in c57bl/6j hfa mice. *Food Funct.* **2016**, *7*, 4956–4966. [CrossRef] [PubMed]

66. Ikarashi, N.; Ogawa, S.; Hirobe, R.; Kon, R.; Kusunoki, Y.; Yamashita, M.; Mizukami, N.; Kaneko, M.; Wakui, N.; Machida, Y.; et al. Epigallocatechin gallate induces a hepatospecific decrease in the cyp3a expression level by altering intestinal flora. *Eur. J. Pharm. Sci.* **2017**, *100*, 211–218. [CrossRef] [PubMed]
67. Plovier, H.; Everard, A.; Druart, C.; Depommier, C.; Van Hul, M.; Geurts, L.; Chilloux, J.; Ottman, N.; Duparc, T.; Lichtenstein, L.; et al. A purified membrane protein from akkermansia muciniphila or the pasteurized bacterium improves metabolism in obese and diabetic mice. *Nat. Med.* **2017**, *23*, 107–113. [CrossRef]

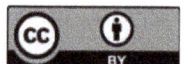

© 2019 by the authors. Licensee MDPI, Basel, Switzerland. This article is an open access article distributed under the terms and conditions of the Creative Commons Attribution (CC BY) license (http://creativecommons.org/licenses/by/4.0/).

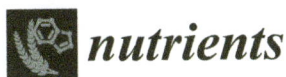

Article

Protein Hydrolysates from Fenugreek (*Trigonella foenum graecum*) as Nutraceutical Molecules in Colon Cancer Treatment

Amine Allaoui [1], Sonia Gascón [2], Souhila Benomar [1], Javier Quero [2], Jesús Osada [3], Moncef Nasri [4], María Jesús Rodríguez-Yoldi [2,*] and Ahmed Boualga [1,*]

[1] Laboratoire de Nutrition Clinique et Métabolique, Faculté des Sciences de la Nature et de la Vie, Université Oran1, 31000 Oran, Algeria; amn.allaoui@gmail.com (A.A.); souhila-13@hotmail.fr (S.B.)
[2] Departamento de Farmacología y Fisiología, Unidad de Fisiología, Facultad de Veterinaria, Universidad de Zaragoza, CIBERobn (ISCIII), IIS Aragón, IA2, 50013 Zaragoza, Spain; gasconmsonia@hotmail.com (S.G.); javierquero94@gmail.com (J.Q.)
[3] Departamento de Bioquímica y Biología Molecular y Celular, Facultad de Veterinaria, Universidad de Zaragoza, CIBERobn (ISCIII), IIS Aragón, IA2, 50013 Zaragoza, Spain; josada@unizar.es
[4] Laboratoire de Génie Enzymatique et de Microbiologie—Ecole Nationale d'Ingénieurs de Sfax, 3038 Sfax, Tunisia; mon_nasri@yahoo.fr
* Correspondence: mjrodyol@unizar.es (M.J.R.-Y.); boualga.ahmed@univ-oran1.dz (A.B.); Tel.: +213-772599943 (A.B.)

Received: 8 March 2019; Accepted: 23 March 2019; Published: 28 March 2019

Abstract: The application of plant extracts for therapeutic purposes has been used in traditional medicine since the plants are a source of a great variety of chemical compounds that possess biological activity. Actually, the effect of these extracts on diseases such as cancer is being widely studied. Colorectal adenocarcinoma is one of the main causes of cancer related to death and the second most prevalent carcinoma in Western countries. The aim of this work is to study the possible effect of two fenugreek (*Trigonella foenum graecum*) protein hydrolysates on treatment and progression of colorectal cancer. Fenugreek proteins from seeds were hydrolysed by using two enzymes separately, which are named Purafect and Esperase, and were then tested on differentiated and undifferentiated human colonic adenocarcinoma Caco2/TC7 cells. Both hydrolysates did not affect the growth of differentiated cells, while they caused a decrease in undifferentiated cell proliferation by early apoptosis and cell cycle arrest in phase G1. This was triggered by a mitochondrial membrane permeabilization, cytochrome C release to cytoplasm, and caspase-3 activation. In addition, the hydrolysates of fenugreek proteins displayed antioxidant activity since they reduce the intracellular levels of ROS. These findings suggest that fenugreek protein hydrolysates could be used as nutraceutical molecules in colorectal cancer treatment.

Keywords: fenugreek; protein hydrolysate; antiproliferative; apoptosis; antioxidant; Caco2 cells

1. Introduction

Fenugreek is one of the oldest plants used in traditional medicine. It has been used for a long time due to its beneficial properties in the treatment of wounds, abscesses, arthritis, bronchitis, and digestive disorders [1]. The seeds are the most important and useful part of the fenugreek plant [1]. Many of the functional and medicinal properties of fenugreek are attributed to its chemical composition (20–25% protein, 45–50% dietary fiber, 20–25% mucilaginous soluble fiber, 6–8% fatty acids and essential oils, and 2–5% steroidal saponins) [2].

Belguith-Hadriche, et al. [3] and Subhashini, et al. [4] demonstrated that seed fenugreek extracts are effective against free radical mediated diseases. In addition, Madhava Naidu et al. [5] observed that fenugreek husk, which is more rich in fiber, exhibits an important antioxidant property. However, the proteins of fenugreek seeds, unlike other plants, have been barely investigated.

Legume proteins have become a topic of many studies on health being and certain disease treatments. They are associated with a reduction in the incidence of various cancers, cholesterol, type-2 diabetes, and heart disease [6]. Furthermore, protein hydrolysate has the additional advantage of having improved functional properties as compared to the original protein isolates from which they are prepared. This is due to the release of certain bioactive peptides, which are encoded in the native protein molecule. More recently, potential health-promoting properties of peptides in these hydrolysates have been discovered [7].

The antiproliferative property is among the numerous biological activities attributed to hydrolysates. Effectively, several peptides with anticancer activity have been found in food protein hydrolysates as well as colon antitumor activity of egg yolk proteins or the cytotoxic activity on human colon carcinomas and mouse lymphoma cell lines of hydrophobic peptides extracted from soy [8]. The same findings have been reported in many other studies on *Vicia faba* protein hydrolysate [9], common beans peptides [10], and rice brain peptides [11].

Even if the mechanisms underpinning the antiproliferative effect of the protein hydrolysates is not well established, some hypotheses are proposed. For example, Ortiz-Martinez et al. [12] suggest that the antiproliferative effect on HepG2 cells of peptide fractions isolated from maize albumin hydrolysate is based on the induction of apoptosis due to the decrease of antiapoptotic factors expression. However, Xue et al. [13] reported that a chickpea-derived peptide inhibits the proliferation of breast cancer cells by increasing the p53 expression. Yet, Gao et al. [14] found that peptides derived from soy Vglycin activate the expression levels of pro-apoptotic proteins and caspase-3.

Since colorectal cancer is one of the most commonly diagnosed cancers, and it is strongly influenced by diet [8], the aim of this work has been to study the functional properties of the hydrolysed proteins of fenugreek seeds in relation to the treatment of colon cancer. For this, we have measured the possible antiproliferative and antioxidant effect of these hydrolysates on Caco-2 cells, and determined its mechanism of action.

2. Materials and Methods

2.1. Fenugreek Protein Hydrolysates Preparation

Fenugreek was purchased from a local spices market in the city of Tiaret (Algeria). Seeds were cleaned, grounded to a fine powder, and defatted in Soxhlet, (Labotech LT-6, Rosdorf, Germany), using *n*-hexane for 12 cycles and their proteins were extracted at an isoelectric point (pH 4.5) according to Boye et al. [15], as detailed previously [16]. The protein isolate was freeze dried and then hydrolyzed.

2.2. Preparation of FP Hydrolysates (FPHs)

Two hydrolysates were prepared from fenugreek proteins using Esperase® 0.8L (Sigma Chemical, St. Louis, MO, USA) (pH 9; 50 °C) or Purafect® 2000E (Genencor International, Palo Alto, CA, USA) (pH 10; 50 °C). FP were dissolved in distilled water at a proportion of 5% (*w/v*). Mixture pH and temperature were adjusted to optimum enzyme activity prior its incorporation. The enzymes were added to the solution at an enzyme/substrate ratio (E/S) of 5. Once the enzyme added, the mixture pH was maintained constant by a continuous addition of 2N NaOH solution. The degree of hydrolysis (DH) of FP was monitored by using a pH-stat method [17].

$$DH\ (\%) = \frac{h}{h_{tot}} \times 100 = \frac{B \times N_B}{MP} \times \frac{1}{\alpha} \times \frac{1}{h_{tot}} \times 100$$

where B is the amount (mL) of NaOH consumed to keep the pH constant during the reaction, N_B is the normality of NaOH, MP is the mass of protein (g), and α is the average degree of dissociation of the α-NH$_2$ groups released during hydrolysis. h_{tot} is the total number of peptide bonds, which was assumed to be 7.6 meq/g.

Hydrolysis was performed for 5 hours. Afterward, the reaction was stopped by heating the solution at 90 °C for 10 min. Then, the digest was cooled at room temperature and centrifuged at 5000× g for 15 min. The obtained hydrolysates: Esperase-fenugreek proteins hydrolysate (EFPH) and Purafect-fenugreek proteins hydrolysate (PFPH), were collected, freeze dried, and then stored at 4 °C.

2.3. Hydrolysates Proximate Composition

The protein, moisture, lipids, and ash contents in the freeze-dried fenugreek proteins and proteins hydrolysates were determined by using the AOAC methods [18]. A factor of 6.25 was used to convert the nitrogen value to protein. Minerals were analyzed by using Inductively Coupled Plasma-Optical Emission Spectroscopy (ICP-OES, Perkin Elmer 4300DV, Shelton, CT, USA), after dissolving samples in nitric acid (70%).

2.4. Amino Acid Analysis

A total of 50 µL of the sample (1 mg proteins/mL) were first hydrolyzed in a vacuum-sealed glass tube for 24 h at 110 °C in the presence of 6 N HCl and 1% phenol. For tryptophane analysis, samples were hydrolyzed in 4N NaOH, as described by Yust et al. [19]. At the end of hydrolysis, the samples pH was adjusted to 7 and filtered through a 0.45 µm cellulose acetate membrane filter.

The samples were then analyzed by the reversed phase HPLC (Agilent 1100 HPLC system, Wilmington, DE, USA) after automatic precolumn derivatization with a combination of OPA-3MPA (o-phtaldialdehyde-3-mercaptopropionic acid) for primary amino acids and FMOC (9-fluorenylmethylchloroformate) for secondary amino acids, following the manufacturer instructions. The separation was done on a reversed-phase Zorbax Eclipse-AAA column (4.6 × 150 mm, 3.5 µm). The quantification was determined by using norleucine as internal standard. The amino acid composition was expressed as the percent of residues.

2.5. Cell Culture

The biological activity of fenugreek protein hydrolysates was evaluated on the human colonic adenocarcinoma Caco2 cell line TC7 clone, provided by Dr. Edith Brot-Laroche (Université Pierre et Marie Curie-Paris 6, UMR S 872, Les Cordeliers, France). Caco2/TC7 cells were maintained in a humidified atmosphere of 5% CO$_2$ at 37 °C. Cells (passages 38–41) were grown in Dulbecco's Modified Eagles Medium (DMEM) (Gibco Invitrogen, Paisley, UK) supplemented with 20% fetal bovine serum, 1% non-essential amino acids, and 1% amphotericin (250 U/mL). The cells were passaged enzymatically with 0.25% trypsin-1 mM EDTA and sub-cultured on 25 cm^2 plastic flasks at a density of 5 × 10^5 cells per flask. Culture medium was replaced every three days. Cell confluence (80%) was confirmed by the microscopic observance. Experiments were performed in differentiated cells and in cancerous or undifferentiated cells (24 h post-seeding to prevent cell differentiation).

2.6. Cell Treatment and Antiproliferative Property Analysis

EFPH and PFPH were diluted in DMEM to the final concentration of 1 mg/mL. For an antiproliferative experiment, 4 × 10^3 cells were dispensed into each well of a 96-well plate. The culture medium was then replaced after 24 h with fresh medium (without fetal bovine serum, FBS) containing fenugreek protein hydrolysates, with an exposure time of 24, 48, or 72 h. Untreated cells were taken as a control. The anti-proliferative effect was measured with the sulforhodamine B assay, as described by Sánchez-de-Diego et al. [20]. Cells were fixed with 10% trichloroacetic acid (1 h, 4 °C), washed with distilled water, and stained with 4 g/L of sulforhodamine B (20 min, at room temperature). The plates were then washed with 1% acetic acid (v/v) to remove the unbound dye. Protein-bound dye was extracted with 10 mM Tris base (pH 10.5). Untreated cells were taken as a control (C).

The same experiment was done with the differentiated cells. Lastly, the results were obtained by measuring absorbance (A) with a scanning multi-well spectrophotometer (SPECTROstar Nano Microplate Reader—BMG LABTECH, Ortenberg, Germany) at a wavelength of 562 nm. The anti-proliferative effect was expressed as a percentage of living cells compared to the control, and calculated as follows:

$$\text{Viability (\%)} = \frac{A_{sample}}{A_{control}} \times 100$$

2.7. Apoptosis Measurement

Undifferentiated Caco2/TC7 cells were exposed for 24 h to 1 mg/mL of EFPH or PFPH, then collected and stained with AnnexinV-FTIC in combination with propidium iodide (PI), as described by Sánchez-de-Diego et al. [20]. Untreated cells were used as a negative control. After incubation, cells were transferred to flow-cytometry tubes and washed twice with temperate phosphate-buffered saline and re-suspended in 100 µL Annexin V binding buffer (10 mM Hepes/NaOH, pH 7.4, 140 mM NaCl, 2.5 mM $CaCl_2$). Afterward, 5 µL of the Annexin V-FITC and 5 µL of PI were added to each 100 µL of cell suspension. After incubation for 15 min at room temperature in the dark, 400 µL of Annexin binding buffer were added and analyzed by flow cytometry within one hour. The signal intensity was measured using a BD FACSAria (BD Biosciences, Piscataway, NJ, USA) and analyzed using BD FACSDiva (BD Biosciences, San Jose, CA, USA).

2.8. Propidium Iodide Staining of DNA Content and Cell Cycle Analysis

The fenugreek protein hydrolysates treated Caco2/TC7 cells were fixed in 70% ice-cold ethanol and stored at 4 °C for 24 h. After centrifugation (2500 rpm, 5 min), cells were rehydrated in PBS and stained with propidium iodide (PI) solution (50 µg/mL) containing RNase A (100 µg/mL). PI stained cells were analysed for DNA content in a BD FACSArray (BD Biosciences, Piscataway, NJ, USA). The red fluorescence emitted by PI was collected by a 620-nm longer pass filter, as a measure of the amount of DNA-bound PI and displayed on a linear scale. Cell cycle distribution was determined on a linear scale. The results were treated with ModFit LT 3.0 (Verity Software House, Topsham, ME, USA) [20].

2.9. Mitochondrial Membrane Potential Assay by Flow Cytometry

Caco2/TC7 cells were plated in 25 cm^2 flask at a density of 3×10^5 cells per flask and incubated for 24 h under standard cell culture conditions. Afterward, cells were treated with 1 mg/mL of fenugreek hydrolysates and incubated for 24 h. The control cells were incubated with a new medium without treatment and without FBS. Then, cells were washed twice with temperate PBS and re-suspended in temperate PBS at a concentration of 1×10^6 cells/mL. Later, 5 µL of 10 µM cationic dye 1,1′,3,3,3′-hexamethylindodicarbo-cyanine iodide (DiIC1) were added to each sample and the cells were incubated 15 min at 37 °C, 5% CO_2. After the incubation period, 400 µL of PBS were added to each tube and fluorescence was analyzed by flow cytometry using a BD FACSArray equipped with an argon ion laser. Excitation and emission settings were 633 and 658 nm, respectively.

2.10. Determination of Caspase 3 and Cytochrome C

Caco2/TC7 cells were plated in a 25 cm^2 flask at a density of 3×10^5 cells per flask and incubated for 24 h under standard cell culture conditions. Then, 1 mg/mL fenugreek hydrolysate solution was added to the flask and incubated for 24 h.

The caspase-3 analysis were studied as previously described by Sánchez-de-Diego et al. [20]. The cells were fixed in 0.01% formaldehyde for 15 min and centrifuged for 5 min at 300× g. Then, the pellet was suspended in 100 µL digitonin lysis buffer (50 mg/mL digitonin, 100 mM KCl, in 1× PBS) and incubated for 15 min in the dark at room temperature (RT). After incubation, cells were washed with 2 mL of PBS containing 0.1% digitonin and centrifuged at 300× g for 5 min. The supernatant was discarded and the pellet was re-suspended in 200 µL of PBS containing 0.1% digitonin. In addition, 2 µL of diluted caspase-3 antibody (Novus Biologicals, Abingdon, UK) were added to each sample and the resultant mix was incubated for 1 hour. After incubation, cells were centrifuged at 500× g, for 5 min at room temperature, and washed twice with PBS. Lastly, the cells were re-suspended in 400 µL of PBS. Fluorescence was analyzed by flow cytometry (Ex: 494 nm, Em: 520 nm) using a BD FACSArray.

Cells with liberated cytochrome C were analyzed according to Christensen et al. [21] with slight modifications [20]. Cells were initially resuspended thoroughly in 100 µL digitonin permeabilization buffer (50 µg/mL digitonin; 100 mM KCl; in 1× PBS) followed by incubation for 5 min at room temperature. This was followed by fixing the cells with 100 µL of 4% paraformaldehyde (PFA) in PBS for 30 min. Centrifugation (500× g, 5 min) was carried out to remove PFA and cells were washed once with 100 µL 1× PBS. Cells were then incubated with 100 µL blocking buffer (3% bovine serum albumin, 0.05% saponin, in 1× PBS) for 15 min at room temperature. Afterward, 2 µL of diluted cytochrome C antibody 7H8-2C12 (Novus Biologicals, Abingdon, UK) was incubated with cells for 1 h. Cells were washed twice with 1× PBS, then re-suspended in 400 µL of blocking buffer, and samples were analyzed by flow cytometry (Ex: 488 nm, Em: 575 nm) in BD FACSArray.

2.11. Intracellular Levels of Reactive Oxygen Species (ROS)

The cells were seeded in 96-wells plate at a density of 4×10^3 cells/well. The intracellular level of ROS was assessed using the dichlorofluorescein assay [22]. Caco2/TC7 cells were cultured for 24 h before oxidative stress induction, and then incubated with 100 µL of serum-free culture media with 1 mg/mL of EFPH or PFPH for 24 h. After that, the medium was removed, cells were washed twice with phosphate buffered saline, and incubated for 1 h with 100 µL of 20 µM 2′,7′-dichlorofluorescein diacetate (DCFH-DA) in PBS at 37 °C. After this period, cells were washed and re-suspended in PBS supplemented with 20 mM or 500 µM H_2O_2. The formation of the fluorescence oxidized derivative of DCF was monitored at an emission wavelength of 535 nm and an excitation wavelength of 485 nm in a multiplate reader. A measure at time "zero" was performed, cells were then incubated at 37 °C in the multiplate reader, and generation of fluorescence was measured after 20 min. ROS levels were expressed as a percentage of fluorescence (f) compared to the control, and reported using the following formula.

$$\text{ROS levels (\%)} = \frac{f_{\text{sample}}}{f_{\text{Control}}} \times 100 \times \frac{100}{\text{Viability}}$$

2.12. Thioredoxin Reductase 1 (TrxR1) Activity Assay

Undifferentiated cells were seeded in a 96-well plate with different protein hydrolysates for 24 h. The cells were then lysed (5 M NaCl, 1 M Tris-HCl pH 8.0, 0.5 M EDTA pH 8.0, SDS 10%, miliQ water) and incubated in a shaking motion for 20 min. After the incubation time, 25 µL of the reaction mixture (500 µL PBS pH 7.0, 80 µL, 100 mM EDTA pH 7.5, 20 µL 0.05% BSA, 100 µL 20 mM NADPH, 300 µL H_2O) were added to each well. Lastly, the reaction was started by adding 25 µL of 20 mM DTNB in pure ethanol. The absorbance increase was followed at 405 nm every minute for 6 min. Wells with TrxR1 inhibitor (auranofin) were measured in the same conditions to subtract the unspecific activity [20]. Cell protein contents were calculated by the Bradford method [23]. The result is expressed as a percentage of TxrR1 activity of treated cells compared to the TxrR1 activity of C cells.

2.13. Statistical Analysis

Data are presented as mean ±SD. Data were subjected to one-way ANOVA and the LSD-Fisher post hoc test. Differences were considered significant at $p \leq 0.05$.

3. Results

3.1. Kinetic and Degree of Hydrolysis

The hydrolysis curve of fenugreek proteins, illustrated in Figure 1, showed a first fast reaction kinetics characterized by an initial rapid phase (during the first 60 min for Esperase and the first 15 min for Purafect). At the end of the hydrolysis reaction, the DHs of the protein isolate were 9% with Purafect and 19% with Esperase.

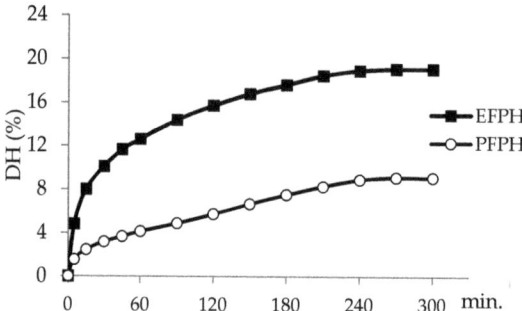

Figure 1. Kinetic of fenugreek proteins hydrolysis. E/S ratio= 5 U/mg proteins. EFPH: Esperase-fenugreek proteins hydrolysate. PFPH: Purafect-fenugreek proteins hydrolysate.

3.2. Chemical and Amino Acids Composition of FP and FPHs

Since the properties of protein hydrolysates depend strongly on their composition, the physicochemical composition of fenugreek protein hydrolysates was first analyzed. The proximate composition of EFPH and PFPH and their amino acid composition are shown in Table 1. Protein and lipids contents in EFPH were higher when compared to PFPH.

Table 1. Chemical composition of fenugreek protein hydrolysates.

	PFPH	EFPH
	(%)	(%)
Proteins	89.9 ± 0.2	92.3 ± 0.5 *
HAA	49.4	49.0
AAA	16.8	17.2
PCAA	12.2	12.5
Lipids	2.8 ± 0.2	3.3 ± 0.4 *
Total fiber	3.0 ± 0.1	2.0 ± 0.1 *
Carbohydrates #	1.5	<1
Moisture	1.0 ± 0.1	1.1 ± 0.1
Ash	1.8 ± 0.2	1.3 ± 0.3
Mineral composition		
Potassium (mg/100 g)	986 ± 5	1001 ± 1 *
Phosphorus (µg/g)	1933 ± 7	1927 ± 11
Sulphide (µg/g)	1128 ± 5	1268 ± 48 *
Magnesium (µg/g)	1013 ± 4	985 ± 9 *
Calcium (µg/g)	636 ± 2	502 ± 14 *
Sodium (µg/g)	122 ± 4	110 ± 3 *
Selenium (µg/kg)	53 ± 1	52 ± 1

PFPH: Purafect fenugreek proteins hydrolysate. EFPH: Esperase fenugreek proteins hydrolysate. HAA: hydrophobic amino acids (Ala, Val, Ile, Leu, Tyr, Phe, Trp, Pro, Met, and Cys). AAA: aromatic amino acids (Phe, Tyr, Trp). PCAA: positively charged amino acids (Arg, His, Lys). Results are presented as mean ± SD ($n = 3$). Superscripted (*) means within a row are significantly different ($p \leq 0.05$). #: Calculated by difference.

The bioactive properties of proteins hydrolysates are tightly related to the nature of their amino acids (Maestri et al., 2018). Aromatic, hydrophobic, and positively charged amino acids were similar in both hydrolysates. The detailed amino acids composition of fenugreek protein hydrolysates is reported in Reference [16].

Potassium, sulphide, and phosphorus were the most abundant minerals in FPHs, while selenium and sodium concentrations represented the less abundant.

3.3. Antiproliferative Activity

We first examined if the exposition of Caco2 TC7 cells to 1 mg/mL of FPH inhibits their proliferation. The treatment of undifferentiated Caco2/TC7 cells with fenugreek proteins hydrolysates exhibited a decrease in their viability. The PFPH anti-proliferative property was time dependent and passed from 27% after 24 h to 55% after 72 h of the incubation period, compared to the control. With EFPH, there was also a cells proliferation inhibitory effect, which varied between 39% and 50%. Nevertheless, it was not significantly time dependent (Figure 2A). In order to demonstrate if the antiproliferative effect of FPH found on Caco2/TC7 cells was specific for the undifferentiated cells or was a cytotoxic mechanism, we tested this property on differentiated cells. There was no difference in differentiated cell growth between the control and the treated cells (Figure 2B).

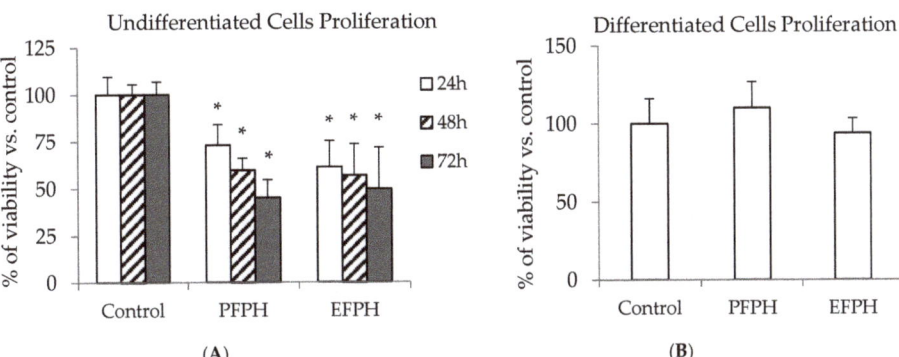

Figure 2. Relative viability of undifferentiated ((**A**): 24 h, 48 h, and 72 h) and differentiated Caco2/TC7 cells (**B**) treated (24 h) or not with fenugreek proteins hydrolysates. Data are presented as mean ± SD. The experiment was done in triplicate (each performed with six determinations). Superscripted (*) means are significantly different ($p \leq 0.05$) compared to their respective control. Control: Untreated cells. PFPH: Purafect fenugreek proteins hydrolysate. EFPH: Esperase fenugreek proteins hydrolysate. The hydrolysates were used at a final concentration of 1 mg/mL.

3.4. Apoptosis Analysis

Two major mechanisms could lead to cell death: necrosis and apoptosis. Necrosis is characterized as passive, with uncontrolled release of inflammatory cellular contents. On the opposite side, apoptosis is considered to be a regulated and controlled process that avoids eliciting inflammation [24]. Thus, we examined which of the two mechanisms was triggered by FPH. After 24 h of incubation with PFPH and EFPH (final concentration 1 mg/mL) vs. untreated cells, undifferentiated Caco2 living cells decreased. Whereas, those with early apoptosis increased by 4.6-fold. There were no significant differences in cells with late apoptosis or necrosis before and after treatment (Figure 3).

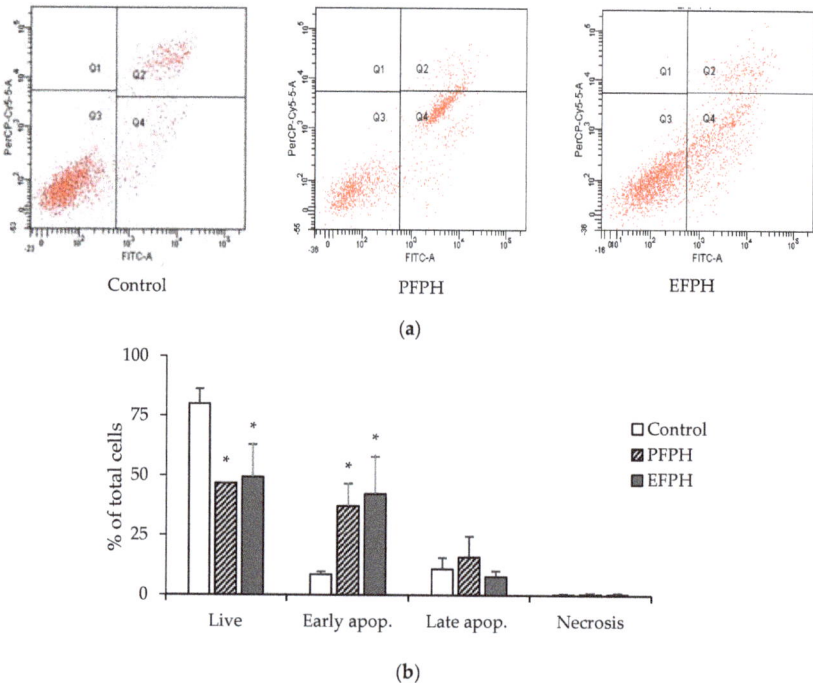

Figure 3. Effect of treating undifferentiated Caco2/TC7 cells with fenugreek proteins hydrolysates (24 h) on apoptosis. (**a**) Representative histogram of cytometry analysis. (**b**) Cell death process repartition. Data are presented as mean ± SD. The experiment was done in duplicate. Superscripted (*) means are significantly different ($p \leq 0.05$) when compared to their respective control. Control: Untreated cells. PFPH: Purafect fenugreek proteins hydrolysate. EFPH: Esperase fenugreek proteins hydrolysate. The hydrolysates were used at a final concentration of 1 mg/mL.

3.5. Cell Cycle Analysis

We subsequently analyzed if the treatment with 1 mg/mL of FPH caused a cell-cycle arrest in Caco2 TC7. Cell-cycle analysis (Figure 4) showed that cells stopped in the G0-G1 phase were, respectively, 1.6-fold and 1.5-fold higher in PFPH and EFPH-treated cells compared to non-treated cells. In the S phase, the cells treated with EFPH, and not those treated with PFPH, decreased by 40% vs. the control cells. Even if there was a reduction in PFPH-treated cells blocked in the G2-M phase (−33%), this difference was not statistically significant.

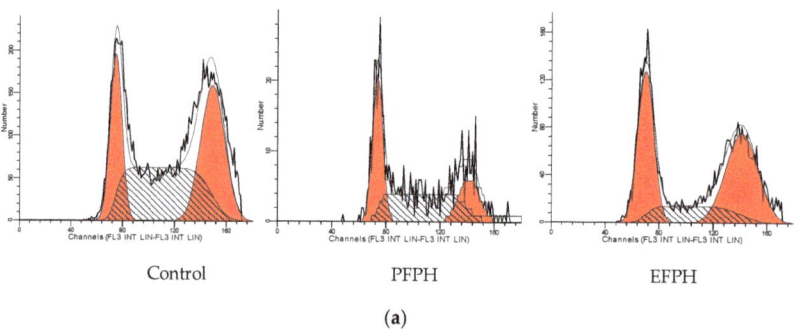

(**a**)

Figure 4. *Cont.*

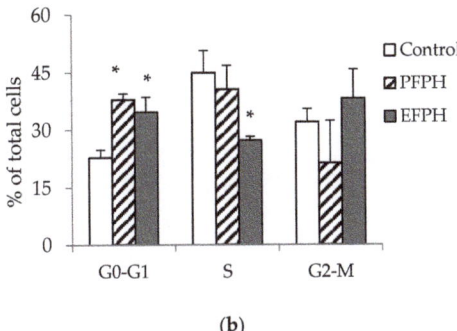

(b)

Figure 4. Cell cycle repartition of undifferentiated Caco2/TC7 treated (24 h) or not with fenugreek proteins hydrolysates. (**a**): a representative cells cycle histogram. (**b**): G1, S, and G2 phases percentage distribution. Data are presented as mean ± SD. The experiment was done in duplicate. Superscripted (*) means are significantly different ($p \leq 0.05$) when compared to their respective control. Control: Untreated cells. PFPH: Purafect fenugreek proteins hydrolysate. EFPH: Esperase fenugreek proteins hydrolysate. The hydrolysates were used at a final concentration of 1 mg/mL.

3.6. Analysis of Mitochondrial Membrane Potential Change, Cytochrome C Release, and Caspase-3 Activation

Since FPH treatment (at 1 mg/mL) caused apoptosis in undifferentiated cells, we hypothesized that it could induce mitochondrial permeabilization and cytochrome C release in Caco-2/TC7 cells. Compared to non-treated cells, the number of cells exhibiting a changed in the mitochondrial membrane potential (ΔΨm) increased by 70% in PFPH-treated and EFPH-treated cells. The results also showed that, in treated cells, mitochondria cytochrome C contents decreased significantly compared to the untreated cells.

The release of cytochrome C can lead to the activation of caspase 3, which is an executor of the apoptosis pathway. The activated caspase-3 concentrations were significantly increased by 24-fold and 13-fold, respectively, in PFPH-treated and EFPH-treated cells when compared to the control (Table 2).

Table 2. Percentage of Caco2/CT7 cells with a positive mitochondrial membrane potential. Cells with mitochondrial cytochrome C and active caspase-3, quantified by flow cytometry in response to fenugreek proteins hydrolysates treatment (24 h).

Number of Cells (/100 Cells)	Control	PFPH	EFPH
Cells with positive MMP	28.7 ± 10.9	69.2 ± 11.4 *	70.4 ± 4.1 *
Cells with mitochondrial cytochrome C	90.7 ± 1.6	71.3 ± 1.2 *	61.0 ± 9.8 *
Cells with active caspase-3	1.4 ± 0.0	33.3 ± 4.3 *	18.5 ± 3.8 *

Data are presented as mean ± SD. The experiment was done in duplicate. Superscripted (*) means within a row are significantly different ($p \leq 0.05$) when compared to their respective control. Control: untreated cells. PFPH: Purafect fenugreek proteins hydrolysate. EFPH: Esperase fenugreek proteins hydrolysate. The hydrolysates were used at a final concentration of 1 mg/mL. MMP: mitochondrial membrane potential.

3.7. Antioxidant Activity of FPH in Caco2 Cells

Oxidative stress is a characteristic state of many cancers, and it is implicated in cancer development and progression. The intracellular ROS levels, in the presence of high concentration of H_2O_2 (20 mM), decreased by 35% in cells incubated with 1 mg/mL of EFPH when compared to the control. PFPH cells did not exhibit any modification. However, in the presence of low concentrations of H_2O_2 (0.5 mM), both treated cells exhibited better antioxidant activity vs. untreated cells. The inhibition reached 39% and 33%, respectively, in EFPH and PFPH treated cells (final concentration 1 mg/mL) (Figure 5).

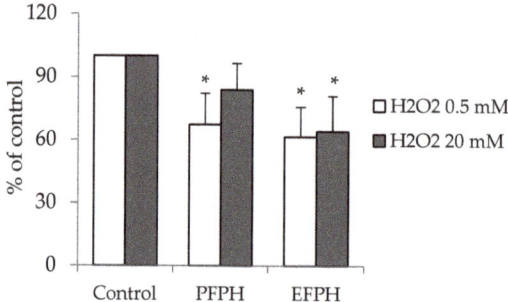

Figure 5. Relative reactive oxygen species levels in undifferentiated Caco2/TC7 cells treated (24 h) or not with fenugreek proteins hydrolysates. Data are presented as mean ± SD. The experiment was done in triplicate (each performed with six determinations). Superscripted (*) means are significantly different ($p \leq 0.05$) compared to their respective control. Control: Untreated cells. PFPH: Purafect fenugreek proteins hydrolysate. EFPH: Esperase fenugreek proteins hydrolysate. The hydrolysates were used at a final concentration of 1 mg/mL.

3.8. Thioredoxin Reductase 1 Activity

Since FPH induced a decrease in intracellular ROS levels in Caco2 TC7, we proposed to study whether this decrease is caused by up-regulated enzyme activities or not. Hence, we proposed to measure the activity of one of the most important cellular antioxidant enzyme: thioredoxin reductase. TrxR1 activity was lower in PFPH (−41%) and EFPH (−12%) treated cells vs. control cells (Figure 6).

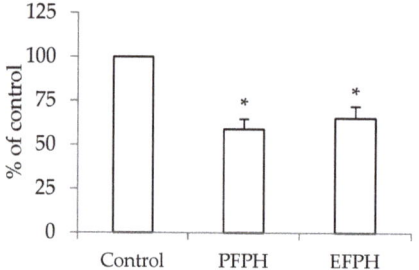

Figure 6. Relative thioredoxin reductase activity in undifferentiated Caco2/TC7 cells treated (24 h) or not with fenugreek proteins hydrolysates. Data are presented as mean ± SD. The experiment was done in duplicate (each performed with six determinations). Superscripted (*) means are significantly different ($p \leq 0.05$) compared to their respective control. Control: Untreated cells. PFPH: Purafect fenugreek proteins hydrolysate. EFPH: Esperase fenugreek proteins hydrolysate. The hydrolysates were used at a final concentration of 1 mg/mL.

4. Discussion

The anticancer property of natural products became one of the most studied topics. In recent years, the studies on plant proteins and peptides have increased, which is motivated by their huge diversity, affordability, and lack of side effects. Legumes are the plant source for which most peptides with anticancer properties are reported [25]. Fenugreek is a legume-rich protein, which could be a potential source of biological active peptides.

The hydrolysis curve of fenugreek proteins was typical of many protein hydrolysates obtained by Sbroggio et al. [26] with okara hydrolysates. The differences in hydrolysis shape and DH values were probably due to the difference in enzyme specificity. On the other hand, the DH could inform the peptides' mean size [17]. Hence, EFPH with DH = 19% could contain smaller peptides than PFPH.

Our results suggest that protein contents of the hydrolysates are important. These findings were in line with Pownall et al. [27] and Mundi and Aluko [28]. The high protein content could be a result of the solubilisation of peptides during hydrolysis. It is speculated that the hydrolysis, especially when alkaline enzymes are used, enhance the solubilisation of proteins and removes insoluble undigested non-protein substances [29].

Even if the amino acids profile showed that aromatic and hydrophobic amino acids did not differ between the hydrolysates, these values are higher than those found by other authors [27,28,30].

After analyzing the FPH composition, we tried to check if FPH possesses an anti-proliferative property in cells. The treatment of undifferentiated Caco2/TC7 cells with FPH exhibited a decrease in their viability, especially with PFPH that was correlated with incubation time. These results are in line with works reporting an anti-proliferative property of peptides and hydrolysates from soy [14], corn [12,31], chickpeas [13], and rice [11] on different cell models. Vglycin, a peptide isolated from soy, inhibited the proliferation of three types of colon cancer cells [14]. Ortiz-Martinez et al. [12] also found that corn peptide fractions decreased HepG2 cells growth by more than 50%. Li et al. [31] noticed that this antiproliferative property was time-dependent. In addition, a pentapeptide from rice brane showed 84% of viability inhibition on colon cancer cells [11].

Caco2/TC7 differentiated cell viability was not influenced by the FPH treatment. Same observation, in normal and cancer oral cells, was also reported by Kumar et al. [32] with a chickpea protein fraction. Ours findings could indicate a possible selective antiproliferative effect of PFPH and EFPH on cancer cells without affecting the normal cells.

One of the possible ways by which FPH inhibited the cancerous cells could be the same mechanism seen with antimicrobial peptides when they act as anticancer agents as well. It is believed that normal cells exhibit an asymmetric composition between the internal and the external layers of their membrane. In cancer cells, this asymmetry is affected principally by the externalization of phosphatidylserine (normally confined to the inner leaflet), and the external layer of cancer cell membranes that will carry a net negative charge. This permits an electrostatic interaction between cationic anticancer peptides and anionic cell membrane components [33].

It seemed interesting to investigate if FPH could induce the anti-proliferative effect by apoptosis. The study with EPFH and PEPH was carried out in undifferentiated cells by flow cytometry analysis after staining with annexin V/propidium iodide. Since cells in early apoptosis express phosphatidylserine in their outer side of the cytoplasmic membrane, they will be stained by Annexin-V labelled with FITC (early apoptosis). However, membranes of dead and damaged cells are permeable to propidium iodide (necrosis) and are also stained with annexin-V (late apoptosis) [20]. It seemed that PFPH and EFPH set off an early apoptosis mechanism, rather than necrosis, in undifferentiated cells. In this way, Ortiz-Martinez et al. [12] showed that HepG2 cells treated with corn peptide fractions have a four-fold increase of both early and late apoptotic events, compared to the untreated cells. Similarly, Li et al. [31] remarked that corn peptides generated apoptosis in 11% to 55% of HepG2 cells in a dose-dependent manner. Moreover, Vglycin treatment for 24 hours caused a significant increase of apoptosis in different colon cancer cells [14].

With apoptotic and no necrotic property, PFPH and EFPH seem to have a beneficial effect against cancer cells. Additionally, in this work, it was found that both FPH stimulated the early apoptosis, which is favored to the late one since it allows early recognition of dead cells [34].

By analyzing the effect of fenugreek proteins hydrolysates on cell cycles, it is suggested that both hydrolysates caused mainly a cell cycle arrest in the G1 phase, which has also been shown in other studies. In this way, Gao et al. [14] deduced that soy Vglycin induced a G1-phase arrest of colorectal cancer cells. Li et al. [31] indicated that corn peptides could induce HepG2 cell cycle arrest in the S phase. The hemagglutinin caused cell cycle arrest in the G2/M phase, as demonstrated by Lam and Ng [35].

Many studies have shown associations between some minerals and carcinogenesis. Mg^{2+} ions are enzyme cofactors involved in DNA repair mechanisms that maintain genomic stability and fidelity.

Magnesium deficiency may also be associated with inflammation and increased levels of free radicals where both inflammatory mediators and free radicals arising could cause oxidative DNA damage and, therefore, tumor formation [36]. There is also evidence that dietary Ca^{2+} loading reduces colon cell proliferation and carcinogenesis [37]. The presence of these two elements in FPH could also be responsible for their anti-proliferative properties. According to Kasprzak [38], the molecular mechanisms involved in the effects of such minerals are likely to include binding at chromatin (e.g., DNA, histones, transcription factors, DNA repair enzymes) and other regulatory molecules in the target cells.

Apoptosis manifests in two major execution programs downstream of the death signal: the caspase pathway and organelle dysfunction of which mitochondrial dysfunction is best characterized [39]. To see if the apoptotic action of FPH was led by these mechanisms, we analyzed, by flow cytometry, the change in mitochondrial membrane potential, cytochrome C in the mitochondria, and the cytoplasmic level of the active form of caspase-3.

Mitochondria play a pivotal role in life and death of the cell since it produces the majority of energy required for survival and regulates the intrinsic pathway of apoptosis. The involvement of mitochondria in cell death is generally measured by following mitochondrial membrane depolarisation [21]. FPH-treated cells showed a higher change in mitochondrial membrane potential. Disruption of the mitochondrial outer membrane permeability leads to the release of proteins confined in the intermembrane space into the cytosol. These proteins include the apoptogenic factors, such as cytochrome C, which plays a crucial role in activating the mitochondrial-dependent death in the cytosol [32].

With the aim to discover whether PFPH and EFPH were able to induce mitochondrial permeabilization and cytochrome C release, we used flow cytometry to analyze the mitochondrial cytochrome C in treated and untreated cells. The results showed that, in treated cells, there was a greater cytochrome C release to cytoplasm than in the untreated cells. Once cytochrome C is released to the cytoplasm, it could activate different proteins of the intrinsic apoptosis pathway such as the effector caspase-3 [40]. Once caspase-3 is activated, it induces the proteolytic cleavage of a large number of essential proteins for apoptosis [41]. Moreover, caspase-3 is a prototypical executioner caspase that, upon activation by extrinsic and intrinsic pathways, cleaves a wide panel of several substrates that are vital for the cell, which precipitates regulated cell death. It is also responsible for modulating some enzyme activities like those required for the exposure of phosphatidylserine (PS) on the outer leaflet of dying cells [42].

Activated caspase-3 concentrations were increased in PFPH and EFPH treated cells. Gao et al. [14] also confirmed that Vglycin promoted caspase-3 activity in colon cancer cells. The same results were obtained by Li et al. [31], with corn peptides on HepG2 cells.

Higher levels of ROS are generated through the increased metabolic activity of cancer cells including enhanced signalling pathways or mitochondrial dysfunction [43]. The ROS levels in Caco2 cells were determined based on the reaction between ROS and DCFH-DA [13].

In our assays, Fenugreek protein hydrolysates showed antioxidant power. EFPH showed a better ROS inhibitory property even though PFPH was not effective with high levels of ROS. In this way, when HepG2 cells were incubated with 100 µM of peroxide, the corn peptides fraction could not decrease the peroxide-ROS generation [12]. In contrast, Xue et al. [13] showed that chickpea peptides decreased the ROS in MCF-7 and MDA-MB-231 cells. Torres-Fuentes et al. [44] and Zhang et al. [45] reported an antioxidant property of chickpea and soy proteins hydrolysates in Caco2 cells.

A study undertaken by Chi et al. [46] confirmed that peptides with a smaller molecular size, the presence of hydrophobic and aromatic amino acid residues, and the amino acid sequences were the key factors that determine the antioxidant activities of hydrolysates and peptides. Fenugreek protein hydrolysates are rich in hydrophobic and aromatic amino acids [16]. Moreover, as the cells incubated with protein hydrolysates were washed, some peptides may be lost since they are not able to cross the cell membrane due to their big size and polarity. However, small hydrophobic peptides are able to cross this membrane and stay in the cytoplasm, where they may exert their antioxidant property [44]. EFPH in which DH is higher than that of PFPH (19% vs. 9%, respectively) has higher ROS inhibition activity.

Because of the increase in ROS production in tumor cells, it is concerted that many antioxidants and redox control systems are up regulated. One of the most important cellular redox systems is the thioredoxin (Trx) system, comprised of Trx, TrxR1, and NADPH [43]. However, in our study, TrxR1 activity was found to be lower in both FPH-treated cells. Since the antioxidant enzymes activities are up-regulated following an increase of ROS production in cancer cells, we supposed that the decrease in TrxR1 could result from the low levels of ROS in treated cells (low stimuli of Trx and TrxR1 expression), and not a direct inhibition of the enzyme by FPH.

5. Conclusions

This data demonstrated that Purafect and Esperase fenugreek protein hydrolysates possess a selective antiproliferative property on colorectal cancer cells, by enhancing intrinsic apoptosis rather than necrosis on Caco2/TC7, and by blocking the cell cycle in the G1 phase. Both hydrolysates induced alteration in mitochondrial membrane permeability, induced cytochrome C release to the cytoplasm, and induced caspase-3 activation. Furthermore, these two hydrolysates exerted an antioxidant activity by inhibiting the reactive oxygen species. In light of these results, fenugreek proteins hydrolysates could represent a promising nutraceutical in the treatment and progression of colon cancer. Future studies will be interesting to perform in order to see if these fenugreek protein hydrolysates are also effective in other types of cancer cells and in vivo animal models.

Author Contributions: A.B. and M.J.R.-Y. were responsible for the overall direction of the research. A.A. performed the experiments, analysis of data, and wrote the manuscript. S.G. performed and supervised the experiments. S.B. and J.Q. performed a part of the experiments. J.O. contributed with materials and analysis results. M.N. supervised the hydrolysis processes. A.A. performed cell culture experiments supervised by M.J.R.-Y. A.B. and M.J.R.-Y. analyzed the obtained data. All authors have given approval to the final version of the manuscript.

Funding: The Spanish Ministry of Economy and Innovation under Grant (SAF 2016-75441-R); Aragón Regional Government (A-32 B16-R17), CIBERobn under Grant (CB06/03/1012) of the Instituto de Salud Carlos III, European Grant Interreg/SUDOE (Redvalue, SOE1/PI/E0123), and the Algerian Ministry of Higher Education, Scientific Research and the Tunisian Ministry of Higher Education and Scientific Research (Joint Research Project Algeria/Tunisia 137/2012) supported this research.

Acknowledgments: Authors thank Centro de Investigation Biomédica de Aragón (Spain) for technical assistance (http://www.iacs.aragon.es). Authors also thank the Regional Laboratory of Quality Control and Fraud Repression of Oran (Algeria) for their help with amino acid composition analysis of fenugreek protein hydrolysates.

Conflicts of Interest: The authors declare no conflict of interest.

References

1. Meghwal, M.; Goswami, T.K. A Review on the functional properties, nutritional content, medicinal utilization and potential application of fenugreek. *J. Food Process. Technol.* **2012**, *3*, 181–190. [CrossRef]
2. Khorshidian, N.; Asli, M.Y.; Arab, M.; Mirzaie, A.A.; Mortazavian, A.M. Fenugreek: Potential applications as a functional food and nutraceutical. *Nutr. Food Sci. Res.* **2016**, *3*, 5–16. [CrossRef]
3. Belguith-Hadriche, O.; Bouaziz, M.; Jamoussia, K.; Simmonds, M.; El Feki, A.; Makni-Ayedi, F. Comparative study on hypocholesterolemic and antioxidant activities of various extracts of fenugreek seeds. *Food Chem.* **2013**, *138*, 1448–1453. [CrossRef] [PubMed]
4. Subhashini, N.; Thangathirupathi, A.; Lavanya, N. Antioxidant activity of *Trigonella foenum graecum* using various in vitro and ex vivo models. *J. Pharm. Pharm. Sci.* **2011**, *3*, 96–102.
5. Madhava Naidu, M.; Shyamala, B.N.; Pura Naik, J.; Sulochanamma, G.; Srinivas, P. Chemical composition and antioxidant activity of the husk and endosperm of fenugreek seeds. *Food Sci. Technol.* **2011**, *44*, 451–456. [CrossRef]
6. Roy, F.; Boye, J.I.; Simpson, B.K. Bioactive proteins and peptides in pulse crops: Pea, chickpea and lentil. *Food Res. Int.* **2010**, *43*, 432–442. [CrossRef]

7. Girón-Calle, J.; Vioque, J.; Pedroche, J.; Alaiz, M.; Yust, M.M.; Megías, C.; Millán, F. Chickpea protein hydrolysate as a substitute for serum in cell culture. *Cytotechnology* **2008**, *57*, 263–272. [CrossRef] [PubMed]
8. Zambrowicz, A.; Timmer, M.; Polanowski, A.; Lubec, G.; Trziszka, T. Manufacturing of peptides exhibiting biological activity. *Amino Acids* **2013**, *44*, 315–320. [CrossRef] [PubMed]
9. León-Espinosa, E.B.; Sánchez-Chino, X.; Garduño-Siciliano, L.; Álvarez-González, R.I.; Dávila-Ortiz, G.; Madrigal-Bujaidar, E.; Téllez-Medina, D.I.; Jiménez-Martínez, C. Hypocholesterolemic and anticarcinogenic effect of *Vicia faba* protein hydrolyzates. *Nutr. Cancer* **2016**, *68*, 856–864. [CrossRef]
10. Luna Vital, D.A.; González de Mejía, E.; Dia, V.P.; Loarca-Piña, G. Peptides in common bean fractions inhibit human colorectal cancer cells. *Food Chem.* **2014**, *157*, 347–355. [CrossRef]
11. Kannan, A.; Hettiarachchy, N.S.; Lay, J.O.; Liyanage, R. Human cancer cell proliferation inhibition by a pentapeptide isolated and characterized from rice bran. *Peptides* **2010**, *31*, 1629–1634. [CrossRef] [PubMed]
12. Ortiz-Martinez, M.; de Mejia, E.G.; García-Lara, S.; Aguilar, O.; Lopez-Castillo, L.M.; Otero-Pappatheodorou, J.T. Antiproliferative effect of peptide fractions isolated from a quality protein maize, a white hybrid maize, and their derived peptides on hepatocarcinoma human HepG2 cells. *J. Funct. Foods* **2017**, *34*, 36–48. [CrossRef]
13. Xue, Z.; Wen, H.; Zhai, L.; Yu, Y.; Li, Y.; Yu, W.; Cheng, A.; Wang, C.; Kou, X. Antioxidant activity and anti-proliferative effect of a bioactive peptide from chickpea (*Cicer arietinum* L.). *Food Res. Int.* **2015**, *77*, 75–81. [CrossRef]
14. Gao, C.; Sun, R.; Xie, Y.R.; Jiang, A.L.; Lin, M.; Li, M.; Chen, Z.W.; Zhang, P.; Jin, H.; Feng, J.P. The soy-derived peptide Vglycin inhibits the growth of colon cancer cells in vitro and in vivo. *Exp. Boil. Med.* **2017**, *242*, 1034–1043. [CrossRef] [PubMed]
15. Boye, J.I.; Aksay, S.; Roufik, S.; Ribéreau, S.; Mondor, M.; Farnworth, E.; Rajamohamed, S.H. Comparison of the functional properties of pea, chickpea and lentil protein concentrates processed using ultrafiltration and isoelectric precipitation techniques. *Food Res. Int.* **2010**, *43*, 537–546. [CrossRef]
16. Allaoui, A.; Barranquero, C.; Yahia, S.; Herrera-Marcos, L.V.; Benomar, S.; Jridi, M.; Navarro-Ferrando, M.Á.; Rodriguez-Yoldi, M.J.; Nasri, M.; Osada, J.; et al. Fenugreek proteins and their hydrolysates prevent hypercholesterolemia and enhance the HDL antioxidant properties in rats. *Nutr. Food Sci.* **2018**, *48*, 973–989. [CrossRef]
17. Adler-Nissen, J. A review of food hydrolysis specific areas. In *Enzymic Hydrolysis of Food Proteins*; Adler-Nissen, J., Ed.; Elsevier Applied Science Publishers: Copenhagen, Dermark, 1986; pp. 57–109.
18. Horwitz, W. Food composition; additives; natural contaminants. In *Official Methods of Analysis of AOAC International*, 17th ed.; Horwitz, W., AOAC International, Eds.; AOAC International: Gaithersburg, MD, USA, 2000; Volume 2.
19. Yust, M.M.; Pedroche, J.; Girón-Calle, J.; Vioque, J.; Millán, F.; Alaiz, M. Determination of tryptophan by high-performance liquid chromatography of alkaline hydrolysates with spectrophotometric detection. *Food Chem.* **2004**, *85*, 317–320. [CrossRef]
20. Sánchez-de-Diego, C.; Mármol, I.; Pérez, R.; Gascón, S.; Rodriguez-Yoldi, M.J.; Cerrada, E. The anticancer effect related to disturbances in redox balance on Caco-2 cells caused by an alkynyl gold(I) complex. *J. Inorg. Biochem.* **2017**, *166*, 108–121. [CrossRef] [PubMed]
21. Christensen, M.E.; Jansen, E.S.; Sanchez, W.; Waterhouse, N.J. Flow cytometry based assays for the measurement of apoptosis-associated mitochondrial membrane depolarisation and cytochrome c release. *Methods* **2013**, *61*, 138–145. [CrossRef] [PubMed]
22. Ruiz-Leal, M.; George, S. An in vitro procedure for evaluation of early stage oxidative stress in an established fish cell line applied to investigation of PHAH and pesticide toxicity. *Mar. Environ. Res.* **2004**, *58*, 631–635. [CrossRef] [PubMed]
23. Bradford, M.M. A rapid and sensitive method for the quantitation of microgram quantities of protein utilizing the principle of protein-dye binding. *Anal. Biochem.* **1976**, *72*, 248–254. [CrossRef]
24. Fink, S.L.; Cookson, B.T. Apoptosis, pyroptosis, and necrosis: Mechanistic description of dead and dying eukaryotic cells. *Infect. Immun.* **2005**, *73*, 1907–1916. [CrossRef]
25. Ortiz-Martinez, M.; Winkler, R.; García-Lara, S. Preventive and therapeutic potential of peptides from cereals against cancer. *J. Proteom.* **2014**, *111*, 165–183. [CrossRef]
26. Sbroggio, M.F.; Montilha, M.S.; de Figueiredo, V.R.G.; Georgetti, S.R.; Kurozawa, L.E. Influence of the degree of hydrolysis and type of enzyme on antioxidant activity of okara protein hydrolysates. *Food Sci. Technol.* **2016**, *36*, 375–381. [CrossRef]

27. Pownall, T.L.; Udenigwe, C.C.; Aluko, R.E. Amino acid composition and antioxidant properties of pea seed (*Pisum sativum* L.) enzymatic protein hydrolysate fractions. *J. Agric. Food Chem.* **2010**, *58*, 4712–4718. [CrossRef]
28. Mundi, S.; Aluko, R.E. Inhibitory properties of kidney bean protein hydrolysate and its membrane fractions against renin, angiotensin converting enzyme, and free radicals. *Austin J. Nutr. Food Sci.* **2014**, *2*, 1008.
29. Kristinsson, H.G.; Rasco, B.A. Fish protein hydrolysates: Production, biochemical, and functional properties. *Crit. Rev. Food Sci. Nutr.* **2000**, *40*, 43–81. [CrossRef]
30. Yust, M.d.M.; Millán-Linares, M.d.C.; Alcaide-Hidalgo, J.M.; Millán, F.; Pedroche, J. Hypocholesterolaemic and antioxidant activities of chickpea (Cicer arietinum L.) protein hydrolysates. *J. Sci. Food Agric.* **2012**, *92*, 1994–2001. [CrossRef]
31. Li, J.T.; Zhang, J.L.; He, H.; Ma, Z.L.; Nie, Z.K.; Wang, Z.Z.; Xu, X.G. Apoptosis in human hepatoma HepG2 cells induced by corn peptides and its anti-tumor efficacy in H22 tumor bearing mice. *Food Chem. Toxicol.* **2013**, *51*, 297–305. [CrossRef]
32. Kumar, S.; Kapoor, V.; Gill, K.; Singh, K.; Xess, I.; Das, S.N.; Dey, S. Antifungal and antiproliferative protein from *Cicer arietinum*: A bioactive compound against emerging pathogens. *BioMed Res. Int.* **2014**, *2014*, 387203. [CrossRef]
33. Hoskin, D.W.; Ramamoorthy, A. Studies on anticancer activities of antimicrobial peptides. *Biochim. Biophys. Acta Biomembr.* **2008**, *1778*, 357–375. [CrossRef]
34. Pistritto, G.; Trisciuoglio, D.; Ceci, C.; Garufi, A.; D'Orazi, G. Apoptosis as anticancer mechanism: Function and dysfunction of its modulators and targeted therapeutic strategies. *Aging* **2016**, *8*, 603–619. [CrossRef]
35. Lam, S.K.; Ng, T.B. Apoptosis of human breast cancer cells induced by hemagglutinin from *Phaseolus vulgaris* cv. Legumi secchi. *Food Chem.* **2011**, *126*, 595–602. [CrossRef]
36. Blaszczyk, U.; Duda-Chodak, A. Magnesium: Its role in nutrition and carcinogenesis. *Roczniki Państwowego Zakładu Hig.* **2013**, *64*, 165–171.
37. Whitfield, J. Calcium, calcium-sensing receptor and colon cancer. *Cancer Lett.* **2009**, *275*, 9–16. [CrossRef]
38. Kasprzak, K.S. Effects of calcium, magnesium, zinc, and iron on nickel carcinogenesis: Inhibition versus enhancement. In *Cytotoxic, Mutagenic and Carcinogenic Potential of Heavy Metals Related to Human Environment*; Hadjiliadis, N.D., Ed.; Springer: Dordrecht, The Netherlands, 1997; Volume 26, pp. 93–106.
39. Zhang, F.L.; Wang, P.; Liu, Y.H.; Liu, L.B.; Liu, X.B.; Li, Z.; Xue, Y.X. Topoisomerase I inhibitors, shikonin and topotecan, inhibit growth and induce apoptosis of glioma cells and glioma stem cells. *PLoS ONE* **2013**, *8*, e81815. [CrossRef]
40. Riedl, S.J.; Shi, Y. Molecular mechanisms of caspase regulation during apoptosis. *Nat. Rev. Mol. Cell Boil.* **2004**, *5*, 897–907. [CrossRef]
41. Slee, E.A.; Adrain, C.; Martin, S.J. Executioner caspase-3, -6, and -7 perform distinct, non-redundant roles during the demolition phase of apoptosis. *J. Boil. Chem.* **2001**, *276*, 7320–7326. [CrossRef]
42. Galluzzi, L.; López-Soto, A.; Kumar, S.; Kroemer, G. Caspases connect cell-death signaling to organismal homeostasis. *Immunity* **2016**, *44*, 221–231. [CrossRef]
43. Bhatia, M.; McGrath, K.L.; Di Trapani, G.; Charoentong, P.; Shah, F.; King, M.M.; Clarke, F.M.; Tonissen, K.F. The thioredoxin system in breast cancer cell invasion and migration. *Redox Biol.* **2016**, *8*, 68–78. [CrossRef]
44. Torres-Fuentes, C.; del María, C.M.; Isidra, R.; Manuel, A.; Javier, V. Identification and characterization of antioxidant peptides from chickpea protein hydrolysates. *Food Chem.* **2015**, *180*, 194–202. [CrossRef] [PubMed]
45. Zhang, Q.; Tong, X.; Sui, X.; Wang, Z.; Qi, B.; Li, Y.; Jiang, L. Antioxidant activity and protective effects of Alcalase-hydrolyzed soybean hydrolysate in human intestinal epithelial Caco-2 cells. *Food Res. Int.* **2018**, *111*, 256–264. [CrossRef] [PubMed]
46. Chi, C.F.; Hu, F.Y.; Wang, B.; Li, Z.R.; Luo, H.Y. Influence of amino acid compositions and peptide profiles on antioxidant capacities of two protein hydrolysates from skipjack tuna (*Katsuwonus pelamis*) dark muscle. *Mar. Drugs* **2015**, *13*, 2580–2601. [CrossRef] [PubMed]

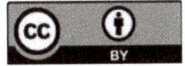

© 2019 by the authors. Licensee MDPI, Basel, Switzerland. This article is an open access article distributed under the terms and conditions of the Creative Commons Attribution (CC BY) license (http://creativecommons.org/licenses/by/4.0/).

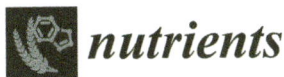

Article

Bioavailability and Sustained Plasma Concentrations of CoQ10 in Healthy Volunteers by a Novel Oral Timed-Release Preparation

Alessio Martucci [1,*], Delia Reurean-Pintilei [2] and Anamaria Manole [2]

[1] Ophthalmology Unit, Department of Experimental Medicine, University of Rome Tor Vergata, 00133 Rome, Italy
[2] Department of Diabetes, Nutrition and Metabolic Diseases, Consultmed Medical Center, 700547 Iasi, Romania; drdeliapintilei@gmail.com (D.R.-P.); anamaria_manole10@yahoo.com (A.M.)
* Correspondence: alessio.martucci@live.it; Tel.: +39-339-3607125

Received: 8 February 2019; Accepted: 25 February 2019; Published: 28 February 2019

Abstract: Coenzyme Q10 (CoQ10) is a natural compound with potent antioxidant properties. Its provision through diet does not always allow adequate levels in the human body, and supplementation is often necessary. This bioavailability study intended to explore the plasma concentration levels of a novel CoQ10 oral preparation (COQUN®, Coenzyme Q10 Miniactives Retard 100 mg capsules) mimicking assumption on a regular basis. Twenty-four healthy adults tested a single dose of CoQ10 100 mg in one day to assess bioavailability. After a one week wash-out period, they were randomly assigned (1:1) to continuous administration for four weeks: Group A (n = 12) 100 mg once a day (OD); and Group B (n = 12) 100 mg twice a day (BID). During the single dose phase, C_{max} was observed at 4 h, and the mean values of AUC_t and T_{max} were 8754 µg/mL·h and 4.29 h, respectively. The multiple dose phase showed increasing plasma levels up to 7 days after the start of administration, and sustained high concentrations during the all administration period. No relevant adverse events were reported. These results show that Miniactives® technology can release CoQ10 to allow high constant blood concentrations without a sharp decrease. This may be the first step of evidence for a potential new antioxidative treatment in human chronic diseases deserving high CoQ10 levels.

Keywords: coenzyme Q10 (CoQ10); bioavailability; intestinal absorption; neuroprotection

1. Introduction

Coenzyme Q (CoQ), or ubiquinone, is a lipophilic, vitamin-like compound with exceptional biochemical properties, synthetized by prokaryotic and eukaryotic cells. CoQ10 is the lipid form produced by the human body, where Q10 indicates the number of isoprenoid subunits in the lipid tail attached to the quinone ring of the coenzyme [1]. CoQ10 can also be obtained from diet, mainly from meat, poultry, and fish, and in much less quantity from fruits, vegetables, cereals, and dairy products [2].

CoQ10 is a physiological component of the human mitochondrial electron transport chain, but its half-reduced and fully reduced forms allow CoQ10 to function as an antioxidant [3]. By virtue of its proven ability to change in a reduced form, CoQ10 has been shown to induce protective effects against lipid peroxidation in a ubiquitous manner in the human body, with special regard in organs and systems' tissues such as cardiovascular, nervous, and metabolic. Over the years, an ever-increasing number of diseases have been associated with mitochondrial dysfunction and oxidative stress.

Significant reduction of cardiovascular mortality, decrease of NT-proBNP blood levels, and improvement of cardiac function has been reported among elderly subjects after five years of combined supplementation of CoQ10 and selenium [4]. The long-term (two years) beneficial effects of CoQ10 supplementation on symptoms improvement and reduction of major adverse cardiovascular events (i.e., cardiovascular and all-cause mortality, and incidence of hospital stay) have also been assessed in patients with chronic heart failure (CHF) [5].

Most of clinical evidence sustains that the glycemic control among individuals with type-2 diabetes mellitus (T2DM) can be improved by CoQ10 supplementation. CoQ10 administration at different daily doses (ranging 60–200 mg/day) and for different periods (eight weeks–six months) can determine increased insulin synthesis and secretion by pancreatic β cells, significant decrease of glycated hemoglobin level, and kidney protection against diabetic nephropathy. However, despite other studies reported, marginal or not significant clinical benefits of CoQ10 in glycemic control, it is now clear that mitochondrial dysfunction is secondary to oxidative stress that, most of time, can be successfully treated by adequate supplementation of CoQ10 in T2DM patients [6].

Promising results have been reported in the treatment of neurodegenerative disorders such as Parkinson disease (PD) and Huntington's disease (HD) with CoQ10. As these are chronic, progressive and non-regressive disorders, the goal of any treatment is to cause a slowing of the disease progression, since improvement and cure are not currently possible. That is why only the highest dose of CoQ10 slowed the functional decline of PD among the three dosages tested of 300, 600 or 1200 mg/day in subjects with the early stage of disease, and not yet requiring treatment for their disability [7]. Conversely, a chronic supplementation with 600 mg/day of CoQ10 did not produce any significant slowing in functional decline in patients with early HD [8].

An interesting field of CoQ10 neuroprotective research against reactive oxygen species focused on promoting mitochondrial functions and retinal ganglion cell (RGC) survival in ischemic retina under conditions of intraocular pressure elevation (glaucoma). Glaucoma is a progressive neurodegenerative disease of RGCs associated with axon degeneration in the optic nerve. During recent years, researchers became aware that traditional strategies of lowering intraocular pressure were often unsatisfactory to prevent progressive vision loss. Thus, the current trend of using neuroprotective strategies for the treatment of glaucoma is sustained by the growing evidence that glaucomatous neurodegeneration is analogous to other neurodegenerative disorders in the central nervous system [9,10]. Consistently, CoQ10 showed to significantly block activation of astroglial and microglial cells and apoptosis in ischemic retina in addition to protecting RGCs in animals [11], and to improving inner retinal function and visual cortical responses in humans [12].

Combination of appropriate formulations and dosages is a key factor to allow optimal absorption and achieve adequate blood concentration of CoQ10 to exert the expected clinical benefits. The importance of achieving an optimal CoQ10 bioavailability is justified by the possible risk of exposing treated subjects to a lack of efficacy in the case of underdosing. On the other hand, too high concentrations can induce toxic effects or increase the rate of adverse events. The clinical evidence suggests that CoQ10 bioavailability can greatly vary not only after different daily doses or dose strategies, but especially belongs to formulations used [13–17]. For instance, it was shown that an emulsified CoQ10 preparation can increase the intestinal absorption, being more permeable across cellular membranes and allowing a relatively low-dose administration [13]. Despite many other factors can influence plasma CoQ10 concentrations, such as serum lipoproteins levels, i.e., cholesterol, High Density Lipoprotein (HDL), and Low Density Lipoprotein (LDL)/Very Low Density Lipoprotein (VLDL) are carriers of CoQ10 in the circulation–diet, daily motion, time of day, human race, age, and gender, and some authors indicated that dissolution is probably the more important factor rather than release and absorption rate [14,15]. Lu and coworkers [14] administered the same single daily dose of CoQ10 (50 mg/day) to a small group of healthy Asian volunteers using two different formulations. The baseline plasma values, and after day 15 of treatment of CoQ10, were similar to the respective values observed in European subjects, but CoQ10 bioavailability was higher in subjects treated with the sustained release tablets compared to regular tablets. Another colloidal CoQ10 preparation achieved astonishingly higher plasma levels compared to the same doses (120 mg/day) of other more conventional formulations [15].

Good intestinal absorption and the achievement of high peak plasma concentrations should not be the only objectives of an oral formulation of CoQ10. It is important to ensure that plasma concentrations remain constant over time, avoiding excessive fluctuations in bioavailability, especially if once-daily dosing is clinically required. The authors of Reference [16] showed that the plasma concentrations of the five formulations used, following a high peak reached after 2–4 h, returned to the same initial levels after 12 h from the administration. Moreover, the dosing strategy is another major important cause to reach adequately high plasma CoQ10 concentrations. A divided dose administration (e.g., BID) improves absorption by almost double, as compared with the same amount of active substance taken in one single dose [16]. The dose fractionation strategy should be carefully considered when high doses have to be administered or when high bioavailability should be achieved with a relatively small daily dose.

The aim of this bioavailability study was to determine the single (100 mg) and multidose dose (100 mg/day vs. 2 × 100 mg/day) pharmacokinetics (i.e., dosage effect and dosage strategy) of a novel CoQ10 preparation based on neutral micro-particles dissolution technology (i.e., formulation effects), a prolonged-release capsule administered orally to healthy volunteers. Bioavailability intended to explore the plasma concentration levels which might assure antioxidant effect if the novel CoQ10 preparation were taken on a regular basis.

2. Materials and Methods

2.1. Study Design

This was a single-center (Consultmed Iasi, IASI, Romania), open-label, single and multi-dose bioavailability study of an innovative CoQ10 oral formulation in 24 healthy adults. All subjects tested a single dose of 100 mg of CoQ10 in 1 day to assess bioavailability. Then, the subjects followed a 1 week wash-out period after which they were randomly assigned (1:1) to a 4 week period of continuous administration of CoQ10: Group A of 12 subjects with intake of 100 mg OD (after dinner); Group B of 12 subjects with intake of 100 mg BID (after lunch and dinner). The primary objective was to evaluate the best dosage between 100 mg OD or 100 mg BID of the novel CoQ10 oral formulation in order to reach a level of plasma concentration which might assure its antioxidant effect if taken on a regular basis. The secondary objectives were to evaluate the safety and tolerability of both the single 100 mg oral dose and the multiple doses of 100 mg OD and BID during the 1 month daily dose phase.

In order to participate in the study, each subject had to meet all major inclusion and exclusion criteria at screening and at check-in visits. Inclusion criteria: informed consent form (ICF) signed, both gender aged between 25–75 years, body mass index (BMI) between 20–29 kg/m^2, fasting the night before enrolment for at least 10 h, healthy status, abstention from consumption of any food supplements except vitamin D and calcium at least 2 weeks before and during the study, consumption of dairy and cereal products, and willing to follow all study procedures. Exclusion criteria: intake of any prescribed medication within 2 weeks of the beginning of the study, hypotension, any clinically significant history of serious digestive tract, liver, kidney, cardiovascular or hematological disease, diabetes, gastrointestinal disorders, or other serious acute or chronic diseases, known lactose/gluten intolerances/food allergies, inadequate veins, or known contraindication to placement of a dedicated peripheral line for venous blood withdrawal, known drug and/or alcohol abuse, use of any form of nicotine or tobacco, mental incapacity precluding adequate understanding or cooperation, participation in another investigational study or blood donation within 3 months prior to or during this study.

During the study the following procedures were performed: Physical examination, vital signs recording (blood pressure, heart rate, temperature, and respiratory rate), body measurements (height and weight), 12 lead electrocardiogram (ECG), safety laboratory analysis (Haematology: Red blood cells, white blood cells, platelet, haemoglobin, and haematocrit; Biochemistry: hepatic transaminases, alcalin phosphatase, total cholesterol, LDL, and HDL cholesterol), concomitant medication recording, and adverse events monitoring. With special regard to the latter, mild insomnia, elevated levels of liver enzymes, rash, nausea, upper abdominal pain, dizziness, sensitivity to light, irritability, headache, heartburn, and fatigue were closely monitored.

2.2. Pharmacokinetic Timing and Assessments

When they arrived at the study center, subjects were hospitalized for at least 12 h for the single dose phase, and they remained at study site for approximately 24 h. At the end of this visit (visit 1), if no serious adverse event (SAE) occurred, subjects were dismissed and requested to return after 1 week (wash-out period) for the second study visit (visit 2), in order to initiate the multidose phase. Besides, subjects received a diary and were requested to report any possible adverse event experienced between V1 and V2, as well as any treatment taken for treating adverse events (AEs), if applicable. In the wash-out period subjects had to respect the same lifestyle regimen and no medication had to be taken, if not necessary.

During the single-dose phase plasma CoQ10 levels were measured before dosing (0 h) and over the next 12 h after intake: at 1, 2, 4, 8, and 12 h. Pharmacokinetic properties were measured accordingly: Area under the curve until the last observation (AUC_t) (µg/mL·h), maximum plasma concentration (C_{max}) (µg/L), time at which the C_{max} was observed (T_{max}) (hours), and elimination half-life ($T_{\frac{1}{2}}$) (hours). During the multidose-dose phase, plasma CoQ10 concentrations were measured once at the following timepoints: V2 (day 0), V3 (day 7), V4 (day 14), and V5 (day 28) (Figure 1). The pharmacokinetic properties measured were AUC_t, C_{max}, T_{max}. Samples were analyzed for plasma CoQ10 using an immunosorbent assay (ELISA; enzyme-linked immunosorbent assay) validated at the analytical laboratory (Consultmed Iasi Laboratory, IASI, Iasi county, Romania).

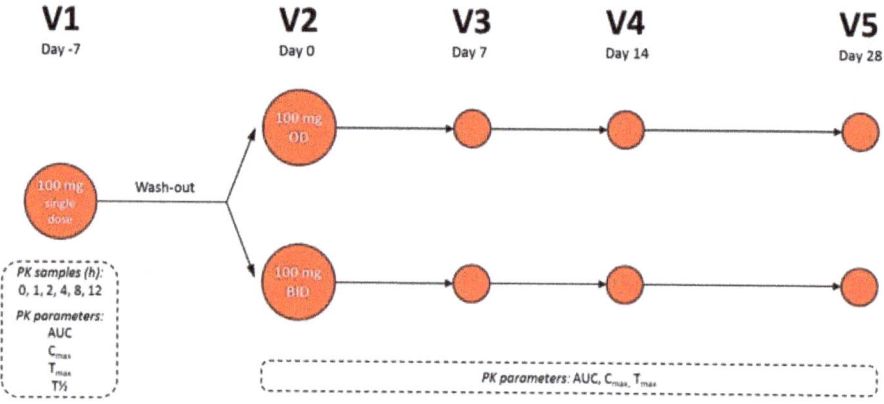

Figure 1. Flow-chart of blood sampling times (●) for the bioavailability assessment after a single dose of 100 mg and after multiple doses of 100 mg once a day (OD) or twice a day (BID) of CoQ10. During visits, V2, V3, V4, and V5 (multiple dose phase) only had one sample (at one timepoint) was collected. AUC: area under the curve; PK: pharmacokinetic; Cmax: maximum concentration; Tmax: the time at which the Cmax is observed; T1/2: half-life.

For pharmacokinetic analyses 4 mL of blood were collected in blood collection tubes. Each blood sample was allowed to clot for 20–25 min at room temperature. Then, they were centrifuged for 15 min at 1300 g at 4 °C. Afterwards the plasma was separated into the secondary sample tubes as follows: 0.5 mL plasma into two cryotubes, one to be sent to the pharmacokinetic laboratory and one as back-up. The plasma cryotubes were appropriately labeled (study code, treatment period, subject number, sampling time) and stored at −20 °C to −80 °C at the study center until shipment to the specified laboratory. The backup cryotubes were kept at the study center at least until the confirmation from the pharmacokinetic laboratory that the samples arrived in good conditions.

2.3. Formulation Administered

The CoQ10 formulation administered (COQUN®, Coenzyme Q10 Miniactives Retard 100 mg capsules, Visufarma S.p.A.) is a novel oral preparation based on an innovative modified release technology of active principles at certain time intervals. The basis in Miniactives® form is neutral microparticles of round shape, with dimensions between 400 and 500 microns. Each single particle is covered with one or more concentric layers of the active ingredients, and subsequently coated with a polymeric membrane suitable for obtaining a pre-established timed release. This technology leaves the time of the active ingredients absorption unchanged. This formulation gradually releases the active ingredients by diffusion, in a pre-determined time, thanks to a polymeric permeable and insoluble membrane coating each single particle, thus assuring a constant release.

2.4. Ethical Conduct of the Study

All subjects gave their informed consent for inclusion before they participated in the study. The study was conducted in accordance with the Declaration of Helsinki revised in 2013, and the protocol was approved by the local Ethics Committee Comisia Locala de Etica Consultmed, Sos Paracurari n. 70, bl 550, parter, Iasi, Romania (Project identification code: VF-BAQ10/2018) on May 31st, 2018, and also approved by Romanian Ministry of Health (Ministerul Sanatatii, Str Cristian Popisteanu, n. 1–3, Bucaresti, Romania) on June 19th, 2018.

The study was registered at ClinicalTrials.gov (Internet). Bethesda (MD): National Library of Medicine (US) (Identifier NCT03819491).

2.5. Statistical Analysis

Due to the explorative aim of the study no formal power calculation has been attempted, and no hypotheses were pre-specified. Twenty-four subjects (12 for each arm) have been considered sufficient to obtain reliable results for the exploratory purposes of the study. Descriptive statistics and confidence intervals (CI) at 95% level are provided. In particular, continuous variables are presented as arithmetic mean values ± standard deviation (SD), median values with interquartile range, minimum, maximum, and coefficient of variation (CV); for categorical variables, the absolute and percentage frequencies are provided. When normality assumption hold, results of Student t-tests are presented in order to compare pharmacokinetics parameters in subjects assigned to the two treatment groups. The statistical software package used was SAS version 9.4.

The following analysis sets were considered in the study: Safety Population (SP), all randomized subjects who signed the informed consent and took at least one dose of study product; Intention-To-Treat Population (ITT), all randomized subjects; and Protocol Population (PP), all subjects who met all inclusion/exclusion criteria and who did not have any major protocol deviation.

3. Results

Twenty-seven subjects were screened in the study but 3 were screening failures. A total of 24 subjects entered the study, half (n = 12) allocated to CoQ10 100 mg OD oral intake and half (n = 12) to CoQ10 100 mg BID. All randomized subjects completed the study. The SP, ITT- and PP-population were composed of 24 subjects. The two treatment groups were comparable for baseline characteristics (Table 1). A complete listing of all demographic variables of each participating subject is reported in Table S1.

Table 1. Demographic features of subjects randomized in each CoQ10 treatment group.

	Group A (CoQ10 100 mg OD)	Group B (CoQ10 100 mg BID)	Total
Gender			
Female n (%)	8 (66.67)	8 (66.67)	16
Male n (%)	4 (33.33)	4 (33.33)	8
Ethnic Group			
Caucasian n (%)	12 (100.00)	12 (100.00)	24
Age (years)			
Mean (SD)	35 (7.08)	43 (6.61)	39 (7.69)
Median	35	43	39
Range	26–46	30–50	26–50
Height (cm)			
Mean (SD)	168.08 (5.85)	165.92 (8.51)	167.00 (7.23)
Median	169.50	162.50	167.00
Range	156.00–178.00	154.00–185.00	154.00–185.00
Weight (kg)			
Mean (SD)	70.88 (9.59)	70.24 (13.87)	70.56 (11.67)
Median	71.50	76.20	72.50
Range	58.00–85.00	48.00–87.00	48.00–87.00
BMI (kg/m^2)			
Mean (SD)	25.05 (2.84)	25.16 (3.37)	25.11 (3.05)
Median	25.02	25.80	25.47
Range	20.79–28.81	20.23–28.86	20.23–28.86

SD: standard deviation.

3.1. Single Dose Phase

The plasma concentration curve of CoQ10 over time is shown in Figure 2. The distribution of plasma concentrations was wide as well as standard deviations, indicating quite different levels of plasma concentration among subjects. The mean baseline plasma CoQ10 concentration (0 h) was 649.8 (191.8) µg/L. However, a slightly increasing absorption phase of CoQ10 mean plasma values was observed until 4 h (772.1 µg/L), followed by a slow terminal decline until 12 h (696.3 µg/L) (Table S2A. Plasma concentration of CoQ10 by time (0, 1, 2, 4, 8, 12 h) during the single dose phase (V1)—ITT population; Table S2B. Individual plasma concentrations of CoQ10 (µg/L) in the single dose oral administration phase—ITT population).

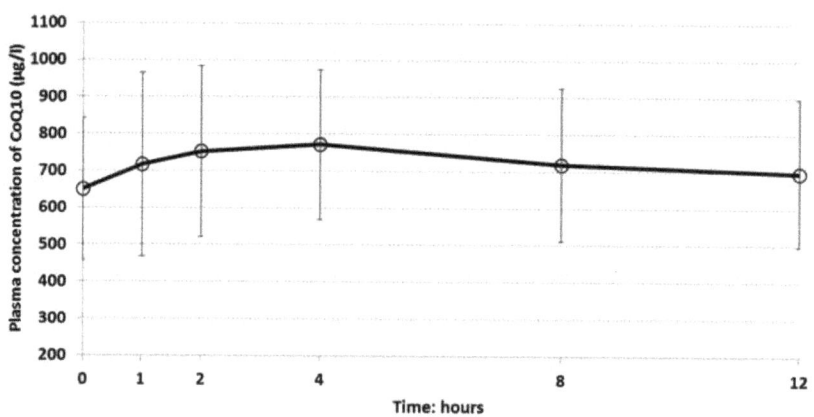

Figure 2. Single dose phase: mean plasma concentrations of CoQ10 by time after 100 mg single dose oral administration— Intention-To-Treat Population (ITT) population.

The descriptive statistics for pharmacokinetic parameters in the single dose phase are reported in Table 2. The mean AUC_t was 8754 µg/mL·h. The maximum registered value was almost the double the mean (15,394.54 µg/mL·h) while the minimum was 5277.62 µg/mL·h. Among other parameters, T_{max} values showed very high fluctuation with a minimum of 0 h (i.e., the maximum concentration was reached before CoQ10 oral intake) and a maximum of 12 h. The standard deviation was 3.58 h and the coefficient of variation was 83%, indicating that subjects registered very different time of maximum concentration (Table S3. Individual pharmacokinetic parameters of CoQ10 in the single dose oral administration phase—ITT population).

Males showed higher mean plasma concentrations compared to females at each time point (i.e., males: 759.79, 894.74, 844.33, 915.58, 840.01, and 772.41 µg/mL; females: 594.79, 628.38, 706.88, 700.34, 657.84, and 658.28 µg/mL, at 0, 1, 2, 4, 8, and 12 h, respectively). In the samples, significantly different plasma concentrations of CoQ10 between males and females were registered ($p < 0.001$); on average, females had a plasma concentration of 182.16 µg/L lower than men.

Table 2. Descriptive statistics for pharmacokinetic parameters of CoQ10 in the single and multiple phase—ITT population.

Pharmacokinetic Parameters		Single Dose Phase (n = 24)	Multiple Dose Phase	
			Group A 100 mg OD (n = 12)	Group B 100 mg BID (n = 12)
AUC_t (µg/mL·h)	Mean (SD)	8754.34 (2382.03)	2657.45 (681.74)	3459.05 (1026.66)
	CI 95%	7748.41–9760.1	2224.29–3090.6	2806.75–4111.36
	Median	8319.91	2490.96	3520.28
	Range	5277.62–15,394.54	1671.77–3778.37	2173.31–6068.15
	Coefficient of variation (%)	27	26	30
	Interquartile range	2920.10	1025.78	1073.09
C_{max} (µg/L)	Mean (SD)	828.92 (233.09)	1163.99 (354.95)	1501.89 (474.64)
	CI 95%	730.49–927.35	938.46–1389.51	1200.32–1803.47
	Median	830.37	1131.38	1495.78
	Range	482.54–1438.45	679.81–1826.85	906.43–2441.84
	Coefficient of variation (%)	28	30	32
	Interquartile range	283.69	542.84	759.72
T_{max} (h */day **)	Mean (SD)	4.29 (3.58)	17.5 (10.12)	16.92 (8.68)
	CI 95%	2.78–5.80	11.07–23.93	11.4–22.43
	Median	4.00	14.00	14.00
	Range	0–12	0–28	7–28
	Coefficient of variation (%)	83	58	51
	Interquartile range	2.50	17.50	17.50
$T_{\frac{1}{2}}$ (h)	Mean (SD)	8.88 (2.40)		
	CI 95%	7.87–9.90		
	Median	8.14		
	Range	6.77–16.26		
	Coefficient of variation (%)	27		
	Interquartile range	0.79		

* h: Tmax during single dose phase, ** day: Tmax during multiple dose phase.

3.2. Multiple Dose Phase

The mean plasma concentrations of CoQ10 increased over time in both treatment groups (Figure 3). At each study visit subjects who were assigned to 100 mg BID (Group B) had higher mean values than subjects in Group A, indicating that the assumption CoQ10 twice a day gave a higher concentration in the body.

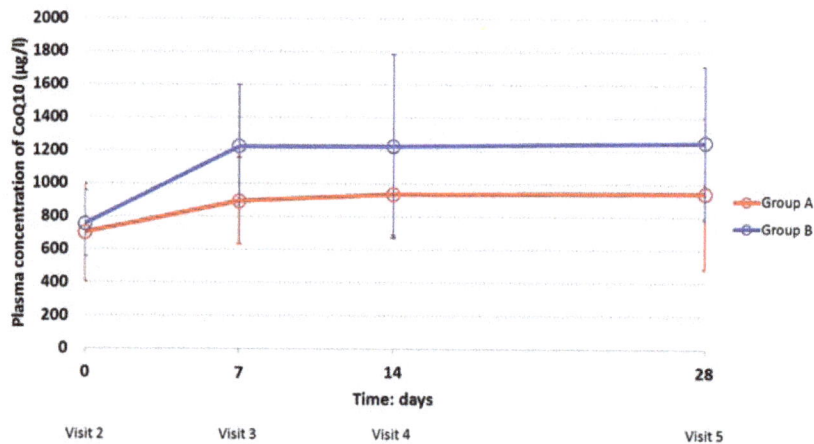

Figure 3. Multiple dose phase: plasma concentrations of CoQ10 by visit and by treatment group (Group A: 100 mg OD; Group B: 100 mg BID)—ITT population.

The two dosages of the same CoQ10 oral formulation followed the same pattern over time. In both groups, the mean values of plasma concentrations increased considerably from Visit 2 (Day 0) to Visit 3 (Day 7). At Visit 2 (Day 0), the mean plasma CoQ10 concentrations in Group A and B (701.95 ± 295.17 μg/L and 756.96 ± 201.17 μg/L, respectively) represent the mean plasma values after the end of the washout period. After day 7 (Visit 3), constant trends of high plasma levels were observed, which remained high during the rest of the multidose phase (21 days), with higher values for the Group taking 100 mg BID.

Additionally, in the multidose phase males showed higher plasma concentration of CoQ10 compared to females at each study visit. As in the single dose phase, the pattern over time was the same for men and women. The distribution of plasma concentration was very wide: Standard deviations and coefficients of variation—showing the extent of variability in relation to the mean of the population—were quite large indicating that levels of plasma concentration were different among individuals. The high inter-individual variability observed in this study could be probably due to a series of physiological conditions such as age, gender, and multiple administration time, which makes a subject very different from another. More likely, by reviewing the pharmacokinetics profile of each subject randomized in this study, exceptionally high pharmacokinetic values were observed. They belong to a 36-year-old man randomized to Group B, who registered values of plasma concentration far above from the mean of the total set of subjects. By considering this individual as an outlier and by excluding him from the analysis ($n = 23$), mean plasma concentration values (and SD) were smaller for Group B, as follows (μg/L): 743.83 (205.53), 1153.86 (290.86), 1118.12 (421.44), and 1155.94 (338.48) at visit 2, visit 3, visit 4, and visit 5, respectively (Table S4. Individual plasma concentrations of CoQ10 (μg/mL) in the multiple dose oral administration phase—ITT population).

The descriptive statistics for pharmacokinetic parameters by treatment group are reported in Table 2. The mean CoQ10 bioavailability (AUC_t) in Group B (3459.05 μg/mL·h) was statistically higher than in Group A (2657.45 μg/mL·h) ($p = 0.0345$). Despite values of the other pharmacokinetics parameters (C_{max}, T_{max}) remained higher for subjects treated by CoQ10 100 mg BID compared to ones with the OD dosing scheme, no statistically significant differences between groups were detected. As previously described, by excluding the outlier subject from the analysis, the difference between the AUC_t values of the two groups was no more statistically significant ($p = 0.0548$) (Table S5. Individual pharmacokinetic parameters of CoQ10 in the multiple dose oral administration phase—ITT population). In the scenario without this subject, there is evidence of a difference in the CoQ10 bioavailability (AUC_t) between the two dosages of the novel oral formulation of CoQ10, but the low power of the study due to the small sample size did not allow highlighting, albeit slightly, a significant difference when excluding him.

3.3. Adverse Events

The oral formulation of CoQ10 was well tolerated in all 24 healthy subjects; only 3 non-serious, moderate intensity AEs were reported during all the study period. The 3 AEs occurred in 2 subjects, both enrolled in the Group B (100 mg BID): (1) Intermittent dizziness of 5 days duration, possibly related to the oral preparation, and spontaneously resolved; (2) 1 day respiratory virosis, adequately treated, but unrelated to the study product; and (3) pultaceous angina of 5 days duration, unrelated to the CoQ10 oral preparation.

During the multiple dose phase (at visit 2 and visit 5), 21 subjects (9 in Group A and 12 in Group B) showed some biochemical values out of normal ranges, but none was considered clinically significant. Only 5 subjects—2 in Group A and 3 in Group B—showed clinically not significant out-of-range liver biochemical values. The ranges of values considered outside the normal ranges are shown in Table 3.

Table 3. Range of values of liver biochemical parameters outside the normal ranges observed during the multiple dose phase in both treatment groups—ITT population.

Biochemistry (Normal Ranges)	Group A (n. of Subjects) *		Group B (n. of Subjects) *	
AST (<32 U/L)	39–42	(2)	34–40	(2)
ALT (<33 U/L)	43–48	(2)	42–96	(3)
ALP (35–104 U/L)	---		27–237	(2)
TC (<200 mg/dL)	203–235	(3)	200–251	(5)
HDL (≥60 mg/dL)	39	(1)	36–40	(2)
LDL (<100 mg/dL)	100–186	(8)	101–200	(11)
TGs (<100 mg/dL)	---		257	(1)

AST = Aspartate Aminotransferase; ALT = Alanine Aminotransferase; ALP = Alkaline Phosphatase; TC = Total Cholesterol; HDL = High-Density Lipoprotein; LDL = Low-Density Lipoprotein; and TGs = Triglycerides. * Some subjects experienced more than one biochemical value outside the normal range of the reference laboratory.

Subjects randomized to treatment with 100 mg BID of CoQ10 did not show higher out-of-range liver values compared to subjects treated with the halved dose (100 mg OD). Both doses were safely tolerated. However, renal function tests were not monitored during the study because they were not included in the protocol requirements, and no blood samples were taken for the evaluation of basic plasma biochemistry.

4. Discussion

These results demonstrate that in human plasma high levels of CoQ10 can be achieved by administrating relatively low oral doses by the use of a novel timed-release oral formulation determining optimal intestinal absorption and sustained plasma concentrations over time. The combination of bioavailability and safety results obtained with two oral dosages of CoQ10 (100 mg OD and BID) contribute to the construction of a rationale for a clinical use of this novel formulation of CoQ10. The information can help clinicians to protect patients from the negative effects of lipid peroxidation, on the one hand preventing possible therapeutic failures due to CoQ10 underdosing, and on the other, the possible development of toxicity following administration of too high doses.

In the experience of Joshi and coll. the pharmacokinetic properties of two new oral CoQ10 formulations (i.e., fast-melting tablet and effervescent tablet) were not statistically different compared with those of commercial formulations (i.e., soft gelatin capsule and powder-filled hard shell) when administered at 60 mg in single dose fashion [16]. The mean C_{max} values of the four formulations (around 80 µg/mL) measured over 12 h were essentially similar to the one of CoQ10 Miniactives Retard capsule we studied (83 µg/mL), but the mean T_{max} values were almost halved (1.3 and 2.0 h for fast-melting and effervescent tablets, respectively) compared to the one of Miniactives capsule (4.29 h). It is hard to believe that the more rapid delivery of the two fast melting formulations can play a significant role in the clinical cure of diseases in which the main feature of long-term treatment should be to ensure consistently high levels of CoQ10 over time. Furthermore, the bioavailabilities of the four formulations (ranging 4.9–5.5 µg/mL·h) were far below the bioavailability of the one we tested (8.754 µg/mL·h). This can be probably explained mainly by the dissolution properties of the Miniactives® technology that allows more sustained plasma concentrations over time (until 12 h after dosing), as well as by the higher dose administered (100 mg) in our study.

When supplemented at 100 mg/day by oral formulation consisting of soya oil in soft gelatin capsule (Myoqinon® 100 mg CoQ10), CoQ10 achieved median plasma concentration of 2.5 mg/L (2500 µg/L) after a 2 month administration period [18], far above the median plasma level achieved at day 28 with Miniactives capsule (773.35 µg/L) administered at 100 mg/day in Group A. It is difficult to draw conclusions when comparing our results with those of Zita and coll. [18] due to the profound difference between the durations of oral administration of CoQ10 in the two studies (2 months vs. 1 month). In addition to this, no other pharmacokinetic parameters were reported by the authors of Reference [18]. Astonishingly, in another study [17], the same 100 mg/day CoQ10 soya oil in soft gelatin capsule (Myoqinon® 100 mg CoQ10) did not generate comparable pharmacokinetic results to those reported by Zita. After 20 days CoQ10 plasma concentration was approximately 0.9 mg/L (900 µg/L), a result much below the 2.5 mg/L reported in the study [18]. The mean plasma concentrations of CoQ10 after administration of oil/soft gel formulation used by Singh [17] are closer to those observed in our study after 28 days of CoQ10 100 mg/day administration (944.8 µg/L). Moreover, the author also highlighted the importance of the dosing strategy in addition to the daily dose. Divided dosages (2 × 100 mg) of oil/soft gel CoQ10 formulation caused a larger increase in plasma levels of CoQ10 (approximately >1.9 mg/L) than a single dose of 200 mg (approximately >1.3 mg/L) [17]. Our results show that, after 28 days of supplementation of Miniactives®, formulation 2 × 100 mg the mean plasma concentration was a little higher than 1200 µg/L.

With the aim to overcome the poor intestinal absorption, the bioavailability of a CoQ10 colloidal oral preparation was determined versus one oil-based formulation and two solubilizates in a single dose (120 mg) study. The mean C_{max} colloidal formulation was the highest among the four formulations studied (6890 µg/L), as well as its $AUC_{(0-10)}$ (30,620 µg/mL·h). Nevertheless, the oil-based formulation and the two solubilizates showed rather high bioavailability (i.e., 4900, 6100, 10,700 µg/mL·h, respectively) [15]. When comparing the pharmacokinetic profiles of the four formulations with Miniactives® capsule, all achieved the peak of plasma concentration 4 h after the administration and maintained sustained levels afterwards. Once again, it is difficult to compare the results of different studies, since several factors may have contributed to the achievement of a particular bioavailability profile (e.g., study design, selection criteria, diet, analytical procedures, etc.). In the case of colloidal preparation, it is undoubted that it has favored the intestinal absorption of the conveyed CoQ10.

Very recently, a pharmacokinetic study highlighted the importance of inter-subjects variability in the plasma level of CoQ10 caused by significant variation of intestinal absorption of CoQ10 between subjects and irrespective of the oral formulation or molecular form administered [19]. The three commercial preparations tested (i.e., ubiquinol 150 mg capsule, ubiquinone 150 mg capsule and liposome ubiquinone 40 mg/2 sprays) showed plasma levels of CoQ10 ranging 5000–6000 µg/L at the 2 h interval, with ubiquinol preparation having the highest response, but a high inter-individual variation was observed for each preparation at every time interval. In our experience, this phenomenon has also been observed in both the single and multiple dose phase. After the single dose phase, the mean AUC_t (8754.34 ± 2382.03 µg/mL·h) showed a very wide range (5277.62–15,394.54 µg/mL·h) and also mean T_{max} had a high fluctuation, indicating different times of maximum concentration between subjects (coefficient of variation: 83%). During the multidose phase a very wide distribution of plasma concentration was observed, indicating quite different levels among individuals. Particularly, the exceptionally high pharmacokinetic values of a single subject (36-year-old man) randomized in the group of 2 × 100 mg CoQ10 dose contributed to increase in the overall variability of pharmacokinetic results of the entire subject population. Despite the bioavailability values of CoQ10 of the two groups (Group A and Group B), they were not statistically different after exclusion of the outlier subject ($p = 0.0548$), however, there is evidence of a difference at limits of the significance threshold ($p < 0.05$) between the two groups. Probably, a clear difference did not emerge due to the small sample size studied.

During both single and multiple dose phases, males showed higher plasma CoQ10 concentration than females at each time point. CoQ10 baseline is naturally higher in men than in women [14,20], ranging 0.40–1.72 µmol/L (345.34–1484.94 µg/L) for males and 0.43–1.47 µmol/L (371.24–1269.11 µg/L) for females in European (Finnish) population [20]. Our results on baseline CoQ10 plasma levels (0 h) in both sexes are included in these normal ranges (males 759.79 ± 198.09; females 594.79 ± 168.63). During the multidose phase, the same pattern of plasma CoQ10 concentration was observed between genders (e.g., males 909.79 ± 241.54 µg/L, females 639.29 ± 203.81 µg/L at Visit 2; males 1173.32 ± 524.40 µg/L, and females 1061.03 ± 464.98 µg/L at Visit 5). In this study, the proportion between genders was unbalanced (i.e., 8 males/16 females). However, this disproportion did not appear to have influenced the plasma concentrations of CoQ10 according to the expected levels in males and females. In addition, another pharmacokinetic study reported the same numerical disproportion between the two genders, without any reported influence on the observed results [15]. Regarding the difference between genders in CoQ10 plasma concentrations, our results are in line with previous studies. The present experience and others in the literature support the conclusions that men can have better absorption and/or lower clearance than women [13].

The results presented in our bioavailability study suggest that Miniactives® timed release formulation of CoQ10 gradually released the active ingredient by diffusion, in a pre-determined time, thanks to a polymeric permeable and insoluble membrane coating each single particle, thus assuring a constant release. After having achieved the peak at 4 h, CoQ10 plasma concentrations did not undergo a sharp decrease and remained constantly high. The development of this technology was supported with the aim of creating an oral formulation able to ensure consistently high CoQ10 blood concentrations, useful for supporting a treatment strategy in the neuroprotection of RGC. In glaucoma, retinal neuroprotection can be significantly improved through maintenance of mitochondrial functions and survival of RGC by CoQ10, one of the most powerful antioxidant compounds. The potential clinical significance of this finding should be further evaluated.

In conclusion, based on the obtained results and on data available in literature regarding the expected average plasma levels of CoQ10, this exploratory study highlighted that both 100 mg OD or BID are safe and assure a plasma concentration of CoQ10 that remains high for the duration of the intake and that 100 mg COQUN® Miniactives® BID would be preferred than OD in reaching a higher plasma concentration of CoQ10. These positive results suggest that further studies are needed in order to investigate the antioxidative effects of COQUN® OS oral formulation in patients with specific diseases like glaucoma where the antioxidative effect of the CoQ10 is expected to be seen at the target organ.

Supplementary Materials: The following are available online at http://www.mdpi.com/2072-6643/11/3/527/s1, Table S1: Individual demographic variables—ITT population; Table S2A. Plasma concentration of CoQ10 by time (0, 1, 2, 4, 8, 12 h) during the single dose phase (V1)—ITT population, Table S2B. Individual plasma concentrations of CoQ10 (µg/L) in the single dose oral administration phase—ITT population; Table S3. Individual pharmacokinetic parameters of CoQ10 in the single dose oral administration phase—ITT population; Table S4. Individual plasma concentrations of CoQ10 (µg/L) in the multiple dose oral administration phase—ITT population; Table S5. Individual pharmacokinetic parameters of CoQ10 in the multiple dose oral administration phase—ITT population.

Author Contributions: Conceptualization, clinical study design and writing—original draft preparation, A.M. (Alessio Martucci) and D.R.-P.; plasma separation, performance of ELISA testing, collection of laboratory data, reading, amendment, and approval of the final version of the manuscript A.M. (Anamaria Manole) and D.R.-P.

Funding: This research and the APC were funded by VISUFARMA S.p.A., Via Canino 21, 00191 Rome–Italy.

Acknowledgments: CRO 1MED Via Campagna, 13 6982 Agno–CH managed the study.

Conflicts of Interest: A.M. (Alessio Martucci) is medical consultant for Visufarma S.p.A.; D.R.-P. and M.A. (Anamaria Manole) received a grant for the conduction of the study. The authors have no further conflicts of interest relevant to the content of this manuscript. The funders had no role in the collection, analyses, interpretation of data, in the writing of the manuscript, or in the decision to publish the results.

References

1. Stefely, J.A.; Pagliarini, D.J. Biochemistry of mitochondrial coenzyme q biosynthesis. *Trends Biochem. Sci.* **2017**, *42*, 824–843. [CrossRef] [PubMed]
2. Pravst, I.; Zmitek, K.; Zmitek, J. Coenzyme Q10 contents in foods and fortification strategies. *Crit. Rev. Food Sci. Nutr.* **2010**, *50*, 269–280. [CrossRef] [PubMed]
3. Ernster, L.; Dallner, G. Biochemical, physiological and medical aspects of ubiquinone function. *Biochim. Biophys. Acta* **1995**, *1271*, 195–204. [CrossRef]
4. Alehagen, U.; Johansson, P.; Björnstedt, M.; Rosén, A.; Dahlström, U. Cardiovascular mortality and N-terminal-proBNP reduced after combined selenium and coenzyme Q10 supplementation: A 5-year prospective randomized double-blind placebo-controlled trial among elderly Swedish citizens. *Int. J. Cardiol.* **2013**, *167*, 1860–1866. [CrossRef] [PubMed]
5. Mortensen, S.A.; Rosenfeldt, F.; Kumar, A.; Dolliner, P.; Filipiak, K.J.; Pella, D.; Alehagen, U.; Steurer, G.; Littarru, G.P.; Q-SYMBIO Study Investigators. The Effect of Coenzyme Q10 on morbidity and mortality in chronic heart failure. Results from Q-SYMBIO: A randomized double-blind trial. *JACC Heart Fail.* **2014**, *2*, 641–649. [CrossRef] [PubMed]
6. Shen, Q.; Pierce, J.D. Supplementation of Coenzyme Q10 among Patients with Type 2 Diabetes Mellitus. *Healthcare* **2015**, *3*, 296–309. [CrossRef] [PubMed]
7. Shults, C.W.; Oakes, D.; Kieburtz, K.; Beal, M.F.; Haas, R.; Plumb, S.; Juncos, J.L.; Nutt, J.; Shoulson, I.; Carter, J.; et al. Effects of coenzyme Q10 in early parkinson disease. evidence of slowing of the functional decline. *Arch. Neurol.* **2002**, *59*, 1541–1550. [CrossRef] [PubMed]
8. Huntington Study Group. A randomized, placebo-controlled trial of coenzyme Q10 and remacemide in Huntington's disease. *Neurology* **2001**, *57*, 397–404. [CrossRef]
9. Martucci, A.; Nucci, C. Evidence on neuroprotective properties of coenzyme Q10 in the treatment of glaucoma. *Neural Regen. Res.* **2019**, *14*, 197–200. [CrossRef] [PubMed]
10. Nucci, C.; Martucci, A.; Cesareo, M.; Mancino, R.; Russo, R.; Bagetta, G.; Cerulli, L.; Garaci, F.G. Brain involvement in glaucoma: Advanced neuroimaging for understanding and monitoring a new target for therapy. *Curr. Opin. Pharmacol.* **2013**, *13*, 128–133. [CrossRef] [PubMed]
11. Lee, D.; Kim, K.-Y.; Shim, M.S.; Kim, S.Y.; Ellisman, M.H.; Weinreb, R.N.; Ju, W.-K. Coenzyme Q10 ameliorates oxidative stress and prevents mitochondrial alteration in ischemic retinal injury. *Apoptosis* **2014**, *19*, 603–614. [CrossRef] [PubMed]
12. Parisi, V.; Centofanti, M.; Gandolfi, S.; Marangoni, D.; Rossetti, L.; Tanga, L.; Tardini, M.; Traina, S.; Ungaro, N.; Vetrugno, M.; et al. Effects of coenzyme Q10 in conjunction with vitamin E on retinal-evoked and cortical-evoked responses in patients with open-angle glaucoma. *J. Glaucoma* **2014**, *23*, 391–404. [CrossRef] [PubMed]
13. Wahlqvist, M.L.; Wattanapenpaiboon, N.; Savige, G.S.; Kannar, D. Bioavailability of two different formulations of coenzyme Q10 in healthy subjects. *Asia Pac. J. Clin. Nutr.* **1998**, *7*, 37–40. [PubMed]
14. Lu, W.-L.; Zhang, Q.; Lee, H.-S.; Zhou, T.-Y.; Sun, H.-D.; Zhang, D.-W.; Zheng, L.; Lee, M.; Wong, S.-M. Total coenzyme Q10 concentrations in Asian men following multiple oral 50-mg doses administered as coenzyme Q10 sustained release tablets or regular tablets. *Biol. Pharm. Bull.* **2003**, *26*, 52–55. [CrossRef] [PubMed]
15. Liu, Z.-X.; Artmann, C. Relative bioavailability comparison of different coenzyme Q10 formulations with a novel delivery system. *Altern. Ther. Health Med.* **2009**, *15*, 42–46. [PubMed]
16. Joshi, S.S.; Sawant, S.V.; Shedge, A.; Halpner, A.D. Comparative bioavailability of two novel coenzyme Q10 preparations in humans. *Int. J. Clin. Pharmacol. Ther.* **2003**, *41*, 42–48. [CrossRef] [PubMed]
17. Singh, R.B.; Niaz, M.A.; Kumar, A.; Sindberg, C.D.; Moesgaard, S.; Littarru, G.P. Effect on absorption and oxidative stress of different oral Coenzyme Q10 dosages and intake strategy in healthy men. *BioFactors* **2005**, *25*, 219–224. [CrossRef] [PubMed]

18. Zita, C.; Overvad, K.; Mortensen, S.A.; Sindberg, C.D.; Moesgaard, S.; Hunter, D.A. Serum coenzyme Q10 concentrations in healthy men supplemented with 30 mg or 100 mg coenzyme Q10 for two months in a randomised controlled study. *BioFactors* **2003**, *18*, 185–193. [CrossRef] [PubMed]
19. Vitetta, L.; Leong, A.; Zhou, J.; Dal Forno, S.; Hall, S.; Rutolo, D. The plasma bioavailability of coenzyme Q10 absorbed from the gut and the oral mucosa. *J. Funct. Biomater.* **2018**, *9*, 73. [CrossRef] [PubMed]
20. Bhagavan, H.N.; Chopra, R.K. Coenzyme Q10: Absorption, tissue uptake, metabolism and pharmacokinetics. *Free Radic. Res.* **2006**, *40*, 445–453. [CrossRef] [PubMed]

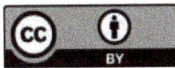

© 2019 by the authors. Licensee MDPI, Basel, Switzerland. This article is an open access article distributed under the terms and conditions of the Creative Commons Attribution (CC BY) license (http://creativecommons.org/licenses/by/4.0/).

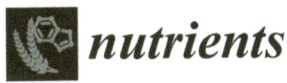

Review

Pharmacological Properties of *Morus nigra* L. (Black Mulberry) as A Promising Nutraceutical Resource

Sung Ho Lim and Chang-Ik Choi *

College of Pharmacy, Dongguk University-Seoul, Goyang 10326, Korea; teruai0608@naver.com
* Correspondence: cichoi@dongguk.edu; Tel.: +82-31-961-5230

Received: 30 January 2019; Accepted: 18 February 2019; Published: 20 February 2019

Abstract: Mulberry plants belonging to the Moraceae family have been grown for the purpose of being the nutrient source for silk worm and raw materials for the preparation of jams, marmalades, vinegars, juices, wines, and cosmetics. *Morus nigra* L. (black mulberry) is native to Southwestern Asia, and it has been used as a traditional herbal medicine for animals and humans. In this article, recent research progress on various biological and pharmacological properties of extracts, fractions, and isolated active constituents from different parts of *M. nigra* are reviewed. *M. nigra* exhibited a wide-spectrum of biological and pharmacological therapeutic effects including antinociceptive, anti-inflammatory, antimicrobial, anti-melanogenic, antidiabetic, anti-obesity, anti-hyperlipidemic, and anticancer activities. *M. nigra* also showed protective effects against various human organs and systems, mainly based on its antioxidant capacity. These findings strongly suggest that *M. nigra* can be used as a promising nutraceutical resource to control and prevent various chronic diseases.

Keywords: *Morus nigra* L.; black mulberry; nutraceutical; pharmacological properties

---

1. Introduction

Morus, commonly known as mulberry, is the genus of a flowering plant belonging to the Moraceae family. They are widely distributed into subtropic regions of Asia (including Korea, Japan, China, and India), North America, and Africa [1]. In Asian countries, mulberry plants have been grown for the production of silk worms (*Bombyx mori* L.), because their leaves are a major and important nutrient source for silk worms [2]. Meanwhile, most European countries have usually used mulberry fruits to prepare jams, marmalades, vinegars, juices, wine, and cosmetic products [3]. Various parts of mulberry plants have also been used as traditional herbal medicines [4]. Diels-Alder-type adducts, flavonoids, benzofurans, stilbenes, and polyhydroxylated alkaloids are the most representative bioactive compounds identified from Sang-Bai-Pi (Chinese name for root barks of *Morus* species) [5]. Some previous review articles on *Morus alba* L. (*M. alba*), one of the most valuable plants rich in natural ingredients, have demonstrated that extracts, fractions and major constituents from *M. alba* exhibit numerous pharmacological activities such as antioxidant, anti-inflammatory, anticancer, antimicrobial, antifungal, skin-whitening, antidiabetic, anti-hyperlipidemic, anti-atherosclerotic, anti-obesity, cardioprotective, cognitive enhancing, hepatoprotective, anti-platelet, anxiolytic, anti-asthmatic, anthelmintic, antidepressant, and immunomodulatory activities [6–8].

Morus nigra L. (*M. nigra*), also called black mulberry, is native to Southwestern Asia. It has been grown throughout Europe and around the Mediterranean for centuries. Although biological and/or pharmacological activities of *M. nigra* have been relatively less studied compared to those of *M. alba*, several bioactive compounds isolated from *M. nigra* have also been used as herbal medicines for animals and humans due to their analgesic and anti-inflammatory effects [1]. Budiman et al. [9] briefly summarized chemical compounds isolated from various parts of *M. nigra* and their pharmacological activities. In this review article, we extensively covered recent research progress on biological and

2. Antinociceptive Activity

In 2000, de Souza et al. [10] firstly reported on the antinociceptive effect of morusin, the main prenylflavonoid of M. nigra isolated from acetonic extract of its root barks. Morusin showed a significant inhibitory effect on acetic acid-induced abdominal constriction responses and formalin-induced pain, and it also resulted in prolongation of the latency period in a hot plate test in mice. Because morusin is also purified from other mulberry plants, such as M. alba [11], M. australis [12] and M. lhou [13], this study result alone is insufficient to fully reflect the analgesic activity of M. nigra. Nine years later, Padilha et al. [14] investigated the antinociceptive effect of methylene chloride extract of M. nigra leaves in mice. Similar to the results of de Souza et al. [10], M. nigra leaves extract showed significantly and dose-dependently reduced acetic acid-induced writhing and formalin-induced pain and increased response latency period in a tail-immersion test and hot plate test without any acute toxicity when the dose of the extract was up to 300 mg/kg.

Two studies by Chen et al. [15,16] recently evaluated the antinociceptive properties of total flavonoid extracts and main active ingredients from fresh fruits of M. nigra. In the first study [15], total flavonoids from M. nigra showed dose-dependent decreases in the duration of formalin-induced pain-response behaviors. In the second study, three different mulberry fruits (M. alba, M. nigra and M. mongolia) were compared [16]. M. nigra fruits had more anthocyanin and flavonol contents than other species. The duration of the formalin-induced secondary pain phase (inflammatory phase) in the group treated with total flavonoid extract from M. nigra was significantly shorter than that in the control group. Reduced development of inflammatory cytokine interleukin-6 (IL-6) and an increased level of an anti-inflammatory cytokine IL-10 associated with the nuclear factor kappa-light-chain-enhancer of activated B cells (NF-κB) and nitric oxide (NO) pathways were observed after treatment with M. nigra extract, suggesting the possible mechanism of its antinociceptive effects. Interestingly, the three main flavonoid ingredients (cyanidin-3-O-glucoside, rutin and isoquercetin) from M. nigra did not reduce the duration of formalin-induced pain individually, although they significantly decreased such duration when they were used as a mixture.

3. Anti-Inflammatory Activity

Inflammation is defined as a set of physiological defense mechanisms taking place in the body. However, inflammation is also considered an initial event of major chronic diseases such as cardiovascular, autoimmune, eye, age-related, neurodegenerative diseases, and cancers [17]. In this respect, inhibiting and controlling inflammatory responses in the human body can be one of fundamental approaches for treating chronic diseases.

As a follow-up research of a previous study on antinociceptive activity, Padilha et al. [18] evaluated the anti-inflammatory effects of methylene chloride extract of M. nigra leaves in male rats. M. nigra leaves extract significantly inhibited the volume of paw edema induced by intraplantar injection of carrageenan at a half-maximal inhibitory concentration (IC_{50}) value of 15.2 mg/kg. M. nigra leaves also significantly inhibited the formation of granulomatous tissues in the chronic inflammation status using a cotton pellet-induced granuloma rat model (IC_{50} of 71.1 mg/kg). In the same year, Wang et al. [19] isolated three new compounds (mornigrol D, G and H) with six other known compounds (norartocarpetin, dihydrokaempferol, albanin A, albanin E, moracin M, and albafuran C) from the stem bark of M. nigra and assessed their anti-inflammatory activities by calculating the inhibition of releasing β-glucuronidase from rat polymorphonuclear leukocytes induced by platelet-activating factor. At a concentration of 10^{-5} M, mornigrol D and norartocarpetin showed potent anti-inflammatory properties, showing inhibition rates of 65.9% and 67.7%, respectively. In 2014, Zelová et al. [20] investigated into the anti-inflammatory activities of two Diels-Alder adducts (soroceal and sanggenon E) isolated from the root bark of M. nigra, by determining the attenuation of secretion of pro-inflammatory cytokines, tumor necrosis factor-alpha (TNF-α) and IL-1β, in lipopolysaccharide (LPS)-stimulated macrophages. Although sanggenon E significantly reduced the production of TNF-α compared to the vehicle control, both compounds failed to significantly affect the level of IL-1β.

Chen et al. [15] reported that the total flavonoid extract of M. nigra fruits can dose-dependently inhibit xylene-induced ear edema (edema rate 60.1% at a concentration of 200 mg/20 mL/kg) and carrageenan-induced paw edema (edema rate 9.5% at a concentration of 100 mg/20 mL/kg; 8.6% at a concentration of 200 mg/20 mL/kg) in mice. Levels of pro-inflammatory cytokines including IL-1β, TNF-α, NO, and interferon-gamma (IFN-γ) were also significantly decreased after the treatment of M. nigra fruit extract in mice with xylene-induced inflammation. In addition, M. nigra fruits extract significantly reduced levels of NO in LPS-stimulated RAW 264.7 cells without showing the cytotoxicity effect at the concentration of 50 to 100 μg/mL.

A very recent study [21] has shown that extracts of M. nigra pulps and leaves can improve survival rate and decrease the number of total leukocytes in bronchoalveolar lavage fluid in LPS-induced septic mice, indicating the reduction of inflammatory infiltrate in the lung. Although most hepatic and serum cytokine levels were not changed by the administration of M. nigra extracts, serum levels of TNF, an important mediator of sepsis, were significantly lower in the M. nigra extract-treated group than those in the septic animal group.

4. Antimicrobial Activity

Antibacterial activities of M. nigra leaves have been investigated in various organic fractions. Tahir et al. [22] reported that the ethyl acetate fraction of M. nigra leaves is active against four dental caries-causing bacterial strains: Streptococcus mutans, Escherichia coli (E. coli), Staphylococcus aureus (S. aureus), and Bacillus subtilis (B. subtilis). Also, the chloroform fraction showed antibacterial properties against Pseudomonas aeruginosa (P. aeruginosa) and B. subtilis, while the methanol fraction was only active against B. subtilis. No activity was observed for n-hexane or aqueous fraction. The inhibition rate of streptococcal biofilm formation (anti-adherence effect) by M. nigra ethyl acetate fraction was 87%. In another study conducted by Souza et al. [23], crude ethanol extract of M. nigra leaves exhibited bactericidal activities against Bacillus cereus (B. cereus), Enterococcus faecalis (E. faecalis), and E. coli, with minimal inhibitory concentration (MIC) and minimum bactericidal concentration (MBC) less than 0.195 mg/mL for all. Potent antibacterial activities against B. cereus and E. faecalis were also observed for hexane, chloroform and ethyl acetate extracts (MIC values < 0.195 mg/mL for all). However, their measured MBCs were over 6 mg/mL. It was noted that chloroform extract exclusively showed a bactericidal effect against Salmonella choleraesuis (MIC and MBC value < 0.195 mg/mL, respectively). The antibacterial activities of the total flavonoid extract of M. nigra fruits were evaluated against three inflammatory pain-causing bacteria, E. coli, P. aeruginosa and S. aureus. Its fruit extract strongly inhibited all three strains, with MBC values of 2 mg/mL or less [16].

The antimicrobial activities of fresh juice of M. nigra fruits against five Gram-positive and three Gram-negative bacterial strains have been compared with conventional antibiotics [24]. Although 100 μL of M. nigra fruits juice produced generally smaller zones of inhibition (ranging from 9.98 to 19.87 mm) than other antibiotics treated at their standard doses, it showed a broad-spectrum antimicrobial effect against both Gram-positive and Gram-negative bacteria, having the highest inhibition against P. aeruginosa. Minhas et al. [25] investigated into the antimicrobial effect of five M. nigra fruits extracts classified by different solvents against 16 bacterial and 2 fungal strains in comparison with conventional antibiotics and antifungal agent nystatin. Ethanolic and acetone extracts of M. nigra fruits showed highly-sensitive inhibition (defined as 20 mm or more longer diameter of zone of inhibition) against E. coli, S. aureus, and Neisseria spp.; methanolic extract against Klebsiella pneumoniae and Neisseria spp.; and chloroform extract against Serratia marcesscens, Staphylococcus epidermidis (S. epidermidis), P. aeruginosa, and S. aureus. Similar to the results of Khalid et al. [24], M. nigra extracts had smaller zones of inhibition than those observed with conventional drugs.

In a recent study assessing antibacterial activities against two strains causing acne, *S. epidermidis* and *Propionibacterium acnes* (*P. acnes*), the ethanolic extract of *M. nigra* fruits had MIC values of 2.5% for both strains and MBC values of 2.5% and 5%, respectively [26]. As a follow-up approach, a comparative study was performed for extracts from three parts (stem barks, fruits and leaves) of *M. nigra* on their antibacterial effects against *S. epidermidis* and *P. acnes* [27]. *M. nigra* stem barks possessed the most potent antibacterial activities against both strains, with an MIC value of 4 mg/mL for *S. epidermidis* and 2 mg/mL for *P. acnes*. In addition, *M. nigra* stem barks extract induced nucleic acid, protein, and ion leakages and cellular membrane damages against *P. acnes*. These results suggest that the antibacterial effect of *M. nigra* stem bark is related to reduced cell membrane fluidity and bacterial cell wall destruction.

Mazzimba et al. [28] reported that six isolated constituents (oxyresveratrol, moracin M, cyclomorusin, morusin, kuwanon C, and a derivative of kuwanon C) from aerial parts of *M. nigra* show antibacterial activities against *S. aureus*, *B. subtilis*, *Micrococcus flavus*, *S. faecalis*, *Salmonella abony*, and *P. aeruginosa*, with morusin having the most potent activity against *B. subtilis* (MIC value 3.91 µg/mL).

Tuberculosis (TB), an infectious disease caused by *Mycobacterium tuberculosis* (*M. tuberculosis*), is one of the top 10 causes of death in the world. TB is a curable and preventive disease, but resistance against conventional antibiotic medications for *M. tuberculosis* has increased the number of cases of multidrug-resistant or extensively drug-resistant TB [29]. In this respect, demand for new medications with novel therapeutic targets such as protein tyrosinase phosphatases (PTPs) is growing [30,31]. Mascarello et al. [32] evaluated the anti-tuberculosis activity of Diel–Alder-type adducts from *M. nigra* root bark to determine their potential as candidates for *M. tuberculosis* PTP inhibitor. A total of eight compounds (Kuwanon L, G, and H; cudraflavanone A; morusin, oxyresveratrol; chalcomoracin; and norartocarpetin) were isolated from *M. nigra*. They all significantly inhibited *M. tuberculosis* PTP-B (Mtb PtpB) with IC_{50} values ranging from 0.36 to 8.42 µM. Further enzyme kinetic analyses for Kuwanon G and H, two of the most potent compounds, showed that both compounds competitively inhibited Mtb PtpB, with inhibitory constant (K_i) values of 0.39 ± 0.27 µM and 0.20 ± 0.01 µM, respectively. In addition, Kuwanon G inhibited the growth of *M. tuberculosis* inside macrophages by 61.3% at a non-cytotoxic concentration (10 µg/mL, corresponding to 14.4 µM of Kuwanon G), indicating that it is the most promising anti-tuberculosis constituent isolated from *M. nigra*.

Antimicrobial activity of *M. nigra* against *Candida* spp., the most common cause of fungal infections around the world [33], was assessed with aqueous and methanol extracts of its fruits, by using a disc-diffusion assay [34]. Of nine selected *Candida* spp., both extracts exhibited anticandidal effect against *Candida* (*C.*) *albicans*, *C. parapsilosis*, *C. tropicalis*, and *Geotricum candidum*, with lower MIC values observed for the methanol extract (0.625–2.5 mg/mL) than those for the aqueous extract (1.25–5 mg/mL).

5. Anti-Melanogenic (Skin-Whitening) Activity

Although melanin pigmentation in the skin is an important defense mechanism against ultraviolet radiation, abnormal melanin hyperpigmentation catalyzed by tyrosinase can cause several serious aesthetic problems [35–37]. As an anti-melanogenic strategy, tyrosinase inhibitors have become increasingly important for treating skin disorders associated with pigmentation and to improve skin-whitening.

Zhang et al. [38] investigated the inhibitory effect of 2,4,2',4'-tetrahydroxy-3-(3-methyl-2-butenyl)-chalcone (TMBC) isolated from the stem of *M. nigra* on tyrosinase activity and melanin biosynthesis. TMBC dose-dependently and competitively inhibited mushroom tyrosinase-mediated L-dopa oxidation (IC_{50} value 0.95 ± 0.04 µM), which was more potent than kojic acid (IC_{50} value 24.88 ± 1.13 µM), a well-known skin depigmenting agent. Furthermore, TMBC significantly reduced the melanin content and cellular tyrosinase activity in B16 melanoma cells, although it increased mRNA levels of cellular tyrosinase. Zheng et al. [39] screened tyrosinase inhibitory properties of a total of 29 constituents isolated from roots of *M. nigra*. Among them, nine compounds (5'-geranyl-5,7,2',4'-tetrahydroxyflavone, steppogenin-7-O-β-D-glucoside, 2,4,2',4'-tetrahydroxychalcone, moracin N, kuwanon H, mulberrofuran G, morachalcone A, oxyresveratrol-3'-O-β-D-glucopyranoside and oxyresveratrol-2-O-β-D-glucopyranoside) showed better tyrosinase inhibitory activities than kojic acid (IC_{50} value 46.95 ± 1.72 µM, with 2,4,2′,4′-tetrahydroxychalcone having the highest activity (IC_{50} value 0.062 ± 0.002 µM, 757-fold lower IC_{50} than kojic acid). More recently, de Freitas et al. [40] reported that five different batches of standardized ethanolic extracts of *M. nigra* leaves all exhibited tyrosinase inhibitory activities, with IC_{50} ranging from 5.00 to 8.49 µg/mL.

Koyu et al. [41] tested the microwave-assisted extraction of fresh fruits of *M. nigra* in variable conditions for optimizing and maximizing tyrosinase inhibitory activity. Consequently, the highest tyrosinase inhibitory activity (IC_{50} value 1.44 mg/mL) was observed in the optimum microwave extraction system yielding the highest amount of anthocyanin content (13.28 mg/g cyanidin-3-glucoside equivalent), suggesting the important potential of anthocyanins on tyrosinase inhibition.

6. Antidiabetic and Anti-Obesity Activity

Diabetes mellitus is a chronic endocrine disorder characterized by hyperglycemia related to metabolic impairment of insulin production, secretion, and/or utilization. It is closely associated with the development of several important complications in cardiovascular, neurological and renal systems that can lead to increased morbidity and mortality in diabetic patients [42]. Various classes of antihyperglycemic agents are now available. However, some undesirable adverse effects such as hypoglycemia, gastrointestinal symptoms, weight gain and hepato-renal toxicity caused by the administration of these medications have been arousing interests on the discovery of new effective and safer naturally-occurring antidiabetic agents with different therapeutic pathophysiological mechanisms and targets [43–45].

M. nigra has also shown good antidiabetic effects on extracts and active constituents from some parts of this plant. Abd El-Mawla et al. [46] investigated the hypoglycemic efficacy of *M. nigra* leaf extracts and its cell suspension cultures treated with methyl jasmonate to induce accumulation of flavonoid contents in cell cultures. Extracts from *M. nigra* leaves dose-dependently decreased plasma glucose concentrations and increased insulin levels up to 500 mg/kg/day in streptozotocin (STZ)-treated diabetic rats. In addition, a slightly higher hypoglycemic effect was observed when rats were treated with extracts from cultured cells, indicating the additive action of flavonoids induced by methyl jasmonate. Hydroethanolic extracts of *M. nigra* leaves also significantly decreased serum fasting and 2-h glucose concentrations (at dose of 50 mg/kg) and increased serum insulin level (at dose of 10 mg/kg) in nicotinamide-STZ-induced type 2 diabetic rats [47]. Diabetes-induced changes in blood vessels may enhance the pathophysiological activity of metalloproteinases (MMPs). It is known that the inhibition of MMPs can improve insulin resistance and oxidative stress [48,49]. Araujo et al. [49] demonstrated the hypoglycemic potential of *M. nigra* leaves via reduction of expression and activity of MMP-2 in livers of diabetic rats. In addition, several phenolic compounds and isoprenylated flavonoids isolated from extracts of *M. nigra* twigs showed good antidiabetic activities, involving mechanisms of peroxisome proliferators-activated receptor gamma (PPARγ) activation [50] and α-glucosidase inhibition [51]. On the other hand, 3-week treatment of aqueous extract of *M. nigra* leaves failed to affect serum glucose levels in non-diabetic or diabetic pregnant rats [52].

Although there is no published report on the antidiabetic activity of black mulberry fruit yet, its effects on obesity, associated with increased risk of many chronic adverse health effects including cardiovascular diseases, dyslipidemia, non-alcoholic hepatic disease, cancer, and type 2 diabetes [53,54] have been evaluated by Fabroni et al. [55]. They demonstrated that 80% hydroethanolic freeze-dried extract of fruits of *M. nigra* had moderate total anthocyanin and total phenolic contents, with an IC_{50} value for pancreatic lipase inhibition at 6.32 ± 0.01 mg/mL.

7. Anti-Hyperlipidemic and Anti-Atherosclerotic Activity

Cholesterol is a lipid molecule that acts as a structural component of cell membrane modulating fluidity and permeability, and as a precursor for steroid hormone and bile acid synthesis [56]. At the same time, hypercholesterolemia, a typical type of hyperlipidemia characterized by excessive accumulation of cholesterol in serum, is one of the crucial risk factors for coronary heart disease and atherosclerotic progression [57]. It has also been reported that reduction of low-density lipoprotein cholesterol (LDL-C) and improvement in levels of high-density lipoprotein cholesterol (HDL-C) can contribute to the anti-atherogenic condition [58,59].

Results from biochemical profile studies conducted by Volpato et al. [52] and Mahmoud [60] demonstrated that *M. nigra* extracts can decrease total cholesterol, triglyceride, LDL-C, and very low-density lipoprotein cholesterol (VLDL-C) levels and increase HDL-C in diabetic pregnant rats [52] and rats fed a high-fat diet [60]. Zeni et al. [61] evaluated the lipid-lowering effect of *M. nigra* leaf extract using Triton WR-1339-induced hyperlipidemic rats. The LDL-C level had significantly decreased after treatment with 100 mg/kg *M. nigra* infusion extract and HDL-C levels were restored in all groups treated with *M. nigra* extract at three different concentrations (100, 200 and 400 mg/kg), compared to those in the group only treated with Triton WR-1339. Atherogenic index and cardiac risk factor, indicators of likelihood of cardiovascular diseases associated with hyperlipidemia, were also decreased by *M. nigra* leaf extract. In another study by Jiang et al. [62], a high dose (210 mg/kg) of ethanolic extract of *M. nigra* fruit (EEBM) resulted in lowering mean body weight in rats fed a 6-week high-fat diet, which is comparable to the effect observed in the group treated with 5 mg/kg simvastatin. EEBM also dose-dependently improved serum lipid profiles, atherosclerosis indexes and lipid peroxidation compared to the control (high-fat diet-induced hyperlipidemic model) group. Histopathological changes in rat liver and thoracic aorta with reduction in the intima-media thickness of rat aortic arch after treatment with EEBM suggest that *M. nigra* fruit can effectively suppress the development and deterioration of atherosclerosis.

8. Organ-Protective Activity

8.1. Neuroprotective Effect

Turgut et al. [63] investigated the effect of *M. nigra* leaves extract on D-galactose-induced cognitive impairment and oxidative stress in mice. The results from the Morris water maze test showed significant and dose-dependent decreases in mean escape latency and time required to reach the target quadrant. Time spent in the target quadrant and number of times crossed the platform location were increased after the administration of lyophilized *M. nigra* extract, suggesting its potential neuroprotective role by preventing D-galactose-induced learning dysfunction and memory loss. *M. nigra* extract also showed DNA damage protection, reduced malondialdehyde (MDA) levels and augmented activities of three anti-oxidant enzymes, superoxide dismutase (SOD), glutathione peroxidase (GPx), and catalase (CAT) in the serum, brain and liver of D-galactose-treated mice. These antioxidant and anti-aging properties are considered as one of key mechanisms of *M. nigra* in delaying neurodegenerative processes.

Dalmagro et al. [64] performed a forced swimming test (FST) and tail suspension test (TST) to evaluate antidepressant-like activities of *M. nigra* and its major phenolic compounds syringic acid in mice. Acute and subchronic oral administration of aqueous extract of *M. nigra* leaves significantly decreased the immobility time in FST and TST except for acute administration at a dose of 100 mg/kg extract in TST. Acute treatment with 1 mg/kg and 10 mg/kg and subchronic treatment with 1 mg/kg of syringic acid also significantly decreased immobility time in TST. Nitro-oxidative stress in the serum and brain was assessed by measuring thiobarbituric acid reactive substances (TBARS), nitrite, protein carbonyl content (PC) and non-protein thiol groups (NPSH) levels, with some inconsistent and controversial study results. A significant decrease of TBARS level was observed at acute doses of 3 mg/kg *M. nigra* extract. However, TBARS levels were oppositely increased at subchronic doses of 3, 10, and 100 mg/kg extract in the serum and at a subchronic dose of 3 mg/kg extract in the brain. Levels of nitrites in the serum were significantly decreased after subchronic administration of 10, 30 and 100 mg/kg extracts of *M. nigra* leaves, and nitrites in the brain were also decreased after subchronic treatment with the extract at doses of 30 and 100 mg/kg. In addition, subchronic treatment with 1 mg/kg syringic acid resulted in significant changes in TBARS and nitrite levels in the serum and brain (all decreased, except TBARS level was increased in the brain). PC level was decreased after treatment with 30 mg/kg *M. nigra* extract and syringic acid. There was no significant change in NPSH level at all treatment conditions. Nevertheless, *M. nigra* leaf extract and syringic acid both exhibited good cell viabilities in hippocampal and cerebral cortex slices incubated with 100 mM glutamate, suggesting their proper neuroprotective effect against glutamate-induced toxicity.

8.2. Hepatoprotective Effect

Tag et al. [65] evaluated the hepatoprotective effect of the ethanolic extract of *M. nigra* leaves. With an IC_{50} value at 14.5 µg/mL in in vitro cytotoxicity to HepG2 (a well-differentiated human hepatocellular carcinoma) cell line, *M. nigra* leaf extract also significantly decreased levels of liver enzymes alanine aminotransaminase (ALT), aspartate aminotransaminase (AST), alkaline phosphatase (ALP), and lactate dehydrogenase (LDH) in male albino rats with methotrexate-induced hepatotoxicity. Hematosomatic index, defined as the ratio between liver- and body-weight and considered as an indicator for hepatic damage and liver inflammation, in the group co-treated with *M. nigra* extract and methotrexate, was also apparently decreased compared to that in methotrexate-only treated group. In histopathological studies, *M. nigra* treatment resulted in moderate enhancement in the hepatoprotection from methotrexate-related injury. Microscopic damage scores (hepatocyte degeneration, congestion, leukocyte infiltration, fibrosis, and total histopathology score) were significantly decreased when *M. nigra* extract was simultaneously administered compared to those in the group treated with methotrexate alone. In addition, methotrexate-induced progressive increases in collagen deposition of liver tissue were normalized by treatment with *M. nigra* leaf extract. Another study performed by Hassanalilou et al. [66] also showed that *M. nigra* leaf extract can lead to less fatty degeneration in liver tissue and smaller distension of hepatic cytoplasm due to fatty droplets in STZ-induced diabetic rats along with reduced fasting blood glucose, compared to glibenclamide, a well-known sulfonylurea antihyperglycemic agent.

Hepatoprotective activity of *M. nigra* fruits in carbon tetrachloride (CCl_4, a well-known potent hepatotoxin)-treated HepG2 cells [67] and adult male Sprague-Dawley rats [68] have been reported. Extracts of *M. nigra* fruits dose-dependently and significantly reduced levels of hepatic enzymes AST, ALT and gamma-glutamyl transferase (GGT) compared to control (CCl_4-treated group). At the same time, they significantly increased SOD and gluatathione peroxidase (GPx) enzymatic capacities and decreased expression levels and activities hepatic capsase-3 (a biomarker for cell apoptosis) and 8-oxo-2'-deoxyguanosine (a biomarker for oxidative stress) in rat liver tissues, indicating that the hepatoprotective effect of *M. nigra* fruits might be closely associated with its antioxidant activity [67,68].

8.3. Renal-Protective Effect

The effects of hydroalcoholic extract of *M. nigra* fruits on biochemical and histopathological changes in serum and kidney tissues have been evaluated in alloxan-induced diabetic rats [69]. Milder glomerular damage and no mesenchymal tissue expansion into renal glomerular vessels were observed in the group after 8 weeks of treatment with 800 mg/kg *M. nigra* fruit extract compared to those in diabetic and positive control (150 mg/kg metformin) groups. Although an increase in serum creatinine level was observed in the group treated with 800 mg/kg *M. nigra* extract, this group had lower serum glucose and urea levels compared to diabetic and positive control groups. These results suggest that *M. nigra* fruits have a protective effect on diabetic nephropathy and related kidney tissue injury. The extract of *M. nigra* leaves also significantly improved biochemical parameters reflecting kidney functions (serum creatinine, urea, and uric acid) and exhibited milder histopathological glycogen accumulation, fatty degeneration, and lymphocyte infiltration of renal convoluted tubules in STZ-induced diabetic rats compared to non-treated and glibenclamide-treated groups [66].

8.4. Gastroprotective Effect

Nesello et al. [70] reported that oral administration of methanolic extract from *M. nigra* fruits at a high dose (300 mg/kg) can protect gastric mucosa against acidified ethanol-induced acute gastric ulcer in female mice. This study result was confirmed by macroscopic and microscopic representative images, showing that the degree of epithelial damage in gastric tissue was decreased. To further investigate the underlying mechanisms for the gastroprotective effect, levels of lipid hydroperoxide (LOOH) and glutathione (GSH) in ulcerated gastric mucosa were quantified. *M. nigra* fruits extract prevented GSH depletion and promoted partial reduction of LOOH, suggesting its ability to ameliorate oxidative stress involved in the development of gastric injury by acidified ethanol. Because *M. nigra* fruits did not affect the activity of H^+/K^+-ATPase in their study, they have pharmacological advantages of being free from the risk of several side effects such as rebound acid hypersecretion, hypergastrinemia, gastric polyps, or atrophic gastritis [71] known to be associated with suppressed gastric acid secretion.

9. Activity on Female Reproductive System

De Queiroz et al. [72] investigated the estrogenic effect of *M. nigra* on the female reproductive system and embryonic development. Five different concentrations (25, 50, 75, 350, and 700 mg/kg) of hydroalcoholic extract of dried *M. nigra* leaves were administered in female Wistar rats for 15 days and their biological and clinical features were compared with the control group, in which distilled water instead of *M. nigra* extract was used as treatment. There were no significant differences in the number of deaths, clinical signs of toxicity, changes in food consumption, or body weight between groups, suggesting that *M. nigra* leaves did not cause maternal reproductive toxicity. Histological changes in ovarian structures, signs of edema, cystic follicles, retained oocytes, or thickened uterine epithelium were not observed. The number of corpora lutea, live fetuses, implants, resorptions, implantation, and pre- or post-implantation loss were not affected by the administration of *M. nigra* leaf extract either. Consequently, *M. nigra* exhibited no estrogenic effect or toxicity on the female reproductive system.

Another study conducted by Cavalcante et al. [73] showed that ethanolic extract of *M. nigra* fresh leaves at 0.1 mg/mL can improve percentages of follicular morphology, antrum formation, and fully grown oocytes, as well as the diameter of follicles compared to control group at 12 days after treatment. Furthermore, additive effects on follicular growth (described as follicular diameter increase and higher daily growth rate) were observed when *M. nigra* extract with supplemented medium and follicle-stimulating hormone (FSH) were used as co-treatment, indicating its capacity on ovine secondary follicle development.

10. Anticancer Activity

Cancer is a life-threatening disease state characterized by unregulated and permanent cell growth and proliferation [74]. Because of its ability to avoid programmed cell death (apoptosis) as one of the main driving forces for maintaining cancer cell proliferation, induction of apoptosis in cancer has been considered a reasonable strategy to treat cancer [75,76].

Morniga M, a mannose-specific jacalin-related lectin from the bark of *M. nigra*, can preferentially trigger the proliferation and activation of human T- and natural killer- (NK-)lymphocytes and dose-dependently induce cell death of α-CD3 activated T lymphocytes when compared with concanavalin A (Con A), a well-known mannose-specific legume leptin from *Canavalia ensiformis* [77]. Results from flow cytometry analysis have demonstrated that morniga M-induced cell death is probably associated with the apoptotic mechanism, suggesting the anticancer potential of morniga M via cell-death induction and immunomodulation as reported in previous studies with Con A [78,79]. Anticancer activities of morniga M were further investigated by Çakıroğlu et al. [80], in which they demonstrated that both *M. nigra* fruit extract and morniga M significantly and dose-dependently decreased cell viability against HT-29 cell line (human colorectal cancer). Another brief research by Qadir et al. [81] the demonstrated dose-dependent anticancer activity of n-hexane and aqueous methanol extract of *M. nigra* leaves against HeLa cell line (human cervical cancer), with IC_{50} values of 185.9 ± 8.3 µg/mL and 56.0 ± 1.7 µg/mL, respectively.

Anti-proliferative and apoptotic effects of *M. nigra* fruits against several human adenocarcinoma cell lines have been reported [80,82,83]. Ahmed et al. [82] compared the anticancer effects between fresh and dried fruit extracts of *M. nigra* on MCF-7 cell line (human breast cancer). Study results have shown that both ethanolic extracts dose- and time-dependently inhibit cellular growth of MCF-7 cells; exhibit apoptotic morphological changes in their cytoplasmic membranes, cell bodies, and nuclei; induce DNA fragmentations and single strand breaks; and decrease mitotic indexes, with better pharmacological properties in fresh fruit of *M. nigra*. Turan et al. [83] evaluated the anticancer activities of *M. nigra* fruit extract on PC-3 cells (human prostate cancer). Dimethyl sulfoxide (DMSO) extract of *M. nigra* exhibited moderate cytotoxicity against PC-3 cells with an IC_{50} value of 370.1 ± 5.8 µg/mL. It significantly increased the cell number at G_0/G_1 phase and decreased the cell number at S phase, indicating that *M. nigra* fruits inhibited the progression of the cell cycle at the G_0/G_1 phase. *M. nigra* fruit extract at a high dose (666 µg/mL) significantly increased the number of necrotic, early apoptotic and late apoptotic cells compared to the untreated control group. It also dose-dependently decreased mitochondrial membrane potential and increased activities of caspase 3 and 7 (key mediators of apoptosis) in PC-3 cells [83].

11. Antioxidant Activity

Oxidative stress is characterized by an excessive increase in intracellular oxidizing species such as reactive oxygen species (ROS) involved in the loss of antioxidant defense capacity. It plays a critical role in various clinical conditions including aging, cancer, diabetes, atherosclerosis, chronic inflammation, neurodegenerative diseases, rheumatoid arthritis, human immunodeficiency virus (HIV) infection, ischemia and reperfusion injury, and obstructive sleep apnea [84,85]. Many researchers are interested in the antioxidant activity of naturally-occurring ingredients because phenolic compounds and flavonoids, the largest phytochemical molecules from natural resources, possess a variety of biological properties including antioxidant activity [86–89]. It has also been widely reported that mulberries are rich in anthocyanin constituents having remarkable antioxidant activities and other health benefits such as anti-inflammatory, antimicrobial, anti-obesity, antidiabetic, anti-hyperlipidemic, antihypertensive, cardioprotective (reduced risk of coronary heart disease and stroke), and anticancer effects [90–92].

Numerous researches have proven antioxidant properties of *M. nigra* with different in vitro methods, including DPPH (2,2-diphenyl-1-picrylhydrazyl) radical scavenging assay [15,23–26,28,61,70,93–113], ABTS (2,2'-azino-bis(3-ethylbenzothiazoline)-6-sulfonic acid) radical scavenging assay [15,91,94,99–103, 107,110,112–117], reducing power assay [15,99,113,118,119], superoxide anion radical (O_2^-) scavenging assay [15,118,120], hydroxyl radical (OH-) scavenging assay [15,113,120], lipid peroxidation assay [19, 52,60,62–64,70,121,122], antioxidant enzyme activity assay [21,49,52,62,63,67], β-carotene bleaching assay [23,119,123], ferric-reducing antioxidant power (FRAP) assay [24,85,91,95,100,102,104,107,110,111], protein carbonyl assay [49,64,96], GSH measurement [67,70,112], hydrogen peroxide ($H2O2$)-induced injury assay [113,121], NO radical scavenging assay [111,118], SOD-like activity [96], cupric-ion reducing antioxidant capacity (CUPRAC) assay [102,107,108,110], H_2O_2 scavenging assay [108,119], phosphomolybdenum assay [108,119], and ROS measurement [112].

12. Other Pharmacological Activities

Malik et al. [124] investigated the cardiovascular activity of aqueous methanolic extract of *M. nigra* fruit in frogs. Treatment of *M. nigra* fruit extract showed significant and dose-dependent decreases in heart rate without direct effects on the contractility of frog's heart. Results of phytochemical analysis revealed the presence of cardiac glycosides in *M. nigra* fruit, along with other active constituents including saponins, alkaloids, phenolic compounds, and flavonoids.

Crude extract and fractions of *M. nigra* fruits exhibit both in vitro and in vivo prokinetic, laxative, and antidiarrheal effects [125]. *M. nigra* extract significantly promoted the transit of charcoal meal through the small intestine, increased gastric emptying rate and the mean number of wet feces, and decreased castor oil-induced diarrhea in mice. In in vitro studies, chloroform and petroleum ether fractions of *M. nigra* fruits dose-dependently inhibited carbachol- and potassium ion-induced contractions of rabbit jejunum while aqueous and ethyl acetate fractions showed stimulatory effects on guinea-pig ileum. Suppression of maximum responses of acetylcholine and calcium ion (Ca^{2+}) by *M. nigra* fruits was also observed, and most gastrointestinal effects were conversely affected by concomitant administration of atropine, suggesting that the underlying mechanisms of these prokinetic, laxative, and antidiarrheal activities might be associated with cholinergic control and Ca^{2+} channel antagonism [125].

Fahimi and Jahromy [126] described the effects of *M. nigra* fruit juice on levodopa-induced dyskinesia in mice with 1-methyl-4-phenyl-1,2,3,6-tetrahydropyridine (MPTP)-induced Parkinson's disease. After 14 days of levodopa treatment, administration of 10 or 15 mL/kg of *M. nigra* fruit juice significantly decreased abnormal involuntary movement scale (AIMS) scores compared to levodopa treatment only.

13. Drug-Food Interaction and Toxicity

Food ingredients can cause drug-food interactions, most of which are pharmacokinetic interactions associated with the alteration in activities of drug-metabolizing enzymes or drug transporters [127]. A brief experimental report by Kim et al. [128] demonstrated that the fruit juice of *M. nigra* has a potent inhibitory effect of human liver microsomal cytochrome P450 3A (CYP3A) activity, with IC_{50} values for midazolam (a probe drug for CYP3A) 1'-hydroxylation of 2.96 ± 0.33% (v/v, with 20-min preincubation) and 6.22 ± 0.47% (no preincubation). Because approximately 30% of clinically used drugs including macrolide antibiotics, antiarrhythmics, benzodiazepines, immune modulators, human immunodeficiency virus (HIV) antivirals, antihistamines, calcium channel blockers, and statins are metabolized by CYP3A [129,130], concomitant intake of CYP3A substrates with *M. nigra* fruit can lead to an increase in plasma drug exposure.

Figueredo et al. [131] assessed the acute and subacute toxicities of *M. nigra* leaves extract in Wistar rats. A single or 28-day oral dose of ethanolic extract of *M. nigra* leaves did not cause any adverse effects. It did not induce abnormal behaviors or mortality. *M. nigra* extract resulted in some significant but non-toxic changes in biochemical profiles (decreased urea and AST in males; decreased total cholesterol and AST in females) and leukocyte parameters (increased neutrophils in males; decreased white blood cell in females). *M. nigra* leaves did not affect lipid peroxidation and changes in renal and hepatic CAT enzymatic activities.

Table 1. Summary of major biological and pharmacological therapeutic activities of *M. nigra*.

Pharmacological Activity	Study Model	Used Part	SampleType [a]	Ref.
Antinociceptive	Swiss mice	Root bark	C	[10]
	Male Swiss mice	Leaf	E	[14]
	Male Kunming mice	Fruit	E	[15]
	Male Kunming mice	Fruit	E,C	[16]
Anti-inflammatory	Kunming male mice; RAW 264.7 cell	Fruit	E	[15]
	Adult male rats	Leaf	E	[18]
	Rat polymorphonuclear leukocytes	Bark	C	[19]
	THP-1 human monocytic leukemia cell line	Root	C	[20]
	Male C57BL/6 mice	Pulp; leaf	E	[21]
Antimicrobial	In vitro assay	Fruit	E	[16]
	In vitro assay	Leaf	E,F	[22]
	In vitro assay	Leaf	E,F	[23]
	In vitro assay	Fruit	J	[24]
	In vitro assay	Fruit	E	[25]
	In vitro assay	Fruit	E	[26]
	In vitro assay	Stem bark; fruit; leaf	E	[27]
	In vitro assay	Stem bark; stem wood	E,C	[28]
	In vitro assay; THP-1 cell line	Root	E,C	[32]
	In vitro assay	Fruit	E	[34]

Table 1. *Cont.*

Pharmacological Activity	Study Model	Used Part	SampleType [a]	Ref.
Anti-melanogenic (Skin-whitening)	In vitro assay; B16 melanoma cells	Stem	C	[38]
	In vitro assay	Root; twig	C	[39]
	In vitro assay	Leaf	E	[40]
	In vitro assay	Fruit	E	[41]
Antidiabetic	Male Wistar rats	Leaf	E [b]	[46]
	Male albino mice	Leaf	E	[47]
	Female albino Fischer rats	Pulp; leaf	E	[49]
	PPARγ-transfected HEK293 cells	Twig	C	[50]
	In vitro assay	Twig	C	[51]
Anti-obesity	In vitro assay	Fruit	E	[55]
Anti-hyperlipidemic	Wistar rats	Leaf	E	[52]
	Adult male albino Sprague-Dawley rats	Fruit	E	[60]
	Male Wistar rats	Leaf	E	[61]
	Male Sprague-Dawley rats	Fruit	E	[62]
Organ-protective	Male BALB/c mice	Leaf	E	[63]
	Male Swiss mice	Leaf	E,C	[64]
	HepG2 human hepatocellular carcinoma cell line; male albino rats	Leaf	E	[65]
	Male Wistar rats	Leaf	E	[66]
	HepG2 cells	Fruit	E	[67]
	Adult male Sprague-Dawley rats	Fruit	E	[68]
	Male Wistar rats	Fruit	E	[69]
	Female Swiss mice	Fruit	E	[70]
Anticancer	Peripheral blood mononuclear cells (PBMCs); peripheral blood T lymphocytes; Jurkat T leukemia cells	Bark	C	[77]
	HT-29 human colorectal adenocarcinoma cell line	Fruit	E,C	[80]
	HeLa human cervical cancer cell line	Leaf	E	[81]
	MCF-7 human breast cancer cell line	Fruit	E	[82]
	PC-3 human prostate adenocarcinoma cells	Fruit	E	[83]

[a], E, extract; F, fraction; C, isolated compound; J, juice. [b], Cell suspension cultures of *M. nigra* extract were used.

14. Conclusions

M. nigra, especially its leaf and fruit parts, exhibited various pharmacological properties including antinociceptive, anti-inflammatory, antimicrobial, anti-melanogenic, antidiabetic, anti-obesity, anti-hyperlipidemic, and anticancer activities. *M. nigra* also showed protective and therapeutic effects on the central nervous system, liver, kidney, gastrointestinal tract, and female reproductive system. Most of these features were attributable to its antioxidant capacity due to abundant phytochemical constituents such as polyphenols, flavonoids and anthocyanins. These findings suggest that *M. nigra* can be used as a promising nutraceutical resource to control and prevent various chronic diseases. Given that most researches are performed in vitro and in animal models, further studies at the clinical level are required to establish the efficacy and safety of *M. nigra* in the human body.

Author Contributions: S.H.L. was responsible for collecting and summarizing literature data. C.-I.C. wrote and edited the manuscript.

Funding: This research was supported by Basic Science Research Program through the National Research Foundation of Korea (NRF) funded by the Ministry of Education (No. 2016R1D1A1B03933963).

Conflicts of Interest: The authors declare no conflict of interest.

References

1. Hussain, F.; Rana, Z.; Shafique, H.; Malik, A.; Hussain, Z. Phytopharmacological potential of different species of *Morus alba* and their bioactive phytochemicals: A review. *Asian Pac. J. Trop. Biomed.* **2017**, *7*, 950–956. [CrossRef]
2. Vijayan, K.; Chauhan, S.; Das, N.K.; Chakraborti, S.P.; Roy, B.N. Leaf yield component combining abilities in mulberry (*Morus* spp.). *Euphytica* **1997**, *98*, 47–52. [CrossRef]
3. Natić, M.M.; Dabić, D.Č.; Papetti, A.; Fotirić Akšić, M.M.; Ognjanov, V.; Ljubojević, M.; Tešić, Ž. Analysis and characterisation of phytochemicals in mulberry (*Morus alba* L.) fruits grown in Vojvodina, North Serbia. *Food Chem.* **2014**, *171*, 128–136. [CrossRef] [PubMed]
4. Sánchez-Salcedo, E.M.; Sendra, E.; Carbonell-Barrachina, Á.A.; Martínez, J.J.; Hernández, F. Fatty acids composition of Spanish black (*Morus nigra* L.) and white (*Morus alba* L.) mulberries. *Food Chem.* **2016**, *190*, 566–571. [CrossRef] [PubMed]
5. Wei, H.; Zhu, J.J.; Liu, X.Q.; Feng, W.H.; Wang, Z.M.; Yan, L.H. Review of bioactive compounds from root barks of *Morus* plants (Sang-Bai-Pi) and their pharmacological effects. *Cogent. Chem.* **2016**, *2*, 1212320. [CrossRef]
6. Yang, Y.; Tan, Y.X.; Chen, R.Y.; Kang, J. The latest review on the polyphenols and their bioactivities of Chinese *Morus* plants. *J. Asian Nat. Prod. Res.* **2014**, *16*, 690–702. [CrossRef] [PubMed]
7. Chan, E.W.; Lye, P.Y.; Wong, S.K. Phytochemistry, pharmacology, and clinical trials of *Morus alba*. *Chin. J. Nat. Med.* **2016**, *14*, 17–30.
8. Gryn-Rynko, A.; Bazylak, G.; Olszewska-Slonina, D. New potential phytotherapeutics obtained from white mulberry (*Morus alba* L.) leaves. *Biomed. Pharmacother.* **2016**, *84*, 628–636. [CrossRef]
9. Budiman, A.; Sulastri, A.; Alfauziah, T.Q. Chemical compounds and pharmacological activity of *Morus nigra* as a potential product of drug: A review. *Int. Res. J. Pharm.* **2018**, *9*, 76–81. [CrossRef]
10. De Souza, M.M.; Bittar, M.; Cechinel-Filho, V.; Yunes, R.A.; Messana, I.; Delle Monache, F.; Ferrari, F. Antinociceptive properties of morusin, a prenylflavonoid isolated from *Morus nigra* root bark. *Z. Naturforsch. C.* **2000**, *55*, 256–260. [CrossRef]
11. Nomura, T.; Fukai, T.; Yamada, S.; Katayanagi, M. Studies on the constituents of the cultivated mulberry tree. I. Three new prenylflavones from the root bark of *Morus alba* L. *Chem. Pharm. Bull.* **1978**, *26*, 1394–1402. [CrossRef]
12. Ko, H.H.; Yu, S.M.; Ko, F.N.; Teng, C.M.; Lin, C.N. Bioactive constituents of *Morus australis* and *Broussonetia papyrifera*. *J. Nat. Prod.* **1997**, *60*, 1008–1011. [CrossRef] [PubMed]
13. Ryu, Y.B.; Ha, T.J.; Curtis-Long, M.J.; Ryu, H.W.; Gal, S.W.; Park, K.H. Inhibitory effects on mushroom tyrosinase by flavones from the stem barks of *Morus lhou* (S.) Koidz. *J. Enzyme Inhib. Med. Chem.* **2008**, *23*, 922–930. [CrossRef] [PubMed]
14. Padilha, M.M.; Vilela, F.C.; da Silva, M.J.; dos Santos, M.H.; Alves-da-Silva, G.; Giusti-Paiva, A. Antinociceptive Effect of the extract of *Morus nigra* leaves in mice. *J. Med. Food* **2009**, *12*, 1381–1385. [CrossRef] [PubMed]
15. Chen, H.; Pu, J.; Liu, D.; Yu, W.; Shao, Y.; Yang, G.; Xiang, Z.; He, N. Anti-Inflammatory and Antinociceptive Properties of Flavonoids from the Fruits of Black Mulberry (*Morus nigra* L.). *PLoS ONE* **2016**, *11*, e0153080. [CrossRef] [PubMed]
16. Chen, H.; Yu, W.; Chen, G.; Meng, S.; Xiang, Z.; He, N. Antinociceptive and Antibacterial Properties of Anthocyanins and Flavonols from Fruits of Black and Non-Black Mulberries. *Molecules* **2018**, *23*, 4. [CrossRef] [PubMed]
17. Chalons, P.; Amor, S.; Courtaut, F.; Cantos-Villar, E.; Richard, T.; Auger, C.; Chabert, P.; Schni-Kerth, V.; Aires, V.; Delmas, D. Study of Potential Anti-Inflammatory Effects of Red Wine Extract and Resveratrol through a Modulation of Interleukin-1-Beta in Macrophages. *Nutrients* **2018**, *10*, 1856. [CrossRef]
18. Padilha, M.M.; Vilela, F.C.; Rocha, C.Q.; Dias, M.J.; Soncini, R.; dos Santos, M.H.; Alves-da-Silva, G.; Giusti-Paiva, A. Antiinflammatory properties of *Morus nigra* leaves. *Phytother. Res.* **2010**, *24*, 1496. [CrossRef]
19. Wang, L.; Yang, Y.; Liu, C.; Chen, R.Y. Three new compounds from *Morus nigra* L. *J. Asian Nat. Prod. Res.* **2010**, *12*, 431–437. [CrossRef]

20. Zelová, H.; Hanáková, Z.; Čermáková, Z.; Šmejkal, K.; Dall' Acqua, S.; Babula, P.; Cvačka, J.; Hošek, J. Evaluation of anti-inflammatory activity of prenylated substances isolated from *Morus alba* and *Morus nigra*. *J. Nat. Prod.* **2014**, *77*, 1297–1303. [CrossRef]
21. De Pádua Lúcio, K.; Rabelo, A.C.S.; Araújo, C.M.; Brandão, G.C.; de Souza, G.H.B.; da Silva, R.G.; de Souza, D.M.S.; Talvani, A.; Bezerra, F.S.; Cruz Calsavara, A.J.; et al. Anti-Inflammatory and Antioxidant Properties of Black Mulberry (*Morus nigra* L.) in a Model of LPS-Induced Sepsis. *Oxid. Med. Cell Longev.* **2018**, *2018*, 5048031.
22. Tahir, L.; Aslam, A.; Ahmed, S. Antibacterial activities of *Diospyros blancoi*, *Phoenix dactylifera* and *Morus nigra* against dental caries causing pathogens: An in vitro study. *Pak. J. Pharm. Sci.* **2017**, *30*, 163–169. [PubMed]
23. Souza, G.R.; Oliveira-Junior, R.G.; Diniz, T.C.; Branco, A.; Lima-Saraiva, S.R.G.; Guimarães, A.L.; Oliveira, A.P.; Pacheco, A.G.M.; Silva, M.G.; Moraes-Filho, M.O.; et al. Assessment of the antibacterial, cytotoxic and antioxidant activities of *Morus nigra* L. (Moraceae). *Braz. J. Biol.* **2018**, *78*, 248–254. [CrossRef] [PubMed]
24. Khalid, N.; Fawad, S.A.; Ahmed, I. Antimicrobial activity, phytochemical profile and trace minerals of black mulberry (*Morus nigra* L.) fresh juice. *Pak. J. Bot.* **2011**, *43*, 91–96.
25. Minhas, M.A.; Begum, A.; Hamid, S.; Babar, M.; Ilyas, R.; Ali, S.; Latif, F.; Andleeb, S. Evaluation of Antibiotic and Antioxidant Activity of *Morus nigra* (Black Mulberry) Extracts Against Soil Borne, Food Borne and Clinical Human Pathogens. *Pak. J. Zool.* **2016**, *48*, 1381–1388.
26. Budiman, A.; Aulifa, D.L.; Kusuma, A.S.W.; Sulastri, A. Antibacterial and Antioxidant Activity of Black Mulberry (*Morus nigra* L.) Extract for Acne Treatment. *Pharmacogn. J.* **2017**, *9*, 611–614. [CrossRef]
27. Aulifa, D.L.; Fitriansyah, S.N.; Ardiansyah, S.A.; Wibowo, D.P.; Julata, Y.A.; Christy, D.S. Phytochemical Screening, Antibacterial Activity, and Mode of Action on *Morus nigra*. *Pharmacogn. J.* **2018**, *10*, 167–171. [CrossRef]
28. Mazimba, O.; Majinda, R.R.T.; Motlhanka, D. Antioxidant and antibacterial constituents from *Morus nigra*. *Afr. J. Pharm. Pharmacol.* **2011**, *5*, 751–754. [CrossRef]
29. Tuberculosis: WHO Fact Sheet No. 104. Available online: https://www.who.int/en/news-room/fact-sheets/detail/tuberculosis (accessed on 2 January 2019).
30. Sajid, A.; Arora, G.; Singhal, A.; Kalia, V.C.; Singh, Y. Protein Phosphatases of Pathogenic Bacteria: Role in Physiology and Virulence. *Annu. Rev. Microbiol.* **2015**, *69*, 527–547. [CrossRef]
31. Mascarello, A.; Chiaradia-Delatorre, L.D.; Mori, M.; Terenzi, H.; Botta, B. *Mycobacterium tuberculosis*-Secreted Tyrosine Phosphatases as Targets against Tuberculosis: Exploring Natural Sources in Searching for New Drugs. *Curr. Pharm. Des.* **2016**, *22*, 1561–1569. [CrossRef]
32. Mascarello, A.; Orbem Menegatti, A.C.; Calcaterra, A.; Martins, P.G.A.; Chiaradia-Delatorre, L.D.; D'Acquarica, I.; Ferrari, F.; Pau, V.; Sanna, A.; De Logu, A.; et al. Naturally occurring Diels-Alder-type adducts from *Morus nigra* as potent inhibitors of *Mycobacterium tuberculosis* protein tyrosinase phosphatase B. *Eur. J. Med. Chem.* **2018**, *144*, 277–288. [CrossRef] [PubMed]
33. Manolakaki, D.; Velmahos, G.; Kourkoumpetis, T.; Chang, Y.; Alam, H.B.; De Moya, M.M.; Mylonakis, E. *Candida* infection and colonization among trauma patients. *Virulence* **2010**, *1*, 367–375. [CrossRef] [PubMed]
34. Yiğit, N.; Yiğit, D.; Özgen, U.; Aktaş, A.E. Anticandidal activity of black mulberry (*Morus nigra* L.). *Türk. Mikrobiyol. Cem. Derg.* **2007**, *37*, 169–173.
35. Briganti, S.; Camera, E.; Picardo, M. Chemical and instrumental approaches to treat hyperpigmentation. *Pigment Cell Res.* **2003**, *16*, 101–110. [CrossRef] [PubMed]
36. Slominski, A.; Tobin, D.J.; Shibahara, S.; Wortsman, J. Melanin pigmentation in mammalian skin and its hormonal regulation. *Physiol. Rev.* **2004**, *84*, 1155–1228. [CrossRef] [PubMed]
37. Solano, F.; Briganti, S.; Picardo, M.; Ghanem, G. Hypopigmenting agents: An updated review on biological, chemical and clinical aspects. *Pigment Cell Res.* **2006**, *19*, 550–571. [CrossRef]
38. Zhang, X.; Hu, X.; Hou, A.; Wang, H. Inhibitory effect of 2,4,2',4'-tetrahydroxy-3-(3-methyl-2-butenyl)-chalcone on tyrosinase activity and melanin biosynthesis. *Biol. Pharm. Bull.* **2009**, *32*, 86–90. [CrossRef]
39. Zheng, Z.P.; Cheng, K.W.; Zhu, Q.; Wang, X.C.; Lin, Z.X.; Wang, M. Tyrosinase inhibitory constituents from the roots of *Morus nigra*: A structure-activity relationship study. *J. Agric. Food Chem.* **2010**, *58*, 5368–5373. [CrossRef]

40. De Freitas, M.M.; Fontes, P.R.; Souza, P.M.; William Fagg, C.; Neves Silva Guerra, E.; de Medeiros Nóbrega, Y.K.; Silveira, D.; Fonseca-Bazzo, Y.; Simeoni, L.A.; Homem-de-Mello, M.; et al. Extracts of *Morus nigra* L. Leaves Standardized in Chlorogenic Acid, Rutin and Isoquercitrin: Tyrosinase Inhibition and Cytotoxicity. *PLoS ONE* **2016**, *11*, e0163130. [CrossRef]
41. Koyu, H.; Kazan, A.; Demir, S.; Haznedaroglu, M.Z.; Yesil-Celiktas, O. Optimization of microwave assisted extraction of *Morus nigra* L. fruits maximizing tyrosinase inhibitory activity with isolation of bioactive constituents. *Food Chem.* **2018**, *248*, 183–191. [CrossRef]
42. Baynes, J.W. Role of oxidative stress in development of complications in diabetes. *Diabetes* **1991**, *40*, 405–412. [CrossRef] [PubMed]
43. Hung, H.Y.; Qian, K.; Norris-Natschke, S.L.; Hsu, C.S.; Lee, K.H. Recent discovery of plant-derived anti-diabetic natural products. *Nat. Prod. Rep.* **2012**, *29*, 580–606. [CrossRef] [PubMed]
44. Alkhalidy, H.; Wang, Y.; Liu, D. Dietary Flavonoids in the Prevention of T2D: An Overview. *Nutrients* **2018**, *10*, 438. [CrossRef] [PubMed]
45. Xu, L.; Li, Y.; Dai, Y.; Peng, J. Natural products for the treatment of type 2 diabetes mellitus: Pharmacology and mechanisms. *Pharmacol. Res.* **2018**, *130*, 451–465. [CrossRef] [PubMed]
46. Abd El-Mawla, A.M.; Mohamed, K.M.; Mostafa, A.M. Induction of Biologically Active Flavonoids in Cell Cultures of *Morus nigra* and Testing their Hypoglycemic Efficacy. *Sci. Pharm.* **2011**, *79*, 951–961. [CrossRef] [PubMed]
47. AbouZid, S.F.; Ahmed, O.M.; Ahmed, R.R.; Mahmoud, A.; Abdella, E.; Ashour, M.B. Antihyperglycemic effect of crude extracts of some Egyptian plants and algae. *J. Med. Food* **2014**, *17*, 400–406. [CrossRef] [PubMed]
48. Kłysik, A.B.; Naduk-Kik, J.; Hrabec, Z.; Goś, R.; Hrabec, E. Intraocular matrix metalloproteinase 2 and 9 in patients with diabetes mellitus with and without diabetic retinopathy. *Arch. Med. Sci.* **2010**, *6*, 375–381. [CrossRef] [PubMed]
49. Araujo, C.M.; Lúcio Kde, P.; Silva, M.E.; Isoldi, M.C.; de Souza, G.H.; Brandão, G.C.; Schulz, R.; Costa, D.C. *Morus nigra* leaf extract improves glycemic response and redox profile in the liver of diabetic rats. *Food Funct.* **2015**, *6*, 3490–3499. [CrossRef]
50. Xu, L.J.; Yu, M.H.; Huang, C.Y.; Niu, L.X.; Wang, Y.F.; Wu, C.Z.; Yang, P.M.; Hu, X. Isoprenylated flavonoids from *Morus nigra* and their PPAR γ agonistic activities. *Fitoterapia* **2018**, *127*, 109. [CrossRef]
51. Xu, L.; Yu, M.; Niu, L.; Huang, C.; Wang, Y.; Wu, C.; Yang, P.; Hu, X. Phenolic compounds isolated from *Morus nigra* and their α-glucosidase inhibitory activities. *Nat. Prod. Res.* **2018**. [CrossRef]
52. Volpato, G.T.; Calderson, I.M.P.; Sinzato, S.; Campos, K.E.; Rudge, M.V.C.; Damasceno, D.C. Effect of *Morus nigra* aqueous extract treatment on the maternal-fetal outcome, oxidative stress status and lipid profile of streptozotocin-induced diabetic rats. *J. Ethnopharmacol.* **2011**, *138*, 691–696. [CrossRef] [PubMed]
53. Jung, U.J.; Choi, M.S. Obesity and its metabolic complications: The role of adipokines and the relationship between obesity, inflammation, insulin resistance, dyslipidemia and nonalcoholic fatty liver disease. *Int. J. Mol. Sci.* **2014**, *15*, 6184–6223. [CrossRef] [PubMed]
54. Nakayama, H.; Shimada, Y.; Zang, L.; Terasawa, M.; Nishiura, K.; Matsuda, K.; Toombs, C.; Langdon, C.; Nishimura, N. Novel Anti-Obesity Properties of *Palmaria mollis* in Zebrafish and Mouse Models. *Nutrients* **2018**, *10*, 1401. [CrossRef] [PubMed]
55. Fabroni, S.; Ballistreri, G.; Amenta, M.; Romeo, F.V.; Rapisarda, P. Screening of the anthocyanin profile and in vitro pancreatic lipase inhibition by anthocyanin-containing extracts of fruits, vegetables, legumes and cereals. *J. Sci. Food Agric.* **2016**, *96*, 4713–4723. [CrossRef] [PubMed]
56. Bhagavan, N.V.; Ha, C.E. *Essentials of Medical Biochemistry*, 1st ed.; Academic Press: Cambridge, MA, USA, 2011; pp. 209–223.
57. Kannel, W.B.; Castelli, W.P.; Gordon, T. Choelsterol in the prediction of atherosclerotic disease: New perspectives based on the Framingham study. *Ann. Intern. Med.* **1979**, *90*, 85–91. [CrossRef] [PubMed]
58. Lusis, A.J. Atherosclerosis. *Nature* **2000**, *407*, 233–241. [CrossRef] [PubMed]
59. Assmann, G.; Nofer, J.R. Atheroprotective effects of high-density lipoproteins. *Annu. Rev. Med.* **2003**, *54*, 321–341. [CrossRef]
60. Mahmoud, M.Y. Natural antioxidants effect of mulberry fruits (*Morus nigra* and *Morus alba* L.) on lipids profile and oxidative stress in hypercholestrolemic rats. *Pak. J. Nutr.* **2013**, *12*, 665–672. [CrossRef]

61. Zeni, A.L.B.; Moreira, T.D.; Dalmagro, A.P.; Camargo, A.; Bini, L.A.; Simionatto, E.L.; Scharf, D.R. Evaluation of phenolic compounds and lipid-lowering effect of *Morus nigra* leaves extract. *An. Acad. Bras. Cienc.* **2017**, *89*, 2805–2815. [CrossRef]
62. Jiang, Y.; Dai, M.; Nie, W.J.; Yang, X.R.; Zeng, X.C. Effects of the ethanol extract of black mulberry (*Morus nigra* L.) fruit on experimental atherosclerosis in rats. *J. Ethnopharmacol.* **2017**, *200*, 228–235. [CrossRef]
63. Turgut, N.H.; Mert, D.G.; Kara, H.; Egilmez, H.R.; Arslanbas, E.; Tepe, B.; Gungor, H.; Yilmaz, N.; Tuncel, N.B. Effect of black mulberry (*Morus nigra*) extract treatment on cognitive impairment and oxidative stress status of D-galactose-induced aging mice. *Pharm. Biol.* **2016**, *54*, 1052–1064. [CrossRef] [PubMed]
64. Dalmagro, A.P.; Camargo, A.; Zeni, A.L.B. *Morus nigra* and its major phenolic, syringic acid, have antidepressant-like and neuroprotective effects in mice. *Metab. Brain Dis.* **2017**, *32*, 1963–1973. [CrossRef]
65. Tag, H.M. Hepatoprotective effect of mulberry (*Morus nigra*) leaves extract against methotrexate induced hepatotoxicity in male albino rat. *BMC Complement. Altern. Med.* **2015**, *15*, 252. [CrossRef] [PubMed]
66. Hassanalilou, T.; Payahoo, L.; Shahabi, P.; Abbasi, M.M.; Jafar-abadi, M.A.; Bishak, Y.K.; Khordadmehr, M.; Esnaashari, S.; Barzegar, A. The protective effects of *Morus nigra* L. leaves on the kidney function tests and kidney and liver histological structures in streptozotocin-induced diabetic rats. *Biomed. Res.* **2017**, *28*, 6113–6118.
67. Youssef, F.S.; Labib, R.M.; Eldahshan, O.A.; Singab, A.N.B. Synergistic Hepatoprotective and Antioxidant Effect of Artichoke, Fig, Blackberry Herbal Mixture on HepG2 Cells and Their Metabolic Profiling Using NMR Coupled with Chemometrics. *Chem. Biodivers.* **2017**, *14*, e1700206. [CrossRef] [PubMed]
68. Deniz, G.Y.; Laloglu, E.; Koc, K.; Nadaroglu, H.; Geyikoglu, F. The effect of black mulberry (*Morus nigra*) extract on carbon tetrachloride-induced liver damage. *Arch. Biol. Sci.* **2018**, *70*, 371–378. [CrossRef]
69. Rahimi-Madiseh, M.; Naimi, A.; Heydarian, E.; Rafieian-Kopaei, M. Renal biochemical and histopathological alterations of diabetic rats under treatment with hydro alcoholic *Morus nigra* extract. *J. Renal Inj. Prev.* **2016**, *6*, 56–60. [CrossRef] [PubMed]
70. Nesello, L.A.N.; Beleza, M.L.M.L.; Mariot, M.; Mariano, L.N.B.; de Souza, P.; Campos, A.; Cechinel-Filho, V.; Andrade, S.F.; da Silva, L.M. Gastroprotective Value of Berries: Evidences from Methanolic Extracts of *Morug nigra* and *Rubus niveus* Fruits. *Gastroenterol. Res. Pract.* **2017**, 7089697. [CrossRef] [PubMed]
71. Park, H.W.; Jung, H.Y. Safety profile of acid suppression with proton pump inhibitors. *Korean J. Helicobacter Up. Gastrointest. Res.* **2009**, *9*, 11–17.
72. De Queiroz, G.T.; Santos, T.R.; Macedo, R.; Peters, V.M.; Leite, M.N.; de Cássia da Silveira e Sá, R.; de Oliveira Guerra, M. Efficacy of *Morus nigra* L. on reproduction in female Wistar rats. *Food Chem. Toxicol.* **2012**, *50*, 816–822. [CrossRef] [PubMed]
73. Cavalcante, A.; Lins, T.; Santos, J.; Barros, V.; Monte, A.; Barberino, R.S.; Almeida, J.; Matos, M. Supplemented *Morus nigra* extract-based medium associated with FSH enables the survival and growth of isolated ovine secondary ovarian follicles. *Reprod. Domest. Anim.* **2018**, *53*, 423–432. [CrossRef] [PubMed]
74. Hsu, P.P.; Sabatini, D.M. Cancer cell metabolism: Warburg and beyond. *Cell* **2008**, *134*, 703–707. [CrossRef] [PubMed]
75. Fisher, D.E. Apoptosis in cancer therapy: Crossing the threshold. *Cell* **1994**, *78*, 539–542. [CrossRef]
76. Brown, J.M.; Attardi, L.D. The role of apoptosis in cancer development and treatment response. *Nat. Rev. Cancer* **2005**, *5*, 231–237. [CrossRef] [PubMed]
77. Benoist, H.; Culerrier, R.; Poiroux, G.; Ségui, B.; Jauneau, A.; Van Damme, E.J.; Peumans, W.J.; Barre, A.; Rougé, P. Two structurally identical mannose-specific jacalin-related lectins display different effects on human T lymphocyte activation and cell death. *J. Leukoc. Biol.* **2009**, *86*, 103–114. [CrossRef] [PubMed]
78. Miyagi, T.; Takehara, T.; Tatsumi, T.; Suzuki, T.; Jinushi, M.; Kanazawa, Y.; Hiramatsu, N.; Kanto, T.; Tsuji, S.; Hori, M.; et al. Concanavalin a injection activates intrahepatic innate immune cells to provoke an antitumor effect in murine liver. *Hepatology* **2004**, *40*, 1190–1196. [CrossRef] [PubMed]
79. Amin, A.R.; Paul, R.K.; Thakur, V.S.; Aqarwal, M.L. A novel role for p73 in the regulation of Akt-Foxo1a-Bim signaling and apoptosis induced by the plant lectin, Concanavalin A. *Cancer Res.* **2007**, *67*, 5617–5621. [CrossRef]
80. Çakıroğlu, E.; Uysal, T.; Çalıbaşı Koçal, G.; Aygenli, F.; Baran, G.; Baskın, Y. The role of *Morus nigra* extract and its active compounds as drug candidate on human colorectal adenocarcinoma cell line HT-29. *Int. J. Clin. Oncol. Cancer Res.* **2017**, *2*, 10–14.

81. Qadir, M.I.; Ali, M.; Ibrahim, Z. Anticancer activity of *Morus nigra* leaves extract. *Bangladesh J. Pharmacol.* **2014**, *9*, 496–497. [CrossRef]
82. Ahmed, A.; Ali, M.; El-Kholie, E.; El-Garawani, I.; Sherif, N. Anticancer activity of *Morus nigra* on human breast cancer cell line (MCF-7): The role of fresh and dry fruit extracts. *J. Biosci. Appl. Res.* **2016**, *2*, 352–361.
83. Turan, I.; Demir, S.; Kilinc, K.; Burnaz, N.A.; Yaman, S.O.; Akbulult, K.; Mentese, A.; Aliyazicioglu, Y.; Deger, O. Antiproliferative and apoptotic effect of *Morus nigra* extract on human prostate cancer cells. *Saudi Pharm. J.* **2017**, *25*, 241–248. [CrossRef] [PubMed]
84. Dröge, W. Free radicals in the physiological control of cell function. *Physiol. Rev.* **2002**, *82*, 47–95. [CrossRef] [PubMed]
85. Collins, C.A.; Fry, F.H.; Holme, A.L.; Yiakouvaki, A.; Al-Qenaei, A.; Pourzand, C.; Jacob, C. Towards multifunctional antioxidants: Synthesis, electrochemistry, *in vitro* and cell culture evaluation of compounds with ligand/catalytic properties. *Org. Biomol. Chem.* **2005**, *3*, 1541–1546. [CrossRef] [PubMed]
86. Li, A.N.; Li, S.; Zhang, Y.J.; Xu, X.R.; Chen, Y.M.; Li, H.B. Resources and Biological Activities of Natural Polyphenols. *Nutrients* **2014**, *6*, 6020–6047. [CrossRef] [PubMed]
87. Kumar, S.; Pandey, A.K. Chemistry and Biological Activities of Flavonoids: An Overview. *Sci. World J.* **2013**, 162750. [CrossRef] [PubMed]
88. Saxena, M.; Saxena, J.; Pradhan, A. Flavonoids and phenolic acids as antioxidants in plants and human health. *Int. J. Pharm. Sci. Rev. Res.* **2012**, *16*, 130–134.
89. Huyut, Z.; Beydemir, S.; Gülçin, I. Antioxidant and Antiradical Properties of Selected Flavonoids and Phenolic Compounds. *Biochem. Res. Int.* **2017**, 7616791. [CrossRef]
90. Zafra-Stone, S.; Yasmin, T.; Bagchi, M.; Chatterjee, A.; Vinson, J.A.; Bagchi, D. Berry anthocyanins as novel antioxidants in human health and disease prevention. *Mol. Nutr. Food Res.* **2007**, *51*, 675–683. [CrossRef]
91. Özgen, M.; Serçe, S.; Kaya, C. Phytochemical and antioxidant properties of anthocyanin-rich *Morus nigra* and *Morus alba* fruits. *Sci. Hortic. (Amsterdam)* **2009**, *119*, 275–279. [CrossRef]
92. Lee, Y.M.; Yoon, Y.; Yoon, H.; Park, H.M.; Song, S.; Yeum, K.J. Dietary Anthocyanins against Obesity and Inflammation. *Nutrients* **2017**, *9*, 1089. [CrossRef]
93. Kalkan Yildirim, H. Evaluation of colour parameters and antioxidant activities of fruit wines. *Int. J. Food Sci. Nutr.* **2006**, *57*, 47–63. [CrossRef] [PubMed]
94. Al-Mustafa, A.H.; Al-Thunibat, O.Y. Antioxidant activity of some Jordanian medicinal plants used traditionally for treatment of diabetes. *Pak. J. Biol. Sci.* **2008**, *11*, 351–358. [CrossRef] [PubMed]
95. Ercisli, S.; Tosun, M.; Duralija, B.; Voća, S.; Sengul, M.; Turan, M. Phytochemical content of some black (*Morus nigra* L.) and purple (*Morus rubra* L.) mulberry genotypes. *Food Technol. Biotechnol.* **2010**, *48*, 102–106.
96. El-Khawaga, O.Y.; Abou-Seif, M.A. Biochemical studies on antioxidant and oxidant activities of some plant extracts. *Eur. Rev. Med. Pharmacol. Sci.* **2010**, *14*, 731–738. [PubMed]
97. Imran, M.; Khan, H.; Shah, M.; Khan, R.; Khan, F. Chemical composition and antioxidant activity of certain *Morus* species. *J. Zhejiang Univ. Sci. B* **2010**, *11*, 973–980. [CrossRef] [PubMed]
98. Thabti, I.; Marzougui, N.; Elfalleh, W.; Ferchichi, A. Antioxidant composition and antioxidant activity of white (*Morus alba* L.), black (*Morus nigra* L.) and red (*Morus rubra* L.) mulberry leaves. *Acta Bot. Gallica* **2011**, *158*, 205–214. [CrossRef]
99. Arfan, M.; Khan, R.; Rybarczyk, A.; Amarowicz, R. Antioxidant activity of mulberry fruit extracts. *Int. J. Mol. Sci.* **2012**, *13*, 2472–2480. [CrossRef]
100. Iqbal, S.; Younas, U.; Sirajuddin; Chan, K.W.; Sarfraz, R.A.; Uddin, K. Proximate composition and antioxidant potential of leaves from three varieties of Mulberry (*Morus* sp.): A comparative study. *Int. J. Mol. Sci.* **2012**, *13*, 6651–6664. [CrossRef]
101. Kostić, D.A.; Dimitrijević, D.S.; Mitić, S.S.; Mitić, M.N.; Stojanović, G.S.; Živanović, A.V. Phenolic content and antioxidant activities of fruit extracts of *Morus nigra* L (Moraceae) from Southeast Serbia. *Trop. J. Pharm. Res.* **2013**, *12*, 105–110. [CrossRef]
102. Kamiloglu, S.; Serali, O.; Unal, N.; Capanoglu, E. Antioxidant activity and polyphenol composition of black mulberry (*Morus nigra* L.) products. *J. Berry Res.* **2013**, *3*, 41–51.
103. Sánchez-Salcedo, E.M.; Mena, P.; García-Viguera, C.; Hernández, F.; Martínez, J.J. (Poly)phenolic compounds and antioxidant activity of white (*Morus alba*) and black (*Morus nigra*) mulberry leaves: Their potential for new products rich in phytochemicals. *J. Funct. Foods* **2015**, *18*, 1039–1046. [CrossRef]

104. Dimitrova, M.P.; Petkova, N.T.; Denev, P.P.; Aleksieva, I.N. Carbohydrate composition and antioxidant activity of certain *Morus* species. *Int. J. Pharmacogn. Phytochem. Res.* **2015**, *7*, 621–627.
105. Jiang, B.; Mantri, N.; Hu, Y.; Lu, J.; Jiang, W.; Lu, H. Evaluation of bioactive compounds of black mulberry juice after thermal, microwave, ultrasonic processing, and storage at different temperatures. *Food Sci. Technol. Int.* **2015**, *21*, 392–399. [CrossRef] [PubMed]
106. Khattak, K.F.; Rahman, T.R. Effect of geographical distributions on the nutrient composition, phytochemical profile and antioxidant activity of *Morus nigra*. *Pak. J. Pharm. Sci.* **2015**, *28*, 1671–1678. [PubMed]
107. Tomas, M.; Toydemir, G.; Boyacioglu, D.; Hall, R.; Beekwilder, J.; Capanoglu, E. The effects of juice processing on black mulberry antioxidants. *Food Chem.* **2015**, *186*, 277–284. [CrossRef] [PubMed]
108. Celep, E.; Charehsaz, M.; Akyüz, S.; Acar, E.T.; Yesilada, E. Effect of *in vitro* gastrointestinal digestion on the bioavailability of phenolic components and the antioxidant potentials of some Turkish fruit wines. *Food Res. Int.* **2015**, *78*, 209–215. [CrossRef] [PubMed]
109. Ionica, M.E.; Nour, V.; Trandafir, I. Bioactive compounds and antioxidant capacity of some *Morus* species. *South.-west. J. Hortic. Biol. Environ.* **2017**, *8*, 79–88.
110. Tomas, M.; Toydemir, G.; Boyacioglu, D.; Hall, R.D.; Beekwilder, J.; Capanoglu, E. Processing black mulberry into jam: Effects on antioxidant potential and *in vitro* bioaccessibility. *J. Sci. Food Agric.* **2017**, *97*, 3106–3113. [CrossRef] [PubMed]
111. Montenote, M.C.; Wajsman, V.Z.; Konno, Y.T.; Ferreira, P.C.; Silva, R.M.G.; Therezo, A.L.S.; Silva, L.P.; Martins, L.P.A. Antioxidant effect of *Morus nigra* on Chagas disease progression. *Rev. Inst. Med. Trop. Sao. Paulo* **2017**, *59*, e73. [CrossRef] [PubMed]
112. Li, Y.; Bao, T.; Chen, W. Comparison of the protective effect of black and white mulberry against ethyl carbanate-induced cytotoxicity and oxidative damage. *Food Chem.* **2018**, *243*, 65–73. [CrossRef]
113. Wang, W.; Li, X.; Bao, X.; Gao, L.; Tao, Y. Extraction of polysaccharides from black mulberry fruit and their effect on enhancing antioxidant activity. *Int. J. Biol. Macromol.* **2018**, *120*, 1420–1429. [CrossRef] [PubMed]
114. Calín-Sánchez, A.; Martínez-Nicolás, J.J.; Munera-Picazo, S.; Carbonell-Barrachina, A.A.; Legua, P.; Hernández, F. Bioactive compounds and sensory quality of black and white mulberries grown in Spain. *Plant. Foods Hum. Nutr.* **2013**, *68*, 370–377. [CrossRef] [PubMed]
115. Abbas, G.M.; Abdel Bar, F.M.; Baraka, H.N.; Gohar, A.A.; Lahloub, M.F. A new antioxidant stilbene and other constituents from the stem bark of *Morus nigra* L. *Nat. Prod. Res.* **2014**, *28*, 952–959. [CrossRef]
116. Tarko, T.; Duda-Chodak, A.; Satora, P.; Sroka, P.; Pogoń, P.; Machalica, J. *Chaenomeles japonica*, *Cornus mas*, *Morus nigra* fruits characteristics and their processing potential. *J. Food Sci. Technol.* **2014**, *51*, 3934–3941. [CrossRef] [PubMed]
117. Gundogdu, M.; Tunçtürk, M.; Berk, S.; Şekeroğlu, N.; Gezici, S. Antioxidant capacity and bioactive contents of mulberry species from Eastern Anatolia region of Turkey. *Indian J. Pharm. Educ. Res.* **2018**, *52*, S96–S101. [CrossRef]
118. Nikkhah, E.; Khayami, M.; Heidari, R. In vitro screening for antioxidant activity and cancer suppressive effect of blackberry (*Morus nigra*). *Int. J. Cancer Manag.* **2008**, *1*, e80627.
119. Issa, N.K.; Abd-Aljabar, R.S. Evaluation of antioxidant properties of *Morus nigra* L. fruit extracts [II]. *Jordan J. Biol. Sci.* **2013**, *6*, 258–265. [CrossRef]
120. Feng, R.Z.; Wang, Q.; Tong, W.Z.; Xiong, J.; Wei, Q.; Zhou, W.H.; Yin, Z.Q.; Yin, X.Y.; Wang, L.Y.; Chen, Y.Q.; et al. Extraction and antioxidant activity of flavonoids of *Morus nigra*. *Int. J. Clin. Exp. Med.* **2015**, *8*, 22328–22336.
121. Naderi, G.A.; Asgary, S.; Sarraf-Zadegan, N.; Oroojy, H.; Afshin-Nia, F. Antioxidant activity of three extracts of *Morus nigra*. *Phytother. Res.* **2004**, *18*, 365–369. [CrossRef]
122. Mnaa, S.; Aniess, W.; Olwy, Y.; Shaker, E. Antioxidant activity of white (*Morus alba* L.) and black (*Morus nigra* L.) berries against CCl4 hepatotoxic agent. *Adv. Tech. Biol. Med.* **2014**. [CrossRef]
123. Hassimotto, N.M.; Genovese, M.I.; Lajolo, F.M. Antioxidant activity of dietary fruits, vegetables, and commercial frozen fruit pulps. *J. Agric. Food Chem.* **2005**, *53*, 2928–2935. [CrossRef] [PubMed]
124. Malik, M.N.H.; Alamgeer; Salma, U.; Qayyum, A.; Samreen, S. Phytochemical analysis and cardiac depressant activity of aqueous methanolic extract of Morus nigra L. fruit. *J. Appl. Pharm. Sci.* **2012**, *2*, 39–41.
125. Akhlaq, A.; Mehmood, M.H.; Rehman, A.; Ashraf, Z.; Syed, S.; Bawany, S.A.; Gilani, A.H.; Ilyas, M.; Siddiqui, B.S. The prokinetic, laxative, and antidiarrheal effects of *Morus nigra*: Possible muscarinic, Ca2+ channel blocking, and antimuscarinic mechanisms. *Phytother. Res.* **2016**, *30*, 1362–1376. [CrossRef] [PubMed]

126. Fahimi, Z.; Jahromy, M.H. Effects of blackberry (*Morus nigra*) fruit juice on levodopa-induced dyskinesia in a mice model of Parkinson's disease. *J. Exp. Pharmacol.* **2018**, *10*, 29–35. [CrossRef] [PubMed]
127. Briguglio, M.; Hrelia, S.; Malaguti, M.; Serpe, L.; Canaparo, R.; Dell'Osso, B.; Galentino, R.; De Michele, S.; Dina, C.Z.; Porta, M.; et al. Food Bioactive Compounds and Their Interference in Drug Pharmacokinetic/Pharmacodynamic Profiles. *Pharmaceutics* **2018**, *10*, 277. [CrossRef] [PubMed]
128. Kim, H.; Yoon, Y.J.; Shon, J.H.; Cha, I.J.; Shin, J.G.; Liu, K.H. Inhibitory effects of fruit juices on CYP3A activity. *Drug Metab. Dispos.* **2006**, *34*, 521–523. [CrossRef] [PubMed]
129. Zanger, U.M.; Schwab, M. Cytochrome P450 enzymes in drug metabolism: Regulation of gene expression, enzyme activities, and impact of genetic variation. *Pharmacol. Ther.* **2013**, *138*, 103–141. [CrossRef]
130. Drug Interactions Flockhart Table. Available online: https://drug-interactions.medicine.iu.edu/main-table.aspx (assessed on 11 February 2019).
131. Figueredo, K.C.; Guex, C.G.; Reginato, F.Z.; Haas da Silva, A.R.; Cassanego, G.B.; Lhamas, C.L.; Boligon, A.A.; Lopes, G.H.H.; de Freitas Bauermann, L. Safety assessment of *Morus nigra* L. leaves: Acute and subacute oral toxicity studies in Wistar rats. *J. Ethnopharmacol.* **2018**, *224*, 290–296. [CrossRef]

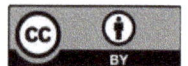

© 2019 by the authors. Licensee MDPI, Basel, Switzerland. This article is an open access article distributed under the terms and conditions of the Creative Commons Attribution (CC BY) license (http://creativecommons.org/licenses/by/4.0/).

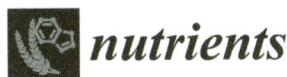

Article

Prevention of Recurrent Acute Otitis Media in Children Through the Use of *Lactobacillus salivarius* PS7, a Target-Specific Probiotic Strain

Nivia Cárdenas [1,†], Virginia Martín [1,‡], Rebeca Arroyo [1], Mario López [2,§], Marta Carrera [3], Carlos Badiola [4], Esther Jiménez [1,†] and Juan M. Rodríguez [1,*]

1. Department of Nutrition and Food Science, Complutense University of Madrid, 28040 Madrid, Spain; niviacu@yahoo.com (N.C.); vmartinmerino@gmail.com (V.M.); rebecaa@vet.ucm.es (R.A.); esther.jimenez@probisearch.com (E.J.)
2. Centro de Salud Bermeo, Tonpoi Kalea, s/n, 48370 Bermeo, Bizkaia, Spain; mario.lopezmateo@osakidetza.eus
3. Centro de Salud Silvano, Av. de Machupichu, 58, 28043 Madrid, Spain; marta.carrera@salud.madrid.org
4. Laboratorios Casen Recordati S.L., Vía de las Dos Castillas, 33, 28224 Pozuelo de Alarcón, Madrid, Spain; cjbadiola@casenrecordati.com
* Correspondence: jmrodrig@ucm.es
† Current address: Probisearch S.L.U., C/Santiago Grisolía, 2, 28760 Tres Cantos, Spain.
‡ Current address: Centro Nacional de Microbiología, Instituto de Salud Carlos III, Ctra. de Pozuelo, 28, 28222 Majadahonda, Madrid, Spain.
§ Current address: Centro de Salud, Donibane Plaza, s/n, 48287 Ea, Bizkaia, Spain.

Received: 8 January 2019; Accepted: 4 February 2019; Published: 12 February 2019

Abstract: Acute otitis media (AOM) is one of the most common bacterial infections in children. Empiric antibiotherapy leads to increasing antimicrobial resistance rates among otopathogens and may impair the correct development of the microbiota in early life. In this context, probiotics seem to be an attractive approach for preventing recurrent AOM (rAOM) through the restoration of the middle ear and nasopharyngeal microbiota. The aim of this study was the selection of a probiotic strain (*Lactobacillus salivarius* PS7), specifically tailored for its antagonism against otopathogens. Since *L. salivarius* PS7 was safe and displayed a strong antimicrobial activity against otopathogens, its efficacy in preventing rAOM was assessed in a trial involving 61 children suffering from rAOM. Children consumed daily ~1×10^9 CFU of *L. salivarius* PS7, and the number of AOM episodes were registered and compared with that observed in the previous 6 and 12 months. The microbiota of samples collected from the external auditory canal samples was quantitatively and qualitatively assessed. The number of AOM episodes during the intervention period decreased significantly (84%) when compared to that reported during the 6 months period before the probiotic intervention. In conclusion, *L. salivarius* PS7 is a promising strain for the prevention of rAOM in infants and children.

Keywords: *Lactobacillus salivarius*; otitis; probiotic; bacteriocin; prevention

1. Introduction

Acute otitis media (AOM) is one of the most common diseases in infancy and childhood, and the leading cause for seeking medical care and for the prescription of antibiotics, both in high-income and low-income countries [1,2]. Approximately 70% of infants experience at least one otitis episode by the age of 2 years, and 20–30% suffer from recurrent AOM (rAOM) [3]. rAOM is a very relevant issue in clinical practice since it causes pain and discomfort in children, causing a strong impact on their families and a relevant economic burden on society [3].

Middle ear and nasopharyngeal colonization with multiple bacterial otopathogens (mainly *Streptococcus pneumoniae*, *Streptococcus pyogenes*, *Haemophilus influenzae* and *Moraxella catarrhalis*) is considered to be the main risk for both AOM and rAOM [4,5]. Recent microbiome studies have revealed that *Alloiococcus otitidis* may also play a relevant role in the pathogenesis of otitis media [6,7], while other species frequently isolated from the middle ear fluid of children experiencing this condition include *Staphylococcus aureus*, *Staphylococcus epidermidis*, *Pseudomonas aeruginosa* and *Escherichia coli* [8].

In practice, eradicating or decreasing the concentration of such species through empiric systemic and topical antibiotherapy is usually considered as the main (and, often, unique) approach for the treatment of rAOM and, also, for providing prophylaxis for this condition [9]. However, a routine antibiotherapy may have negative consequences. First of all, it drives the selection of resistant otopathogens [9,10]. Although rAOM episodes occurring within one month from the completion of an antibiotic therapy may be the result of either a relapse or a new infection, antibiotic pressure seems to be essential for selecting the causal agent(s) in both circumstances [11,12]; in fact, the incidence of antibiotic-resistant *S. pneumoniae* and *H. influenzae* strains in nasopharyngeal samples is higher among children with rAOM than among healthy controls [13,14]. In addition, otopathogens, such as *H. influenzae*, *S. pneumoniae*, *M. catarrhalis* and *A. otitidis*, form polymicrobial biofilms within the middle ear [15–17], and bacteria within these structures have an increased antibiotic resistance [18]. Recently, it was shown that *A. otitidis* promoted *H. influenzae* survival in mixed biofilms by decreasing its antibiotic susceptibility and enhancing its growth under adverse conditions [17]. A Cochrane review [2] aimed to assess the effects of antibiotics for children with AOM revealed that, although they may be useful in children under two years of age with bilateral AOM and otorrhea, their global effect on health outcomes associated to this condition is limited. The same review encouraged the weighing of the benefits of antibiotics against possible harms, including adverse events (such as vomiting, diarrhea or rashes), and suggested that clinical management should provide a limited role for antibiotics, and that a search for new preventive and treatment strategies should be stimulated.

The collateral damage that antibiotics exert on the host's health by eliminating prominent (but sensitive) members of the microbiota must also be taken into account. Our relationship with our microbiota is especially important during the first years of life, when the microbiome is still forming and any strong disturbance can have short, medium and long-term consequences for homeostasis and health [19–24]. The microbiome of the middle ear, ear canal and nasopharynx of healthy children with no history of AOM seems to be characterized by the presence of potentially protective commensal bacteria and the absence or low abundance of classic otopathogens [25].

In this context, probiotics seem to be an attractive approach for preventing rAOM through the restoration of the middle ear and nasopharyngeal microbiota. The lack of specificity of the probiotics used for this target may be one of the main reasons for the limited and contradictory results obtained so far [25,26]. Therefore, the aim of this study was the characterization of a probiotic strain specifically selected for its antagonism against otopathogens. In addition, other potentially properties related to its probiotic potential and safety were investigated, including the assessment of its acute and repeated-doses oral toxicity in a rat model. Finally, the efficacy of the selected strain (*Lactobacillus salivarius* PS7) in preventing rAOM in infants and children was assessed in a pilot clinical trial.

2. Materials and Methods

2.1. Isolation and Identification of the Strain

Strain PS7 was isolated in a de Man, Rogosa, and Sharpe (MRS, Oxoid, Basingstoke, UK) agar plate within the framework of a previous study to evaluate the bacterial diversity of milk from healthy women. Initially, the identification of the strain was performed by PCR amplification and the sequencing of the 16S rRNA gene using the primers pbl16 (5′-AGAGTTTGATCCTGGCTCAG-3′) and mbl16 (5′-GGCTGCTGGCACGTAGTTAG-3′) [27]. The identification was confirmed by Matrix Assisted Laser Desorption Ionization-Time of Flight (MALDI-TOF) mass spectrometry using a

Vitek-MS™ instrument (BioMérieux, Marcy l'Etoile, France) [28]. The strain could be differentiated from other *L. salivarius* strains of our own collection by genotyping using randomly amplified polymorphic DNA (RAPD) analyses, as previously described [29].

2.2. Survival after In Vitro Exposure to Saliva and Gastrointestinal-Like Conditions

The survival of the strain to conditions resembling those found in the human digestive tract (saliva, human stomach and small intestine) was assessed in the in vitro system described by Marteau et al. [30], with the modifications reported by Martín et al. [31]. For this purpose, the strain was vehiculated in UHT-treated milk (25 mL) at a concentration of 10^9 CFU/mL. The values of the pH curve in the stomach-like compartment were those recommended by Conway et al. [32]. Different fractions were taken at 20, 40, 60, and 80 min from this compartment, and exposed for 120 min to a solution with a composition similar to that of human duodenal juice [30]. The survival rate of the strain was determined by culturing the samples on MRS agar plates, which were incubated at 37 °C for 48 h.

2.3. Adhesion to Caco-2/HT-29 Cells

The ability of the strain to adhere to HT-29 and Caco-2 cells was evaluated as described by Coconnier et al. [33] with the modifications reported by Martín et al. [31]. HT-29 and Caco-2 were cultured to confluence in 2 mL of DMEM medium (PAA, Linz, Austria) containing 25 mM of glucose, 1 mM of sodium pyruvate and supplemented with 10% heat-inactivated foetal calf serum, 2 mM of L-glutamine and 1% of a non-essential amino acid preparation. At day 10 after the confluence, 1 mL of the medium was replaced with 1 mL of DMEM containing 10^8 CFU/mL of the PS7 strain. The adherence was measured as the number of lactobacilli adhering to the cells in 20 random microscopic fields. The assay was performed by triplicate.

2.4. Production of Riboflavin, Folate and Cyanocobalamin

The riboflavin, folate and cyanocobalamin production by strain PS7 was determined using the microbiological assays described by Juarez del Valle et al. [34], Laiño et al. [35], and Horwitz [36], respectively. *Lactobacillus rhamnosus* ATCC 7469, *L. rhamnosus* NCIMB 10463 and 7469, and *Lactobacillus delbrueckii* B_{12} were used as the indicator organism for the biosynthesis of the respective vitamins. The riboflavin production in the riboflavin-free medium was confirmed by an HPLC analysis following a procedure described previously [34].

2.5. Antimicrobial Activity of Strain PS7 against AOM-Related Pathogens

Initially, an overlay method was used as previously described [37] to determine the ability of strain PS7 to inhibit the growth of a spectrum of bacterial strains previously isolated from clinical cases of AOM (own collection of the Complutense University of Madrid) including: *A. otitidis* MP02, *S. pneumoniae* MP07, *S. pyogenes* MP03, *Enterococcus faecalis* MP64, *S. aureus* MP29, *S. epidermidis* MP33, *H. influenzae* MP04, *M. catarrhalis* MP08, *P. aeruginosa* MP24 and *E. coli* MP69. Brain Heart Infusion (BHI, Oxoid, Basingstoke, UK), Columbia Nalidixic Acid (CNA, Biomerieux, Marcy-l'Étoile, France) or Trypticase Soy (TSA, Oxoid) agar plates (depending on the indicator strain) were overlaid with bacterial indicators, incubated at 37 °C for 48 h, and they were examined for zones of inhibition around the PS7 streaks.

2.6. Production of Specific Antimicrobials (Bacteriocins, Lactic Acid, Acetic Acid, Hydrogen Peroxide) by Strain PS7

Bacteriocin production was assayed using an agar diffusion method as described by Dodd et al. [38] and modified by Martín et al. [31], using the Gram-positive strains employed for the overlay method as indicator bacteria. Since, at that stage, it was already known that strain PS7 belongs to the *Lactobacillus salivarius* species, the strain was tested by PCR for the presence of the structural genes encoding salivaricins. More specifically, the primer couples used in this study were: (i) SalB-for (5′-TGATAAGAAAGAATTGGCACATATAATTG-3′) and SalB-rev (5′-TCTGTTTAACTACAAATATTTTGATTTGAATG-3′) for salivaricin B [39], and (ii) Abp118A-for (5′-AAACGTGGTCCTAACTGTGTAGG-3′) and Abp118B-rev (5′-AACGGCAACTTGTAAAACCACCAG-3′) for bacteriocin Abp-118 [40]. The PCR reactions were carried out as indicated in the respective articles.

L-and D-lactic acid and acetic acid production by the strain PS7 was quantified in MRS cultures using enzymatic kits (Roche Diagnostics, Mannheim, Germany), as previously reported [31]. The assays were performed in triplicate and the values were expressed as the mean ± SD. The pH values of the supernatants were also measured. Finally, hydrogen peroxide production by the strain PS7 was assayed using the procedures described by Song et al. [41] and by Yap and Gilliland [42]. *L. johnsonii* La1 was used as a positive control in both assays.

2.7. Coagregation Assays

The ability of the strain to aggregate with cells of the otitis-related strains cited above was investigated following the procedure of Reid et al. [43], as adapted by Younes et al. [44].

2.8. Co-Culture Studies

Broth co-cultures of strain PS7 and some of the otitis-related strains cited above were performed in a BHI broth, since it was observed that this medium allowed most of their growth. The tubes were initially inoculated at a concentration of ~1×10^8 CFU/mL for each of the bacterial strains (PS7 and the corresponding otitis-related strain) and incubated overnight at 37 °C in aerobic conditions. BHI monocultures of each of the strains used in these assays were performed as control cultures. After incubation, samples of all the co-cultures and monocultures were seeded onto MRS, CNA, TSA and BHI agar plates for a selective enumeration based on the ability of the strains to growth and to display differential colony morphologies when inoculated on such media.

2.9. Sensitivity to Antibiotics

The sensitivity of the strain PS7 to antibiotics was tested using the lactic acid bacteria susceptibility test medium (LSM) [45] and the microtiter VetMIC plates for lactic acid bacteria (National Veterinary Institute of Sweden, Uppsala, Sweden), as described previously [46]. Parallel, minimum inhibitory concentrations (MICs) were also determined by the E-test (AB BIODISK, Solna, Sweden) following the instructions of the manufacturer. The results were compared to the cut-off levels proposed by the European Food Safety Authority [47].

2.10. Formation of Biogenic Amines and Degradation of Mucin

The capacity of the strain PS7 to synthesize biogenic amines (tyramine, histamine, putrescine and cadaverine) from their respective precursor amino acids (tyrosine, histidine, ornithine and lysine; Sigma-Aldrich) was evaluated using the method described by Bover-Cid and Holzapfel [48]. The potential of the strain to degrade gastric mucine (HGM; Sigma, St. Louis, MO, USA) was evaluated in vitro as indicated by Zhou et al. [49].

2.11. Acute and Repeated Dose (4-Weeks) Oral Toxicity Studies in a Rat Model

Wistar male and female rats (Charles River Inc., Marget, Kent, UK) were used to study the acute and repeated dose (4-weeks) oral toxicity of the strain PS7 in a rat model. The acclimatization, housing and management (including feeding) of the rats was performed as previously described [50]. The rats were 56-days old at the initiation of treatment. Acute (limit test) and repeated dose (4 weeks) studies were conducted in accordance with the European Union guidelines (EC Council Regulation No. 440) and authorized by the Ethical Committee on Animal Research of the Complutense University of Madrid (protocol 270111).

In the acute (limit test) study, 24 rats (12 males, 12 females) were distributed into two groups of 6 males and 6 females each. After an overnight fasting, each rat received skim milk (500 µL) orally (control group or Group 1), or a single oral dose of 1×10^{10} CFU of *L. salivarius* PS7 dissolved in 500 µL of skim milk (treated group or Group 2). The doses of the test and control products were administered by gavage. At the end of a 14-day observation period, the rats were weighed, euthanized by CO_2 inhalation, exsanguinated, and necropsied.

The repeated dose (4 weeks) (limit test) study was conducted in 48 rats (24 males, 24 females) divided in four groups of 6 males and 6 females each (control group or Group 3; treated group or Group 4; satellite control group or Group 5; and satellite treated group or Group 6). Rats either received a daily oral dose of skim milk (Groups 3 and 5) or of 1×10^9 CFU of *L. salivarius* PS7 dissolved in 500 µL of skim milk (Groups 4 and 6) over 4 weeks. All rats of Groups 3 and 4 were deprived of food for 18 h, weighed, euthanized by CO_2 inhalation, exsanguinated, and necropsied on day 29. All animals of the satellite groups (Groups 5 and 6) were kept for a further 14-day period without treatment to detect delayed occurrence, persistence or recovery from potential toxic effects. All rats from Groups 5 and 6 were deprived of food for 18 h, weighed, euthanized by CO_2 inhalation, exsanguinated, and necropsied on day 42.

The behavior and clinical observations, blood biochemistry and haematology analysis, organ weight ratios and histopathological analysis were conducted as described previously [50]. The bacterial translocation to the blood, liver or spleen, and the total liver glutathione (GSH) concentration was evaluated following the methods described by Lara-Villoslada et al. [51].

2.12. Pilot Clinical Trial: Prevention of rAOM in Children

In this prospective pilot clinical assay, 64 children (aged 10 months to 6 years) with a previous history of rAOM were recruited between September 2012 and April 2015. The primary outcome variables were the occurrence and duration of the AOM episodes. The secondary end point was the frequency of an otitis-related pathogen carriage in the external auditory canal. The inclusion criteria were at least four episodes of AOM during the preceding 12 months or at least three episodes during the preceding 6 months [52]. The exclusion criteria included chronic medication, chronic illnesses, lip or palatal cleft, programmed tympanostomy or adenoidectomy during the study, and lactose intolerance or cow's milk protein allergy (because of the excipient used to administer the strain). Those children who had undergone tympanostomy or adenoidectomy during the preceding 6 months were also excluded. The data on the occurrence of AOM episodes from a similar population (age, gender) of otitis-prone children ($n = 60$), who were attended by the same pediatrician but did not receive the tested strain, were used for comparison purposes. Written informed consent was obtained from the parents or legal tutorsin accordance with the Declaration of Helsinki. The protocol was approved by the Ethical Committee on Clinical Research of Hospital Universitario Clínico San Carlos (Madrid, Spain), under protocol B12/262.

During the 6-month intervention period, the recruited children consumed daily ~1×10^9 CFU of *L. salivarius* PS7. The parents recorded whether the child had or had not received the daily dose. Compliance was expressed as the percentage of days in which the child received the dose. The use of antibiotics (except for the treatment of an AOM episode) or other probiotics was not allowed during the study. A physical examination was performed by a pediatrician for each suspected AOM episode. AOM was diagnosed according to defined clinical criteria [52,53], including evidence of middle ear effusion, inflammation of the tympanic membrane and any other sign of an acute infection (fever, ear ache, otorrhoea, etc.). The number of AOM episodes and the duration of each episode were also recorded and compared to the same data obtained in the 6 months preceding the probiotic treatment.

Samples from the external auditory canal were collected with a sterile swab at the baseline and at the end (6 months) of the study and submitted for a bacterial analysis following the guidelines recommended by the Spanish Society of Infectious Diseases and Clinical Microbiology [53]. Microbial isolates were identified by a MALDI-TOF analysis as previously reported.

2.13. Statistical Analysis

All the quantitative assays included in this study were performed at least in triplicate. The quantitative data were expressed as the mean and standard deviation (SD). When not normally distributed, the data were presented as the median and interquartile range (IQR). For the murine assays, the data were expressed as the means ± standard error of the mean (SEM) of the determinations. The differences between the control and treated groups were evaluated with a one-way analysis of variance (ANOVA) followed by Dunnett's test. A Wilcoxon signed rank test was used to compare paired microbiological data before and after the probiotic intake and the χ^2 test was used to find differences in the detection frequencies of the bacterial species in the external auditory canal samples. For all the comparisons, differences were considered significant at $p < 0.05$. The statistical analyses were conducted using R (version 3.0.2, R-project) software [54].

3. Results

3.1. Identification and In Vitro Characterization of the Strain

Strain PS7 was identified as a member of the *L. salivarius* species (from now, *L. salivarius* PS7). A RAPD genotyping analysis showed that the profile of this strain was different to those of other *L. salivarius* strains from our own collection. Subsequently, the strain was deposited at the Spanish Type Culture Collection (CECT; Burjassot, Spain) under accession number CECT 9422.

In relation to the survival of *L. salivarius* PS7 after exposition to conditions resembling those found in the human digestive tract, an exposure to a saliva-like solution had no deleterious effect on the strain while the survival rate after a transit through the stomach- and small intestine-like compartments was at approximately 52% of the population initially inoculated.

The strain produced neither folates nor cyanocobalamin under the assayed conditions. In contrast, it was able to produce riboflavin at a total concentration of ~200 ng/mL (intracellular riboflavin: 165.00 ± 0.52 ng/mL; extracellular riboflavin: 34.74 ± 3.06 ng/mL).

L. salivarius PS7 showed a high ability to adhere to both Caco-2 and HT-29 cells. The mean ± SD of the number of adhered lactobacilli in 20 random microscopic fields was 697.1 ± 297.6 and 251.7 ± 82.3, respectively.

L. salivarius PS7 showed a clear antimicrobial activity (inhibition zone >2 mm around the streak) against most of the otitis-related indicator organisms used in this study (Table 1). Subsequently, and to try to elucidate the compound(s) responsible for the antimicrobial activity, the strain was screened for production of bacteriocins, organic acids (D-and L-lactic acid, acetic acid) and hydrogen peroxide. The strain displayed bacteriocin activity against the Gram-positive strains included as indicator organisms in this study (Table 1). A PCR analysis for structural genes of known salivaricins revealed that this strain produced the bacteriocin Abp-118 (both structural genes were identical) (Figure 1). *L. salivarius* PS7 produced a high concentration of L-lactic acid in the MRS broth while it did not produce the D-lactic acid isomer (Table 2). A significant concentration of acetic acid could also be detected in the culture supernatants of the strain (0.68 ± 0.17 mg/mL). This strain did not produce hydrogen peroxide.

L. salivarius PS7 showed a high potential for co-aggregating with bacterial strains involved in AOM cases, particularly with those belonging to the genera *Streptococcus*, *Alloiococcus*, *Enterococcus* and *Staphylococcus*. In addition, most of the otitis-related Gram-positive pathogens could not be detected, or their concentrations decreased notably after their overnight co-culture with the strain PS7 in the BHI broth (Table 1).

The antibiotic sensitivity assays showed that all the MIC values were below the cut-off values recommended by EFSA for all antibiotics, with the exception of kanamycin (MIC in this study: 128 µg/mL; EFSA cut-off value: 64 µg/mL) (Table 3). However, recent reports suggest that *L. salivarius* may be intrinsically resistant to kanamycin, and this aspect will be discussed below. Finally, *L. salivarius* PS7 was able neither to degrade gastric mucin in vitro nor to produce biogenic amines.

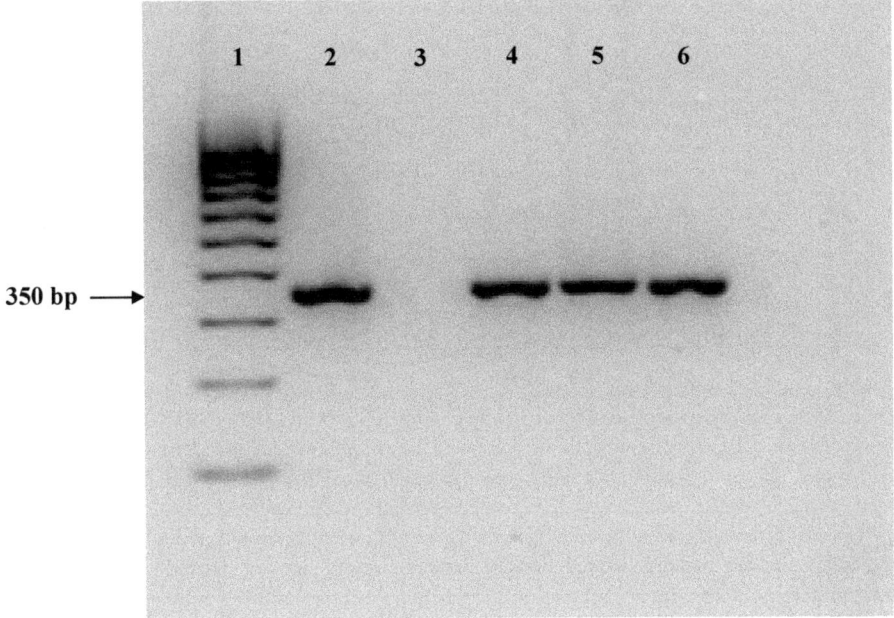

Figure 1. PCR assay for the detection of the bacteriocin Abp118 structural gene. Lane 1: marker (Hyperladder™ 100 bp, BIOLINE, London, UK). Lane 2: positive control. Lane 3: negative control. Lanes 4, 5 and 6: *L. salivarius* PS7.

Table 1. Antimicrobial activity of *L. salivarius* PS7 against bacterial strains isolated from clinical cases of AOM, as assessed by different assays.

Indicator Strain	Overlay Method (cm)	Well Diffusion Assay (cm)		Co-Cultures (CFU/mL)	
		Non-Adjusted pH	pH 6.2	Initial Load	Final Load
S. pneumoniae MP07	3.6	1.1	1.1	7.40	Nd [a]
S. pyogenes MP03	2.0	1.2	0.7	7.74	Nd [a]
S. aureus MP29	1.6	1.3	1.2	7.52	4.81 [a]
S. epidermidis MP33	2.3	1.1	1.0	7.53	5.90 [a]
A. otitidis MP02	1.0	1.2	1.2	–	–
E. faecalis MP64	0.5	0.4	0.4	8.02	8.78 [b]
H. influenzae MP04	2.2	–	–	–	–
M. catarrhalis MP08	2.1	–	–	–	–
P. aeruginosa MP24	1.5	–	–	–	–
E. coli MP69	1.4	–	–	7.70	5.74 [a]

[a] $p < 0.01$. [b] $p = 0.29$; Nd, no growth detected; – not assayed. AOM: Acute otitis media; CFU: colony-forming unit.

Table 2. Final pH and production of organic acids (mg/mL; mean ± SD) in an MRS broth by *L. salivarius* PS7.

pH	L–Lactic Acid	D-Lactic Acid	Acetic Acid
4.01 ± 0.04	10.29 ± 0.70	Nd	0.68 ± 0.17

Nd, not detectable.

Table 3. Minimum inhibitory concentrations (MICs) and cut-off values (µg/mL) of a variety of antibiotics for *L. salivarius* PS7.

Antibiotics	Cut-Off Values *	MIC (*L. salivarius* PS7)
Ampicillin	4	0.5
Clindamycin	4	0.5
Chloramphenicol	4	2
Erythromycin	1	0.25
Streptomycin	64	32
Gentamicin	16	2
Kanamycin	64	128
Tetracyclin	8	2
Vancomycin	n.r.	>128
Linezolid	2	1
Penicillin	1	0.25

* EFSA (2018), except for linezolid and penicillin (Klare et al., 2007). n.r.: not required.

3.2. Acute and Repeated Dose (4-Weeks) oral Toxicity Studies in a Rat Model

All animals survived both oral toxicity trials. The development of the treated animals during the experimental periods corresponded to their species and age. At no time point of the experimental period were there any significant differences in body weight or body weight gain among the groups treated with *L. salivarius* PS7 (including the satellite ones) in comparison to the control groups. No abnormal clinical signs, behavioural changes, body weight changes, haematological and clinical chemistry parameters, macroscopic or histological findings, or organ weight changes were observed. There were no statistical differences in body weights among the groups. Similarly, no statistically significant differences in body weight gain, or in food and water consumption were observed between the groups.

No significant differences in the liver GSH concentration were observed between the control and treated groups (9.67 ± 1.42 vs. 9.71 ± 1.56 mmol/g, $p > 0.1$), and lactobacilli could not be isolated from the blood, liver or spleen of the treated rats.

3.3. Pilot Clinical Trial: Prevention of AOM in Children

A total of 64 children who fulfilled the inclusion criteria were enrolled and received the probiotic treatment (Table 4). Three children (~4.6%) dropped out (one due to antibiotic intake; one due to tympanostomy; one due to a previously unadvertized allergy to cow's milk protein); thus, 61 children completed the study. Compliance during the study was very high ($\geq 96\%$). Twenty-two out of the 61 recruited children (36%) suffered at least one episode of AOM (median [25Q–75Q]), with a median duration of 4 days (Table 4). In contrast, ~70% of the children with rAOM who were attended by the same pediatrician in the same period but did not receive the probiotic strain suffered at least one AOM episode with a median duration of 6 days. The number of AOM episodes during the 6-month intervention period decreased by 84% when compared to the number registered in the 6 months that preceded the intervention (Figure 2). Although any child suffering an AOM episode received an antibiotic treatment, the number of antimicrobial treatments decreased by ~60% in the children receiving the probiotic strain with respect to the other otitis-prone children treated by the same pediatrician.

Globally, the microbial density in the external auditory canal decreased notably along the intervention period, from $\geq 3.5 \log_{10}$ CFU at the baseline (all the cultures were positive at this sampling time) to $\leq 2 \log_{10}$ CFU at the end of the intervention (with 22% of the cultures being negative). At time 0, *M. catarralis*, coagulase-negative staphylococci and *A. otitidis* were the dominant bacteria in swabs taken from the external auditory canal of the recruited children, while coagulase-negative staphylococci and viridans streptococci dominated after 6 months of the probiotic treatment (Table 5). *A. otitidis*, *H. haemolyticus*, *H. influenzae*, *M. catharralis*, *Neisseria* spp, *P. aeruginosa*, *S. aureus*, *S. pneumoniae* and *S.*

pyogenes, which were relatively common in the samples obtained at time 0, were not detected or their frequency of detection decreased notably at the end of the intervention (Table 5).

Table 4. Main demographic characteristics of the infants and children recruited in the pilot trial (*n* = 61), and main outcomes of the study.

Characteristic	Sex	n	Mean ± SD or Median *	p-Value
Age (Years) and Gender			3.31 ± 1.7	
<3 years (*n* = 30)	Males	16		
	Females	14		
≥3 years (*n* = 31)	Males	15		
	Females	16		
Inclusion months:				
September		7		
October		5		
November		6		
December		7		
January		6		
February		10		
March		9		
April		6		
May		3		
June		2		
History of AOM episodes/child				
Preceding 6 months			4 (3–4) *	<0.001 ¥
Preceding 12 months			5 (5–6) *	<0.001 ¥
During the study			0 (0–1) *	

n, number of children; * Median (25Q–75Q); ¥ Wilcoxon rank sum test paired comparison.

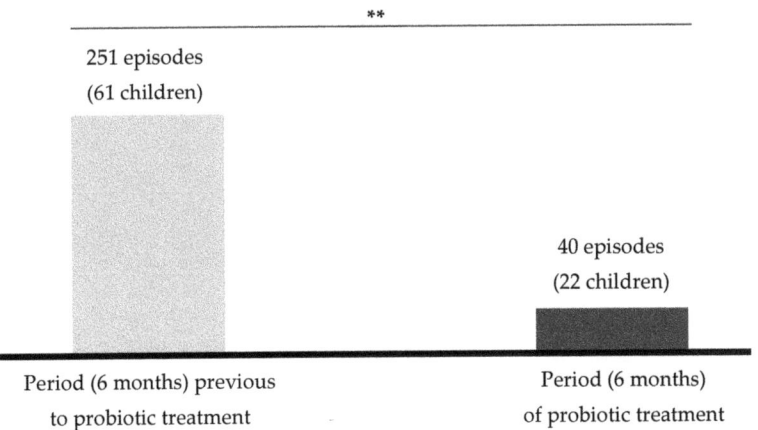

Figure 2. Comparison between the number of AOM episodes reported during the 6 months of the probiotic treatment and those reported during the previous 6 months. **, statistically significant change ($p < 0.05$; χ^2 test).

Table 5. Results of the microbiological analysis of the samples from the external auditory canal taken at day 0 before the probiotic intervention and at the end of the 6-month treatment period.

	Time 0	After 6 Months	p-Value
Number of positive samples (bacterial growth)	61	17	< 0.001 [¥]
Median $\log_{10}$ CFU (per swab)	4 (3.5–5)	2 (1.5–2)	0.012 *
Number of samples with the presence of:			
Actinomyces europaeus	2	0	
Alloiococcus otitidis	12	2	
Coagulase-negative staphylococci	14	15	
Haemophilus haemolyticus	11	1	
Haemophilus influenza	7	1	
Moraxella catharralis	14	3	
Neisseria spp.	6	0	
Pseudomonas aeruginosa	4	0	
Rhodococcus ruber	2	0	
Staphylococcus aureus	11	3	
Streptococcus pneumoniae	9	3	
Streptococcus pyogenes	10	6	
Group viridans streptococci	9	11	

[¥] Chi-squared test. * Wilcoxon rank sum test.

4. Discussion

In the present study, the probiotic potential of L. salivarius PS7 was characterized by using a wide variety of in vitro and in vivo assays, including its ability to antagonize otopathogens, its toxicological assessment in rats, and a pilot clinical trial for the initial evaluation of its efficacy for preventing rAOM in infants and children. The characterization scheme of this strain followed the guidelines for the evaluation of probiotics provided by FAO and WHO [55].

Both the survival rate (52%) of L. salivarius PS7 when exposed to conditions similar to those found in the digestive tract and its capacity for adhesion to intestinal cells were similar or higher than those found for commercial probiotic strains in previous studies using the same in vitro models [31,56]. These properties indicate that a high concentration of the strain can reach the pharynx and the gut mucosal surfaces and adhere to them. The adhesion ability of this strain may allow the competitive exclusion of pathogenic bacteria [57]. While its presence in the pharynx may facilitate its direct interaction with otopathogens, its presence in the gut might also have positive consequences. It has been shown that exposure (after swallowing) of the gut to upper respiratory pathogens involved in otitis media provides a potent modulation of the immune responses in the middle ear [58]. The potential ear-related immunomodulatory properties of L. salivarius PS7 were not addressed in this work but deserve future research.

In order to select a strain for the prevention of otitis, its ability to exert antagonism against otopathogens seems an essential property. The results of the in vitro assays to evaluate the antimicrobial activity of L. salivarius PS7 against a wide variety of strains and species previously isolated from clinical rAOM cases confirmed that it was a suitable candidate for such a target. All the otitis-related indicator strains were inhibited when the overlay method was used and, among them, all the Gram-positive strains were sensitive to the bacteriocin-like compound produced by L. salivarius PS7. The PCR analyses revealed that L. salivarius PS7 produces Abp-118. This is a potent broad-spectrum class II bacteriocin, which was originally described in L. salivarius UCC118 [59]. A previous study demonstrated that Abp-118 is produced in vivo and that it was the primary mediator conferring protection against infection by Listeria monocytogenes in mice [60]. The lack of inhibition of a few otopathogens (E. faecalis MP64) in the co-culture assay may be due to the fact that Abp-118 is not expressed when the bacteriocinogenic strain grows in a BHI medium. In addition, L. salivarius PS7 produced high amounts of L-lacic acid in the MRS cultures, and this is in agreement with the results obtained with other L. salivarius strains in previous studies [31,56]. Smaller concentrations of acetic acid were also present in the MRS cultures. The fact that L. salivarius PS7 cells were able to co-aggregate with most of the otopathogenic strains tested in this work may facilitate the exposure of otopathogens to the antimicrobial substances produced by *L. salivarius* PS7 [44]. Recently, it was shown that, to exert antimicrobial activity in mucosal surfaces, physical contact between lactobacilli and pathogens may be required [61]. Interestingly, the presence of lactobacilli in the nasopharynx has been associated with a reduced risk of respiratory conditions in children [62]. Unfortunately, the presence of *Lactobacillus* in ear or nasopharynx samples was not tested in this study.

Although *L. salivarius* is a species included among those with the "qualified presumption of safety" (QPS) status [63], *L. salivarius* PS7 was submitted to a thorough safety assessment. In relation to its pattern of antibiotic sensitivity, all the MIC values were below the cut-off values recommended by EFSA [47], with the exception of kanamycin. A resistance of lactobacilli to kanamycin is a common finding among *L. salivarius* strains [64–66] due to the lack of a transport system for this antibiotic. This type of intrinsic resistance does not represent a human health risk [47]. In a previous study, the MIC value of *L. salivarius* CECT 5713 (a commercial probiotic strain) for kanamycin (128 µg/mL) [46] was the same as the one obtained with *L. salivarius* PS7 in this study. The analysis of the genome of *L. salivarius* CECT 5713 revealed the absence of transmissible genes involved in kanamycin resistance. Moreover, *L. salivarius* PS7 did not produce biogenic amines and did not show any ability for mucin degradation. These results are also similar to those reported for other *L. salivarius* strains using the same assays [31,56]. An acute and repeated-dose oral toxicity assessment in rats showed that *L. salivarius* PS7 was completely safe in this animal model when administrated in doses ranging from 9 to 10 $\log_{10}$ CFU daily. No significant differences in the liver GSH concentration were observed between the control and treated groups, indicating that the treatment did not cause oxidative stress to rats. This result is consistent with the absence of bacteremia since no lactobacilli could be isolated from the blood, liver or spleen of the rats, indicating that the tested strains do not cause either a local or a systemic infection in rats. These findings are in agreement with those previously reported for another *L. salivarius* strain also isolated from human milk [51].

Because of the wide antimicrobial activity of *L. salivarius* PS7 against otopathogens and its safety, a pilot clinical trial was carried out to assess its efficacy in preventing rAOM in infants and children. Oral intakes of *L. salivarius* PS7 over 6 months led to a statistically significant reduction (84%) in the number of episodes of AOM in comparison to those observed in the same population during the 6 months preceding the probiotic intervention. Such a percentage is higher than that observed in previous studies after oral or nasal administration of other probiotic strains, such as *Lactobacillus rhamnosus* GG and LC705, *Bifidobacterium breve* 99 and *Propionibacterium freudenreichii* JS [67,68], and *Streptococcus salivarius* 24SMB or *Streptococcus oralis* 89a [69,70]. When AOM occurred, the median duration of AOM episodes was 4 days, which is lower than the value obtained in previous probiotic trials (5.6 days) [68].

The external ear canal may act as a bacterial reservoir for the same otopathogens usually found in the middle ear during AOM [17,25,71]. Therefore, ear canal samples were analyzed before and after the probiotic intake period. The probiotic treatment led to a statistically significant decrease in the number of ear canal samples that were positive for bacterial growth and in the bacterial density of the positive samples (Table 5). The frequency of detection of potential otopathogens (*A.otitidis*, *Haemophilus haemolyticus*, *H. influenzae*, *M. catharralis*, *Neisseria* spp., *P. aeruginosa*, *S. aureus*, *S. pneumoniae* and *S. pyogenes*) in the samples also decreased notably after the trial (Table 5). The only bacterial groups whose detection frequency remained similar before and after the probiotic treatment were coagulase-negative staphylococci and viridans streptococci. This change in the composition of the ear canal microbiota seems to be closely associated with the decrease in the number of AOM episodes. In previous studies, otopathogens were more frequently detected in children with otitis than in healthy controls [10,72,73]. In fact, a failure to erradicate otopathogens from the ear and/or nasoparhyngeal surfaces has been viewed as an explanation for rAOM episodes after treatments with antibiotics [4] or with generic non-otitis-targeted probiotics [68,74]. A lack of specificity may explain the conflicting evidence on the effectiveness of probiotics in preventing AOM [75,76]. In contrast, the presence of coagulase-negative staphylococci and viridans streptococci seems to be a feature of a healthy ear and nasopharynx [13,77].

We acknowledge that the clinical trial performed in this study must be considered as a preliminary "proof of concept" trial since it faces some design limitations (e.g., lack of a placebo group and randomization). However, the results have shown that, while antibiotics may still play a relevant role in treatment of AOM, a target-specific probiotic strain may have a preventive role, significantly reducing the number of episodes in children with rAOM and the number of antibiotic doses required to treat them. This is a relevant finding within the context both of the present "antibiotic resistance crisis" and of the steady rise in autoimmune diseases associated with host microbiota disturbances. Additional work is in progress in order to initiate a well-designed multicenter clinical trial to further confirm the results obtained in this work.

Author Contributions: J.M.R. and C.B. designed the study; N.C., V.M., R.A. and E.J. characterized the strain and performed the microbial analyses. M.L. and M.C. were the pediatricians involved in this study. J.M.R. and E.J. wrote, edited and revised the manuscript. All the authors approved the final version of the manuscript.

Funding: This work was supported by Laboratorios Casen Recordati SL. The funding agency had no role in study design, data collection and analysis.

Acknowledgments: We acknowledge all the families that participated in this study. We are grateful to Leónides Fernández for the critical reading of the manuscript.

Conflicts of Interest: E.J. and N.C. are employees of Probisearch S.L.U. C.B. is employee of Casen Recordati SL. The remaining authors declare that the research was conducted in the absence of any commercial or financial relationships that could be construed as a potential conflict of interest.

References

1. Rovers, M.M. The burden of otitis media. *Vaccine* **2008**, *26*, G2–G4. [CrossRef] [PubMed]
2. Venekamp, R.P.; Sanders, S.L.; Glasziou, P.P.; Del Mar, C.B.; Rovers, M.M. Antibiotics for acute otitis media in children. *Cochrane Database Syst. Rev.* **2015**, CD000219. [CrossRef]
3. Klein, J.O. The burden of otitis media. *Vaccine* **2000**, *19*, S2–S8. [CrossRef]
4. Pelton, S.I.; Leibovitz, E. Recent advances in otitis media. *Pediatr. Infect. Dis. J.* **2009**, *28*, S133–S137. [CrossRef] [PubMed]
5. Pichichero, M.E. Ten-year study of acute otitis media in Rochester, NY. *Pediatr. Infect. Dis. J.* **2016**, *35*, 1027–1032. [CrossRef] [PubMed]
6. Jervis-Bardy, J.; Rogers, G.B.; Morris, P.S.; Smith-Vaughan, H.C.; Nosworthy, E.; Leong, L.E.; Smith, R.J.; Weyrich, L.S.; de Haan, J.; Carney, A.S.; et al. The microbiome of otitis media with effusion in Indigenous Australian children. *Int. J. Pediatr. Otorhinolaryngol.* **2015**, *79*, 1548–1555. [CrossRef] [PubMed]
7. Chan, C.L.; Wabnitz, D.; Bardy, J.J.; Bassiouni, A.; Wormald, P.J.; Vreugde, S.; Psaltis, A.J. The microbiome of otitis media with effusion. *Laryngoscope* **2016**, *126*, 2844–2851. [CrossRef]
8. Ngo, C.C.; Massa, H.M.; Thornton, R.B.; Cripps, A.W. Predominant bacteria detected from the middle ear fluid of children experiencing otitis media: A systematic review. *PLoS ONE* **2016**, *11*, e0150949. [CrossRef]
9. Granath, A. Recurrent acute otitis media: What are the options for treatment and prevention? *Curr. Otorrhinolatyngol. Rep.* **2017**, *5*, 93–100. [CrossRef]
10. Karlidağ, T.; Demirdağ, K.; Kaygusuz, I.; Ozden, M.; Yalçin, S.; Oztürk, L. Resistant bacteria in the adenoid tissues of children with otitis media with effusion. *Int. J. Pediatr. Otorhinolaryngol.* **2002**, *64*, 35–40. [CrossRef]
11. Brook, I.; Gober, A.E. In vitro bacterial interference in the nasopharynx of otitis media-prone and non-otitis media-prone children. *Arch. Otolaryngol. Head Neck Surg.* **2000**, *126*, 1011–1013. [CrossRef] [PubMed]
12. Leibovitz, E.; Greenberg, D.; Piglansky, L.; Raiz, S.; Porat, N.; Press, J.; Leiberman, A.; Dagan, R. Recurrent acute otitis media occurring within one month from completion of antibiotictherapy: Relationship to the original pathogen. *Pediatr. Infect. Dis. J.* **2003**, *22*, 209–216. [CrossRef] [PubMed]
13. Marchisio, P.; Claut, L.; Rognoni, A.; Esposito, S.; Passali, D.; Bellussi, L.; Drago, L.; Pozzi, G.; Mannelli, S.; Schito, G.; et al. Differences in nasopharyngeal bacterial flora in children with nonsevere recurrent acute otitis media and chronic otitis media with effusion: Implications for management. *Pediatr. Infect. Dis. J.* **2003**, *22*, 262–268. [CrossRef]

14. Klein, J.O. Bacterial resistance and antimicrobial drug selection. In *Evidence Based Otitis Media*; BC Decker: Hamilton, ON, Canada, 2003; pp. 429–437.
15. Hall-Stoodley, L.; Hu, F.Z.; Gieseke, A.; Nistico, L.; Nguyen, D.; Hayes, J. Direct detection of bacterial biofilms on the middle-ear mucosa of children with chronic otitis media. *JAMA* **2006**, *296*, 202–211. [CrossRef] [PubMed]
16. Thornton, R.B.; Rigby, P.J.; Wiertsema, S.P.; Filion, P.; Langlands, J.; Coates, H.L.; Vijayasekaran, S.; Keil, A.D.; Richmond, P.C. Multi-species bacterial biofilm and intracellular infection in otitis media. *BMC Pediatr.* **2011**, *11*, 94. [CrossRef] [PubMed]
17. Chan, C.L.; Richter, K.; Wormald, P.J.; Psaltis, A.J.; Vreugde, S. *Alloiococcus otitidis* forms multispecies biofilm with *Haemophilus influenzae*: Effects on antibiotic susceptibility and growth in adverse conditions. *Front. Cell Infect. Microbiol.* **2017**, *7*, 344. [CrossRef] [PubMed]
18. Fergie, N.; Bayston, R.; Pearson, J.P.; Birchall, J.P. Is otitis media with effusion a biofilm infection? *Clin. Otolaryngol. Allied Sci.* **2004**, *29*, 38–46. [CrossRef]
19. Tanaka, S.; Kobayashi, T.; Songjinda, P.; Tateyama, A.; Tsubouchi, M.; Kiyohara, C.; Shirakawa, T.; Sonomoto, K.; Nakayama, J. Influence of antibiotic exposure in the early postnatal period on the development of intestinal microbiota. *FEMS Immunol. Med. Microbiol.* **2009**, *56*, 80–87. [CrossRef]
20. Blaser, M.J.; Falkow, S. What are the consequences of the disappearing human microbiota? *Nat. Rev. Microbiol.* **2009**, *7*, 887–894. [CrossRef]
21. Rutten, N.B.; Rijkers, G.T.; Meijssen, C.B.; Crijns, C.E.; Oudshoorn, J.H.; van der Ent, C.K.; Vlieger, A.M. Intestinal microbiota composition after antibiotic treatment in early life: The INCA study. *BMC Pediatr.* **2015**, *15*, 204. [CrossRef]
22. Azad, M.B.; Konya, T.; Persaud, R.R.; Guttman, D.S.; Chari, R.S.; Field, C.J.; Sears, M.R.; Mandhane, P.J.; Turvey, S.E.; Subbarao, P.; et al. Impact of maternal intrapartum antibiotics, method of birth and breastfeeding on gut microbiota during the first year of life: A prospective cohort study. *BJOG* **2016**, *123*, 983–993. [CrossRef] [PubMed]
23. Lewis, J.D.; Chen, E.Z.; Baldassano, R.N.; Otley, A.R.; Griffiths, A.M.; Lee, D.; Bittinger, K.; Bailey, A.; Friedman, E.S.; Hoffmann, C.; et al. Inflammation, antibiotics, and diet as environmental stressors of the gut microbiome in pediatric Crohn's disease. *Cell Host Microbe* **2015**, *18*, 489–500. [CrossRef] [PubMed]
24. Zeissig, S.; Blumberg, R.S. Life at the beginning: Perturbation of the microbiota by antibiotics in early life and its role in health and disease. *Nat. Immunol.* **2014**, *15*, 307–310. [CrossRef] [PubMed]
25. Lappan, R.; Imbrogno, K.; Sikazwe, C.; Anderson, D.; Mok, D.; Coates, H.; Vijayasekaran, S.; Bumbak, P.; Blyth, C.C.; Jamieson, S.E.; et al. A microbiome case-control study of recurrent acute otitis media identified potentially protective bacterial genera. *BMC Microbiol.* **2018**, *18*, 13. [CrossRef] [PubMed]
26. Niittynen, L.; Pitkäranta, A.; Korpela, R. Probiotics and otitis media in children. *Int. J. Pediatr. Otorhinolaryngol.* **2012**, *76*, 465–470. [CrossRef] [PubMed]
27. Kullen, M.J.; Sanozky-Dawes, R.B.; Crowell, D.C.; Klaenhammer, T.R. Use of DNA sequence of variable regions of the 16SrRNA gene for rapid and accurate identification of bacteria in the *Lactobacillus acidophilus* complex. *J. Appl. Microbiol.* **2000**, *89*, 511–518. [CrossRef] [PubMed]
28. Marín, M.; Arroyo, R.; Espinosa-Martos, I.; Fernández, L.; Rodríguez, J.M. Identification of emerging human mastitis pathogens by MALDI-TOF and assessment of their antibiotic resistance patterns. *Front. Microbiol.* **2017**, *8*, 1258. [CrossRef] [PubMed]
29. Martín, V.; Maldonado-Barragán, A.; Moles, L.; Rodriguez-Baños, M.; Campo, R.D.; Fernández, L.; Rodríguez, J.M.; Jiménez, E. Sharing of bacterial strains between breast milk and infant feces. *J. Hum. Lact.* **2012**, *28*, 36–44. [CrossRef]
30. Marteau, P.; Minekus, M.; Havenaar, R.; Huis In't Veld, J.H.J. Survival of lactic acid bacteria in a dynamic model of the stomach and small intestine: Validation and the effects of bile. *J. Dairy Sci.* **1997**, *80*, 1031–1037. [CrossRef]
31. Martín, R.; Olivares, M.; Marín, M.L.; Fernández, L.; Xaus, J.; Rodríguez, J.M. Probiotic potential of 3 Lactobacilli strains isolated from breast milk. *J. Hum. Lact.* **2005**, *21*, 8–17. [CrossRef]
32. Conway, P.L.; Gorbach, S.L.; Goldin, B.R. Survival of lactic acid bacteria in the human stomach and adhesion to intestinal cells. *J. Dairy Sci.* **1987**, *70*, 1–12. [CrossRef]

33. Coconnier, M.H.; Klaenhammer, T.R.; Kernéis, S.; Bernet, M.F.; Servin, A.L. Protein-mediated adhesion of *Lactobacillus acidophilus* BG2FO4 on human enterocyte and mucus-secreting cell lines in culture. *Appl. Environ. Microbiol.* **1992**, *58*, 2034–2039. [PubMed]
34. Juarez del Valle, M.; Laiño, J.; Savoy de Giori, G.; LeBlanc, J.G. Riboflavin producing lactic acid bacteria as a biotechnological strategy to obtain bio-enriched soymilk. *Food Res. Int.* **2014**, *62*, 1015–1019. [CrossRef]
35. Laiño, J.E.; LeBlanc, J.G.; Savoy de Giori, G. Production of natural folates by lactic acid bacteria starter cultures isolated from artisanal Argentinean yogurts. *Can. J. Microbiol.* **2012**, *58*, 581–588. [CrossRef] [PubMed]
36. Horwitz, W. *Official Methods of Analysis of AOAC International*; AOAC International: Gaithersburg, MD, USA, 2000.
37. Magnusson, J.; Schnürer, J. *Lactobacillus coryniformis* subsp. *coryniformis* strain Si3 produces a broad-spectrum proteinaceous antifungal compound. *Appl. Environ. Microbiol.* **2001**, *67*, 1–5. [CrossRef] [PubMed]
38. Dodd, H.M.; Horn, N.; Zhang, H.; Gasson, M.J. A lactococcal expression system for engineered nisins. *Appl. Environ. Microbiol.* **1992**, *58*, 3683–3693. [PubMed]
39. Çataloluk, O. Molecular characterization of the gene encoding for salivaricin B activity and its flanking sequences. *Turk. J. Biol.* **2001**, *25*, 379–386.
40. Flynn, S.; van Sinderen, D.; Thornton, G.M.; Holo, H.; Nes, I.F.; Collins, J.K. Characterization of the genetic locus responsible for the production of ABP-118, a novel bacteriocin produced by the probiotic bacterium *Lactobacillus salivarius* subsp. *salivarius* UCC118. *Microbiology* **2002**, *148*, 973–984. [CrossRef]
41. Song, Y.L.; Kato, N.; Matsumiy, Y.; Lu, C.X.; Kato, H.; Watanabe, K. Identification of an hydrogen peroxide production by fecal and vaginal lactobacilli isolated from Japanese women and newborn infants. *J. Clin. Microbiol.* **1999**, *37*, 3062–3064.
42. Yap, P.S.; Gilliland, S.E. Comparison of newly isolated strains of *Lactobacillus delbrueckii* susp. *lactis* for hydrogen peroxide production at 5 °C. *J. Dairy Sci.* **2000**, *83*, 628–632. [CrossRef]
43. Reid, G.; McGroarty, J.A.; Gil Domingue, P.A.; Chow, A.W.; Bruce, A.W.; Eisen, A.; Costerton, J.W. Coaggregation of urogenital bacterial in vitro and in vivo. *Curr. Microbiol.* **1990**, *20*, 47–52. [CrossRef]
44. Younes, J.A.; van der Mei, H.C.; van den Heuvel, E.; Busscher, H.J.; Reid, G. Adhesion forces and coaggregation between vaginal staphylococci and lactobacilli. *PLoS ONE* **2012**, *7*, e36917. [CrossRef] [PubMed]
45. Klare, I.; Konstabel, C.; Müller-Bertling, S.; Reissbrodt, R.; Huys, G.; Vancanneyt, M.; Swings, J.; Goossens, H.; Witte, W. Evaluation of new broth media for microdilution antibiotic susceptibility testing of lactobacilli, lactococci, pediococci, and bifidobacteria. *Appl. Environ. Microbiol.* **2005**, *71*, 8982–8986. [CrossRef] [PubMed]
46. Langa, S.; Maldonado-Barragán, A.; Delgado, S.; Martín, R.; Martín, V.; Jiménez, E.; Ruíz-Barba, J.L.; Mayo, B.; Connor, R.I.; Suárez, J.E.; et al. Characterization of *Lactobacillus salivarius* CECT 5713, a strain isolated from human milk: From genotype to phenotype. *Appl. Microbiol. Biotechnol.* **2012**, *94*, 1279–1287. [CrossRef] [PubMed]
47. EFSA Guidance on the characterisation of microorganisms used as feed additives or as production organisms. *EFSA J.* **2018**, *16*, e05206.
48. Bover-Cid, S.; Holzapfel, W.H. Improved screening procedure for biogenic amine production by lactic acid bacteria. *Int. J. Food Microbiol.* **1999**, *53*, 33–41. [CrossRef]
49. Zhou, J.S.; Gopal, P.K.; Hill, H.S. Potential probiotic lactic acid bacteria *Lactobacillus rhamnosus* (HN001), *Lactobacillus acidophilus* (HN017) and *Bifidobacterium lactis* (HN019) do not degrade gastric mucin in vitro. *Int. J. Food Microbiol.* **2001**, *63*, 81–90. [CrossRef]
50. Anadón, A.; Martínez, M.A.; Ares, I.; Ramos, E.; Martínez-Larrañaga, M.R.; Contreras, M.M.; Ramos, M.; Recio, I. Acute and repeated dose (4 weeks) oral toxicity studies of two antihypertensive peptides, RYLGY and AYFYPEL, that correspond to fragments (90-94) and (143-149) from alpha(s1)-casein. *Food Chem. Toxicol.* **2010**, *48*, 1836–1845. [CrossRef]
51. Lara-Villoslada, F.; Sierra, S.; Martín, R.; Delgado, S.; Rodríguez, J.M.; Olivares, M.; Xaus, J. Safety assessment of two probiotic strains, *Lactobacillus coryniformis* CECT5711 and *Lactobacillus gasseri* CECT5714. *J. Appl. Microbiol.* **2007**, *103*, 175–184. [CrossRef]
52. Del Castillo, F.; Baquero, F.; de la Calle, T.; López, M.V.; Ruiz-Canela, J.; Alfayate, S.; Llop, F.M.; Ortega, M.J.C.; Rey, C.C. Documento de consenso sobre etiología, diagnóstico y tratamiento de la otitis media aguda. *Rev. Pediatr. Aten. Primaria* **2012**, *14*, 195–205. [CrossRef]

53. Díez, O.; Batista, N.; Bordes, A.; Lecuona, M.; Lara, M. Microbiological diagnosis of upper respiratory tract infections. *Enferm. Infecc. Microbiol. Clin.* **2007**, *25*, 387–393. [CrossRef] [PubMed]
54. The R Project for Statistical Computing. Available online: http:www.R-project.org (accessed on 29 July 2016).
55. FAO; WHO. *Guidelines for the Evaluation of Probiotics in Food*; Report of a Joint FAO/WHO Working Group on Drafting Guidelines for the Evaluation of Probiotics in Food; Joint FAO/WHO Working Group: London, ON, Canada, 2002.
56. Martín, R.; Jiménez, E.; Olivares, M.; Marín, M.; Fernández, L.; Xaus, J. *Lactobacillus salivarius* CECT 5713, a potential probiotic strain isolated from infant feces and breast milk of a mother-child pair. *Int. J. Food Microbiol.* **2006**, *112*, 35–43. [CrossRef] [PubMed]
57. Lee, Y.K.; Puong, K.Y.; Ouwehand, A.C.; Salminen, S. Displacement of bacterial pathogens from mucus and Caco-2 cell surface by lactobacilli. *J. Med. Microbiol.* **2003**, *52*, 925–930. [CrossRef] [PubMed]
58. Bresnick, S.D.; Ryan, A.F. Modulation of middle ear immune response by gut immunization. *Laryngoscope* **1989**, *99*, 1293–1298. [CrossRef] [PubMed]
59. Claesson, M.J.; Li, Y.; Leahy, S.; Canchaya, C.; van Pijkeren, J.P.; Cerdeño-Tárraga, A.M.; Parkhill, J.; Flynn, S.; O'Sullivan, G.C.; Collins, J.K.; et al. Multireplicon genome architecture of *Lactobacillus salivarius*. *Proc. Natl. Acad. Sci. USA* **2006**, *103*, 6718–6723. [CrossRef] [PubMed]
60. Corr, S.C.; Li, Y.; Riedel, C.U.; O'Toole, P.W.; Hill, C.; Gahan, C.G. Bacteriocin production as a mechanism for the antiinfective activity of *Lactobacillus salivarius* UCC118. *Proc. Natl. Acad. Sci. USA* **2007**, *104*, 7617–7621. [CrossRef] [PubMed]
61. Younes, J.A.; Reid, G.; van der Mei, H.C.; Busscher, H.J. Lactobacilli require physical contact to reduce staphylococcal TSST-1 secretion and vaginal epithelial inflammatory response. *Pathog. Dis.* **2016**, *74*, ftw029. [CrossRef]
62. Rosas-Salazar, C.; Shilts, M.H.; Tovchigrechko, A.; Schobel, S.; Chappell, J.D.; Larkin, E.K.; Gebretsadik, T.; Halpin, R.A.; Nelson, K.E.; Moore, M.L.; et al. Nasopharyngeal *Lactobacillus* is associated with a reduced risk of childhood wheezing illnesses following acute respiratory syncytial virus infection in infancy. *J. Allergy Clin. Immunol.* **2018**, *142*, 1447–1456. [CrossRef]
63. EFSA. Scientific opinion on the update of the list of QPS-recommended biological agents intentionally added to food or feed as notified to EFSA. *EFSA J.* **2017**, *15*, 4664.
64. Danielsen, M.; Wind, A. Susceptibility of *Lactobacillus* spp. to antimicrobial agents. *Int. J. Food Microbiol.* **2003**, *26*, 1–11. [CrossRef]
65. Zhou, J.S.; Pillidge, C.J.; Gopal, P.K.; Gill, H.S. Antibiotic susceptibility profiles of new probiotic *Lactobacillus* and *Bifidobacterium* strains. *Int. J. Food Microbiol.* **2005**, *98*, 211–217. [CrossRef] [PubMed]
66. Klare, I.; Konstabel, C.; Werner, G.; Huys, G.; Vankerckhoven, V.; Kahlmeter, G.; Hildebrandt, B.; Müller-Bertling, S.; Witte, W.; Goossens, H. Antimicrobial susceptibilities of *Lactobacillus*; *Pediococcus* and *Lactococcus* human isolates and cultures intended for probiotic or nutritional use. *J. Antimicrob. Chemother.* **2007**, *59*, 900–912. [CrossRef] [PubMed]
67. Tapiovaara, L.; Lehtoranta, L.; Swanljung, E.; Mäkivuokko, H.; Laakso, S.; Roivainen, M.; Korpela, R.; Pitkäranta, A. *Lactobacillus rhamnosus* GG in the middle ear after randomized, double-blind, placebo-controlled oral administration. *Int. J. Pediatr. Otorhinolaryngol.* **2014**, *78*, 1637–1641. [CrossRef] [PubMed]
68. Hatakka, K.; Blomgren, K.; Pohjavuori, S.; Kaijalainen, T.; Poussa, T.; Leinonen, M.; Korpela, R.; Pitkäranta, A. Treatment of acute otitis media with probiotics in otitis-prone children-a double-blind, placebo-controlled randomised study. *Clin. Nutr.* **2007**, *26*, 314–321. [CrossRef] [PubMed]
69. Marchisio, P.; Santagati, M.; Scillato, M.; Baggi, E.; Fattizzo, M.; Rosazza, C. *Streptococcus salivarius* 24SMB administered by nasal spray for the prevention of acute otitis media in otitis-prone children. *Eur. J. Clin. Microbiol. Infect. Dis.* **2015**, *34*, 2377–2383. [CrossRef] [PubMed]
70. La Mantia, I.; Varricchio, A.; Ciprandi, G. Bacteriotherapy with *Streptococcus salivarius* 24SMB and *Streptococcus oralis* 89a nasal spray for preventing recurrent acute otitis media in children: A real-life clinical experience. *Int. J. Gen. Med.* **2017**, *10*, 171–175. [CrossRef] [PubMed]
71. Chan, C.L.; Wabnitz, D.; Bassiouni, A.; Wormald, P.J.; Vreugde, S.; Psaltis, A.J. Identification of the bacterial reservoirs for the middle ear using phylogenic analysis. *JAMA Otolaryngol. Head Neck Surg.* **2017**, *143*, 155–161. [CrossRef] [PubMed]

72. Torretta, S.; Marchisio, P.; Drago, L.; Baggi, E.; De Vecchi, E.; Garavello, W.; Nazzari, E.; Pignataro, L.; Esposito, S. Nasopharyngeal biofilm-producing otopathogens in children with nonsevere recurrent acute otitis media. *Otolaryngol. Head Neck Surg.* **2012**, *146*, 991–996. [CrossRef] [PubMed]
73. Buzatto, G.P.; Tamashiro, E.; Proenca-Modena, J.L.; Saturno, T.H.; Prates, M.C.; Gagliardi, T.B.; Carenzi, L.R.; Massuda, E.T.; Hyppolito, M.A.; Valera, F.C.P.; et al. The pathogens profile in children with otitis media with effusion and adenoid hypertrophy. *PLoS ONE* **2017**, *12*, e0171049. [CrossRef] [PubMed]
74. Cohen, R.; Martin, E.; de La Rocque, F.; Thollot, F.; Pecquet, S.; Werner, A.; Boucherat, M.; Varon, E.; Bingen, E.; Levy, C. Probiotics and prebiotics in preventing episodes of acute otitis media in high-risk children: A randomized, double-blind, placebo-controlled study. *Pediatr. Infect. Dis. J.* **2013**, *32*, 810–814. [CrossRef] [PubMed]
75. Popova, M.; Molimard, P.; Courau, S.; Crociani, J.; Dufour, C.; Le Vacon, F.; Carton, T. Beneficial effects of probiotics in upperrespiratory tract infections and their mechanical actions to antagonize pathogens. *J. Appl. Microbiol.* **2012**, *113*, 1305–1318. [CrossRef] [PubMed]
76. Levi, J.R.; Brody, R.M.; McKee-Cole, K.; Pribitkin, E.; O'Reilly, R. Complementary and alternative medicine for pediatric otitis media. *Int. J. Pediatr. Otorhinolaryngol.* **2013**, *77*, 926–931. [CrossRef] [PubMed]
77. Tano, K.; Grahn Håkansson, E.; Holm, S.E.; Hellström, S. A nasal spray with alpha haemolytic streptococci as long term prophylaxis against recurrent otitis media. *Int. J. Pediatr. Otorhinolaryngol.* **2002**, *62*, 17–23. [CrossRef]

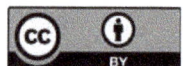

© 2019 by the authors. Licensee MDPI, Basel, Switzerland. This article is an open access article distributed under the terms and conditions of the Creative Commons Attribution (CC BY) license (http://creativecommons.org/licenses/by/4.0/).

MDPI
St. Alban-Anlage 66
4052 Basel
Switzerland
Tel. +41 61 683 77 34
Fax +41 61 302 89 18
www.mdpi.com

Nutrients Editorial Office
E-mail: nutrients@mdpi.com
www.mdpi.com/journal/nutrients

www.ingramcontent.com/pod-product-compliance
Lightning Source LLC
LaVergne TN
LVHW070225100526
838202LV00015B/2094